D0073759

15th EDITION

Lifetime Physical Fitness & Wellness

A Personalized Program

Werner W. K. Hoeger
Boise State University

Sharon A. Hoeger
Cherie I. Hoeger
Amber L. Fawson
Fitness & Wellness, Inc.

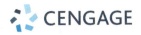

CENGAGE

Australia • Brazil • Mexico • Singapore • United Kingdom • United States

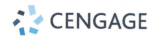

Lifetime Physical Fitness and Wellness:
A Personalized Program, 15e
Werner Hoeger, Sharon Hoeger, Cherie
Hoeger, Amber Fawson

Product Director: Dawn Giovaniello

Product Manager: Krista Mastroianni

Content Developer: Elesha Hyde

Product Assistant: Marina Starkey

Content Project Manager: Carol Samet

Art Director: Michael Cook

Manufacturing Planner: Karen Hunt

Composition and Production Service:
MPS Limited

Photo Researcher: Lumina Datamatics

Text Researcher: Lumina Datamatics

Cover Designer: Michael Cook

Cover Image: Mint Images RF/Getty Images

© 2019, 2017, Cengage Learning, Inc.

Unless otherwise noted, all content is © Cengage.

ALL RIGHTS RESERVED. No part of this work covered by the copyright herein may be reproduced or distributed in any form or by any means, except as permitted by U.S. copyright law, without the prior written permission of the copyright owner.

For product information and technology assistance, contact us at
Cengage Customer & Sales Support, 1-800-354-9706.

For permission to use material from this text or product,
submit all requests online at **www.cengage.com/permissions.**
Further permissions questions can be e-mailed to
permissionrequest@cengage.com.

Library of Congress Control Number: 2017953129

Student Edition:
ISBN: 978-1-337-392686

Cengage
20 Channel Center Street
Boston, MA 02210
USA

Cengage is a leading provider of customized learning solutions with employees residing in nearly 40 different countries and sales in more than 125 countries around the world. Find your local representative at **www.cengage.com.**

Cengage products are represented in Canada by
Nelson Education, Ltd.

To learn more about Cengage platforms and services, visit **www.cengage.com.** To register or access your online learning solution or purchase materials for your course, visit **www.cengagebrain.com.**

Printed at CLDPC, USA, 03-19

Contents

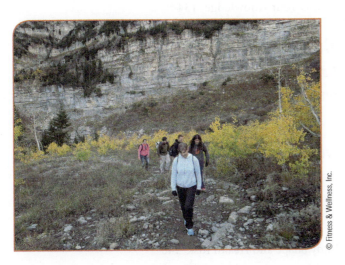

© Fitness & Wellness, Inc.

Chapter 3

Nutrition for Wellness 78

Chapter 4

Body Composition 135

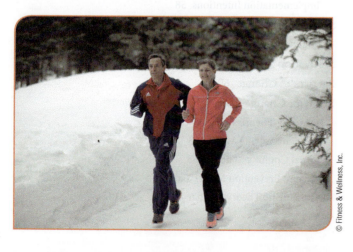

© Fitness & Wellness, Inc.

Chapter 5

Weight Management 161

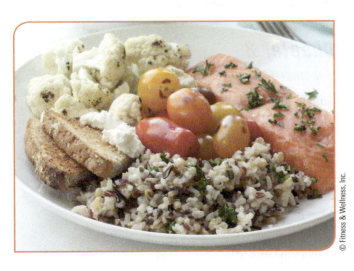

© Fitness & Wellness, Inc.

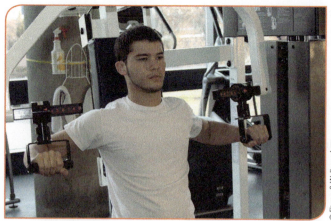

© Fitness & Wellness, Inc.

Chapter 9
Personal Fitness Programming 331

Chapter 10
Preventing Cardiovascular Disease 377

Chapter 11
Cancer Prevention 411

Chapter 12
Stress Assessment and Management Techniques 446

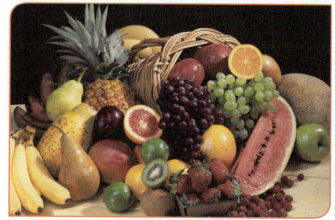

© Fitness & Wellness, Inc.

Chapter 13

Addictive Behavior 484

Chapter 14

Preventing Sexually Transmitted Infections 520

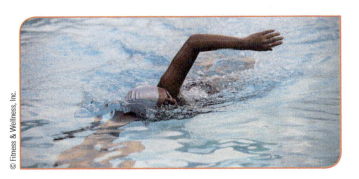

© Fitness & Wellness, Inc.

Chapter 15
Lifetime Fitness and Wellness 542

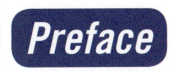

Preface

The American lifestyle does not provide the human body with sufficient physical activity to enhance or maintain adequate health. In reality, our way of life is a serious threat to our health that increases the deterioration rate of the human body and leads to premature illness and mortality.

People in the United States say they believe that physical activity and positive lifestyle habits promote better health, but most do not reap these benefits because they simply do not know how to implement and maintain a sound physical fitness and wellness program that will yield the desired results. About one-half of the adults in the United States do not achieve the recommended daily amount of aerobic activity and an ever lower amount meet the guidelines for muscular (strength) and flexibility fitness, thereby placing themselves at risk for premature morbidity, injury, and early death.

Furthermore, the energy (caloric) expenditure that used to result from activities other than planned daily exercise and basic body functions has also substantially decreased during the last century (known as nonexercise activity thermogenesis or NEAT). Examples of these activities include standing and walking while performing tasks, yard work, housecleaning, gardening, taking stairs, walking to and from stores or offices, or using a bicycle as the primary mode of transportation, and so on. NEAT used to represent a major portion of daily energy expenditure. Currently, however, people spend about eight hours per day or more of their waking time sitting. Excessive sitting is unnatural to the body and is detrimental to human health. This overall decline in physical activity accelerates aging, obesity, and loss of physical function, and further contributes to the development of chronic disease and premature mortality.

A regular exercise program is as close as we get to the miracle pill that people look for to enjoy good health and quality of life over a now longer lifespan. Myriad benefits of exercise include enhanced functional capacity; increased energy; weight loss; improved mood, self-esteem, and physical appearance; and decreased risk for many chronic ailments, including obesity, cardiovascular disease, cancer, and diabetes. As stated as far back as 1982 in the prestigious *Journal of the American Medical Association*, "There is no drug in current or prospective use that holds as much promise for sustained health as a lifetime program of physical exercise."

The benefits of exercise along with healthy lifestyle habits are only reaped through action. Along with the most up-to-date health, fitness, and nutrition guidelines, the information in this book provides extensive behavior modification strategies to help you abandon negative habits and adopt and maintain healthy behaviors.

Many of the behaviors we adopt are a product of our environment and value system. Unfortunately, we live in a "toxic" health/fitness environment. Becoming aware of how the environment affects our health is vital if we wish to achieve and maintain wellness. Yet we are so habituated to this modern-day environment that we miss the subtle ways it influences our behaviors, personal lifestyle, and health every day. As you study and assess physical fitness and wellness parameters, you will need to take a critical look at your behaviors and lifestyle—and most likely make selected lifetime changes to promote overall health and wellness. As you understand and live the concepts presented in this book, your value system will change and you'll be prepared to embark on a lifetime physical fitness and wellness journey.

The book is organized in the most efficient manner possible for students to derive the greatest benefit from its contents. Each chapter starts with the chapter objectives, followed by *Frequently Asked Questions (FAQ)*, a *Real Life Story*, and a *Personal Profile* based on chapter contents that will pique the reader's interest in the chapter's topic. The chapter contents are presented next, with extensive use of graphs, charts, tables, activities, critical thinking questions, keys to wellness, informational boxes, behavior modification boxes, definitions of key terms, and photographs to maximize student learning, content retention, and motivation for healthy lifetime behavioral change. As no other textbook, the Hoegers' *Fitness & Wellness* series makes exceptional use of these special pedagogical aids and high-interest features.

A unique feature of *Lifetime Physical Fitness & Wellness* is the activity experiences provided as key information is addressed in each chapter. These activities allow each student to develop *A Personalized Program* according to individual needs. All chapters highlight key wellness concepts throughout the text and conclude with *Assess Your Behavior* and *Assess Your Knowledge* sections so that students may evaluate the impact of the subject matter on their personal lifestyle and their understanding of the chapter contents through 10 multiple-choice questions.

Scientific evidence has clearly shown that improving the quality—and most likely the longevity—of our lives is a matter of personal choice. The biggest challenge we face in this century is to learn how to take control of our personal health habits to ensure a better, healthier, happier, and more productive life. The information presented in this book has been written with this goal in mind and provides students with the necessary tools and guidelines to implement and adhere to a *Lifetime Physical Fitness and Wellness Program*. The emphasis throughout the book is on teaching the students how to take control of their personal lifestyle habits so that they can do what is necessary to stay healthy and realize their highest potential for well-being.

New in the 15th Edition

For this new edition of *Lifetime Physical Fitness & Wellness: A Personalized Program* we have attempted to provide a more modern and visually stimulating layout throughout the book by including many new figures, graphs, informational boxes, and/or photos in each chapter. These changes in the book are introduced to better help students understand and implement a wellness way of life.

All chapters in the 15th edition have been revised and updated according to recent advances and recommendations in the field, including information reported in the literature and at professional health, fitness, and sports medicine conferences. Furthermore, chapters have been rethought and reorganized with new headings and enhanced introductory text. Chapter 1, for example, includes a new focus on the ways daily physical activity and exercise work together to increase lifetime wellness. Chapter 4 has been reorganized to help students better understand how body weight and shape affect lifetime health outcomes. Chapter 5 has been reorganized with new material to help students understand how thoughts and feelings affect weight maintenance. Chapter 9 has been restructured to be the capstone chapter of exercise programming—to sum up all students have learned about cardiorespiratory, strength, and flexibility training—and to give them complete confidence to write their own exercise programs throughout their lifetime. A new quick reference flow chart, the "Hoeger Values-Based Quick-Reference Guide to Exercise Prescription," has also been added to Chapter 9, so that students can apply correct exercise prescription principles and see fitness progress through their exercise efforts.

In addition to selected new photography, figures, and keys to wellness and insert boxes, the following are the most significant changes to this edition.

Chapter Updates

Chapter 1, Physical Fitness and Wellness

- New figures and features that highlight the importance of daily physical activity and nonexercise activity thermogenesis (NEAT)
- Redesigned figures illustrating the leading causes of death for specific age groups, along with new information about medical error, a prominent and underreported cause of death
- A description and new feature explaining types of scientific studies
- A new feature that explains the connection between light, moderate, and vigorous-intensity exercise and metabolic equivalents (METs)
- All facts and statistics have been updated according to the latest research

Chapter 2, Behavior Modification

- New figures and updated data on the health risks of modern work and leisure habits, community design, and food quality and abundance
- A new feature explaining the mechanisms behind cravings
- Addition of the latest research about willpower, planning, and the use of "implementation intentions" for changing behavior
- A new feature offering tools for using positive self-talk for goal achievement
- The latest information from behavioral science including new information about loss aversion and on choosing a growth versus a fixed mindset

Chapter 3, Nutrition for Wellness

- Editorial changes throughout the chapter to update nutrition concepts based on the most current research and reports in the field
- A more thorough description of the differences between refined and whole grains
- An enhanced description of types of fat based on the degree of hydrogen saturation
- Updates and new information are included throughout the chapter and in particular in the sections on *Simple Carbohydrates (sugars), Saturated Fats, Proteins,* phytonutrients, and *Nuts*
- Inclusion of the *2015–2020 Dietary Guidelines for Americans*

Chapter 4, Body Composition

- Reorganization of chapter material to better emphasize the risks of android obesity and the benefits of regular body composition assessments
- A new feature titled "Can I Influence My Bodyshape?"
- A new figure emphasizing the connection between physical activity and android obesity
- A new section describing white, brown, and beige fat and implications to health
- Expanded discussion on WHtR and the way it is used to more accurately predict disease in public health measures

Chapter 5, Weight Management

- Updated data on the obesity epidemic in the United States
- Updates on the detrimental consequences of excessive body weight and *yo-yo dieting*
- An introduction to the principle of *dynamic energy balance* and its role in the *energy–balancing equation*
- Additional information on the misleading rule of thumb that to lose one pound of fat all a person has to do is produce a caloric deficit of 3,500 calories

- Foods that are most commonly associated with weight gain and weight loss and the principle that "*a calorie may not always be a calorie*"

- New information on the critical role of exercise, both aerobic and strength training, to maintain energy expenditure following weight loss

- An introduction to weight gain and fat cell size and number increase in the lower body and abdominal areas

- The various-calorie diet plans (daily food logs) have been revised to emphasize the importance of sufficient protein intake throughout the day and minimize/eliminate the use of processed foods in the diet

- Additional suggestions for weight-loss strategies

Chapter 6, Cardiorespiratory Endurance

- The cardiorespiratory endurance assessment and exercise prescription principles conform with the newly released 2018 Guidelines for Exercise Testing and Prescription by the American College of Sports Medicine (ACSM)

- Updates on tips to increase daily physical activity and for people who have been physically inactive

Chapter 7, Muscular Fitness

- An update on the mounting evidence of cardioprotective health benefits obtained through proper strength-training

- The effects of strength training and improved muscle mass on blood sugar control

- Benefits of strength training and muscle mass maintenance throughout the lifespan

- The association between grip strength and cardiovascular disease and premature mortality

- The provided strength-training exercise prescription is up-to-date with the current 2018 guidelines by the American College of Sports Medicine

- Effectiveness of light-to-moderate isometric strength training in both normotensive and hypertensive individuals

- An answer to the concern of heavy-resistance strength-training and arterial stiffness

Chapter 8, Muscular Flexibility

- The FITT-VP Flexibility Guidelines within the text and figures also conform with the 2018 Guidelines for Exercise Testing and Prescription by the American College of Sports Medicine

- Expanded information on the benefits of flexibility and introductory information on factors that affect flexibility: joint structure, genetics, age, gender, and other factors

- Expanded section on the most common causes of back pain and methods to prevent back pain from becoming chronic

Chapter 9, Personal Fitness Programming

- Complete reorganization of the chapter to give students added confidence in their ability to understand and apply exercise prescription in their own lives

- Added review of basic exercise prescription principles and new quick-reference flow chart titled "Hoeger Values-Based Quick-Reference Guide to Exercise Prescription," making Chapter 9 the capstone chapter of exercise prescription, topping off material from the cardiorespiratory, muscular, and flexibility chapters

- New information about exercise and behavior modification

- New suggestions to guide students in choosing fitness solutions that fit personal values

- A new Activity titled "Personal Reflection on Exercise and Enjoyment"

- New suggestions for attending a group exercise class for the first time or trying a new sport for the first time

- Presentation of new research about popular ultra-short workouts

Chapter 10, Preventing Cardiovascular Disease

- Up-to-date data on the prevalence of cardiovascular disease

- An update on exercise (both low aerobic and low muscular fitness at age 18), nutrition, and type 2 diabetes

- Updates on most of the cardiovascular disease risk factors based on new evidence reported in the literature, including the impact of fruit and vegetable consumption on blood cholesterol and stress on coronary heart disease

- Foods that either promote or prevent premature mortality

- New information has been added to the section on other, lesser known potential risk factors for coronary heart disease, including too much or too little sleep, depression, lack of laughter, and an excessively long work schedule

Chapter 11, Cancer Prevention

- New feature on cancer research agencies that provide lists of carcinogenic items

- Updated information and illustrations about processed and red meat as risk factors for cancer

- Updated explanation on guidelines for mammography and breast cancer screenings, arming students with information on this controversial topic

- Updated data on the incidence and mortality rates of cancer, along with the most common site-specific cancer risk factors

Chapter 12, Stress Assessment and Management Techniques

- New figure detailing the real-time effects of the fight-or-flight mechanism on the body and the long-term physiological risks of repeated activation of this mechanism due to chronic stress

- New key term, "allostatic load," defined and explained in accordance with current research as the primary cause of disease vulnerability during the exhaustion stage of the general adaptation syndrome

- Expanded information on the role of mindfulness meditation for stress management and the role adequate sleep plays in managing stress

Chapter 13, Addictive Behavior

- New figures reflecting data specific to addictive behaviors most prevalent in college students, including marijuana, heroin, and alcohol abuse

- Expanded section on the addictive and physiological effects of high caffeine intake

- New figure detailing the immediate and long-term benefits of smoking cessation

- Updated data on the most recent trends in substance abuse reported in the *National Survey on Drug Use and Health* by the U.S. Department of Health and Human Services

Chapter 14, Preventing Sexually Transmitted Infections

- New information on the success of pre-exposure prophylaxis (PrEP) in reducing the risk of HIV among those at highest risk for infection

- Current data and graphs on the prevalence of STIs have been added and updated according to the newest data from the Centers for Disease Control and Prevention (CDC)

- Updated HPV vaccination schedule recommendations for adolescents according to recently published CDC guidelines

Chapter 15, Lifetime Fitness and Wellness

- New information on the growing trend of integrative medicine in hospitals, practices, and treatment centers

- Updated resources for students to access credible research on health and wellness topics

Additional Course Resources

- **Health MindTap for Lifetime *Physical Fitness & Wellness.*** MindTap is well beyond an e-Book, a homework solution or digital supplement, a resource center website, a course delivery platform, or a learning management system. More than 70 percent of students surveyed said it was unlike anything they have seen before. MindTap is a personal learning experience that combines all your digital assets—readings, multimedia, activities, and assessments—into a singular learning path to improve student outcomes.

- **Diet & Wellness Plus.** The Diet & Wellness Plus App in MindTap helps you gain a better understanding of how nutrition relates to your personal health goals. It enables you to track your diet and activity, generate reports, and analyze the nutritional value of the food you eat! It includes more than 55,000 foods in the database, custom food and recipe features, and the latest dietary references, as well as your goal and actual percentages of essential nutrients, vitamins, and minerals. It also helps you to identify a problem behavior and make a positive change. After completing a wellness profile questionnaire, Diet & Wellness Plus will rate the level of concern for different areas of wellness, helping you determine the areas where you are most at risk. It then helps you put together a plan for positive change by helping you select a goal to work toward—complete with a reward for all your hard work.

- **Instructor Companion Site.** Everything you need for your course in one place! This collection of book-specific lecture and class tools is available online via http://www.cengage.com/login. Access and download PowerPoint presentations, images, an instructor's manual, videos, and more.

- **Cengage Learning Testing Powered by Cognero.** Cengage Teaming Testing Powered by Cognero is a flexible, online system that allows you to:

  - author, edit, and manage test bank content from multiple Cengage Teaming solutions

  - create multiple test versions in an instant

  - deliver tests from your TMS, your classroom, or wherever you want

Brief Author Biographies

Werner W. K. Hoeger is a professor emeritus of the Department of Kinesiology at Boise State University, where he taught between 1986 and 2009. He had previously taught at the University of the Andes in Venezuela (1978–1982); served as Technical Director of the Fitness Monitoring Preventive Medicine Clinic in Rolling Meadows, Illinois (1982–1983); taught at The University of Texas of the Permian Basin in Odessa, Texas (1983–1986); and briefly taught for one semester in 2012, 2013, and 2016 as an adjunct faculty at Brigham Young University Hawaii in Laie, Hawaii. He remains active in research and continues to lecture in the areas of exercise physiology, physical fitness, health, and wellness.

Dr. Hoeger completed his undergraduate and master's degrees in physical education at the age of 20 and received his doctorate degree with an emphasis in exercise physiology at the age of 24. He is a *Fellow* of the *American College of Sports Medicine* and also of the *Research Consortium* of *SHAPE America (Society of Health and Physical Educators)*. In 2002, he was recognized as the *Outstanding Alumnus* from the *College of Health and Human Performance* at *Brigham Young University*. He is the recipient of the first *Presidential Award for Research and Scholarship* in the *College of Education* at *Boise State University* in 2004.

In 2008, he was asked to be the *keynote speaker* at the *VII Iberoamerican Congress of Sports Medicine and Applied Sciences* in Mérida, Venezuela, and was presented with the *Distinguished Guest of the City* recognition. In 2010, he was also honored as the *keynote speaker* at the *Western Society for Kinesiology and Wellness* in Reno, Nevada.

Using his knowledge and personal experiences, Dr. Hoeger writes engaging, informative books that thoroughly address today's fitness and wellness issues in a format accessible to students. Since 1990, he has been the most widely read fitness and wellness college textbook author in the United States. He has published a total of 63 editions of his nine fitness- and wellness-related titles. Among the textbooks written for Wadsworth/Cengage Learning are *Principles and Labs for Fitness and Wellness: A Personalized Program*, 14th edition; *Fitness & Wellness*, 13th edition; *Principles and Labs for Physical Fitness*, 10th edition; *Wellness: Guidelines for a Healthy Lifestyle*, 4th edition; and *Water Aerobics for Fitness & Wellness*, 4th edition (with Terry-Ann Spitzer Gibson).

Dr. Hoeger was the first author to write a college fitness textbook that incorporated the wellness concept. In 1986, with the release of the first edition of *Lifetime Physical Fitness & Wellness*, he introduced the principle that to truly improve fitness, health, and quality of life and to achieve wellness, a person needed to go beyond the basic health-related components of physical fitness. His work was so well received that every fitness author in the field immediately followed his lead.

As an innovator in the field, Dr. Hoeger has developed many fitness and wellness assessment tools, including fitness tests such as the Modified Sit-and-Reach, Total Body Rotation, Shoulder Rotation, Muscular Endurance, and Muscular Strength and Endurance, and Soda Pop Coordination Tests.

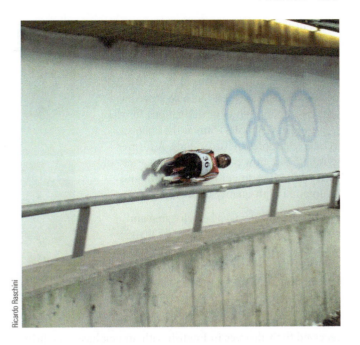

Ricardo Raschini

Proving that he "practices what he preaches," he was the oldest male competitor in the 2002 Winter Olympics in Salt Lake City, Utah, at the age of 48. He raced in the sport of luge along with his then 17-year-old son Christopher. It was the first, and so far only, time in Winter Olympics history that father and son competed in the same event. In 2006, at the age of 52, he was the oldest competitor at the Winter Olympics in Turin, Italy. At different times and in different distances (800 mts, 1,500 mts, and the mile) in 2012, 2014, 2015, and 2016, Dr. Hoeger reached All-American standards for his age group by USA Track and Field (USATF). In 2015, he finished third in the one-mile run at the US-ATF Masters Indoor Track and Field National Championships, and third and fourth, respectively, in the 800- and 1,500-meter events at the Outdoor National Senior Games.

In 2016, he advanced to the finals in both the 800 mts and the 1,500 mts at the World Masters Track and Field Championships held in Perth, Australia. He finished 7th (out of 12 finalists) in the 800 mts and 8th (out of 16 finalists) in the 1,500 mts.

Sharon A. Hoeger is vice president of Fitness & Wellness, Inc., of Boise, Idaho. Sharon received her degree in computer science from Brigham Young University. In the 1980s, she served as a computer science instructor at the University of Texas of the Permian Basin. She is extensively involved in the research process used in retrieving the most current scientific information that goes into the revision of each textbook. She is also the author of the software that was written specifically for the fitness and wellness textbooks. Her innovations in this area since the publication of the first edition of *Lifetime*

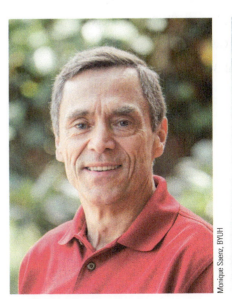

Monique Saenz, BYUH

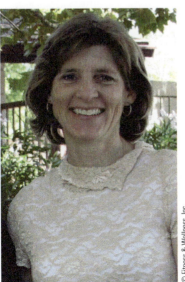

© Fitness & Wellness, Inc.

Physical Fitness & Wellness in 1986 set the standard for fitness and wellness computer software used in this market today.

Sharon is a coauthor of five of the seven fitness and wellness titles. She also served as chef de mission (chief of delegation) for the Venezuelan Olympic Team at the 2006 Winter Olympics in Turin, Italy. A former gymnast, she now participates in a variety of fitness activities to enjoy good health and maintain a high quality of life.

Husband and wife have been jogging and strength training together for more than 41 years. They are the proud parents of five children, all of whom are involved in sports and lifetime fitness activities. Their motto: "Families that exercise together, stay together."

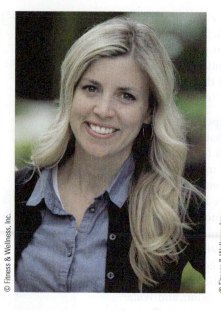 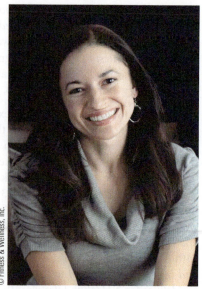

© Fitness & Wellness, Inc.

© Fitness & Wellness, Inc.

Amber L. Fawson and Cherie I. Hoeger

received their degrees in English with an emphasis in editing for publication. For the past 15 years Amber has enjoyed working in the publication industry and has held positions as an Editorial Coordinator for *BYU Studies,* Assistant Editor for Cengage Learning, and freelance writer and editor for tertiary education textbooks and workbooks. During the last decade, Cherie has been working as a freelance writer and editor; writing research and marketing copy for client magazines, newsletters, and websites; and contracting as a textbook copy editor for Cengage Learning (previously under Thomson Learning and the Brooks/Cole brand).

Amber and Cherie have been working for Fitness & Wellness, Inc., for several years as writers and scientific literature reviewers for new editions. They have now taken on a more significant role as co-authors of all fitness & wellness textbooks. Their addition now constitutes an enthusiastic four-person author team to sort through and summarize the extensive literature available in the health, fitness, wellness, and sports medicine fields. Their work has greatly enhanced the excellent quality of these textbooks. They are firm believers in living a health and wellness lifestyle, regularly attend professional meetings in the field, and are active members of the American College of Sports Medicine.

Acknowledgments

We would like to thank Celeste Brown, Alyssa Woo, Gina Jepson, Jessica Eakins, and Inês Almeida for their kind help with new photography used in this book.

The completion of the 15th edition of *Lifetime Physical Fitness & Wellness: A Personalized Program* was made possible through the contributions of many individuals. In particular, we would like to express our gratitude to the reviewers of the 15th edition; their valuable comments and suggestions are most sincerely appreciated.

Reviewers for the 15th edition:

Dr. Stephanie Duguid, Copiah Lincoln Community College

Robert Emery, Plattsburgh State University

Carmen S. Forest, Pratt Community College

Kristen Kane, Ph.D., Morrisville State College

Natalie L. Stickney, Georgia State University

D. Stockton, Coastal Bend College

1

Physical Fitness and Wellness

The human body is extremely resilient during youth—not so during middle and older age. The power of prevention, nonetheless, is yours: It enables you to make healthy lifestyle choices today that will prevent disease in the future and increase the quality and length of your life.

Objectives

1.1 **Understand** the health and fitness consequences of physical inactivity.

1.2 **Identify** the major health problems in the United States.

1.3 **Learn** how to monitor daily physical activity.

1.4 **Learn** the federal Physical Activity Guidelines for Americans.

1.5 **Define** wellness and list its dimensions.

1.6 **Distinguish** between health fitness standards and physical fitness standards.

1.7 **Define** physical fitness and list health-related and skill-related components.

1.8 **Understand** the benefits and significance of participating in a comprehensive wellness program.

1.9 **Determine** if you can safely initiate an exercise program.

1.10 **Learn** to assess resting heart rate and blood pressure.

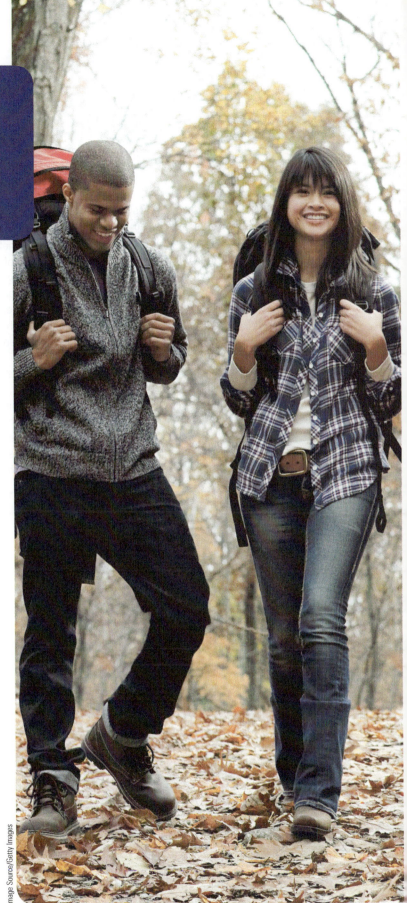

Image Source/Getty Images

1

FAQ

Why should I take a fitness and wellness course?

Most people go to college to learn how to make a living, but a fitness and wellness course will teach you how to live—how to truly live life to its fullest potential. Some people seem to think that success is measured by how much money they make. Making a good living will not help you unless you live a wellness lifestyle that will allow you to enjoy what you earn. You may want to ask yourself: Of what value are a nice income, a beautiful home, and a solid retirement portfolio if, at age 45, I suffer a massive heart attack that will seriously limit my physical capacity or end life itself?

Is the attainment of good physical fitness sufficient to ensure good health?

Regular participation in a sound physical fitness program will provide substantial health benefits and significantly decrease the risk of many chronic diseases. And although good fitness often motivates toward adoption of additional positive lifestyle behaviors, to maximize the benefits for a healthier, more productive, happier, and longer life we have to pay attention to all seven dimensions of wellness: physical, social, mental, emotional, occupational, environmental, and spiritual. These dimensions are interrelated, and one frequently affects the other. A wellness way of life requires a constant and deliberate effort to stay healthy and achieve the highest potential for well-being within all dimensions of wellness.

If a person is going to do only one thing to improve health, what would it be?

This is a common question. It is a mistake to think, though, that you can modify just one factor and enjoy wellness. Wellness requires a constant and deliberate effort to change unhealthy behaviors and reinforce healthy behaviors. Although it is difficult to work on many lifestyle changes all at once, being involved in a regular physical activity program, avoiding excessive sitting, observing proper nutrition, and avoiding addictive behaviour are lifestyle factors to work on first. Others should follow, depending on your current lifestyle behaviours.

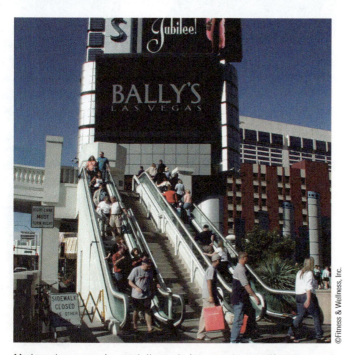

©Fitness & Wellness, Inc.

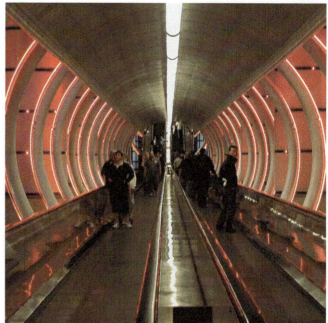

©Fitness & Wellness, Inc.

Modern-day conveniences lull people into a sedentary lifestyle.

Do you ever stop to think about factors that influence your actions on a typical day? As you consider typical moments from this past week, which actions were positive and healthy and which may have been negative or harmful? Did you go for a walk or have a conversation with a friend? Did you buy and eat food that you felt good about? Did you pursue a task that held purpose and meaning for you? Conversely, did you battle ongoing stress and anxiety or allow yourself irregular sleep? Did you settle for highly processed food? Did you struggle with relationship problems? Did you regress to previous, unhealthy behaviors?

Take a moment to consider whether the choices from the past week repeated over years would accumulate to promote

REAL LIFE STORY | Jim's Experience

I am pretty athletic and played baseball and basketball in high school. I also grew up eating well, since my dad is a chef who specializes in healthy cuisine. So when I got to college, I was sure that I was already doing everything necessary to be healthy. However, at the same time that I was congratulating myself for my healthy lifestyle, I was practicing some very unhealthy habits without even thinking about it. My sleep schedule was horrible. I would sometimes only get three to four hours of sleep a night. At times I would pull an "all-nighter" and other times I would crash and sleep for twelve hours. I drank huge amounts of black coffee, diet soda, or energy drinks to stay alert. I was under a lot of stress—I was pre-med and I was struggling in some of my classes. My two roommates and I did not get along, so there was constant fighting and tension between us. I felt isolated and unhappy, and I questioned whether I had made a mistake choosing the college I did. In order to blow off steam, I started going to frat parties and drinking too much. I would often get sick and then suffer a hangover the next morning. I didn't see this as a problem because it seemed to be something a lot of students were

doing. And to add to all that, after months of high-impact running on concrete surfaces, I ended up injuring my knee. I was barely able to move around, let alone work out. I was only in my second year of college when I took a fitness and wellness class. It was then that I really thought about how my lifestyle was affecting my health and wellness. During the course of the class, I made several changes. I tried to even out my sleep schedule and get seven to eight hours a night. To make that happen, I had to work on my procrastination. I could no longer wait to write a paper until the night before it was due and still expect to get eight hours of sleep. This change actually helped me do better in my classes, which relieved some of my stress. The times when I still felt stressed out, I started meditating or listening to relaxing music instead of going out and drinking. I also learned about how to exercise safely and prevent injuries. I took up swimming, since it is a good, low-impact workout. I feel like just how sometimes problems can snowball

Karin Hildebrand Lau/Shutterstock.com

and lead to more problems, small changes for the better can sometimes snowball too, and once you improve one habit, other things in your life become easier to fix. Because of the changes I have made, the rest of my college career has been much healthier and happier than my first year.

I am so glad the fitness course was a required class because I was able to correct my lifestyle before it spiraled out of control and I wasted more time in college. I started to exercise on an almost daily basis, and I learned so much about nutrition and healthy eating. Parties and alcohol were no longer important to me. I had a life to live and prepare for. It felt so good to once again become fit and eat a healthy/balanced diet. I rearranged my activities so that schoolwork and fitness were right at the top of my list. I stopped procrastinating on my schoolwork, and I was doing cardio five times a week and lifting twice per week. My goal is to keep this up for the rest of my life. I now understand that if I want to enjoy wellness, I have to make fitness and healthy living a top priority in my life.

PERSONAL PROFILE: General Understanding of Fitness and Wellness

To the best of your ability, answer the following questions. If you do not know the answer(s), this chapter will guide you through them.

I. What have you done to make yourself aware of potential risk factors in your life that may increase your chances of developing disease? What do you know about your family's health history? Is there any other information that you feel you need to know?

II. Do you know the top two leading causes of death in your age group? What steps do you take to protect yourself and set a good example for others?

III. When are you most physically active throughout the day? Is there a season of the year or day of the week when you are most active? What can you do to become more active on a regular basis?

IV. Of the seven dimensions of wellness, which dimension do you ignore most? Which dimension do you follow best?

V. What steps are you taking toward financial wellness?

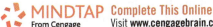

MINDTAP From Cengage **Complete This Online**
Visit **www.cengagebrain.com** to access MindTap, a complete digital course that includes interactive quizzes, videos, and more.

wellness or to cause disease. Your health is a product of complex intertwined physical, mental, inherited, and environmental factors that directly influence your state of wellness. This book will help you navigate through these factors that influence your behavior and will provide you with the necessary

tools to make changes that are right for your life. We will begin this chapter by looking at the big picture and will then use a personalized approach throughout the book to help you create a program aimed at helping you develop a lifetime fitness and wellness lifestyle.

1.1 *The Wellness Challenge for You Today*

There are three basic factors that determine our health and longevity: genetics, the environment, and our behavior. In most cases, we cannot change our genetic circumstances, though the budding field of epigenetics is showing us that select genes can be switched on and off by lifestyle choices and environment. (For a more in-depth discussion on epigenetics see "Epigenetics," Chapter 11, page 417.) We can certainly, however, exert control over the environment and our health behaviors so that we may reach our full physical potential based on our genetic code (see Figure 1.1).

At the beginning of the 20th century, **life expectancy** for a child born in the United States was only 47 years. The most common health problems in the Western world were infectious diseases, such as tuberculosis, diphtheria, influenza, kidney disease, polio, and other diseases of infancy. Progress in the medical field largely eliminated these diseases. Then, as more people started to enjoy the ease and excesses of modern life, we saw a parallel increase in the incidence of **chronic diseases** such as cardiovascular disease, cancer, diabetes, and chronic respiratory diseases (Figure 1.2).

The underlying causes of death attributable to leading **risk factors** in the United States (Figure 1.3) indicate that most factors are related to lifestyle choices we make. Of the approximately 2.6 million yearly deaths in the United States, the "big five" factors—tobacco smoking, high blood pressure, overweight and obesity, physical inactivity, and high blood glucose—are responsible for almost 1.5 million deaths each year.

Based on estimates, more than half of disease is lifestyle related, a fifth is attributed to the environment, and a tenth is influenced by the health care the individual receives. Only 16 percent is related to genetic factors (Figure 1.4). Thus, the individual controls as much as 80 percent of his or her

Figure 1.2 Causes of death in the United States for selected years.

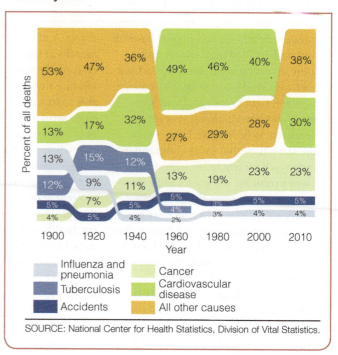

SOURCE: National Center for Health Statistics, Division of Vital Statistics.

vulnerability to disease—and thus quality of life. In essence, most people in the United States are threatened by the very lives they lead today.

As our culture has adopted the ease of Western life, we have undergone profound cultural shifts at a rapid pace. By comparison, advances in past centuries were slow and gradual. Within the last century we have made wide-reaching changes like overhauling our diet to include more processed, refined, sugary, and unhealthy fatty foods. We have become increasingly **sedentary**. We have changed our social interactions so that we are now always online or "plugged in." While it is impossible to completely tease out every cultural shift and its impact on health, we know for certain that some take a heavy toll on our population's overall health and wellness. We will begin by examining one of the most impactful cultural shifts. Let's consider the recent history of physical activity.

Movement is a basic function for which the human body was created, but advances in technology have almost completely eliminated the necessity for physical exertion in daily life. Scientific findings have shown that physical inactivity and a negative lifestyle seriously threaten health and hasten the deterioration rate of the human body. Most nations, both developed and developing, are experiencing an epidemic of physical inactivity. In the United States, physical inactivity is the second greatest threat to public health (after tobacco use) and is often referenced in new concerns about *sitting disease,* **sedentary death syndrome (SeDS),** and **hypokinetic diseases**.

As the populations of the world have adopted a more sedentary lifestyle, the world has seen a steep incline in obesity

Figure 1.1 Factors that affect health and longevity.

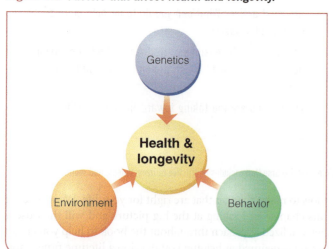

Figure 1.3 Death from all causes attributable to lifestyle-related risk factors for men and women in the United States.

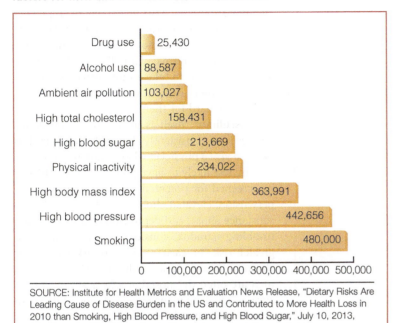

SOURCE: Institute for Health Metrics and Evaluation News Release, "Dietary Risks Are Leading Cause of Disease Burden in the US and Contributed to More Health Loss in 2010 than Smoking, High Blood Pressure, and High Blood Sugar," July 10, 2013, http://www.healthmetricsandevaluation.org/news-events/news-releases.

rates. Before 1980, obesity rates throughout the world remained relatively steady. Then, beginning in the 1980s, obesity rates started to grow rapidly, especially in the United States, Australia, and England. Worldwide, obesity currently claims triple the number of victims as malnutrition. Overweight and obese people are now the majority in the 34 countries that make up the Organization for Economic Cooperation and Development (OECD).

Around the same time that incidence of chronic diseases climbed, we recognized that prevention is the best medicine. Consequently, a fitness and wellness movement developed

gradually, beginning in the 1980s. Gyms and fitness centers as we know them began to be common across the country. People began to realize that good health is mostly self-controlled and that the leading causes of premature death and illness can be prevented by adhering to positive lifestyle habits.

Widespread interest in **health** and preventive medicine in recent years is motivating people to reexamine the foods they eat, incorporate more movement into activities of daily life, participate in organized fitness and wellness programs, and seek to reduce stress and increase well-being. We all desire to live a long life, and wellness programs aim to enhance the overall quality of life—for as long as we live.

1.2 *Life Expectancy*

Currently, the average life expectancy in the United States is 78.9 years (76.6 years for men and 81.4 years for women).[1] In the past decade alone, life expectancy has increased by over 1 year—the news, however, is not all good. The data show that people now spend an extra 1.2 years with a serious illness and an extra 2 years of disability. Mortality has been postponed because medical treatments allow people to live longer with chronic ailments.

While the United States was once a world leader in life expectancy, over recent years, the increase in life expectancy in the United States has not kept pace with that of other developed countries. Based on data from the World Health Organization (WHO), the United States ranks 31st in the world for life expectancy (see Figure 1.5).[2] Japan ranks first in the world with an overall life expectancy of 83.7 years.[3]

Several factors may account for the current U.S. life expectancy ranking, including the extremely poor health of some groups. The United States also has fairly high levels of violence (notably, homicides), rates of traffic fatalities, and suicide rates.[4] The current trend is a widening disparity between those in the United States with the highest and lowest life expectancy.

Figure 1.4 Estimated impact of the factors that affect health and well-being.

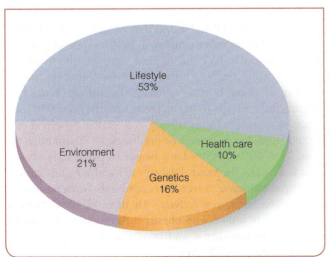

GLOSSARY

Life expectancy Number of years a person is expected to live based on the person's birth year.

Chronic diseases Illnesses that develop as a result of an unhealthy lifestyle and last a long time.

Risk factors Lifestyle and genetic variables that may lead to disease.

Sedentary Description of a person who is relatively inactive

and whose lifestyle is characterized by a lot of sitting.

Sedentary death syndrome (SeDS) Cause of deaths attributed to a lack of regular physical activity.

Hypokinetic diseases *Hypo* denotes "lack of"; therefore, illnesses related to lack of physical activity.

Health State of complete well-being—not just the absence of disease or infirmity.

Figure 1.5 Life expectancy at birth for selected countries: 2005–2015 projections.

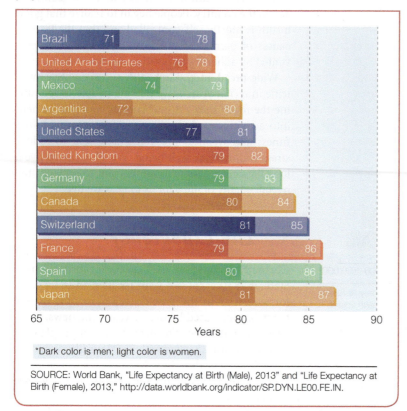

*Dark color is men; light color is women.

SOURCE: World Bank, "Life Expectancy at Birth (Male), 2013" and "Life Expectancy at Birth (Female), 2013," http://data.worldbank.org/indicator/SP.DYN.LE00.FE.IN.

For example, males in Fairfax County, Virginia, can expect to live as long as males in Japan, while those in Bolivar County, Mississippi, have the same life expectancy as males in countries with much lower life expectancies, like Pakistan. People with low socioeconomic status often lead more stressful lives, have more dangerous jobs, have less access to healthy food, are more likely to be exposed to environmental toxins, and live in neighborhoods that are not as safe or as conducive to physical activity. Physical activity trends by U.S. county, in most cases, are aligned with life expectancy trends.[5]

The Gender Gap in Life Expectancy

Life expectancy for men in the United States is almost 5 years lower than for women. For years it had been assumed that the difference is based on biology, but we are learning that most likely the gender gap is related to lifestyle behaviors most commonly observed in men. Around 1980, the gender gap in life expectancy was almost 8 years. The decrease in the gender gap is thought to be due to the fact that women are increasingly taking on jobs, habits, and stressors of men, including drinking and employment outside the home. Women with heavy work schedules, however, are at higher risk than men who have similar work schedules when it comes to heart disease, cancer, and diabetes—most likely because women tend to take on additional stressors at home.[6] Women and men are also becoming more similar to one another in their risk factors for heart disease, such as obesity and diabetes.

Men, nonetheless, still report higher stress on the job and are less likely to engage in stress management programs. Also, 95 percent of employees in the 10 most dangerous jobs are men. Furthermore, men's health is not given the same degree of attention in terms of public health policies. Thus, men need to take a more proactive role in managing their own health, yet, unfortunately, this can be hard for them.

"Masculinity" itself is also partially to blame. Studies have consistently shown that men are less likely to visit a physician when something is wrong and are less likely to have preventive care visits to be screened for potential risk factors such as hypertension, elevated cholesterol, diabetes, obesity, substance abuse, and depression or anxiety. It is a troubling paradox, considering that men are at greater risk for each of the top risk factors for chronic disease. As a result, chronic diseases in men are often diagnosed at a later stage, when a cure or adequate management is more difficult to achieve. Men also drive faster than women and are more likely to engage in risk-taking activities.

The Need to Prevent Disease, Not Only Cure It

The United States has not invested the same resources in preventing disease as it has in treating disease after onset. Ninety-five percent of our health care dollars are spent on treatment strategies, and less than 5 percent are spent on prevention. In contrast, some countries, like Australia, have boosted prevention efforts by arranging primary care to better detect and intervene with hypertension, for example. The latest data indicate that one in four adults in the United States have at least two chronic conditions. Most of these patients do not receive half of the preventative recommendations from the U.S. Preventative Services Task Force. Eva H. DuGoff of Johns Hopkins Bloomberg School of Public Health has said, "Our system is not set up to care for people with so many different illnesses. Each one adds up and makes the burden of disease greater than the sum of its parts."[7]

A report by the OECD found that while the United States far outspent every other country in health care cost per capita, it also easily had the highest rates of obesity of all 34 OECD countries.[8] As a nation, we are seeing the consequences of these numbers unfold. Incidence of diabetes climbed dramatically in parallel step with the increased incidence of obesity.[9] Today, nearly half of the people in the United States have diabetes or prediabetes.[10] Thankfully, the rising U.S. diabetes rates have begun to plateau, as obesity rates have done the same. Diabetes is the third most expensive chronic disease to treat, preceded only by heart disease and hypertension, respectively. All three of these chronic conditions are linked with obesity.[11] Additional information on the obesity epidemic and its detrimental health consequences is given in Chapter 5.

1.3 Leading Health Problems in the United States

The leading causes of death in the United States today are largely related to lifestyle and personal choices (Figure 1.6). The U.S. Centers for Disease Control and Prevention have found that 7 of 10 Americans die of preventable chronic diseases. Specifically, about 48 percent of all deaths in the United States are caused by cardiovascular disease and cancer.[12] Almost 80 percent of the latter deaths could be prevented through a healthy lifestyle program. The third and fourth leading causes of death across all age groups, respectively, are chronic lower respiratory disease and accidents. From the age of 1 to 44, accidents are the leading cause of death, with automobile accidents being the leading cause of death in the 5 to 24 age group.[13]

HOEGER KEY TO WELLNESS

Scientists believe that a healthy lifestyle program has the power to prevent almost 80 percent of deaths from cardiovascular disease and cancer.

Diseases of the Cardiovascular System

The most prevalent degenerative diseases in the United States are those of the cardiovascular system. The umbrella of **cardiovascular diseases** includes such conditions as **coronary heart disease (CHD), heart attacks,** and **strokes** (sometimes referred to as brain attacks because like heart attacks, strokes occur when oxygen-rich blood is blocked from reaching cells). According to the American Heart Association

(AHA), more than one in three adults in the United States is afflicted with diseases of the cardiovascular system, including one in three adults living with hypertension (high blood pressure) and 15.4 million with CHD. (Many of these people have more than one type of cardiovascular disease.) These numbers are devastating but can change. As we gained understanding of the effects of lifestyle on chronic disease during the second half of the 20th century, more people participated in wellness programs, and cardiovascular mortality rates dropped. The decline began in about 1963, and between 1969 and 2013, the incidence of heart disease dropped by 68 percent and the incidence of stroke by 77 percent. This decrease is credited to higher levels of wellness and better treatment modalities in the United States. A complete cardiovascular disease prevention program is outlined in Chapter 10.

---GLOSSARY---

Cardiovascular disease The array of conditions that affect the heart (cardio-) and the blood vessels (-vascular); often used interchangeably with the term *heart disease*. Under the cardiovascular disease umbrella are diseases including stroke and coronary heart disease (CHD). CHD, in turn, is an umbrella term for diseases that affect the heart and coronary arteries, which includes heart attacks.

Coronary heart disease (CHD) A disease in which plaque builds up in the arteries that sup-

ply blood to the heart (these are the coronary arteries; the term "coronary" evolved from the word for "crown or wreath," referring to the arteries that circle the heart).

Heart attack Damage to an area of the myocardium (heart muscle) that is deprived of oxygen, usually due to blockage of a diseased coronary artery.

Stroke A condition in which a blood vessel that feeds the brain is clogged, leading to blood flow disruption to the brain. Sometimes referred to as a brain attack.

Figure 1.6 Leading causes of death in the United States by age.

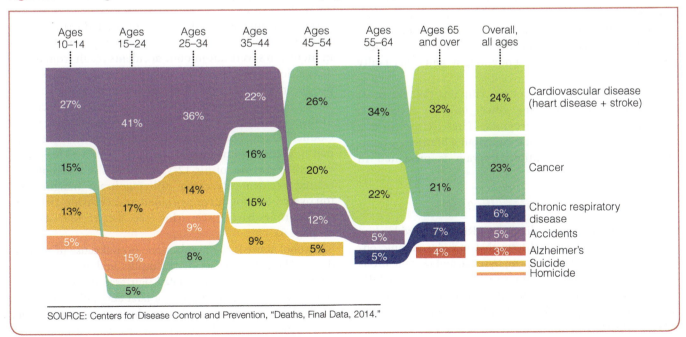

SOURCE: Centers for Disease Control and Prevention, "Deaths, Final Data, 2014."

Healthy Habits That Cut the Risk for Serious Disease

According to the Centers for Disease Control and Prevention, four health habits can reduce your risk of chronic diseases such as heart disease, cancer, and diabetes by almost 80 percent:

- Get at least 30 minutes of daily moderate-intensity physical activity.
- Don't ever smoke.
- Eat a healthy diet (ample fruits and vegetables, whole grain products, and low meat consumption).
- Maintain a body mass index (BMI) of less than 30.

The latest research would add one more crucial life-saving habit: Reduce the amount of time you spend sitting each day.

Cancer

The second overall leading cause of death in the United States is cancer. Cancer is closing the gap to soon become the leading cause of death in the United States as a whole, and it already claims more lives than cardiovascular disease in 22 states. For Americans ages 45 to 64 nationwide, as well as for certain ethnic groups,[14] it is already the leading cause of death. One reason for this change may be that increased rates of obesity lead to increased risk for both cancer and cardiovascular disease, but treatment for cardiovascular disease is not as difficult and complex as cancer treatment. About 23 percent of all deaths in the United States are attributable to cancer.[15]

The major contributor to the increase in the incidence of cancer deaths during the past five decades is lung cancer, of which 90 percent for males and 80 percent for females is caused by tobacco use.[16] Furthermore, smoking accounts for almost 30 percent of all deaths from cancer. More than 30 percent of deaths are related to nutrition, physical inactivity, excessive body weight, and other faulty lifestyle habits.

The American Cancer Society maintains that the most influential factor in fighting cancer today is prevention through health education programs. Lifestyle choices at a young age affect cancer risk throughout a lifetime. A comprehensive cancer-prevention program is presented in Chapter 11.

Chronic Lower Respiratory Disease

Chronic lower respiratory disease (CLRD), the third leading cause of death, is a general term that includes chronic obstructive pulmonary disease, emphysema, and chronic bronchitis (all diseases of the respiratory system). Although CLRD is related mostly to tobacco use (see Chapter 13 for discussion on how to stop smoking), lifetime nonsmokers also can develop CLRD.

Precautions to prevent CLRD include consuming a low-fat, low-sodium, nutrient-dense diet; staying physically active; not smoking and not breathing cigarette smoke; getting a pneumonia vaccine if older than age 50 and a current or ex-smoker; and avoiding swimming pools for individuals sensitive to chlorine vapor.

Accidents

Accidents are the fourth overall leading cause of death and the leading cause of death until age 44. Even though not all accidents are preventable, many are. Consider automobile accidents, the leading cause of death for teens. Across the United States, fewer than 15 percent of people taking trips in automobiles choose not to wear seatbelts, yet these people account for half of all automobile deaths. As for the cause of automobile accidents themselves, fatal accidents are often related to failure to stay in the correct lane or yield the right of way due to driver distraction or alcohol use.[17]

Most people do not perceive accidents as a health problem. Even so, accidents affect the total well-being of millions of Americans each year. Accident prevention and personal safety are part of a health-enhancement program aimed at achieving a better quality of life. Hours spent exercising at the gym are of little help if the person is involved in a disabling or fatal accident as a result of distraction or making a single reckless decision.

Accidents do not just happen. We cause accidents, and we are victims of accidents. Although some factors in life, like natural disasters, are completely beyond our control, more often than not, personal safety and accident prevention are a matter of common sense. Most accidents stem from poor judgment and confused mental states, which occur when people are upset, mentally spent, not paying attention to the task at hand, trying to do too much at once, or abusing alcohol or other drugs.

With the advent of cell phones, distracted driving accidents have climbed. For teens, specifically, 6 in 10 of all moderate to severe automobile accidents result from driver distraction.[18] On an average day in the United States, nine people are killed as a result of distracted driving, and more than 1,000 people are injured. As the Senior Director of Transportation Strategic Initiatives for the National Safety Council, David Teater, put it, "You never think it will happen to you—until it does." Teater's research has been motivated by the loss of his 12-year-old son in a cell phone-related accident. Research utilizing brain imaging has uncovered the cognitive workload and collision risk during multiple driving scenarios (see "Distracted Driving" on page 9).

Alcohol abuse is the number-one overall cause of all accidents. About half of accidental deaths and suicides in the United States are alcohol related. Further, alcohol intoxication remains the leading cause of fatal automobile accidents in the United States by taking the lives of 30 people every day. Other commonly abused drugs alter feelings and

Distracted Driving

Automobile accidents are the number-one cause of death for teens in the United States. Recent studies on distracted driving have used new technology, including real-time brain imaging, to offer new insight about protecting ourselves behind the wheel. Following are insights for drivers.

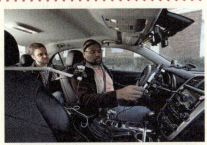
AAA Foundation for Traffic Safety

1. *Listening to the radio is nearly as safe as driving with no distractions.*
2. *Having a cell phone conversation increases collision incidence fourfold.* The risk is identical for a hands-free device and a hand-held phone.[a]
3. *Having a cell phone conversation causes the brain to screen out 50 percent of visual cues.* The ability to look directly at but not "see" an object is termed "inattention blindness." It is not uncommon for a distracted driver running a red light to collide with the second or third car in an intersection, having not "seen" the first cars. Talking on a phone while driving decreases reaction time to pedestrians in a crosswalk by 40 percent.[b]
4. *Having a conversation with an adult passenger is safer than having a conversation on a cell phone.* Passengers who are experienced drivers help the driver by pausing conversation and by pointing out cues as needed. For a teen driver, the incidence of collision resulting in death increases with the number of teen passengers.
5. *Though crash risk is lower when talking with a passenger, cognitive workload can be the same as when talking on a cell phone.* Topic of conversation and emotional involvement affect safety in both types of conversation.
6. *The brain does not multitask, but rather switches attention between tasks.* Some dual tasks do not cause a problem; others do. When driving and holding a conversation, the brain often recognizes conversation as the primary task. Switching is a complex process that requires events to be committed to short-term memory before they can be "encoded," the stage when the brain chooses what to "see." It is not uncommon for switching time to be tenths of a second, the difference of several car lengths when braking. This is termed "reaction time switching costs."
7. *The brain remains somewhat distracted for up to 27 seconds following a phone conversation, text, or voice technology interaction.*[c]
8. *Because the majority of trips do not involve a situation that requires split-second timing, drivers can gain a false sense of security about being able to multitask.*
9. *Making a left turn while talking on a cell phone or hands-free device is among the most dangerous driving activities.*[d]
10. *Reaching for a moving object or turning in your seat increases collision incidence by eight to nine times.*
11. *Texting while driving increases collision incidence by 16 times.* Compared with texting, talking on a cell phone is done by drivers more frequently for longer lengths of time, and so is the cause of more deaths than texting is. Consider using your phone's do not disturb setting or an app that blocks texting while driving. Because our minds are social and curious, we find text alerts difficult to ignore.
12. *Sleepy drivers kill more than half as many Americans as drunk drivers.* More than 6,000 people die each year in the United States in crashes attributed to drowsy drivers. In comparison, roughly 10,000 people die each year because of drunk or buzzed driving.
13. *Parents driving children are just as likely to talk on the phone and use distractions, including navigation systems, as other drivers.*[e]
14. *Using Apple's Siri while driving to get directions, send texts, post to social media, or check appointments can be as dangerous as texting while driving, even when hands-free.*[f]

We cannot control what information our brain chooses to encode and screen out while driving. We can control our decision to use a cell phone or to speak up when a driver is putting passengers in danger.

[a]Training, Research, and Education for Driving Safety, "UC San Diego Joins Nationwide Efforts to Curb Phone Use While Driving," released online December 4, 2013, available at http://health.ucsd.edu/news/releases/Pages /2013-12-04-TREDS-just-drive-program.aspx; J. G. Gaspar, W. M. Street, M. B. Windsor, R. Carbonari, H. Kaczmarski, A. F. Kramer, and K. E. Mathewson, "Providing Conversation Partners Views of the Driving Scene Mitigates Cell Phone-Related Distraction," *Proceedings of the Human Factors and Ergonomics Society Annual Meeting* 57, no. 1 (2013).

[b]Jill U. Adams, "Talking on a Cellphone While Driving Is Risky. But simpler Distractions Can Also Cause Harm," *Washington Post*, February 10, 2014.

[c]"Up to 27 Seconds of Inattention after Talking to Your Car or Smartphone," The University of Utah UNews, October 27, 2015, available at http://unews.utah.edu/up-to-27-seconds -of-inattention-after-talking-to-your-car-or-smart-phone/.

[d]Tom A. Schweizer, Karen Kan, Yuwen Hung, Fred Tarn, Gary Naglie, and Simon J. Graham, "Brain Activity during Driving with Distraction: An Immersive fMRI Study," *Frontiers in Human Neuroscience*, February 28, 2013, doi:10.3389 /fnhum.2013.00053.

[e]Michelle L. Macy, Patrick M. Carter, C. Raymond Bingham, Rebecca M. Cunningham, and Gary L. Freed, "Potential Distractions and Unsafe Driving Behaviors Among Drivers of 1- to 12-Year-Old Children," *Academic Pediatrics* 14, no. 3 (2014): 279.

[f]University of Utah News Center, "Talking to Your Car Is Often Distracting," October 7, 2014, available online at http://unews.utah.edu/news_releases/talking-to-your -car-is-often-distracting/.

perceptions, generate mental confusion, and impair judgment and coordination, greatly enhancing the risk for accidental **morbidity** (Chapter 13).

Medical Error in U.S. Hospitals: An Untracked Mortality Risk

Only recently has attention been brought to the number of deaths that are a direct result of medical error in U.S. Hospitals. When cause of death is recorded by the CDC, medical error is not offered as an option; however, an estimated 250,000 each year are the result of a mistake of omission or commission by medical workers. While nothing can guarantee perfect medical care, it is ideal for every hospitalized patient to have an attentive and vocal advocate, and of course to lead a wellness lifestyle to avoid preventable health complications in the first place.

1.4 Physical Activity Affects Health and Quality of Life

Among the benefits of regular physical activity and exercise are a significant reduction in premature mortality and decreased risks for developing heart disease, stroke, metabolic syndrome, type 2 diabetes, obesity, osteoporosis, colon and breast cancers, high blood pressure, depression, and even dementia and Alzheimer's. But we did not always understand the relationship between physical activity and mortality rates, in particular, the dose-response relationship.

During the second half of the 20th century, scientists began to realize the importance of good fitness and improved lifestyle in the fight against chronic diseases, particularly those of the cardiovascular system. Because of more participation in wellness programs, cardiovascular mortality rates dropped.

Furthermore, several studies showed an inverse relationship between physical activity and premature mortality rates. The first major study in this area was conducted in the 1980s among 16,936 Harvard alumni, and the results linked physical activity habits and mortality rates.[19] As the amount of weekly physical activity increased, the risk for cardiovascular deaths decreased.

A landmark study subsequently conducted at the Aerobics Research Institute in Dallas upheld the findings of the Harvard alumni study.[20] Based on data from 13,344 people followed over an average of 8 years, the study revealed a graded and consistent inverse relationship between physical activity levels and mortality, regardless of age and other risk factors. As illustrated in Figure 1.7, the higher the level of physical activity, the longer the lifespan.

A most significant finding of this landmark study was the large drop in all-cause, cardiovascular, and cancer mortality when individuals went from low fitness to moderate fitness—a clear indication that moderate-intensity physical activity, achievable by most adults, does provide considerable health benefits and extends life. The data also revealed that the participants attained more protection by combining higher fitness levels with reduction in other risk factors such as hypertension, serum cholesterol, cigarette smoking, and excessive body fat. Countless studies since have upheld these results and have established that as physical activity increases, overall mortality rate decreases. Research has also corroborated that the biggest

Figure 1.7 Death rates by physical fitness groups. (Numbers on top of the bars are all-cause death rates per 10,000 person-years of follow-up for each cell; 1 person-year indicates one person who was followed up 1 year later.)

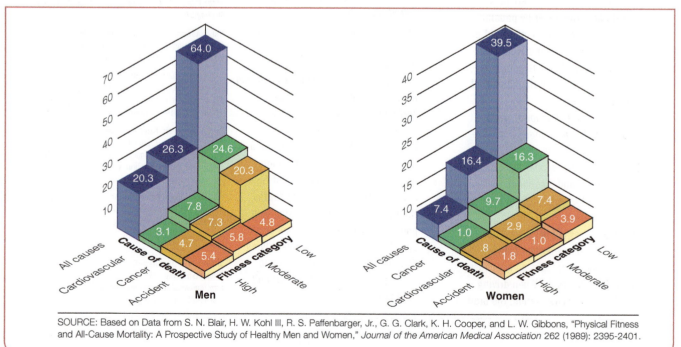

SOURCE: Based on Data from S. N. Blair, H. W. Kohl III, R. S. Paffenbarger, Jr., G. G. Clark, K. H. Cooper, and L. W. Gibbons, "Physical Fitness and All-Cause Mortality: A Prospective Study of Healthy Men and Women," *Journal of the American Medical Association* 262 (1989): 2395-2401.

drop in mortality rate happens when inactive people become moderately active.[21] One recent study found that if the worldwide inactivity rate were to go down by only 20 percent, more than 1 million lives could be saved on a yearly basis and global life expectancy would increase by almost a year.[22]

One study looked to specifically compare the efficacy of commonly prescribed drugs against the impact of regular exercise. The data are based on more than 14,000 patients recovering from stroke, being treated for heart failure, or looking to prevent type 2 diabetes or a second episode of CHD. The study looked at the effectiveness of exercise versus drugs on health outcomes. The results were revealing: Exercise programs were more effective than medical treatment in stroke patients and equally effective as medical treatments in prevention of diabetes and CHD. Only in the prevention of heart failure were diuretic drugs more effective in preventing mortality than exercise.

When physical activity is combined with other healthy lifestyle factors, it becomes clear that individual lifestyle choice is the strongest predictor of longevity. Consider four health-related factors examined in a group of more than 23,000 people.[23] These factors included lifetime nonsmoker, not considered obese (body mass index less than 30), engaging in a minimum of 3.5 hours of weekly physical activity, and adherence to healthy nutrition principles (high consumption of whole-grain breads, fruits, and vegetables and low consumption of red meat). Those who adhered to all four health habits were 78 percent less likely to develop chronic diseases (diabetes, heart disease, stroke, and cancer) during the almost 8-year study. Furthermore, the risk for developing a chronic disease progressively increased as the number of health factors decreased.

While it is clear that moderate-intensity exercise does provide substantial health benefits, research data also show a dose-response relationship between physical activity and health. That is, greater health and fitness benefits occur at higher duration and/or intensity of physical activity. Vigorous activity and longer duration are preferable to the extent of one's capabilities because they are most clearly associated with better health and longer life. Current recommendations suggest that a person accumulate 150 minutes of moderate-intensity physical activity each week. For an inactive person, following this guideline is the most important step toward improving health. Once a person is regularly achieving this weekly minimum, the next step toward improving health through physical activity is to replace at least one-third of weekly moderate physical activity with vigorous physical activity.[24] We are learning that even individuals who feel short on time can gain major ground in their desire to boost physical fitness by participating in high-intensity interval training one to three times per week (for specific recommendations see Chapter 9, pages 340–341). Further, current research indicates that there is no increase in mortality risk when people participate in a large volume of moderate- or vigorous-intensity activity each week. Benefits in decreased mortality risk continue to increase until a person reaches three to five times the recommended weekly minimum of 150 minutes, at which point, benefits in decreased mortality risk plateau.[25]

As compared with prolonged moderate-intensity activity, vigorous-intensity exercise has been shown to provide the best improvements in aerobic capacity, CHD risk reduction, and overall cardiovascular health.[26] A word of caution, however, is in order. Vigorous exercise should be reserved for healthy individuals who have been cleared for it (Activity 1.3).

Exercise Is Medicine

In order to help the public better appreciate the true benefits of exercise, the American College of Sports Medicine (ACSM) and the American Medical Association (AMA) have launched a nationwide "Exercise Is Medicine" program.[27] The initiative calls on all physicians to assess and review every patient's physical activity program at every visit. "Exercise is medicine and it's free." All physicians should be prescribing exercise to all patients and participating in exercise themselves. Currently, physicians and other professionals in the health field receive little training in exercise science and its practical clinical application. The prevalent approach of largely ignoring exercise in the health profession is an outdated way of practicing medicine.

1.5 Additional Benefits of a Comprehensive Fitness Program

Regular physical activity is important for the health of muscles, bones, and joints and has been shown in clinical studies to improve mood, cognitive function, creativity, and short-term memory and enhance one's ability to perform daily tasks throughout life. It also can have a major impact on health care costs and quality of life into old age.

An inspiring story illustrating what fitness can do for a person's health and well-being is that of George Snell from Sandy, Utah. At age 45, Snell weighed approximately 400 pounds, his blood pressure was 220/180, he was blind because of undiagnosed diabetes, and his blood glucose level was 487.

Snell had determined to do something about his physical and medical condition, so he started a walking/jogging program. After about 8 months of conditioning, he had lost almost 200 pounds, his eyesight had returned, his glucose level was down to 67, and he was taken off medication. Just 2 months later—less than 10 months after beginning his personal exercise program—he completed his first marathon, a running course of 26.2 miles!

GLOSSARY

Morbidity A condition related to or caused by illness or disease.

Types of Scientific Studies

Most scientific health studies can be broken down into two basic types: observational studies and experimental studies. Understanding how these types of studies differ will help you better weigh the results of any study and how that study may directly apply to you.

Observational studies are what you would expect from the name: data collected by observing a given population. Scientists do not intervene with the subjects who make up these populations but simply observe trends in the population. Observational studies, therefore, cannot prove cause and effect.

- Among the types of observational studies are *cohort studies,* which follow a group of people over time; *case-control studies,* which compare groups of people who have and do not have a particular condition; *cross-sectional surveys,* which look at one point in time to see how prevalent a given condition is; and *case reports,* which are an in-depth history of a few select cases.

Experimental studies seek to prove cause and effect and, therefore, involve intervention by the researchers followed by an observation of the outcome. Following are common examples of experimental studies.

- *Laboratory studies* can be done using animals or tissue from animals or humans. These studies are also referred to as preclinical research because they are required before clinical research in humans is allowed.

- *Clinical trials* use humans as subjects to test new treatments. It is important when interpreting the results of a clinical trial to know who funded the trial so you can be aware of any bias. Though sponsors of trials cannot affect the outcome, at times, sponsors select researchers whose previous research best aligns with the outcome they prefer to see from the study.

- *Randomized double-blind placebo control studies* are the gold standard of experimental research. These studies employ two groups of subjects who are as similar as possible, with the only

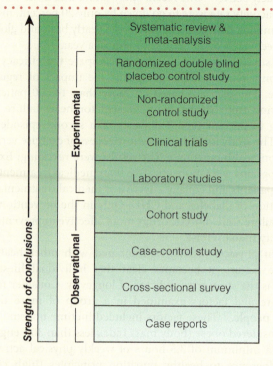

difference being the variable that the scientists are investigating. Neither the researcher(s) nor the participants (or, if applicable, sponsors) know who is being affected by the variable being studied until the full completion of the research.

Systematic reviews gather all of the clinical or observational studies that have already been completed on a particular topic and that fit the criteria the researchers have set out to investigate. The investigators then analyze and combine the data and summarize the results. They often employ a *meta-analysis,* a statistical technique to adjust data from smaller studies so that they are easily comparable with one another and can be combined together.

Health Benefits

Most people exercise because it improves their personal appearance and makes them feel good about themselves. Although many benefits accrue from regular fitness, the greatest benefit of all is that physically fit individuals enjoy a better quality of life. These people live life to its fullest, with far fewer health problems than inactive individuals.

The benefits derived by regularly participating in exercise are so extensive that it is difficult to compile an all-inclusive list. Many of these benefits are summarized in Table 1.1. As far back as 1982, the American Medical Association indicated that "there is no drug in current or prospective use that holds as much promise for sustained health as a lifetime program of physical exercise." Furthermore, researchers and sports medicine leaders have stated that if the benefits of exercise could

be packaged in a pill, it would be the most widely prescribed medication throughout the world today.

While most of the chronic (long-term) benefits of exercise are well-established, what many people fail to realize is that there are immediate benefits derived by participating in just a single bout of exercise. Most of these benefits dissipate within 48 to 72 hours following exercise. The immediate benefits, summarized in Table 1.2, are so striking that they prompted Dr. William L. Haskell of Stanford University to state: "Most of the health benefits of exercise are relatively short term, so people should think of exercise as a medication and take it on a daily basis." Of course, as you regularly exercise a minimum of 30 minutes five times per week and maintain a certain amount of physical activity throughout the day, you will realize the impressive long-term benefits listed in Table 1.1.

Table 1.1 Long-Term Benefits of Exercise

Regular participation in exercise:

- improves and strengthens the cardiorespiratory system.
- maintains better muscle tone, muscular strength, and endurance.
- improves muscular flexibility.
- enhances athletic performance.
- helps maintain recommended body weight.
- helps preserve lean body tissue.
- increases resting metabolic rate.
- improves the body's ability to use fat during physical activity.
- improves posture and physical appearance.
- improves functioning of the immune system.
- lowers the risk for chronic diseases and illnesses (including heart disease, stroke, and certain cancers).
- decreases the mortality rate from chronic diseases.
- thins the blood so that it doesn't clot as readily, thereby decreasing the risk for coronary heart disease and stroke.
- helps the body manage blood lipid (cholesterol and triglyceride) levels more effectively.
- prevents or delays the development of high blood pressure and lowers blood pressure in people with hypertension.
- helps prevent and control type 2 diabetes.
- helps achieve peak bone mass in young adults and maintain bone mass later in life, thereby decreasing the risk for osteoporosis.

- helps people sleep better.
- helps prevent chronic back pain.
- relieves tension and helps in coping with life stresses.
- raises levels of energy and job productivity.
- extends longevity and slows the aging process.
- improves and helps maintain cognitive function, decreasing the risk for dementia and Alzheimer's disease.
- promotes psychological well-being, including higher morale, self-image, and self-esteem.
- reduces feelings of depression and anxiety.
- encourages positive lifestyle changes (improving nutrition, quitting smoking, controlling alcohol and drug use).
- speeds recovery time following physical exertion.
- speeds recovery following injury or disease.
- regulates and improves overall body functions.
- improves physical stamina and counteracts chronic fatigue.
- retards creeping frailty, reduces disability, and helps to maintain independent living in older adults.
- enhances quality of life: People feel better and live a healthier and happier life.

Table 1.2 Immediate (Acute) Benefits of Exercise

You can expect a number of benefits as a result of a single exercise session. Some of these benefits last as long as 72 hours following your workout. Exercise:

- increases heart rate, stroke volume, cardiac output, pulmonary ventilation, and oxygen uptake.
- begins to strengthen the heart, lungs, and muscles.
- enhances metabolic rate or energy production (burning calories for fuel) during exercise and recovery. (For every 100 calories you burn during exercise, you can expect to burn another 15 during recovery.)
- uses blood glucose and muscle glycogen.
- improves insulin sensitivity (decreasing the risk of type 2 diabetes).
- immediately enhances the body's ability to burn fat.
- lowers blood lipids.
- improves joint flexibility.
- reduces low-grade (hidden) inflammation (see pages 397–398 in Chapter 10).
- increases endorphins (hormones), which are naturally occurring opioids that are responsible for exercise-induced euphoria.
- increases fat storage *in muscle,* which can then be burned for energy.

- improves endothelial function. (Endothelial cells line the entire vascular system, which provides a barrier between the vessel lumen and surrounding tissue—endothelial dysfunction contributes to several disease processes, including tissue inflammation and subsequent atherosclerosis.)
- enhances mood and self-worth.
- provides a sense of achievement and satisfaction.
- decreases blood pressure the first few hours following exercise.
- decreases arthritic pain.
- leads to muscle relaxation.
- decreases stress.
- improves brain function.
- promotes better sleep (unless exercise is performed too close to bedtime).
- improves digestion.
- boosts energy levels.
- improves resistance to infections.

Exercise and Brain Function

Exercise affects brain function and academic performance. Physical activity is related to better cognitive health and effective functioning across the lifespan. While much of the research is still in its infancy, even in 400 bc, the Greek philosopher Plato stated: "In order for man to succeed in life, God provided him with two means, education and physical activity. Not separately, one for the soul and the other for the body, but for the two together. With these two means, man can attain perfection."

Data on more than 2.4 million students in the state of Texas have shown consistent and significant associations between physical fitness and various indicators of academic achievement; in particular, higher levels of fitness were associated with better academic grades. Cardiorespiratory fitness was shown to have a dose-response association with academic performance (better fitness and better grades), independent of other sociodemographic and fitness variables.[28] Another analysis looked at the short-term boost of exercise on academics. After reviewing the results from 19 different studies

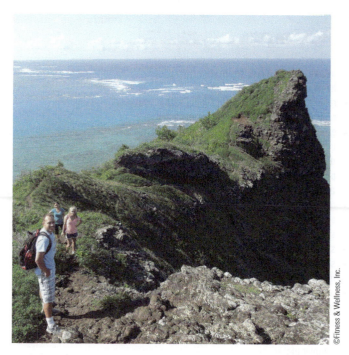

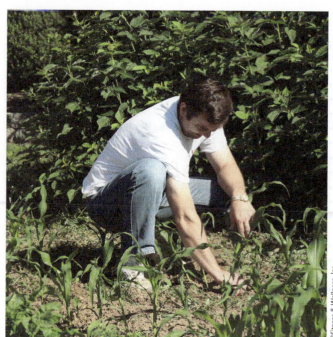

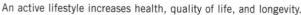

An active lifestyle increases health, quality of life, and longevity.

of children to young adults, researchers found that students who had 20 minutes of exercise immediately preceding a test or giving a speech had higher academic performance and better focus than those who did not exercise.[29] Exercise has proven to make us more clearheaded.

Emerging research shows that exercise allows the brain to function at its best through a combination of biological reactions. First, exercise increases blood flow to the brain, providing oxygen, glucose, and other nutrients and improving the removal of metabolic waste products. The increased blood and oxygen flow also prompt the release of the protein brain-derived neurotrophic factor (BDNF). This protein works by strengthening connections between brain cells and repairing any damage within them. BDNF also stimulates the growth of new neurons in the hippocampus, the portion of the brain involved in memory, planning, learning, and decision-making. The hippocampus is one of only two parts of the adult brain where new cells can be generated. The connections strengthened by BDNF are critical for learning to take place and for memories to be stored. Exercise provides the necessary stimulus for brain neurons to interconnect, creating the perfect environment in which the brain is ready and able to learn.[30]

Exercise also increases the neurotransmitters dopamine, glutamate, norepinephrine, and serotonin, all of which are vital in the generation of thought and emotion. Low levels of serotonin have been linked to depression, and exercise has repeatedly been shown to be effective in treating depression.

The hippocampus tends to shrink in late adulthood, leading to memory impairment. In older adults, regular aerobic exercise has been shown to increase the size of the hippocampus and decrease the rate of brain shrinkage, dramatically minimizing declines in thinking and memory skills. One study found that older adults who followed a regular program of moderate to intense exercise had the cognitive and memory skills that rated a decade younger than sedentary peers of the same age.[31] Physical activity appears to be the most important lifestyle change a person can make to prevent dementia and Alzheimer's later in life. Even light-intensity activities of daily living appear to provide protection against cognitive impairment. The research further shows that as the amount of activity increases, the rate of cognitive decline decreases, and the amount of daily activity performed appears to be more important than the intensity itself in terms of warding off dementia. Additionally, maintaining a high level of physical fitness in mid-life can reduce a person's chances of developing Alzheimer's by half and dementia by 60 percent.[32]

1.6 *Sitting Disease: A 21st-Century Chronic Disease*

The human body requires time to recover (sit and sleep) from labor, tasks, and other typical daily activities. Most Americans, however, sit for way too many hours each day. On *average*, people spend about 8 hours per day or more of their waking time sitting. Prolonged sitting is unnatural to the body, and research now indicates that too much sitting is hazardous to human health and has a direct link to premature mortality.[33] Some organizations have suggested that exposure to sitting time be treated like any other deadly risk factor, such as excessive sun exposure. Although not recognized by the medical community as a diagnosable illness, the scientific community has coined the term "sitting disease" as a chronic 21st-century disease.

The data indicate that the risks that come with sitting are independent from those related to physical activity levels. They suggest that, like the gas or the brake pedal on a car, physical activity or prolonged sitting each act upon human physiology in their own, independent way. Therefore, even individuals who exercise five times per week for at least 30 minutes per session but otherwise spend most of the day sitting are accruing health risks. Some data suggest that as many as 60 to 75 minutes of daily moderate physical activity may counter up to 8 hours of sitting in a day.[34]

There is no question that prolonged sitting is a major risk factor for disease. In one particular study, healthy young men who normally accrued 10,000 steps per day were instructed to become sedentary and keep daily step count under 1,500 for 2 weeks. Within this short 2-week time span, these young men started to develop metabolic problems, including reduced insulin sensitivity and increased abdominal fat (see Chapter 4, pages 141–142 for an overview of health risks associated with increased abdominal fat).[35]

Our bodies are simply not designed for extended periods of sitting. As we sink into inactivity, our biological processes begin to change, down to a cellular and molecular level. Researchers are only beginning to understand all of the factors at work, but studies show, for example, that blood flow becomes sluggish and is more likely to form life-threatening clots in the lungs and legs. Arteries lose flexibility and have a lower capacity to expand and relax.[36] Slower blood flow means less oxygen and glucose delivered to the brain and body and, as a result, cognitive function declines and the feeling of fatigue increases. Additionally, during extended sitting, fat deposits accumulate in muscle cells, which interferes with insulin's ability to transport glucose into muscle cells. (When a person is active, **skeletal muscles** are responsible for 80 percent of glucose disposal.) Thus, insulin resistance increases along with the accompanying risk for diabetes and cardiovascular disease. When you are sitting, the level of triglycerides (a type of fat found in your blood) jumps because inactive muscles also stop producing an enzyme[37] that usually captures these fats from the blood in order to turn them into fuel. Even HDL cholesterol levels (the good cholesterol) drop by 20 percent after as little as 1 hour of uninterrupted sitting.

When we are sitting, some of the largest muscles in our body, including leg and hip muscles, are relaxed and inactive. By simply standing up, we immediately activate these muscles. They work to keep us upright, requiring blood sugar to fuel themselves. They further release the enzyme that captures triglycerides from the blood to help keep cholesterol levels in check and also help regulate other metabolic processes. The simple act of repeatedly standing and moving throughout the day can change disease risk. Further, remaining inactive following meals makes blood glucose levels spike. A slow stroll after a meal can cut this blood glucose spike in half. Inactivity further appears to switch on or off dozens of genes that trigger additional risk factors.

Death rates are high for people who spend most of their day sitting, even though they meet the minimum physical activity recommendations on a weekly basis. The data show that:

- Sitting for more than 3 hours per day cuts off 2 years of life, even if you regularly exercise and avoid unhealthy habits like smoking.
- People who spend most of their day sitting have as much as a 50 percent greater risk of dying prematurely from all causes. Excessive sitting is the "new smoking." The risk of a heart attack in people who sit most of the day is almost the same as that of smokers.
- Inactive adults over age 60 are at almost 50 percent greater odds of disability for each additional hour they sit per day.
- Prolonged daily sitting time is an underestimated risk factor for cancer. Too much sitting has been estimated to cause 91,000 cancer deaths each year in the United States alone (49,000 breast cancers and 42,000 colon cancers).
- Less sitting means greater comfort. Study participants who reduced their sitting time by 66 minutes a day reported feeling less fatigued and more energetic, focused, productive, and comfortable and reported less back and neck pain.[38]

Most people do not realize how much time they spend sitting on a given day. Think about the seats you sit in every day and how much time you spend in each (see Figure 1.8). We can easily accumulate 8 to 12 sitting hours and spend the majority of our day in the seated position, with only the chair beneath us changing.

HOEGER KEY TO WELLNESS

 By being more active throughout the day and avoiding excessive sitting, people can increase their daily energy (caloric) expenditure by the equivalent of a 7-mile run. They will also increase years of healthy life expectancy.

GLOSSARY

Skeletal muscle The type of muscle that powers body movement.

Figure 1.8 **The importance of nonexercise activity thermogenesis (NEAT) and exercise.**

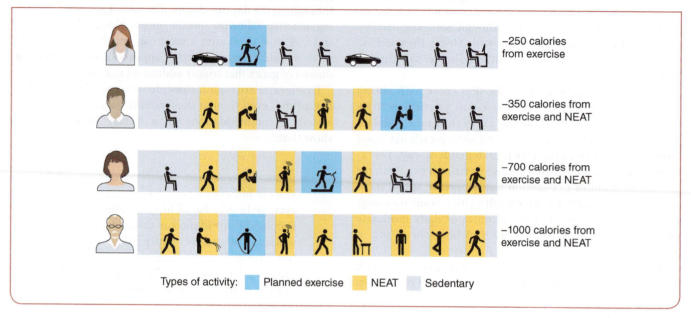

−250 calories from exercise

−350 calories from exercise and NEAT

−700 calories from exercise and NEAT

−1000 calories from exercise and NEAT

Types of activity: Planned exercise   NEAT   Sedentary

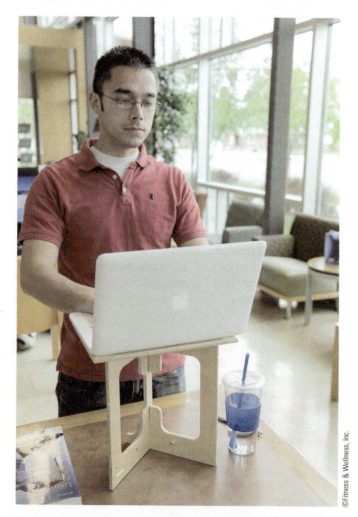

Standing helps prevent the risk factors that result from being sedentary. Portable standing desks like the StandStand can help reduce overall daily sitting time.

©Fitness & Wellness, Inc.

You can fight sitting disease by taking actions to break up periods of inactivity and by becoming more physically active. The key is to sit less and move more. To minimize inactivity when you have limited time and space, look for opportunities to increase daily physical activity:

- Walk or bike instead of drive for short distances.
- Park farther or get off public transit several blocks from the campus or office. At the office, walk to the farthest bathroom rather than the nearest.
- Take a short walk after each meal or snack. Stand up and move for 1 minute every time you take a drink of water.
- Walk faster than usual.
- Take the stairs often.
- When watching a show, stand up and move during each commercial break, or even better, stretch or work out while watching. When working or watching a show, drink plenty of water, which is not only healthy on its own but will give you extra reasons to take a walk for refills and bathroom breaks.
- Do not shy away from housecleaning chores or yard work, even for a minute or two at a time.
- Stand more while working/studying. Place your computer on an elevated stand or shelf.
- Make it a habit to stand or pace while talking on the phone.
- Make it a habit to walk or pace when you need to puzzle through a problem. Put to work the advice of the western philosopher Friedrich Nietzsche: "All truly great thoughts are conceived while walking."

- Break up sitting by closing your office door, if possible, and spending 1 minute doing a full-body exercise, such as holding a plank position or doing slow squats into and out of your chair.
- When you accomplish a difficult task at work or while during homework, stand up and give yourself a mini victory parade or victory dance.
- When reading a book, get up and move after every 6 to 10 pages of the book.
- Use a stability ball for a chair. Such use enhances body stability; balance; and abdominal, low back, and leg strength.
- Whenever feasible, walk while conversing or holding meetings. If meetings are in a conference room, take the initiative to stand. Make telephone conference calls an opportunity for a stroll.
- Walk to classmates' homes or coworkers' offices to study or discuss matters with them instead of using your phone.

Researchers are still working to come to a consensus about the ideal prescription of activity to break up sitting. As little as 2 minutes of gently walking around the room per hour has been shown to cut disease risk by one third.[39] The best current guideline seems to be to stand and stretch after every 20 minutes of inactivity and to take intermittent 5- to 10-minute breaks for every hour that you are at the computer or studying or participating in any type of uninterrupted sitting. Stretching, walking around, or talking to others while standing or walking is beneficial and increases oxygen flow to the brain, making you more effective, creative, and productive.

1.7 Physical Activity and Exercise Defined

Abundant scientific research over the past three decades has established a distinction between physical activity and exercise. **Exercise** is a type of activity that requires planned, structured, and repetitive bodily movement to improve or maintain one or more components of physical fitness. Examples of exercise are walking, running, cycling, doing aerobics, swimming, and strength training. Exercise is usually viewed as an activity that requires a vigorous-intensity effort.

Physical activity is bodily movement produced by skeletal muscles. It requires energy expenditure and produces progressive health benefits. Physical activity can be of light intensity or moderate to vigorous intensity. Examples of daily **light physical activity** include walking to and from work, taking the stairs instead of elevators and escalators, grocery shopping, and doing household chores. Physical inactivity, by contrast, implies a level of activity that is lower than that required to maintain good health.

Extremely light expenditures of energy throughout the day used to walk casually, perform self-care, or do other light work like emptying a dishwasher are of far greater significance in our overall health than we once realized. We now understand the impact of accumulating constant/small movements. Every movement conducted throughout the day matters.

To better understand the impact of all intensities of physical activity, scientists created a new category of movement called **nonexercise activity thermogenesis (NEAT)**.[40] Any energy expenditure that does not come from basic ongoing body functions (such as digesting food) or planned exercise is categorized as NEAT. A person may expend 1,300 calories on an average day simply maintaining vital body functions (the basal metabolic rate) and 200 calories digesting food (thermic effect of food). Any additional energy expended during the day is expended either through exercise or NEAT. For an active person, NEAT accounts for a major portion of energy expended each day. Though it may not increase cardiorespiratory fitness as moderate or vigorous exercise will, NEAT can easily use more calories in a day than a planned exercise session. As a result, NEAT is extremely critical for keeping daily energy balance in check. Especially when beginning or intensifying an exercise program, some individuals tend to adjust other activities of daily living, so they sit more and move less during the remainder of the day. This self-defeating behavior can lead to frustration that exercise is not providing the weight management benefits it should. It is important to keep daily NEAT levels up regardless of exercise levels.

A growing number of studies are showing that the body is much better able to maintain its energy balance—and, therefore, keep body weight at a healthy level—when the overall daily activity level is high. An active person can vary calories from day to day with fewer swings in body weight, while a

---

GLOSSARY

Exercise A type of physical activity that requires planned, structured, and repetitive bodily movement with the intent of improving or maintaining one or more components of physical fitness.

Physical activity Bodily movement produced by skeletal muscles, which requires expenditure of energy and produces progressive health benefits. Examples include walking, taking the stairs, dancing, gardening, working in the yard, cleaning the house, shoveling snow, washing the car, and all forms of structured exercise.

Light physical activity Any activity that uses less than 150 calories of energy per day, such as casual walking and light household chores.

Nonexercise activity thermogenesis (NEAT) Energy expended doing everyday activities not related to exercise.

Light, Moderate, and Vigorous Physical Activity

Adults should do 150 minutes a week of moderate-intensity physical activity, 75 minutes a week of vigorous-intensity physical activity, or an equivalent combination of moderate- and vigorous-intensity aerobic physical activity. Adults should also strive to incorporate light physical activity into daily life as often as possible. Intensity of physical activity can be measured in METs. *MET* stands for *metabolic equivalent*. The baseline measurement is a single MET. One MET is the amount of oxygen utilized by a person when resting. An activity that has the intensity of two METs utilizes double that amount of oxygen. An activity that has the intensity of three METs utilizes triple, and so on.

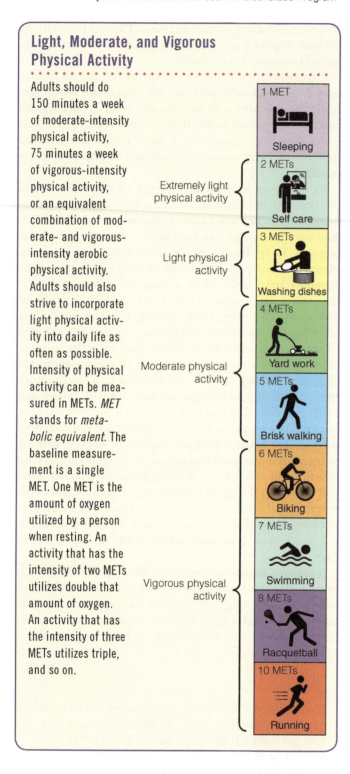

1 MET — Sleeping

Extremely light physical activity
2 METs — Self care

Light physical activity
3 METs — Washing dishes

Moderate physical activity
4 METs — Yard work
5 METs — Brisk walking

Vigorous physical activity
6 METs — Biking
7 METs — Swimming
8 METs — Racquetball
10 METs — Running

expend 700 daily calories more than a person with a sedentary desk job. People with physically demanding jobs, such as construction workers, can easily burn 1,600 daily calories over a sedentary worker.[41]

Beyond the workday are several hours of leisure time that can also be spent quite differently on a vast variety of physical activities, from activities that are light physical activity to sports and exercise that is **vigorous physical activity**. Variations in NEAT add up over days, months, and years and provide substantial benefits with weight management and health.

Regular moderate physical activity provides substantial benefits in health and well-being for the vast majority of people who are not physically active. For those who are already moderately active, even greater health benefits can be achieved by increasing the level of physical activity.

Moderate physical activity has been defined as any activity that requires an energy expenditure of 150 calories per day, or 1,000 calories per week. Examples of moderate physical activity are brisk walking or cycling, playing basketball or volleyball, recreational swimming, dancing fast, pushing a stroller, raking leaves, shoveling snow, and gardening.

Light physical activity (along with moderate physical activities lasting less than 10 minutes in duration) is not included as part of the moderate physical activity recommendation, though it is included as part of one's NEAT for a given day.

1.8 *Types of Physical Fitness*

As the fitness concept grew, it became clear that several specific components contribute to an individual's overall level of fitness. **Physical fitness** is classified into health-related and skill-related fitness.

Health-related fitness relates to the ability to perform activities of daily living without undue fatigue. The health-related fitness components are cardiorespiratory (aerobic) endurance, muscular fitness (muscular strength and endurance), muscular flexibility, and body composition (Figure 1.9).

> **! Critical Thinking**
>
> What role do the four health-related components of physical fitness play in your life? Rank them in order of importance to you and explain the rationale you used.

sedentary person who changes caloric intake will see those changes amplified, observed by greater swings in body weight.

A person with a desk job who has the option to stand and move about throughout the day will expend 300 more calories a day than a person who sits at the desk most of the day. People who spend most of the day working on their feet, such as a medical assistant or a stay-at-home parent,

Skill-related fitness components consist of agility, balance, coordination, reaction time, speed, and power (Figure 1.10). These components are related primarily to successful sports and motor skill performance. Participating in skill-related activities contributes to physical fitness, but in terms of

Figure 1.9 Health-related components of physical fitness.

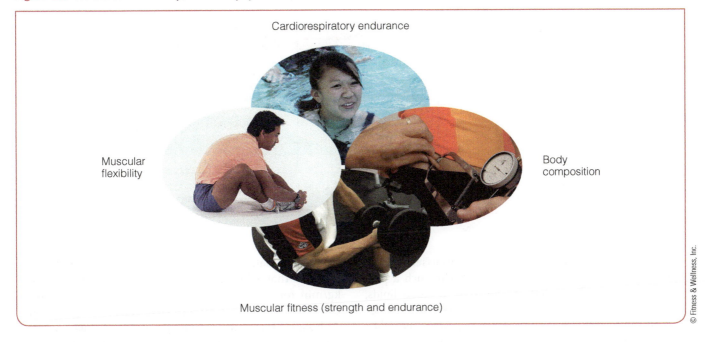

Cardiorespiratory endurance

Muscular flexibility

Body composition

Muscular fitness (strength and endurance)

© Fitness & Wellness, Inc.

Figure 1.10 Motor skill—related components of physical fitness.

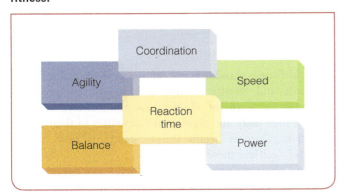

Coordination

Agility

Speed

Reaction time

Balance

Power

general health promotion and wellness, the main emphasis of physical fitness programs should be on the health-related components.

1.9 Fitness Standards: Health versus Physical Fitness

Our bodies adapt to the different types of physical activity we participate in, and the result is different levels of personal fitness. A meaningful debate regarding fitness standards has resulted in two widely recognized categories of fitness: health fitness standards (also referred to as *criterion referenced*) and physical fitness standards. Following are definitions of both. The assessment of health-related fitness is presented in Chapter 4, Chapter 6, Chapter 7, Chapter 8, and Chapter 9, where appropriate physical fitness standards are included for comparison.

Health Fitness Standards

The **health fitness standards** proposed here are based on data linking minimum fitness values to disease prevention and health. Attaining the health fitness standard is conducive to a low risk of premature hypokinetic diseases and requires only moderate physical activity. For example, a 2-mile walk in less than 30 minutes, five or six times a week, seems to be sufficient to achieve the health fitness standard for cardiorespiratory endurance.

---GLOSSARY---

Vigorous physical activity Any exercise that requires a MET level equal to or greater than 6 METs (21 mL/kg/min). One MET is the energy expenditure at rest, 3.5 mL/kg/min, and METs are defined as multiples of this resting metabolic rate. (Examples of activities that require a 6-MET level include aerobics, walking uphill at 3.5 mph, cycling at 10 to 12 mph, playing doubles in tennis, and vigorous strength training.)

Moderate physical activity Activity that uses 150 calories of energy per day, or 1,000 calories per week.

Physical fitness The ability to meet the ordinary, as well as unusual, demands of daily life

safely and effectively without being overly fatigued and still have energy left for leisure and recreational activities.

Health-related fitness Fitness programs prescribed to improve the individual's overall health.

Skill-related fitness Fitness components important for success in skillful activities and athletic events; encompasses agility, balance, coordination, reaction time, speed, and power.

Health fitness standards The lowest fitness requirements for maintaining good health, decreasing the risk for chronic diseases, and lowering the incidence of muscular-skeletal injuries.

Figure 1.11 Health and fitness benefits based on the type of lifestyle and physical activity program.

	Low fitness	Health/metabolic fitness	High physical fitness	
	Sedentary	Active lifestyle	Active lifestyle and exercise	

SOURCE: Fitness & Wellness, Inc. Reprinted by permission.

As illustrated in Figure 1.11 and as discussed earlier, significant health benefits can be reaped with such a program. These benefits include a reduction in blood lipids, lower blood pressure, weight loss, stress release, less risk for diabetes, and lower risk for disease and premature mortality. Fitness improvements, expressed in terms of maximum oxygen uptake, or VO_{2max} (explained next and in Chapter 6), are not as notable. Nevertheless, health improvements are quite striking.

More specifically, improvements in the **metabolic profile** (measured by insulin sensitivity, glucose tolerance, and improved cholesterol levels) can be notable despite little or no weight loss or improvement in aerobic capacity. Metabolic fitness can be attained through an active lifestyle and moderate-intensity physical activity.

One way to determine a person's fitness level is by assessing his or her **cardiorespiratory endurance**, which can be expressed in terms of VO_{2max}. Essentially, as a person moves or exercises more, the body adapts so that it is able to take in more oxygen and better utilize the oxygen it takes in. Specific changes occur in the heart, lungs, and muscles to make this possible (see Chapter 6). The maximum (max) amount of oxygen (O_2) that a person is able to use is measured in volume (V) per minute of exercise. A person's VO_{2max} is commonly expressed in milliliters (mL) of oxygen (volume of oxygen) per kilogram (kg) of body weight per minute (mL/kg/min). Individual values of VO_{2max} can range from about 10 mL/kg/min in cardiac patients to more than 80 mL/kg/min in world-class runners, cyclists, and cross-country skiers.

Research data from the study presented in Figure 1.7 reported that achieving VO_{2max} values of 35 and 32.5 mL/kg/min for men and women, respectively, may be sufficient to lower the risk for all-cause mortality significantly. Although greater improvements in fitness yield an even lower risk for premature death, the largest drop is seen between least fit and moderately fit individuals. Therefore, the 35 and 32.5 mL/kg/min values are selected as the health fitness standards.

Physical Fitness Standards

Physical fitness standards are set higher than health fitness standards and require a more intense exercise program. Physically fit people of all ages have the freedom to enjoy most of life's daily and recreational activities to their fullest potentials. Current health fitness standards may not be enough to achieve these objectives.

Sound physical fitness gives the individual a degree of independence throughout life that many people in the United States no longer enjoy. Most adults should be able to carry out activities similar to those they conducted in their youth, though not with the same intensity. These standards do not require being a championship athlete, but activities such as changing a tire, chopping wood, climbing several flights of stairs, playing basketball, mountain biking, playing soccer with children or grandchildren, walking several miles around a lake, and hiking through a national park do require more than the current "average fitness" level of most Americans.

Which Program Is Best?

Your own personal objectives will determine the fitness program you decide to use. If the main objective of your fitness program is to lower the risk for disease, attaining the health fitness standards will provide substantial health benefits. If, however, you want to participate in vigorous fitness activities, achieving a high physical fitness standard is recommended. This book gives both health fitness and physical fitness standards for each fitness test so that you can personalize your approach.

HOEGER KEY TO WELLNESS

 Individual VO_{2max} values can range from about 10 mL/kg/min in cardiac patients to more than 80 mL/kg/min in world-class athletes. Aim for values of 35 (men) and 32.5 mL/kg/min (women) to reach health fitness standards and benefit from metabolic fitness.

Behavior Modification Planning

Financial Fitness Prescription

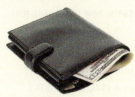

Tatiana Popova/Shutterstock.com

Although not one of the components of physical fitness, taking control of your personal finances is critical for your success and well-being. The sooner you start working on a lifetime personal financial plan, the more successful you will be in becoming financially secure and able to retire early, in comfort, if you choose to do so. Most likely, you have not been taught basic principles to improve personal finance and enjoy "financial fitness." Thus, start today using the following strategies:

1. *Develop a personal financial plan.* Set short-term and long-term financial goals for yourself. If you do not have financial goals, you cannot develop a plan or work toward that end.

2. *Subscribe to a personal finance magazine or newsletter.* In the same way that you should regularly read reputable fitness/wellness journals or newsletters, you should regularly peruse a "financial fitness" magazine. If you don't enjoy reading financial materials, then find a periodical that is quick and to the point; there are many available. You don't have to force yourself to read *The Wall Street Journal* to become financially knowledgeable. Many periodicals have resources to help you develop a financial plan. Educate yourself and stay current on personal finances and investment matters.

3. *Set up a realistic budget and live on less than you make.* Pay your bills on time and keep track of *all* expenses. Then develop your budget so that you spend less than you earn. Your budget may require that you either cut back on expenses and services or figure out a way to increase your income. Balance your checkbook regularly and do not overdraft your checking account. Remind yourself that satisfaction comes from being in control of the money you earn.

4. *Learn to differentiate between wants and needs.* It is fine to reward yourself for goals that you have achieved (see Chapter 2), but limit your spending to items that you truly need. Avoid simple impulse spending because "it's a bargain" or something you just want to have.

5. *Pay yourself first; save 10 percent of your income each month.* Before you take any money out of your paycheck, put 10 percent of your income into a retirement or investment account. If possible, ask for an automatic withdrawal at your bank from your paycheck to avoid the temptation to spend this money. This strategy may allow you to have a solid retirement fund or even provide for an early retirement. If you start putting away $100 a month at age 20, and earn a modest 6 percent interest rate, at age 65 you will have more than $275,000.

6. *Set up an emergency savings fund.* Whether you ultimately work for yourself or for someone else, there may be uncontrollable financial setbacks or even financial disasters in the future. So, as you are able, start an emergency fund equal to 3 to 6 months of normal monthly earnings. Additionally, start a second savings account for expensive purchases such as a car, a down payment on a home, or a vacation.

7. *Use credit, gas, and retail cards responsibly and sparingly.* As soon as you receive new cards, sign them promptly and store them securely. Due to the prevalence of identity theft (someone stealing your creditworthiness), cardholders should even consider a secure post office box, rather than a regular mailbox, for all high-risk mail. Shred your old credit cards, monthly statements, and any and all documents that contain personal information to avoid identity theft. Pay off all credit card debt monthly, and do not purchase on credit unless you have the cash to pay it off when the monthly statement arrives. Develop a plan at this very moment to pay off your debt if you have such. Credit card balances, high interest rates, and frequent credit purchases lead to financial disaster. Credit card debt is the worst enemy to your personal finances!

8. *Understand the terms of your student loans.* Do not borrow more money than you absolutely need for actual educational expenses. Student loans are not for wants but needs (see item 4). Remember, loans must be repaid, with interest, once you leave college. Be informed regarding the repayment process and do not ever default on your loan. If you do, the entire balance (principal, interest, and collection fees) is due immediately and serious financial and credit consequences will follow.

(continued)

---GLOSSARY---

Metabolic profile A measurement of plasma insulin, glucose, lipid, and lipoprotein levels to assess risk for diabetes and cardiovascular disease.

Cardiorespiratory endurance The ability of the lungs, heart, and blood vessels to deliver adequate amounts of oxygen to the cells to meet the demands of prolonged physical activity.

Physical fitness standards A fitness level that allows a person to sustain moderate-to-vigorous physical activity without undue fatigue and to closely maintain this level throughout life.

9. *Complete your college education.* The gap is widening between workers who have and have not graduated from college. On average, those whose education ends with their high school diploma bring home a paycheck that is 62 percent of the paycheck of their peers with a bachelor's degree. Even with rising tuition costs, this investment of time and money is a financially sound choice. Of the two-thirds of students who take on student loans to complete their degree, 86 percent agree the degree pays off.

10. *Eat out infrequently.* Besides saving money that you can then pay to yourself, you will eat healthier and consume fewer calories.

11. *Make the best of tax "motivated" savings and investing opportunities available to you.* For example, once employed, your company may match your voluntary 401(k) contributions (or other retirement plan), so contribute at least up to the match (you may use the 10 percent you "pay yourself first"—see item 5—or part of it). Also, under current tax law, maximize your Roth IRA contribution personally. Always pay attention to current tax rules that provide tax incentives for investing in retirement plans. If at all possible, *never* cash out a retirement account early. You may pay penalties in addition to tax, in most situations. As you are able, employ a tax professional or financial planner to avoid serious missteps in your tax planning.

12. *Stay involved in your financial accumulations.* You may seek professional advice, but you stay in control. Ultimately, no one will look after your interests as well as you. Avoid placing all your trust (and assets) in one individual or institution. Spreading out your assets is one way to diversify your risk.

13. *Protect your assets.* As you start to accumulate assets, get proper insurance coverage (yes, even renter's insurance) in case of an accident or disaster. You have disciplined yourself and worked hard to obtain those assets; now make sure they are protected.

14. *Review your credit report.* The best way to ensure that your credit "identity" is not stolen and ruined is to regularly review your credit report, at least once a year, for accuracy.

15. *Contribute to charity and the needy.* Altruism (doing good for others) is good for heart health and emotional well-being. Remember the less fortunate and donate regularly to some of your favorite charitable organizations and volunteer time to worthy causes.

The Power of Investing Early

Jon and Jim are both 20 years old. Jon begins investing $100 a month starting on his 20th birthday. He stops investing on his 30th birthday (he has set aside a total of $12,000). Jim does not start investing until he's 30. He chooses to invest $100 a month as Jon had done, but he does so for the next 30 years (Jim invests a total of $36,000). Although Jon stopped investing at age 30, assuming an 8 percent annual rate of return in a tax-deferred account, by the time both Jon and Jim are 60, Jon will have accumulated $199,035, whereas Jim will have $150,029. At a 6 percent rate of return, they would both accumulate about $100,000, but Jim invested three times as much as Jon did.

Post these principles of financial fitness in a visible place at home where you can review them often. Start implementing these strategies as soon as you can and watch your financial fitness level increase over the years.

© David Johnson, CPA and Fitness & Wellness, Inc.

1.10 *Federal Guidelines for Physical Activity*

Because of the importance of physical activity to our health, the U.S. Department of Health and Human Services issued *Physical Activity Guidelines for Americans*. These guidelines complement the current *Dietary Guidelines for Americans* (Chapter 3, pages 132–133) and parallel the international recommendations issued by the WHO[42] and recommendations issued by the ACSM and the AHA.[43]

The federal guidelines provide science-based guidance on the importance of being physically active to promote health and reduce the risk for chronic diseases. The federal guidelines include the following recommendations.

Adults between 18 and 64 Years of Age

- Adults should do 150 minutes a week of moderate-intensity aerobic (cardiorespiratory) physical activity, 75 minutes a week of vigorous-intensity aerobic physical activity, or an equivalent combination of moderate- and vigorous-intensity aerobic physical activity (also see Chapter 6). Moderate physical activity should preferably be divided into 30-minute segments over a minimum of 5 days each week (Table 1.3). Although 30 minutes of continuous moderate physical activity is preferred, on days when time is limited, three activity sessions of at least 10 minutes each still provide substantial health benefits. When combining moderate- and vigorous-intensity activities, a person could participate in moderate-intensity activity twice a week for 30 minutes and high-intensity activity for 20 minutes on another 2 days.

- Additional health benefits are provided by increasing to 5 hours (300 minutes) a week of moderate-intensity aerobic physical activity, 2 hours and 30 minutes a week of vigorous-intensity physical activity, or an equivalent combination of both.

- Adults should also do muscle-strengthening activities that involve all major muscle groups on 2 or more days per week.

Table 1.3 Physical Activity Guidelines

Benefits	Duration	Intensity	Frequency per Week	Weekly Time
Health	30 min	MI*	5 times	150 min
Health and fitness	20 min	VI*	3 times	75 min
Health, fitness, and weight gain prevention	60 min	MI/VI†	5–7 times	300 min
Health, fitness, and weight regain prevention	60–90 min	MI/VI†	5–7 times	450 min

*MI = moderate intensity, VI = vigorous intensity

†MI/VI = You may use MI or VI or a combination of the two

Older Adults (ages 65 and older)

- Older adults should follow the adult guidelines. If this is not possible due to limiting chronic conditions, older adults should be as physically active as their abilities allow. They should avoid inactivity. Older adults should do exercises that maintain or improve balance if they are at risk of falling.

Children 6 Years of Age and Older and Adolescents

- Children and adolescents should do 1 hour (60 minutes) or more of physical activity every day. Most of the 1 hour or more a day should be either moderate- or vigorous-intensity aerobic physical activity.
- As part of their daily physical activity, children and adolescents should do vigorous-intensity activity at least 3 days per week. They also should do muscle-strengthening and bone-strengthening activities at least 3 days per week.

Pregnant and Postpartum Women

- Healthy women who are not already doing vigorous-intensity physical activity should get at least 150 minutes of moderate-intensity aerobic activity a week. Preferably, this activity should be spread throughout the week. Women who regularly engage in vigorous-intensity aerobic activity or high amounts of activity can continue their activity provided that their condition remains unchanged and they talk to their health care provider about their activity level throughout their pregnancy.

Because of the ever-growing epidemic of obesity in the United States and the world, adults are encouraged to increase physical activity beyond the minimum requirements and adjust caloric intake until they find their personal balance to maintain a healthy weight.[44] Individuals are also advised that additional physical activity beyond minimum thresholds is necessary for some and can provide additional health benefits for all.

The latest *Physical Activity Guidelines for Americans* issued by the U.S. Department of Health and Human Services have stated that some adults should be able to achieve calorie balance with 150 minutes of moderate physical activity in a week, while others will find they need more than

300 minutes per week.[45] This recommendation was based on evidence indicating that people who maintain healthy weight typically accumulate 1 hour of daily physical activity.[46]

In sum, although health benefits are derived from 30 minutes of physical activity performed on most days of the week, people with a tendency to gain weight need to be physically active for longer, from 60 to as many as 90 minutes daily, to prevent weight gain. This additional activity per day provides additional health benefits, including a lower risk for cardiovascular disease and diabetes.

Critical Thinking

Do you consciously incorporate physical activity throughout the day into your lifestyle? Can you provide examples? Do you think you get sufficient daily physical activity to maintain good health?

1.11 Monitoring Daily Physical Activity

The majority of U.S. adults are not sufficiently physically active to promote good health. The most recent data released in 2014 by the Centers for Disease Control and Prevention (CDC) indicate that only 20.8 percent of U.S. adults 18 and over meet the federal physical activity guidelines for both aerobic and muscular fitness (strength and endurance) activities, whereas 49.2 percent meet the guidelines for aerobic fitness. Another 34 percent of Americans are completely inactive during their leisure time (Figure 1.12).

Pedometers and Activity Trackers

It is important to have an accurate idea of the level of activity you get in a day because this will be the groundwork from which you build your fitness goals. You may face an initial shock, as some of us have, when you see how little daily NEAT you accumulate, but remember that accurate data are the foundation for results. Studies have found that concrete

Figure 1.12 Percentage of adults who met the 2008 federal guidelines for physical activity by gender.

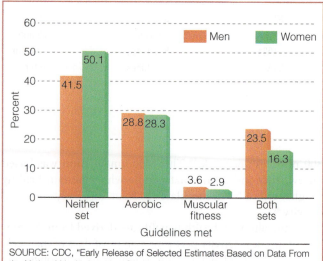

SOURCE: CDC, "Early Release of Selected Estimates Based on Data From the National Health Interview Survey, 2014," available at http://www.cdc.gov/nchs/data/nhis/earlyrelease/earlyrelease201506_07.pdf.

daily step goals inspire individuals to action. The first trick is choosing the method you will use to track your activity, and today's options abound.

Both an **activity tracker** built specifically for this job and the average smartphone contain a device called an accelerometer. The accelerometer itself is an inexpensive device that simply indicates changes in movement (acceleration and deceleration). Activity trackers add an array of features to that functionality. Popular activity trackers not only count your steps and monitor daily movement levels, but also offer features like the ability to vibrate when the user has been sedentary too long, to track sleep, or to check heart rate. Further, accompanying smartphone apps provide feedback on progress, help set goals, and allow support through online social networks. In accuracy tests, accelerometers have shown an

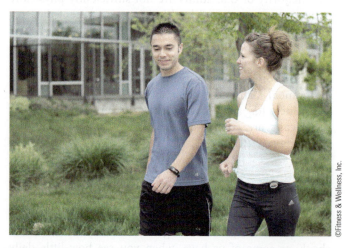

Activity trackers and pedometers can be used to monitor daily physical activity; the recommendation is a minimum of 10,000 steps per day.

©Fitness & Wellness, Inc.

average 15 percent discrepancy from actual activity, a similar accuracy record to a good pedometer. Most are worn on the wrist versus the hip or foot. While wrist placement is not as accurate, most users find it most convenient.

Activity trackers seem to be best at recording straightforward actions that are part of daily physical activity such as brisk walking or jogging. However, they tend to be inaccurate when recording less rhythmic activities, vigorous exercise, overall calories burned, sleep, or other metrics. As you can imagine, a wrist-worn activity tracker will not do well measuring a grueling bike workout. Both accelerometers and pedometers tend to lose accuracy at a very slow walking speed (slower than 30 minutes per mile) because the movement of the wrist or vertical movement of the hip is too small. Users simply need to keep limitations in mind.

In terms of step accuracy, a good pedometer will offer the same information as an activity tracker for the price of about $25 as opposed to $50 or more. For some individuals, the added features of an activity tracker are worth the added price. If you opt for an activity tracker, be sure to check reliable reviews and weigh the features that are most important to you before purchasing. Some companies offer different models depending on whether a user is interested in tracking daily activity or vigorous exercise. Be sure to follow instructions to calibrate the device to your personal stride. In a category all its own is the Apple Watch, which has a higher price point but differentiates among how much you exercise, move, and stand during the day.

Another option is to use the accelerometer in your smartphone with an activity app, which has been shown to be similar in accuracy to an activity tracker. Choose an app from a well-regarded health foundation or university, such as the Mayo Clinic or Johns Hopkins University. If you choose an app created by an independent group or person, be especially wary as spurious information is a possibility. The challenge you may face when using your phone as an activity tracker is carrying it with you consistently throughout the day, dealing with a shorter battery life, and avoiding having the phone in close contact with you if you are concerned about radio frequency waves.

A traditional pedometer is still an excellent option. Before purchasing, however, be sure to verify its accuracy and check ratings available online. Many free and low-cost pedometers are inaccurate, so their use is discouraged.

To test the accuracy of a pedometer or activity tracker, follow these steps: Clip the pedometer on the waist directly above the kneecap or wear the activity tracker as you plan to on a normal day, reset the reading to zero, carefully close the pedometer if using or check your activity tracker reading, walk exactly 50 steps at your normal pace, and look at the number of steps recorded. A reading within 10 percent of the actual steps taken (45 to 55 steps) is acceptable.

Recommended Steps per Day

The typical American man takes about 6,000 steps per day; the typical women takes about 5,300 steps. The general recommendation for adults is 10,000 steps per day, and

Table 1.4 Adult Activity Levels Based on Total Number of Steps Taken per Day

Steps per Day	Category
<5,000	Sedentary lifestyle
5,000–7,499	Low active
7,500–9,999	Somewhat active
10,000–12,499	Active
≥12,500	Highly active

SOURCE: C. Tudor-Locke and D. R. Basset, "How Many Steps/Day Are Enough? Preliminary Pedometer Indices for Public Health," *Sports Medicine* 34 (2004):1–8.

Table 1.4 provides specific activity categories based on the number of daily steps taken.

All daily steps count, but some of your steps should come in bouts of at least 10 minutes so as to meet the national physical activity recommendation. A 10-minute brisk walk (a distance of about 1,200 yards at a 15-minute per mile pace) is approximately 1,300 steps. A 15-minute mile (1,770 yards) walk is about 1,900 steps.[47] Thus, some activity trackers have an "aerobic steps" function that records steps taken in excess of 60 steps per minute over a 10-minute period of time.

If you do not accumulate the recommended 10,000 daily steps, you can refer to Table 1.5 to determine the additional walking or jogging distance required to reach your goal.

Example. If you are 5 feet 8 inches tall and female, and you typically accumulate 5,200 steps per day, you would need an additional 4,800 daily steps to reach your 10,000-steps goal. You can do so by jogging 3 miles at a 10-minute-per-mile pace (1,602 steps × 3 miles = 4,806 steps) on some days, and you can walk 2.5 miles at a 15-minute-per-mile pace (1,941 steps × 2.5 = miles = 4,853 steps) on other days. If you do not find a particular speed (pace) that you typically walk or jog at in Table 1.5, you can estimate the number of steps at that speed using the prediction equations at the bottom of this table.

The first practical application that you can undertake in this course is to determine your current level of daily activity. The log provided in Activity 1.1 will help you do this. Keep a 1- to 7-day log of all physical activities that you do daily. On this log, record the time of day; type and duration of the exercise/activity; and, if possible, steps taken while engaged in the activity. The results will indicate how active you are and serve as a basis to monitor changes in the next few months and years.

HOEGER KEY TO WELLNESS

The general recommendation for adults is to take 10,000 steps per day. A 10-minute brisk walk is approximately 1,300 steps.

GLOSSARY

Activity tracker An electronic device that contains an accelerometer (a unit that measures gravity, detects changes in movement, and counts footsteps). These devices can also determine distance, calories burned, speeds, and time spent being physically active.

Table 1.5 Estimated Number of Steps to Walk, Jog, or Run a Mile Based on Pace, Height, and Gender

	Pace (min/mile)												
	Walking								Jogging/Running				
	20		18		16		15		12	10	8	6	
Height	Women	Men	Women	Men	Women	Men	Women	Men	(both men and women)				
5'0"	2,371	2,338	2,244	2,211	2,117	2,084	2,054	2,021	1,997	1,710	1,423	1,136	
5'2"	2,343	2,310	2,216	2,183	2,089	2,056	2,026	1,993	1,970	1,683	1,396	1,109	
5'4"	2,315	2,282	2,188	2,155	2,061	2,028	1,998	1,965	1,943	1,656	1,369	1,082	
5'6"	2,286	2,253	2,160	2,127	2,033	2,000	1,969	1,937	1,916	1,629	1,342	1,055	
5'8"	2,258	2,225	2,131	2,098	2,005	1,872	1,941	1,908	1,889	1,602	1,315	1,028	
5'10"	2,230	2,197	2,103	2,070	1,976	1,943	1,913	1,880	1,862	1,575	1,288	1,001	
6'0"	2,202	2,169	2,075	2,042	1,948	1,915	1,885	1,852	1,835	1,548	1,261	974	
6'2"	2,174	2,141	2,047	2,014	1,920	1,887	1,857	1,824	1,808	1,521	1,234	947	

Prediction equations (pace in min/mile and height in inches):

Walking

Women: Steps/mile = 1,949 + [(63.4 × pace) − (14.1 × height)]

Men: Steps/mile = 1,916 + [(63.4 × pace) − (14.1 × height)]

Jogging

Women and Men: Steps/mile = 1,084 + [(63.4 × pace) − (14.1 × height)]

Adapted from Werner W. K. Hoeger et al., "One-Mile Step Count at Walking and Running Speeds," *ACSM's Health & Fitness Journal*, Vol 12(1):14–19, 2008.

Activity 1.1   Daily Physical Activity Log*

Name _____ Date _____

Course _____ Section _____ Gender _____ Age _____

Date: [   ]   Day of the Week: [   ]

Time of Day	Exercise/Activity	Duration	Number of Steps	Comments

Totals: [   ] [   ]

Activity category based on steps per day (use Table 1.4, page 25): [   ]

Date: [   ]   Day of the Week: [   ]

Time of Day	Exercise/Activity	Duration	Number of Steps	Comments

Totals: [   ] [   ]

Activity category based on steps per day (use Table 1.4, page 25): [   ]

*Make additional copies of this form as needed.

© Fitness & Wellness, Inc.

MINDTAP From Cengage **Complete This Online** Visit **www.cengagebrain.com** to access MindTap, a complete digital course that includes interactive quizzes, videos, and more.

1.12 *Economic Benefits of Physical Activity*

Sedentary living can have a strong effect on a nation's economy. As the need for physical exertion in Western countries decreased steadily during the past century, health care expenditures increased dramatically. Health care costs in the United States rose from $12 billion in 1950 to $3.2 trillion in 2015 (Figure 1.13), or about 17.1 percent of the country's gross domestic product (GDP). In 1980, health care costs in the

Figure 1.13 U.S. health care cost increments since 1950.

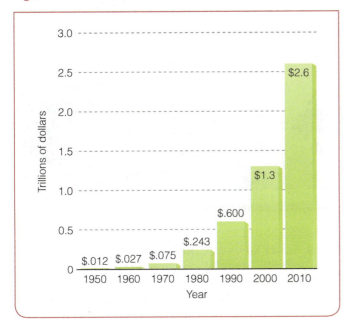

United States represented 8.8 percent of the United States GDP. This ratio far outpaces the spending of all other countries in the OECD. According to the Institute of Medicine, up to a third of health care costs are wasteful or inefficient.

In terms of yearly health care costs per person, the United States ranks in the top three of OECD countries. Per capita U.S. health care costs exceed $9,146 per year. These costs are about 2.5 times the OECD average (Figure 1.14). Furthermore, in terms of health care value, the consumer does not have the needed information to make rational decisions. Costs (prices) and care quality are not readily available as in other markets (automobile, housing, and groceries).

An estimated 5 percent of the people account for 50 percent of health care costs.[48] Half of the people use 84 percent of health care dollars. Without reducing the current burden of disease, real health care reform will not be possible. True health care reform requires a nationwide call for action by everyone against chronic disease.

1.13 *Wellness*

Most people recognize that participating in fitness programs improves their quality of life. At the end of the 20th century, however, we came to realize that physical fitness alone was not always sufficient to lower the risk for disease and ensure better health. For example, individuals who exercise regularly and watch their body weight might be easily classified as having good or excellent fitness. Offsetting these good habits, however, might be risk factors, including high blood pressure, smoking, excessive daily sitting, chronic stress, drinking too much alcohol, and eating too many foods high in saturated and trans fats. These factors place people at risk for cardiovascular disease and other chronic diseases of which they may not be aware.

Even though most people are aware of their unhealthy behaviors, they seem satisfied with life as long as they are free from symptoms of disease or illness. Nevertheless, present lifestyle habits dictate the health and well-being of tomorrow. In particular for some diseases like cancer and Alzheimer's, activity in early- and mid-adulthood affects disease risk for the remainder of the lifespan.

Good health should not be viewed simply as the absence of illness. The notion of good health has evolved considerably and continues to change as scientists learn more about lifestyle factors that bring on illness and affect wellness. Once the idea took hold that fitness by itself would not always decrease the risk for disease and ensure better health, the **wellness** concept followed.

Figure 1.14 Health care expenditure per capita for selected countries, 2014.

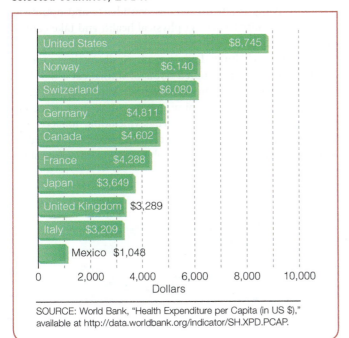

SOURCE: World Bank, "Health Expenditure per Capita (in US $)," available at http://data.worldbank.org/indicator/SH.XPD.PCAP.

GLOSSARY

Wellness The constant and deliberate effort to stay healthy and achieve the highest potential for well-being. It encompasses seven dimensions— physical, emotional, mental, social, environmental, occupational, and spiritual—and integrates them all into a quality life.

Figure 1.15 Dimensions of wellness.

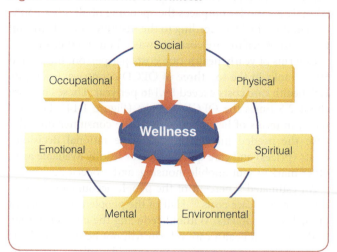

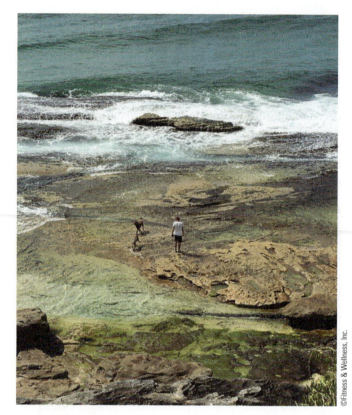

Time spent in natural settings has been clinically shown to improve wellness.

Wellness implies a constant and deliberate effort to stay healthy and achieve the highest potential for well-being. Living a wellness way of life is a personal choice, but you may need additional support to achieve wellness goals. Thus, **health promotion** programs have been developed to educate people regarding healthy lifestyles and provide the necessary support to achieve wellness. To some extent, a person's environment limits choices. Hence, the availability of a health promotion program would provide the much-needed support to get started and implement a wellness way of life.

The Seven Dimensions of Wellness

Wellness has seven dimensions: physical, emotional, mental, social, environmental, occupational, and spiritual (Figure 1.15). These dimensions are interrelated: One frequently affects the others. For example, a person who is emotionally "down" often has no desire to exercise, study, socialize with friends, or attend church, and he or she may be more susceptible to illness and disease.

The seven dimensions show how the concept of wellness clearly goes beyond the absence of disease. Wellness incorporates factors such as adequate fitness, proper nutrition, stress management, disease prevention, spirituality, not smoking or abusing drugs, personal safety, regular physical examinations, health education, and environmental support.

For a wellness way of life, individuals must be physically fit and manifest no signs of disease, and they also must be free

of risk factors for disease (such as hypertension, hyperlipidemia, cigarette smoking, negative stress, faulty nutrition, careless sex). The relationship between adequate fitness and wellness is illustrated in the continuum in Figure 1.16.

Physical Wellness

Physical wellness is the dimension most commonly associated with being healthy. It entails confidence and optimism about one's ability to protect physical health and take care of health problems.

Physically well individuals are physically active, exercise regularly, avoid uninterrupted bouts of sitting, eat a well-balanced diet, maintain recommended body weight, get sufficient sleep, practice safe sex, minimize exposure to environmental contaminants, avoid harmful drugs (including tobacco and excessive alcohol), and seek medical care and exams as needed. Physically well people also exhibit good cardiorespiratory

Figure 1.16 Wellness continuum.

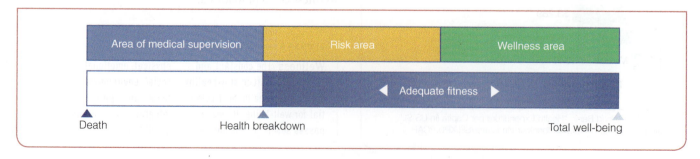

endurance, adequate muscular strength and flexibility, proper body composition, and the ability to carry out ordinary and unusual demands of daily life safely and effectively.

Emotional Wellness

Emotional wellness involves the ability to understand your own feelings, accept your limitations, and achieve emotional stability. Furthermore, it implies the ability to express emotions appropriately, adjust to change, cope with stress in a healthy way, and enjoy life despite its occasional disappointments and frustrations.

Emotional wellness brings with it a certain stability, an ability to look both success and failure squarely in the face and keep moving along a predetermined course. When success is evident, the emotionally well person radiates the expected joy and confidence. When failure seems evident, the emotionally well person responds by making the best of circumstances and moving beyond the failure. Wellness enables you to move ahead with optimism and energy instead of spending time and talent worrying about failure. You learn from it, identify ways to avoid it in the future, and then go on with the business at hand.

Emotional wellness also involves happiness—an emotional anchor that gives meaning and joy to life. Happiness is a long-term state of mind that permeates the various facets of life and influences our outlook. Although there is no simple recipe for creating happiness, researchers agree that happy people are usually participants in some category of a supportive family unit where they feel loved. Healthy, happy people enjoy friends, work hard at something fulfilling, get plenty of exercise, and enjoy play and leisure time. They know how to laugh, and they laugh often. They give of themselves freely to others and seem to have found deep meaning in life.

An attitude of true happiness signals freedom from the tension and depression that many people endure. Emotionally well people are obviously subject to the same kinds of depression and unhappiness that occasionally plague us all, but the difference lies in the ability to bounce back. Well people take minor setbacks in stride and have the ability to enjoy life despite it all. They don't waste energy or time recounting the situation, wondering how they could have changed it, or dwelling on the past.

Mental Wellness

Mental wellness, also referred to as intellectual wellness, implies that you can apply the things you have learned, create opportunities to learn more, and engage your mind in lively interaction with the world around you. When you are mentally well, you are not intimidated by facts and figures with which you are unfamiliar, but you embrace the chance to learn something new. Your confidence and enthusiasm enable you to approach any learning situation with eagerness that leads to success.

Mental wellness brings with it vision and promise. More than anything else, mentally well people are open-minded and accepting of others. Instead of being threatened by people who are different from themselves, they show respect and curiosity without feeling they have to conform. They are faithful to their own ideas and philosophies and allow others the same privilege. Their self-confidence guarantees that they can take their place among others in the world without having to give up part of themselves and without requiring others to do the same.

Social Wellness

Social wellness, with its accompanying positive self-image, endows you with the ease and confidence to be outgoing, friendly, and affectionate toward others. Social wellness involves a concern for oneself and also an interest in humanity and the environment as a whole.

One of the hallmarks of social wellness is the ability to relate to others and to reach out to other people, both within one's family and outside it. Similar to emotional wellness, it involves being comfortable with your emotions and thus helps you understand and accept the emotions of others. Your own balance and sense of self allow you to extend respect and tolerance to others. Healthy people are honest and loyal. This dimension of wellness leads to the ability to maintain close relationships with other people.

Environmental Wellness

Environmental wellness refers to the effect that our surroundings have on our well-being. Our planet is a delicate **ecosystem**, and its health depends on the continuous recycling of its elements. Environmental wellness implies a lifestyle that maximizes harmony with the earth and takes action to protect the world around us.

Environmental threats include air pollution, chemicals, ultraviolet radiation in the sunlight, water and food contamination, secondhand smoke, noise, inadequate shelter, unsatisfactory work conditions, lack of personal safety, and unhealthy relationships. Health is affected negatively when we live in a polluted, toxic, unkind, and unsafe environment.

Polls show that most first-year college students are not concerned about the health of the environment.[49] To enjoy environmental wellness, we are responsible for educating and

---

GLOSSARY

Health promotion The science and art of enabling people to increase control over their lifestyle to move toward a state of wellness.

Physical wellness Good physical fitness and confidence in your personal ability to take care of health problems.

Emotional wellness The ability to understand your own feelings, accept your limitations, and achieve emotional stability.

Mental wellness A state in which your mind is engaged in lively interaction with the world around you.

Social wellness The ability to relate well to others, both within and outside the family unit.

Environmental wellness The capability to live in a clean and safe environment that is not detrimental to health.

Ecosystem A community of organisms interacting with each other in an environment.

protecting ourselves against environmental hazards and also protecting the environment so that we, our children, and future generations can enjoy a safe and clean environment.

Steps that you can take to live an environmentally conscious life include conserving energy; recycling; conserving paper and water; not polluting the air, water, or Earth if you can avoid doing so; not smoking; planting trees and keeping plants and shrubs alive; evaluating purchases and conveniences based on their environmental impact; donating old clothes; and spending leisure time enjoying and appreciating the outdoors. Time spent in natural settings has been clinically shown to improve one's long-term sense of peacefulness, fulfillment, spirituality, and appreciation for nature's wonders.[50]

Occupational Wellness

Occupational wellness is not tied to high salary, prestigious position, or extravagant working conditions. Any job can bring occupational wellness if it provides rewards that are important to the individual. To one person, salary might be the most important factor, whereas another might place much greater value on creativity. Those who are occupationally well have their own "ideal" job, which allows them to thrive.

One school of thought, developed by psychologist Fredrick Herzberg, suggests that the factors of a job that cause dissatisfaction lie on a completely separate continuum than factors that provide satisfaction. Dissatisfaction can be reduced with what Herzberg calls hygiene factors, including a good relationship with supervisors, fair compensation, and reasonable company policies, while satisfaction can be improved with motivating factors such as recognition for accomplishments or work the employee finds purposeful and satisfying. A situation in which employees enjoy both positive hygiene factors and positive motivating factors results in occupational wellness.

People with occupational wellness face demands on the job, but they also have some say over demands placed on them. Any job has routine demands, but in occupational wellness, routine demands are mixed with new, unpredictable challenges that keep a job exciting. Occupationally well people are able to maximize their skills, and they have the opportunity to broaden their existing skills or gain new ones. Their occupation offers the opportunity for advancement and recognition for achievement. Occupational wellness encourages collaboration and interaction among coworkers, which fosters a sense of teamwork and support.

Spiritual Wellness

Spiritual wellness provides a unifying power that integrates all dimensions of wellness. Basic characteristics of spiritual people include a sense of meaning and direction in life and a relationship to a higher being. Pursuing these avenues may lead to personal freedom, including prayer, faith, love, closeness to others, peace, joy, fulfillment, and altruism.

Several studies have reported positive relationships among spiritual well-being, emotional well-being, and satisfaction with life. Spiritual health is somehow intertwined with physical health. People who attend church and regularly participate in religious organizations enjoy better health, have a lower incidence of chronic diseases, are more socially integrated, handle stress more effectively, and appear to live longer.[51] Other studies have shown that spirituality strengthens the immune system, is good for mental health, prevents age-related memory loss, decreases the incidence of depression, leads to fewer episodes of chronic inflammation, and decreases the risk of death and suicide. For example, can you recall feeling awe and amazement during a time of spirituality or while taking in a spectacular scene in nature or a beautiful piece of artwork or music? That sense of wonder has been shown to lower inflammation-inducing compounds and increase life expectancy.[52]

Prayer is a signpost of spirituality at the core of most spiritual experiences. It is communication with a higher power. At least 200 studies have been conducted on the effects of prayer on health. About two-thirds of these studies have linked prayer to positive health outcomes—as long as these prayers are offered with sincerity, humility, love, empathy, and compassion.[53]

Altruism, a key attribute of spiritual people, seems to enhance health and longevity. Studies indicate that people who regularly volunteer live longer. Research has found that health benefits of altruism are so powerful that doing good for others is good for oneself, especially for the immune system.

Researchers believe that there seems to be a strong connection among the mind, spirit, and body. As one improves, the others follow. The relationship between spirituality and

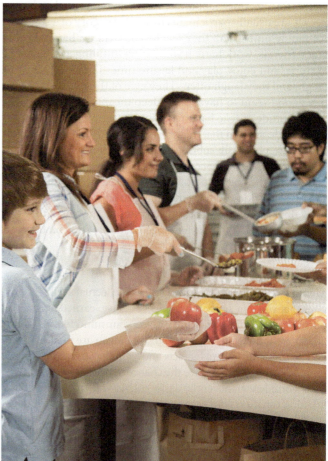

Altruism enhances health and well-being.

fstop123/Getty Images

wellness is meaningful in our quest for a better quality of life. As with the other dimensions, development of the spiritual dimension to its fullest potential contributes to wellness. Wellness requires a balance among all seven dimensions.

Critical Thinking

Now that you understand the seven dimensions of wellness, rank them in order of importance to you and explain your rationale in doing so.

1.14 Meeting the Challenge for Our Day

Because a better and healthier life is something that every person should strive for, our biggest health challenge today is to teach people how to take control of their personal health habits and adhere to a positive lifestyle. A wealth of information on the benefits of fitness and wellness programs indicates that improving the quality and possible length of our lives is a matter of personal choice.

Even though people in the United States believe a positive lifestyle has a great impact on health and longevity, most people do not reap the benefits because they simply do not know how to implement a safe and effective fitness and wellness program. Others are exercising incorrectly and, therefore, are not reaping the full benefits of their program. How, then, can we meet the health challenges of the 21st century? That is the focus of this book—to provide the necessary tools that will enable you to write, implement, and regularly update your personal lifetime fitness and wellness program.

Critical Thinking

What are your thoughts about lifestyle habits that enhance health and longevity? How important are they to you? What obstacles keep you from adhering to these habits or incorporating new habits into your life?

1.15 Wellness Education: Using This Book

Although everyone would like to enjoy good health and wellness, most people don't know how to reach this objective. Lifestyle is the most important factor affecting personal well-being. Granted, some people live long because of genetic factors, but quality of life during middle age and the "golden years" is more often related to wise choices initiated during youth and continued throughout life. In a few short years, lack of wellness can lead to a loss of vitality and gusto for life, as well as premature morbidity and mortality.

A Personalized Approach

Because fitness and wellness needs vary significantly from one individual to another, all exercise and wellness prescriptions must be personalized to obtain the best results. The Wellness Lifestyle Questionnaire in Activity 1.2 will provide an initial rating of your current efforts to stay healthy and well. Subsequent chapters of this book and their respective activities discuss the components of a wellness lifestyle and set forth the necessary guidelines that will allow you to develop a personal lifetime program to improve fitness and promote your own preventive health care and personal wellness.

As you study this book you will learn to:

- Implement motivational and behavior modification techniques to help you adhere to a lifetime fitness and wellness program.
- Determine whether medical clearance is needed for your safe participation in exercise.
- Conduct nutritional analyses and follow the recommendations for adequate nutrition.
- Write sound diet and weight-control programs.
- Assess the health-related components of fitness.
- Write exercise prescriptions for cardiorespiratory endurance, muscular fitness, and muscular flexibility.
- Understand the relationship between fitness and aging.
- Determine your levels of tension and stress, reduce your vulnerability to stress, and implement a stress management program if necessary.
- Determine your potential risk for cardiovascular disease and implement a risk-reduction program.
- Follow a cancer risk-reduction program.
- Implement a smoking cessation program, if applicable.
- Avoid chemical dependency and know where to find assistance if needed.
- Recognize the health consequences of sexually transmitted infections (STIs), including human immunodeficiency virus (HIV)/acquired immune deficiency syndrome (AIDS), and guidelines for preventing STIs.
- Write goals and objectives to improve your fitness and wellness and learn how to chart a wellness program for the future.
- Differentiate myths from facts about exercise and health-related concepts.

> **GLOSSARY**
>
> **Occupational wellness** The ability to perform your job skillfully and effectively under conditions that provide personal and team satisfaction and adequately reward each individual.
>
> **Spiritual wellness** The sense that life is meaningful and has purpose and that some power brings all humanity together; the ethics, values, and morals that guide you and give meaning and direction to life.
>
> **Prayer** Sincere and humble communication with a higher power.
>
> **Altruism** Unselfish concern for the welfare of others.

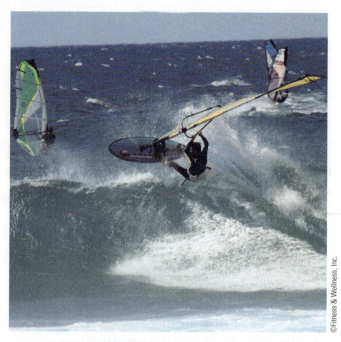

©Fitness & Wellness, Inc.

Good health-related fitness and skill-related fitness are required to participate in highly skilled activities.

Exercise Safety

Even though testing and participation in exercise are relatively safe for most apparently healthy individuals, the reaction of the cardiovascular system to higher levels of physical activity cannot be totally predicted. Consequently, a small but real risk exists for exercise-induced abnormalities in people with a history of cardiovascular problems, those with certain chronic conditions, and those who are at higher risk for disease. Among the exercise-induced abnormalities are abnormal blood pressure; irregular heart rhythm; fainting; and, in rare instances, a heart attack or cardiac arrest.

Before you engage in an exercise program or participate in any exercise testing, at a minimum you should fill out the Physical Activity Readiness Questionnaire (PAR-Q) found in Activity 1.3. Additional information can be obtained by filling out the Health History Questionnaire also given in Activity 1.3. Exercise testing and participation are not wise under some of the conditions listed in this activity and may require a medical evaluation, including a stress electrocardiogram (ECG) test for a few individuals. If you have any questions regarding your current health status, consult your doctor before initiating, continuing, or increasing your level of physical activity.

Now that you are about to embark on a wellness lifestyle program, sit down and subjectively determine where you are at on each of the seven dimensions of wellness. Use Activity 1.5 to help you with this exercise. Record the date at the top of the respective column. Next, write a goal for each wellness dimension to accomplish prior to the end of this course. Also, list three specific objectives that will help you accomplish each goal.

As you continue to study the content of this book, use this same form to monitor your progress. About once a month, reassess your status and make adjustments in your specific objectives so you may reach the desired goals. Modifying unhealthy behaviors and developing new positive habits take time. The plan of action that you are about to develop will help you achieve the desired outcomes.

1.16 Assessment of Resting Heart Rate and Blood Pressure

Heart rate can be obtained by counting your pulse either on the wrist over the radial artery or over the carotid artery in the neck (Chapter 6, page 227). In Activity 1.4, you will have an opportunity to determine your heart rate and blood pressure and calculate the extra heart rate life years an increase in exercise may produce.

You may count your pulse for 30 seconds and multiply by 2 or take it for a full minute. The heart rate usually is at its lowest point (resting heart rate) late in the evening after you have been sitting quietly for about half an hour watching a relaxing TV show or reading in bed or early in the morning just before you get out of bed. Your pulse should have a consistent (regular) rhythm. A pulse that misses beats or speeds up or slows down may be an indication of heart problems and should be followed up by a physician.

Unless you have a pathological condition, a lower resting heart rate indicates a stronger heart. To adapt to cardiorespiratory or aerobic exercise, blood volume increases, the heart enlarges, and the muscle gets stronger. A stronger heart can pump more blood with fewer strokes.

Resting heart rate categories are given in Table 1.6. Although resting heart rate decreases with training, the extent of

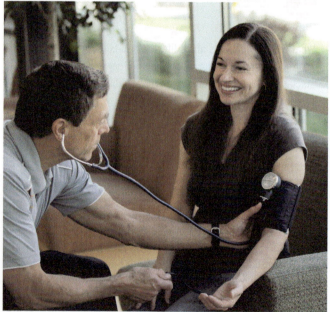

© Fitness & Wellness, Inc.

Assessment of resting blood pressure with an aneroid manometer.

Behavior Modification Planning

Healthy Lifestyle Habits

Research indicates that adherence to the following 12 lifestyle habits will significantly improve health and extend life:

1. *Participate in a lifetime physical activity program and avoid being sedentary for extended periods.* Attempt to accumulate 60 minutes of moderate-intensity physical activity most days of the week. The 60 minutes should include 20 to 30 minutes of aerobic exercise (vigorous-intensity) at least three times per week, along with other routine activities of daily living, and strengthening and stretching exercises two to three times per week. Furthermore, keep moving throughout the day. Do not sit for more than an hour at a time without getting up to move or stretch for 5 to 10 minutes.

2. *Do not smoke cigarettes.* Cigarette smoking is the largest preventable cause of illness and premature death in the United States. If we include all related deaths, smoking is responsible for about 480,000 unnecessary deaths each year.

3. *Eat right.* Eat a good breakfast and two additional well-balanced meals every day. Avoid eating too many calories; processed foods; and foods with a lot of sugar, saturated fat, and salt. Increase your daily consumption of fruits, vegetables, and whole-grain products.

4. *Avoid snacking.* Refrain from frequent high-sugar snacks between meals. Insulin is released to remove sugar from the blood, and frequent spikes in insulin may contribute to the development of diabetes and heart disease.

5. *Maintain recommended body weight through adequate nutrition and exercise.* This is important in preventing chronic diseases and in developing a higher level of fitness.

6. *Sleep 7 to 8 hours every night.*

7. *Lower your stress levels.* Reduce your vulnerability to stress and practice stress management techniques as needed.

8. *Be wary of alcohol.* Drink alcohol moderately or not at all. Alcohol abuse leads to mental, emotional, physical, and social problems.

9. *Surround yourself with healthy friendships.* Unhealthy friendships contribute to destructive behaviors and low self-esteem. Associating with people who strive to maintain good fitness and health reinforces a positive outlook in life and encourages positive behaviors. Mortality rates are much higher among people who are socially isolated.

10. *Be informed about the environment.* Seek clean air, clean water, and a clean environment. Be aware of pollutants and occupational hazards: asbestos fibers, nickel dust, chromate, uranium dust, and so on. Take precautions when using pesticides and insecticides.

11. *Increase education.* Data indicate that people who are more educated live longer. As education increases, so do the number of connections between nerve cells. An increased number of connections help the individual make better survival (i.e., healthy lifestyle) choices.

12. *Take personal safety measures.* Although not all accidents are preventable, many are. Taking simple precautionary measures—such as using seat belts and keeping electrical appliances away from water—lessens the risk for avoidable accidents.

Try It

Look at the previous list and indicate which habits are already a part of your lifestyle. What changes could you make to incorporate some additional healthy habits into your daily life?

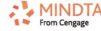 **MINDTAP** From Cengage **Complete This Online**
Visit **www.cengagebrain.com** to access MindTap, a complete digital course that includes interactive quizzes, videos, and more.

Table 1.6 Resting Heart Rate Ratings

Heart Rate (bpm)	Rating
≤59	Excellent
60–69	Good
70–79	Average
80–89	Fair
≥90	Poor

bradycardia depends not only on the amount of training, but also on genetic factors. Although most highly trained athletes have a resting heart rate around 40 beats per minute, occasionally one of these athletes has a resting heart rate in the 60s

or 70s, even during peak training months of the season. For most individuals, however, the resting heart rate decreases as the level of cardiorespiratory endurance increases.

Blood pressure is assessed using a **sphygmomanometer** and a stethoscope. Use a cuff of the appropriate size to get accurate readings. Size is determined by the width of the inflatable bladder, which should be about 80 percent of the circumference of the midpoint of the arm.

GLOSSARY

Bradycardia Slower heart rate than normal.

Sphygmomanometer Inflatable bladder contained within a cuff and a mercury gravity manometer (or aneroid manometer) from which blood pressure is read.

Blood pressure usually is measured while the person is in the sitting position, with the forearm and the manometer at the same level as the heart. The arm should be flexed slightly and placed on a flat surface. At first, the pressure is recorded from each arm and after that from the arm with the highest reading.

The cuff should be applied approximately an inch above the antecubital space (natural crease of the elbow), with the center of the bladder directly over the medial (inner) surface of the arm. The stethoscope head should be applied firmly, but with little pressure, over the brachial artery in the antecubital space.

To determine how high the cuff should be inflated, the person recording the blood pressure monitors the subject's radial pulse with one hand and, with the other hand, inflates the manometer's bladder to about 30 to 40 mm Hg above the point at which the feeling of the pulse in the wrist disappears. Next, the pressure is released, followed by a wait of about 1 minute, then the bladder is inflated to the predetermined level to take the blood pressure reading. The cuff should not be overinflated because this may cause blood vessel spasm, resulting in higher blood pressure readings. The pressure should be released at a rate of 2 to 4 mm Hg per second. As the pressure is released, **systolic blood pressure (SBP)** is recorded as the point where the sound of the pulse becomes audible. The **diastolic blood pressure (DBP)** is the point where the sound disappears. The recordings should be expressed as systolic over diastolic pressure—for example, 124/80.

Whenever possible, blood pressure should be measured in both arms. Readings for both arms will be similar in most people. A large difference in systolic blood pressure between arms, 10 points or more, signals an increased risk for cardiovascular disease. In this case, the individual should follow up with a physician to further discuss disease risk and, if necessary, create a prevention plan.

When you take more than one reading, be sure the bladder is completely deflated between readings and allow at least a full minute before making the next recording. The person measuring the pressure also should note whether the pressure was recorded from the left or the right arm. Resting blood pressure ratings are given in Table 1.7.

In some cases, the pulse sounds become less intense (point of muffling sounds) but still can be heard at a lower pressure (50 or 40 mm Hg) or even all the way down to

Table 1.7 Resting Blood Pressure Guidelines (expressed in mm Hg)

Rating	Systolic	Diastolic
Normal	≤120	≤80
Prehypertension	120–139	80–89
Hypertension	≥140	≥90

SOURCE: National Heart, Lung, and Blood Institute.

zero. In this situation, the diastolic pressure is recorded at the point of a clear, definite change in the loudness of the sound (also referred to as fourth phase) and at complete disappearance of the sound (fifth phase) (e.g., 120/78/60 or 120/82/0).

Mean Blood Pressure

During a normal resting contraction/relaxation cycle of the heart, the heart spends more time in the relaxation (diastolic) phase than in the contraction (systolic) phase. Accordingly, mean blood pressure (MBP) cannot be computed by taking an average of the SBP and DBP blood pressures. The equations used to determine MBP are shown in Activity 1.4.

When measuring blood pressure, be aware that a single reading may not be an accurate value because of the various factors (rest, stress, physical activity, food) that can affect blood pressure. Thus, if you are able, ask different people to take several readings at different times of the day to establish the real values. You can record the results of your resting heart rate and your SBP, DBP, and MBP assessments in Activity 1.4. You can also calculate the effects of aerobic activity on resting heart rate in this activity.

GLOSSARY

Systolic blood pressure (SBP) Pressure exerted by blood against walls of arteries during forceful contraction (systole) of the heart.

Diastolic blood pressure (DBP) Pressure exerted by the blood against the walls of the arteries during the relaxation phase (diastole) of the heart.

Assess Your Behavior

1. Are you aware of your family health history and lifestyle factors that may negatively affect your health?

2. Do you accumulate at least 30 minutes of moderate-intensity physical activity 5 days per week and avoid excessive periods of daily sitting?

3. Do you make a constant and deliberate effort to stay healthy and achieve the highest potential for well-being?

Assess Your Knowledge

1. Advances in modern technology
   a. help people achieve higher fitness levels.
   b. have led to a decrease in chronic diseases.
   c. have almost completely eliminated the necessity for physical exertion in daily life.
   d. help fight hypokinetic disease.
   e. make it easier to achieve good aerobic fitness.

2. The category of movement called nonexercise activity thermogenesis (NEAT) includes
   a. extremely light expenditures of energy like performing self-care.
   b. light physical activity like walking to work.
   c. moderate physical activity like raking leaves.
   d. energy expenditure that does not come from basic ongoing body functions.
   e. All are correct choices.

3. The leading cause of death in the United States is
   a. cancer.
   b. accidents.
   c. CLRD.
   d. diseases of the cardiovascular system.
   e. drug abuse.

4. Bodily movement produced by skeletal muscles is called
   a. physical activity.
   b. kinesiology.
   c. exercise.
   d. aerobic exercise.
   e. muscle strength.

5. Among the long-term benefits of regular physical activity and exercise are significantly reduced risks for developing or dying from
   a. heart disease.
   b. type 2 diabetes.
   c. colon and breast cancers.
   d. osteoporotic fractures.
   e. All are correct choices.

6. To be ranked in the "active" category, an adult has to take between
   a. 3,500 and 4,999 steps per day.
   b. 5,000 and 7,499 steps per day.
   c. 7,500 and 9,999 steps per day.
   d. 10,000 and 12,499 steps per day.
   e. 12,500 and 15,000 steps per day.

7. The constant and deliberate effort to stay healthy and achieve the highest potential for well-being is defined as
   a. health.
   b. physical fitness.
   c. wellness.
   d. health-related fitness.
   e. physiological fitness.

8. Research on the effects of fitness on mortality indicates that the largest drop in premature mortality is seen between
   a. the average and excellent fitness groups.
   b. the low and moderate fitness groups.
   c. the high and excellent fitness groups.
   d. the moderate and good fitness groups.
   e. The drop is similar among all fitness groups.

9. Metabolic fitness can be achieved through
   a. a moderate-intensity exercise program.
   b. a high-intensity speed-training program.
   c. an increased basal metabolic rate.
   d. anaerobic training.
   e. an increase in lean body mass.

10. What is the greatest benefit of being physically fit?
    a. Absence of disease
    b. A higher quality of life
    c. Improved sports performance
    d. Better personal appearance
    e. Maintenance of recommended body weight

Correct answers can be found at the back of the book.

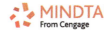 **Complete This Online**
From Cengage   Visit **www.cengagebrain.com** to access MindTap, a complete digital course that includes interactive quizzes, videos, and more.

Activity 1.2 Wellness Lifestyle Questionnaire

Name _____ Date _____

Course _____ Section _____ Gender _____ Age _____

> The purpose of this questionnaire is to analyze current lifestyle habits and help determine changes necessary for future health and wellness. Check the appropriate answer to each question, and obtain a final score according to the guidelines provided at the end of the questionnaire.

		ALWAYS	NEARLY ALWAYS	OFTEN	SELDOM	NEVER
1.	I participate in vigorous-intensity aerobic activity for 20 minutes on 3 or more days per week, and I accumulate at least 30 minutes of moderate-intensity physical activity on a minimum of two additional days per week.	5	4	3	2	1
2.	I avoid uninterrupted sitting for more than an hour at a time and accumulate less than 6 hours of sitting time in a 24-hour time period.	5	4	3	2	1
3.	I participate in strength-training exercises, using a minimum of eight different exercises, two or more days per week.	5	4	3	2	1
4.	I maintain recommended body weight (includes avoidance of excessive body fat, excessive thinness, or frequent fluctuations in body weight).	5	4	3	2	1
5.	Every day, I eat three regular meals that include a wide variety of foods.	5	4	3	2	1
6.	I limit the amount of saturated fat and trans fats in my diet on most days of the week.	5	4	3	2	1
7.	I eat a minimum of five servings of fruits and vegetables and six servings from grain products daily.	5	4	3	2	1
8.	I regularly avoid snacks, especially those that are high in calories, sugar, and fat and low in nutrients and fiber.	5	4	3	2	1
9.	I avoid cigarettes or tobacco in any other form.	5	4	3	2	1
10.	I avoid alcoholic beverages. If I drink, I do so in moderation (one daily drink for womenand two for men), and I do not combine alcohol with other drugs.	5	4	3	2	1
11.	I avoid addictive drugs and needles that have been used by others.	5	4	3	2	1
12.	I use prescription drugs and over-the-counter drugs sparingly (only when needed), and I follow all directions for their proper use.	5	4	3	2	1
13.	I readily recognize and act on it when I am under excessive tension and stress (distress).	5	4	3	2	1
14.	I am able to perform effective stress-management techniques.	5	4	3	2	1
15.	I have close friends and relatives with whom I can discuss personal problems and approach for help when needed, and with whom I can express my feelings freely.	5	4	3	2	1
16.	I spend most of my daily leisure time in wholesome recreational activities.	5	4	3	2	1
17.	I sleep 7 to 8 hours each night.	5	4	3	2	1
18.	I floss my teeth every day and brush them at least twice daily.	5	4	3	2	1

© Fitness & Wellness, Inc.

Activity 1.2 Wellness Lifestyle Questionnaire *(continued)*

	ALWAYS	NEARLY ALWAYS	OFTEN	SELDOM	NEVER
19. I get "safe sun" exposure (that is, 10 to 20 minutes unprotected sun exposure to the face, neck, and arms, on most days of the week between hours of 10:00 a.m. and 4:00 p.m.), I avoid overexposure to the sun, and I use sunscreen and appropriate clothing when I am out in the sun for an extended time.	5	4	3	2	1
20. I avoid using products that have not been shown by science to be safe and effective. (This includes drugs and unproven nutrient and weight loss supplements.)	5	4	3	2	1
21. I stay current with the warning signs for heart attack, stroke, and cancer.	5	4	3	2	1
22. I practice monthly breast/testicle self-exams, get recommended screening tests (blood lipids, blood pressure, Pap tests), and seek a medical evaluation when I am not well or disease symptoms arise.	5	4	3	2	1
23. I have a dental checkup at least once a year, and I get regular medical exams according to age recommendations.	5	4	3	2	1
24. I am not sexually active. / I practice safe sex.	5	4	3	2	1
25. I can deal effectively with disappointments and temporary feelings of sadness, loneliness, and depression. If I am unable to deal with these feelings, I seek professional help.	5	4	3	2	1
26. I can work out emotional problems without turning to alcohol, other drugs, or violent behavior.	5	4	3	2	1
27. I associate with people who have a positive attitude about life.	5	4	3	2	1
28. I respond to temporary setbacks by making the best of the circumstances and by moving ahead with optimism and energy. I do not spend time and talent worrying about failures.	5	4	3	2	1
29. I wear a seat belt whenever I am in a car, I ask others in my vehicle to do the same, and I make sure that children are in an infant seat or wear a shoulder harness.	5	4	3	2	1
30. I do not drive under the influence of alcohol or other drugs, and I make an effort to keep others from doing the same.	5	4	3	2	1
31. I avoid being alone in public places, especially after dark; I seek escorts when I visit or exercise in unfamiliar places.	5	4	3	2	1
32. I seek to make my living quarters accident-free, and I keep doors and windows locked, especially when I am home alone.	5	4	3	2	1
33. I try to minimize environmental pollutants, and I support community efforts to minimize pollution.	5	4	3	2	1
34. I use energy conservation strategies and encourage others to do the same.	5	4	3	2	1
35. I study and/or work in a clean environment (including avoidance of secondhand smoke).	5	4	3	2	1
36. I participate in recycling programs for paper, cardboard, glass, plastic, and aluminum.	5	4	3	2	1

© Fitness & Wellness, Inc.

Activity 1.2 Wellness Lifestyle Questionnaire *(continued)*

How to Score

Enter the score you have marked for each question in the spaces provided below. Next, total the score for each specific wellness lifestyle category and obtain a rating for each category according to the criteria provided below.

	Health-Related Fitness		Nutrition		Avoiding Chemical Dependency		Stress Management		Personal Hygiene/ Health		Disease Prevention		Emotional Well-being		Personal Safety		Environmental Health & Protection
1.		5.		9.		13.		17.		21.		25.		29.		33.	
2.		6.		10.		14.		18.		22.		26.		30.		34.	
3.		7.		11.		15.		19.		23.		27.		31.		35.	
4.		8.		12.		16.		20.		24.		28.		32.		36.	
Total:																	
Rating:																	

Category Rating

Excellent (E) = ≥17 Your answers show that you are aware of the importance of this category to your health and wellness. You are putting your knowledge to work for you by practicing good habits. As long as you continue to do so, this category should not pose a health risk. You are also setting a good example for family and friends to follow. Because you got a very high score on this part of the test, you may want to consider other categories in which your score indicates room for improvement.

Good (G) = 13–16 Your health practices in this area are good, but you have room for improvement. Look again at the items you answered with a 4 or lower and identify changes that you can make to improve your lifestyle. Even small changes often can help you achieve better health.

Needs Improvement (NI) = ≤12 Your health risks are showing. You may be taking serious and unnecessary risks with your health. Perhaps you are not aware of the risks or what to do about them. Most likely you need additional information and help in deciding how to successfully make the changes you desire. You can easily get the information that you need to improve, if you wish. The next step is up to you.

Please note that no final overall rating is provided for the entire questionnaire, because it may not be indicative of your overall wellness. For example, an excellent rating in most categories will not offset the immediate health risks and life-threatening consequences of using addictive drugs or not wearing a seat belt.

© Fitness & Wellness, Inc.

MINDTAP From Cengage **Complete This Online**
Visit **www.cengagebrain.com** to access MindTap, a complete digital course that includes interactive quizzes, videos, and more.

Activity 1.3 PAR-Q and Health History Questionnaire

2015 PAR-Q+

The Physical Activity Readiness Questionnaire for Everyone

The health benefits of regular physical activity are clear; more people should engage in physical activity every day of the week. Participating in physical activity is very safe for MOST people. This questionnaire will tell you whether it is necessary for you to seek further advice from your doctor OR a qualified exercise professional before becoming more physically active.

GENERAL HEALTH QUESTIONS

Please read the 7 questions below carefully and answer each one honestly: check YES or NO.	YES	NO
1) Has your doctor ever said that you have a heart condition ☐ OR high blood pressure ☐?	☐	☐
2) Do you feel pain in your chest at rest, during your daily activities of living, **OR** when you do physical activity?	☐	☐
3) Do you lose balance because of dizziness **OR** have you lost consciousness in the last 12 months? Please answer **NO** if your dizziness was associated with over-breathing (including during vigorous exercise).	☐	☐
4) Have you ever been diagnosed with another chronic medical condition (other than heart disease or high blood pressure)? **PLEASE LIST CONDITION(S) HERE:** _____	☐	☐
5) Are you currently taking prescribed medications for a chronic medical condition? **PLEASE LIST CONDITION(S) AND MEDICATIONS HERE:** _____	☐	☐
6) Do you currently have (or have had within the past 12 months) a bone, joint, or soft tissue (muscle, ligament, or tendon) problem that could be made worse by becoming more physically active? Please answer **NO** if you had a problem in the past, but it *does not limit your current ability* to be physically active. **PLEASE LIST CONDITION(S) HERE:** _____	☐	☐
7) Has your doctor ever said that you should only do medically supervised physical activity?	☐	☐

☑ **If you answered NO to all of the questions above, you are cleared for physical activity.**
Go to Page 4 to sign the PARTICIPANT DECLARATION. You do not need to complete Pages 2 and 3.

▶ Start becoming much more physically active – start slowly and build up gradually.

▶ Follow International Physical Activity Guidelines for your age (www.who.int/dietphysicalactivity/en/).

▶ You may take part in a health and fitness appraisal.

▶ If you are over the age of 45 years and **NOT** accustomed to regular vigorous to maximal effort exercise, consult a qualified exercise professional before engaging in this intensity of exercise.

▶ If you have any further questions, contact a qualified exercise professional.

🛑 **If you answered YES to one or more of the questions above, COMPLETE PAGES 2 AND 3.**

⚠ **Delay becoming more active if:**

✓ You have a temporary illness such as a cold or fever; it is best to wait until you feel better.

✓ You are pregnant – talk to your health care practitioner, your physician, a qualified exercise professional, and/or complete the ePARmed-X+ at **www.eparmedx.com** before becoming more physically active.

✓ Your health changes – answer the questions on Pages 2 and 3 of this document and/or talk to your doctor or a qualified exercise professional before continuing with any physical activity program.

OSHF
Ontario Society for Health and Fitness

Copyright © 2015 PAR-Q+ Collaboration   1 / 4
08-01-2014

PAR-Q+ Collaboration

Activity 1.3 PAR-Q and Health History Questionnaire (*continued*)

2015 PAR-Q+

FOLLOW-UP QUESTIONS ABOUT YOUR MEDICAL CONDITION(S)

1. **Do you have Arthritis, Osteoporosis, or Back Problems?**

If the above condition(s) is/are present, answer questions 1a-1c   If **NO** ☐ go to question 2

1a. Do you have difficulty controlling your condition with medications or other physician-prescribed therapies? (Answer **NO** if you are not currently taking medications or other treatments)   YES☐ NO☐

1b. Do you have joint problems causing pain, a recent fracture or fracture caused by osteoporosis or cancer, displaced vertebra (e.g., spondylolisthesis), and/or spondylolysis/pars defect (a crack in the bony ring on the back of the spinal column)?   YES☐ NO☐

1c. Have you had steroid injections or taken steroid tablets regularly for more than 3 months?   YES☐ NO☐

2. **Do you have Cancer of any kind?**

If the above condition(s) is/are present, answer questions 2a-2b   If **NO** ☐ go to question 3

2a. Does your cancer diagnosis include any of the following types: lung/bronchogenic, multiple myeloma (cancer of plasma cells), head, and neck?   YES☐ NO☐

2b. Are you currently receiving cancer therapy (such as chemotheraphy or radiotherapy)?   YES☐ NO☐

3. **Do you have a Heart or Cardiovascular Condition?** *This includes Coronary Artery Disease, Heart Failure, Diagnosed Abnormality of Heart Rhythm*

If the above condition(s) is/are present, answer questions 3a-3d   If **NO** ☐ go to question 4

3a. Do you have difficulty controlling your condition with medications or other physician-prescribed therapies? (Answer **NO** if you are not currently taking medications or other treatments)   YES☐ NO☐

3b. Do you have an irregular heart beat that requires medical management? **(e.g., atrial fibrillation, premature ventricular contraction)**   YES☐ NO☐

3c. Do you have chronic heart failure?   YES☐ NO☐

3d. Do you have diagnosed coronary artery (cardiovascular) disease and have not participated in regular physical activity in the last 2 months?   YES☐ NO☐

4. **Do you have High Blood Pressure?**

If the above condition(s) is/are present, answer questions 4a-4b   If **NO** ☐ go to question 5

4a. Do you have difficulty controlling your condition with medications or other physician-prescribed therapies? (Answer **NO** if you are not currently taking medications or other treatments)   YES☐ NO☐

4b. Do you have a resting blood pressure equal to or greater than 160/90 mmHg with or without medication? (Answer **YES** if you do not know your resting blood pressure)   YES☐ NO☐

5. **Do you have any Metabolic Conditions?** *This includes Type 1 Diabetes, Type 2 Diabetes, Pre-Diabetes*

If the above condition(s) is/are present, answer questions 5a-5e   If **NO** ☐ go to question 6

5a. Do you often have difficulty controlling your blood sugar levels with foods, medications, or other physician-prescribed therapies?   YES☐ NO☐

5b. Do you often suffer from signs and symptoms of low blood sugar (hypoglycemia) following exercise and/or during activities of daily living? Signs of hypoglycemia may include shakiness, nervousness, unusual irritability, abnormal sweating, dizziness or light-headedness, mental confusion, difficulty speaking, weakness, or sleepiness.   YES☐ NO☐

5c. Do you have any signs or symptoms of diabetes complications such as heart or vascular disease and/or complications affecting your eyes, kidneys, **OR** the sensation in your toes and feet?   YES☐ NO☐

5d. Do you have other metabolic conditions (such as current pregnancy-related diabetes, chronic kidney disease, or liver problems)?   YES☐ NO☐

5e. Are you planning to engage in what for you is unusually high (or vigorous) intensity exercise in the near future?   YES☐ NO☐

Activity 1.3 **PAR-Q and Health History Questionnaire** *(continued)*

2015 PAR-Q+

6. **Do you have any Mental Health Problems or Learning Difficulties?** *This includes Alzheimer's, Dementia, Depression, Anxiety Disorder, Eating Disorder, Psychotic Disorder, Intellectual Disability, Down Syndrome*

If the above condition(s) is/are present, answer questions 6a-6b   If **NO** ☐ go to question 7

6a. Do you have difficulty controlling your condition with medications or other physician-prescribed therapies? (Answer **NO** if you are not currently taking medications or other treatments)   YES☐ NO☐

6b. Do you **ALSO** have back problems affecting nerves or muscles?   YES☐ NO☐

---

7. **Do you have a Respiratory Disease?** *This includes Chronic Obstructive Pulmonary Disease, Asthma, Pulmonary High Blood Pressure*

If the above condition(s) is/are present, answer questions 7a-7d   If **NO** ☐ go to question 8

7a. Do you have difficulty controlling your condition with medications or other physician-prescribed therapies? (Answer **NO** if you are not currently taking medications or other treatments)   YES☐ NO☐

7b. Has your doctor ever said your blood oxygen level is low at rest or during exercise and/or that you require supplemental oxygen therapy?   YES☐ NO☐

7c. If asthmatic, do you currently have symptoms of chest tightness, wheezing, laboured breathing, consistent cough (more than 2 days/week), or have you used your rescue medication more than twice in the last week?   YES☐ NO☐

7d. Has your doctor ever said you have high blood pressure in the blood vessels of your lungs?   YES☐ NO☐

---

8. **Do you have a Spinal Cord Injury?** *This includes Tetraplegia and Paraplegia*

If the above condition(s) is/are present, answer questions 8a-8c   If **NO** ☐ go to question 9

8a. Do you have difficulty controlling your condition with medications or other physician-prescribed therapies? (Answer **NO** if you are not currently taking medications or other treatments)   YES☐ NO☐

8b. Do you commonly exhibit low resting blood pressure significant enough to cause dizziness, light-headedness, and/or fainting?   YES☐ NO☐

8c. Has your physician indicated that you exhibit sudden bouts of high blood pressure (known as Autonomic Dysreflexia)?   YES☐ NO☐

---

9. **Have you had a Stroke?** *This includes Transient Ischemic Attack (TIA) or Cerebrovascular Event*

If the above condition(s) is/are present, answer questions 9a-9c   If **NO** ☐ go to question 10

9a. Do you have difficulty controlling your condition with medications or other physician-prescribed therapies? (Answer **NO** if you are not currently taking medications or other treatments)   YES☐ NO☐

9b. Do you have any impairment in walking or mobility?   YES☐ NO☐

9c. Have you experienced a stroke or impairment in nerves or muscles in the past 6 months?   YES☐ NO☐

---

10. **Do you have any other medical condition not listed above or do you have two or more medical conditions?**

If you have other medical conditions, answer questions 10a-10c   If **NO** ☐ read the Page 4 recommendations

10a. Have you experienced a blackout, fainted, or lost consciousness as a result of a head injury within the last 12 months **OR** have you had a diagnosed concussion within the last 12 months?   YES☐ NO☐

10b. Do you have a medical condition that is not listed (such as epilepsy, neurological conditions, kidney problems)?   YES☐ NO☐

10c. Do you currently live with two or more medical conditions?   YES☐ NO☐

PLEASE LIST YOUR MEDICAL CONDITION(S) AND ANY RELATED MEDICATIONS HERE: _____

_____

GO to Page 4 for recommendations about your current medical condition(s) and sign the PARTICIPANT DECLARATION.

Activity 1.3 **PAR-Q and Health History Questionnaire** *(continued)*

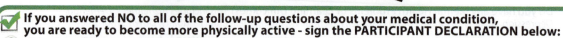

2015 PAR-Q+

☑ **If you answered NO to all of the follow-up questions about your medical condition, you are ready to become more physically active - sign the PARTICIPANT DECLARATION below:**

▸ It is advised that you consult a qualified exercise professional to help you develop a safe and effective physical activity plan to meet your health needs.

▸ You are encouraged to start slowly and build up gradually – 20 to 60 minutes of low to moderate intensity exercise, 3-5 days per week including aerobic and muscle strengthening exercises.

▸ As you progress, you should aim to accumulate 150 minutes or more of moderate intensity physical activity per week.

▸ If you are over the age of 45 years and **NOT** accustomed to regular vigorous to maximal effort exercise, consult a qualified exercise professional before engaging in this intensity of exercise.

🛑 **If you answered YES to one or more of the follow-up questions about your medical condition:**

You should seek further information before becoming more physically active or engaging in a fitness appraisal. You should complete the specially designed online screening and exercise recommendations program - the **ePARmed-X+** at www.eparmedx.com and/or visit a qualified exercise professional to work through the ePARmed-X+ and for further information.

⚠ **Delay becoming more active if:**

✓ You have a temporary illness such as a cold or fever; it is best to wait until you feel better.

✓ You are pregnant – talk to your health care practitioner, your physician, a qualified exercise professional, and/or complete the ePARmed-X+ **at www.eparmedx.com** before becoming more physically active.

✓ Your health changes – talk to your doctor or a qualified exercise professional before continuing with any physical activity program.

● You are encouraged to photocopy the PAR-Q+. You must use the entire questionnaire and NO changes are permitted.
● The authors, the PAR-Q+ Collaboration, partner organizations, and their agents assume no liability for persons who undertake physical activity and/or make use of the PAR-Q+ or ePARmed-X+. If in doubt after completing the questionnaire, consult your doctor prior to physical activity.

PARTICIPANT DECLARATION

● All persons who have completed the PAR-Q+ please read and sign the declaration below.

● If you are less than the legal age required for consent or require the assent of a care provider, your parent, guardian or care provider must also sign this form.

I, the undersigned, have read, understood to my full satisfaction and completed this questionnaire. I acknowledge that this physical activity clearance is valid for a maximum of 12 months from the date it is completed and becomes invalid if my condition changes. I also acknowledge that a Trustee (such as my employer, community/fitness centre, health care provider, or other designate) may retain a copy of this form for their records. In these instances, the Trustee will be required to adhere to local, national, and international guidelines regarding the storage of personal health information ensuring that the Trustee maintains the privacy of the information and does not misuse or wrongfully disclose such information.

NAME _____   DATE _____

SIGNATURE _____   WITNESS _____

SIGNATURE OF PARENT/GUARDIAN/CARE PROVIDER _____

──────── **For more information, please contact** ────────
www.eparmedx.com
Email: eparmedx@gmail.com

Citation for PAR-Q+
Warburton DER, Jamnik VK, Bredin SSD, and Gledhill N on behalf of the PAR-Q+ Collaboration. The Physical Activity Readiness Questionnaire for Everyone (PAR-Q+) and Electronic Physical Activity Readiness Medical Examination (ePARmed-X+). Health & Fitness Journal of Canada 4(2):3-23, 2011.
Key References
1. Jamnik VK, Warburton DER, Makarski J, McKenzie DC, Shephard RJ, Stone J, and Gledhill N. Enhancing the effectiveness of clearance for physical activity participation; background and overall process. APNM 36(S1):S3-S13, 2011.
2. Warburton DER, Gledhill N, Jamnik VK, Bredin SSD, McKenzie DC, Stone J, Charlesworth S, and Shephard RJ. Evidence-based risk assessment and recommendations for physical activity clearance; Consensus Document. APNM 36(S1):S266-s298, 2011.

The PAR-Q+ was created using the evidence-based AGREE process (1) by the PAR-Q+ Collaboration chaired by Dr. Darren E. R. Warburton with Dr. Norman Gledhill, Dr. Veronica Jamnik, and Dr. Donald C. McKenzie (2). Production of this document has been made possible through financial contributions from the Public Health Agency of Canada and the BC Ministry of Health Services. The views expressed herein do not necessarily represent the views of the Public Health Agency of Canada or the BC Ministry of Health Services.

 OSHF
Ontario Society for Health and Fitness

Activity 1.4   **Resting Heart Rate and Blood Pressure**

Name _____   Date _____

Course _____   Section _____   Gender _____   Age _____

Resting Heart Rate and Blood Pressure

Determine your resting heart rate and blood pressure in the right and left arms while sitting comfortably in a chair.

Resting Heart Rate: [   ]   Rating: [   ]   (see Table 1.6, page 33)

Blood Pressure:	Right Arm	Rating (from Table 1.7, page 34)	Left Arm	Rating (from Table 1.7, page 34)
Systolic	[ ]	[ ]	[ ]	[ ]
Diastolic	[ ]	[ ]	[ ]	[ ]

Mean Blood Pressure Computation

The following equation is used to determine MBP:

$MBP = DBP + \frac{1}{3} PP$ Where PP = pulse pressure or the difference between the systolic and diastolic pressures.

1. Compute your MBP using your own blood pressure results:

   PP = _____ (systolic) − _____ (diastolic) = _____ mm Hg

   MBP = _____ (DBP) + $\dfrac{\text{_____ (PP)}}{3}$ = _____ mm Hg

2. Determine the MBP for a person with a BP of 130/80 and a second person with a BP of 120/90.

   _____

   _____

   _____

   _____

   Which subject has the lower MBP? _____

Computing the Effects of Aerobic Activity on Resting Heart Rate

Using your actual resting heart rate (RHR) from Part I of this lab, compute the total number of times your heart beats each day and each year:

A. Beats per day = _____ (RHR bpm) × 60 (min per hour) × 24 (hours per day) = _____ beats per day

B. Beats per year = _____ (heart rate in beats per day, use item A) × 365 = _____ beats per year

If your RHR dropped 20 bpm through an aerobic exercise program, determine the number of beats that your heart would save each year at that lower RHR:

C. Beats per day = _____ (your current RHR − 20) × 60 × 24 = _____ beats per day

D. Beats per year = _____ (heart rate in beats per day, use item C) × 365 = _____ beats per year

E. Number of beats saved per year (B − D) _____ − _____ = _____ beats saved per year

Assuming that you will reach the average U.S. life expectancy of 81 years for women or 76 for men, determine the additional number of "heart rate life years" available to you if your RHR were 20 bpm lower:

F. Years of life ahead = _____ (use 81 for women and 76 for men) − _____ (current age) = _____ years

G. Number of beats saved = _____ (use item E) × _____ (use item F) = _____ beats saved

H. Number of heart rate life years based on the lower RHR = _____ (use item G) ÷ _____ (use item D) = _____ years

© Fitness & Wellness, Inc.

Activity 1.5   Dimensions of Wellness—Setting Your Goal

Name _____   **Date** _____

Course _____   **Section** _____   **Gender** _____   **Age** _____

Instructions

1. In the Wellness Dimension chart below, record the date at the top of the first column, then fill in that column using the following scale to indicate your wellness rating for each dimension:

   poor = 5, fair = 4, average = 3, good = 2, excellent = 1

2. Next, write a goal that you want to accomplish prior to the end of this course for each wellness dimension, and list three specific objectives that will help you accomplish each goal.

3. Once a month, review this form, fill in another column of self-evaluation, and adjust your objectives as necessary.

Here's an example:

Social goal: | To improve my social life at school |

Specific objectives

1. _Find study buddies. Ask each instructor and counselor about study groups._
2. _Attend Friday night discussion groups in Student Center._
3. _Locate activities I enjoy—basketball, chess, dancing—and start a conversation._

Date

Wellness Dimension					
Physical					
Emotional					
Social					
Environmental					
Mental					
Spiritual					
Occupational					

Goals and Objectives

Physical goal: | |

Specific objectives

1. _____
2. _____
3. _____

Emotional goal: | |

Specific objectives

1. _____
2. _____
3. _____

Social goal: | |

Specific objectives

1. _____
2. _____
3. _____

Environmental goal: | |

Specific objectives

1. _____
2. _____
3. _____

Mental goal: | |

Specific objectives

1. _____
2. _____
3. _____

Spiritual goal: | |

Specific objectives

1. _____
2. _____
3. _____

Occupational goal: | |

Specific objectives

1. _____
2. _____
3. _____

© Fitness & Wellness, Inc.

MINDTAP From Cengage   **Complete This Online**
Visit **www.cengagebrain.com** to access MindTap, a complete digital course that includes interactive quizzes, videos, and more.

2

Behavior Modification

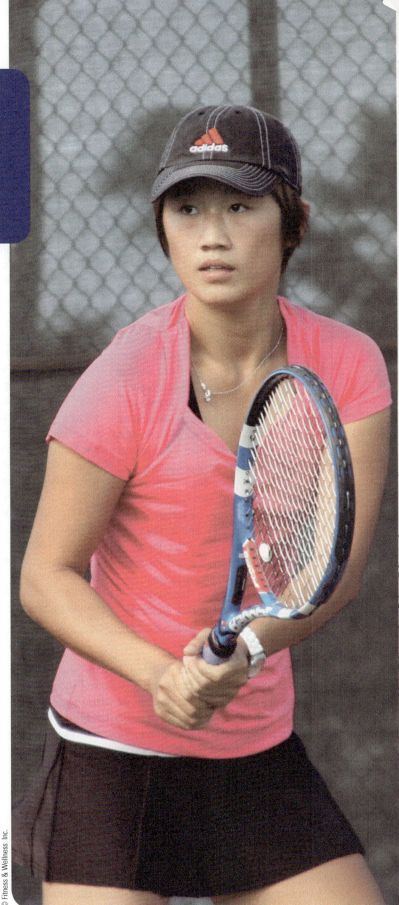

"To reach a goal you have never before attained, you must do things you have never before done."
—Richard G. Scott

Objectives

2.1 **Learn** the effects of environment on human behavior.

2.2 **Understand** obstacles that hinder the ability to change behavior.

2.3 **Describe** how habits are formed and changed.

2.4 **Explain** the importance of personal values and long-term goals.

2.5 **Learn** the techniques for positive self-talk.

2.6 **Explain** the concepts of motivation and locus of control.

2.7 **Identify** the stages of change.

2.8 **Describe** the processes of change.

2.9 **Explain** techniques that will facilitate the process of change.

2.10 **Describe** the role of SMART goal setting in the process of change.

2.11 **Be able to write** specific actions for behavioral change.

© Fitness & Wellness, Inc.

FAQ

Why is it so hard to change?

Change is incredibly difficult for most people. Our behaviors are based on our core values, our personal nature, and actions that are rewarded. Whether we are trying to increase physical activity, quit smoking, change unhealthy eating habits, or get to bed on time, it is human nature to resist change that isn't immediately rewarded, even when we know that change will provide substantial benefits in the near future. We are familiar with the outcomes of our usual daily choices, which gives those choices an aura of comfort and safety. These choices may even help us understand how we fit in with the people around us and how those choices make us predictable to those people. This is one reason we may endure occasional comments from others when we begin to initiate a change in our lives. That is because people around us may be surprised by our change in choices, and it may take them some time to adjust to our new choices. Furthermore, many behavioral scientists believe that people are more affected by the negative information, thoughts, and emotions they encounter than they are by the positive. This tendency, commonly referred to as a "negativity bias," is hardwired into our biology. In every spoken language, there is a ratio of three pessimistic adjectives to one positive adjective. Thus, linguistically, psychologically, and emotionally, we focus on what can go wrong and we lose motivation before we even start.

What triggers the desire to change?

Motivation comes from within. In most instances, no amount of pressure, reasoning, or fear will inspire people to take action. Change in behavior is most likely to occur when people either receive instant gratification for their actions or when people's feelings are addressed. People pursue change—or start contemplating change—when there is a change in core values that will make them feel uncomfortable with the present behavior. Core values change when feelings are addressed. The challenge is to find ways that will help people understand the problems and solutions in a manner that will influence emotions and not just the thought process. Once the problem behavior is understood and "felt," the person may become uncomfortable with the situation and will be more inclined to address the problem behavior or adopt a healthy behavior.

Discomfort can also be a great motivator. People tolerate any situation until it becomes too uncomfortable for them, at which point they become open to alternatives, even when alternatives may bring change in their lives. It is at this point that the skills presented in this chapter will help you implement a successful plan for change. Keep in mind that, as you make lifestyle changes, your relationships and friendships also need to be addressed. You need to distance yourself from those individuals who share your bad habits (e.g., smoking, drinking, and sedentary lifestyle) and associate with people who practice healthy habits. Are you prepared to do so?

Adapted from K. Jenkins, "Why Is Change So Hard?" http://www.healthnexus.ca/projects/articles/change.htm, downloaded March 12, 2011.

The benefits of regular physical activity and living a healthy lifestyle to achieve wellness are well documented. Most people who fail to exercise, eat well, and get regular sleep do not do so because of lack of understanding or interest. Most people see a need to incorporate these choices into their lives, but making change is difficult. Seventy percent of new and returning exercisers, for example, are at risk for early dropout.[1] As the scientific evidence continues to mount each day, most people still are not adhering to a healthy lifestyle program.

Let's look at a common occurrence on college campuses. Most students understand that they should be exercising, and they contemplate enrolling in a fitness course. The motivating factor might be improved physical appearance, health benefits, or simply fulfillment of a college requirement. They sign up for the course, participate for a few months, finish the course, and stop exercising! They offer a wide array of excuses: too busy, no one to exercise with, inconvenient gym hours, job conflicts, and so on. A few months later they realize once again that exercise is vital, and they repeat the cycle (Figure 2.1).

The ability to create positive change in your life, to learn from your mistakes, and to adjust your course for the future is

Figure 2.1 Exercise/exercise dropout cycle.

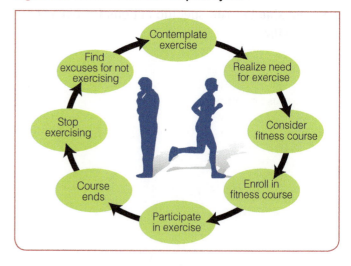

a reward in itself. Small successes are important. They empower you to address additional behaviors that will increase your quality of life. The information in this book will be of little

REAL LIFE STORY | Sharon's Experience

Prior to my marriage, I had never really tried jogging. But then I became convinced that aerobic exercise would improve my fitness and help me maintain a healthy weight. My fiancé was really serious about fitness and had been jogging regularly for several years. We wrote out an exercise prescription and started jogging together. Exercise helped me to accomplish my health goals through my first two pregnancies. The feeling of being physically fit was a reward in itself, but jogging 2 consecutive miles was rarely truly enjoyable. With young children at home, my husband and I were forced to take turns jogging so that one of us would always be home. My jogging program consisted of a 20-minute jog: 1 mile out and 1 mile back, five to six times per week.

Five years later, on one particular day, 25 minutes went by and I wasn't ready to stop jogging. At 30 minutes, I went and knocked on the door: "Honey, I feel great; I'll be back in 10 minutes." I did this again at 40 and 50 minutes.

I ended up jogging for a full 60 minutes for the first time in my life, and the experience was genuinely joyful! That day, I finally reached "the top of the mountain" (the termination/adoption stage of change) and truly experienced the joy of being physically fit. Jogging became as easy as a "bird in flight." I have not stopped jogging in more than 36 years! It wasn't easy at first, but knowledge, commitment, support, action, and perseverance paid off.

Fitness also was the factor that led to improvements in other wellness components in our lives (continuing health education, good nutrition, stress reduction, and chronic disease prevention). Fitness is the daily "bread and butter" that enhances our quality of life. Our children now also follow our active lifestyle. We always say: "A family that exercises together stays together."

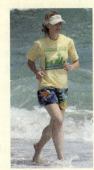

© Fitness & Wellness, Inc.

PERSONAL PROFILE: Personal Behavior Modification Profile

Are you able to answer the following questions regarding behavior change? If you are unable to do so, the chapter contents will help you do so.

I. Can you list the processes of change that most helped Sharon adhere to her fitness program? _____

II. Can you identify behavioral changes that you have consciously made in your life and the process that you went through to do so? _____

III. Would you categorize yourself as having an internal or external locus of control? (Do you believe you can take charge of your own life [internal locus of control] or do you feel victim to forces beyond your control [external locus of control]?) _____

IV. Can you identify your current stage of change for physical activity? How about exercise? (Are you not yet ready to consider exercise? Contemplating exercise? Making preparations to fit exercise in your life? Currently exercising regularly? Or have you exercised regularly for five years or more?) _____

MINDTAP From Cengage **Complete This Online**
Visit **www.cengagebrain.com** to access MindTap, a complete digital course that includes interactive quizzes, videos, and more.

value to you if you are unable to adopt and maintain healthy behaviors. Before looking at any physical fitness and wellness guidelines, take a critical look at your behaviors and lifestyle—consider the permanent changes you need to make to promote your own wellness. This chapter will help you understand and apply **behavior modification** techniques.

2.1 *Living in a Toxic Health and Fitness Environment*

Most of the behaviors we adopt are a product of our environment—the forces of social influences we encounter and the thought processes we go through. This environment includes families, friends, peers, homes, schools, workplaces, and media, as well as our communities, country, and culture in general.

Unfortunately, when it comes to fitness and wellness, we live in a "toxic" environment. Becoming aware of how the environment affects us is vital if we wish to achieve and maintain wellness. Yet, we are so habituated to the environment that we miss the subtle ways it influences our behaviors. From a young age, we observe, we emulate, and without realizing it, we internalize social norms. Receiving validation about our behavior from the people around us makes us feel encouraged and accepted. A group of studies carried out in the United Kingdom, for example, found that something as

GLOSSARY

Behavior modification The process of permanently changing negative behaviors to positive behaviors that will lead to better health and well-being.

simple as informing diners of what their fellow diners were choosing changed eating behavior.[2]

If you examine your own environment, you should be able to identify two types of external obstacles to healthy behavior: physical obstacles and social obstacles. We grow up in communities that lack sidewalks, bike lanes, or amenities that are near enough to walk to. We go about life being transported by car, and we are driven walkable distances to save time, to avoid unpleasant weather, or to keep clothes and appearance pristine. We may not own weather-protective clothes because we go from home to car to school or work. We shop in grocery stores where unhealthy choices are plentiful and well marketed, and we observe those around us choose food for convenience and price point over nutritional value. Classrooms and workplaces are built for sitting. Professionals often prioritize work over sleep and physical activity, and at the end of the day, especially in winter months, we observe as family and friends unwind with hours of uninterrupted sitting. Others engage in risky behaviors by checking their phone while driving, by driving after having a drink, and by having unprotected sex. These social norms are referred to as **anchor points**. Researchers believe that people make decisions not only according to the absolute value of what is good for them, but according to how the decision compares to the social norms or anchor points the individual is accustomed to. Unhealthy social norms can be passed along, unquestioned, to the next generation.

You may have experienced different social norms when moving from one place to another. Everything from driving etiquette, to formality of clothing, to how interactive neighbors are with one another may change. Individuals may also change what they consider to be normal for themselves personally during their own lifetime. Weight gain is an especially common example. Most people do not start life with a weight problem. By age 20, a man may weigh 160 pounds. A few years later, the weight starts to climb and may reach 170 pounds. He now adapts and accepts 170 pounds as his weight. He may go on a diet but not make the necessary lifestyle changes. Gradually his weight climbs to 180, 190, and 200 pounds. Although he may not like it and would like to weigh less, once again he adapts and accepts 200 pounds as his stable weight.

Environmental Influence on Physical Activity

Not a single country has made meaningful progress against the worldwide obesity epidemic of the last 30 years. Change and progress are needed, especially in the United States, which has one of the highest obesity rates in the world and the highest among all OECD countries (see Chapter 1, page 5). In the United States 30 years ago, the state with the highest obesity rate still had a lower prevalence than the state with the lowest obesity rate today. We have adopted a new norm.

Among the leading underlying causes of death in the United States are physical inactivity and poor diet. Light physical activities that go on continually throughout the day (like housecleaning and acts of self-care) accumulate to have a substantial impact on health. Unfortunately, activities that a few decades ago required movement or physical activity now require almost no effort and negatively affect health. Health experts recommend 5 to 6 miles of walking per day. This level of activity equates to about 10,000 to 12,000 daily steps. If you have never tracked your step count, try to do so. When you look at the total number of steps you have taken at the end of the day, you may be surprised to find that the number is lower than expected.

As indicated in Chapter 1, individuals who spend an excessive amount of daily time sitting have an increased risk for all-cause and cardiovascular disease mortality, independent of leisure-time physical activity and excessive body weight.[3] The greater the amount of sitting time per day, the greater the risk of premature disability and mortality.

Work and Leisure Time

The requirement for physical movement has been engineered out of many leisure and work environments. The percentage of U.S. jobs that are sedentary in nature is double what it was in the 1950s.[4] Even during lunch breaks, the majority of office workers spend the break sitting, with many taking lunch at their desk while continuing to check off work tasks.

Unfortunately, when people find a few free minutes during the day or arrive home after work, they often are drawn to a screen. Americans spend an average of 4.4 hours of their leisure time each day on a screen.[5] The average American school child, when graduating from high school, will have spent more time watching TV and viewing screens than they will have spent in school, with time peaking in the summer.[6] The physical activity level of American youth now reaches its peak around age 10, and in some cases as young as age 2. One study sought to examine the current cardiorespiratory fitness of American youth ages 12 to 15, an age when activity should still come naturally. Researchers utilized treadmill tests and were surprised to discover that the cardiorespiratory fitness level of this age group had dropped 10 percent in 8 years, a disquieting statistic foretelling a jump in future disease risk. Ethnicity and income had no effect on test results.[7]

After several large-scale studies about uninterrupted sitting, researchers agree that excessive TV watching appears to heap on an additional risk for earlier death.[8] Excessive TV viewing appears to be more detrimental than other sedentary activities such as reading, studying, or doing homework. A total of 8,800 adults with no history of heart disease were followed for more than 6 years. As compared to individuals who only watched 2 hours of TV per day, those who watched 4 or more daily hours were 80 percent more likely to die from heart disease and 46 percent more likely to die from all causes.[9] Both excessive TV viewing and excessive sitting are associated with a loss of life that is as severe as other disease risk factors such as physical inactivity, smoking, and obesity. Television viewing has further been shown to reduce the number of fruits and vegetables some people consume. A similar result has been observed in those playing video games. Calorie intake has been found to go up regardless of the individual's hunger cues.[10]

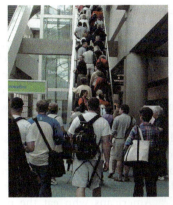
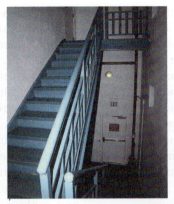
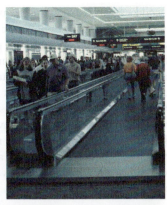
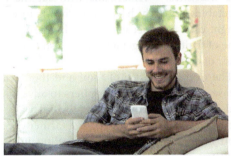
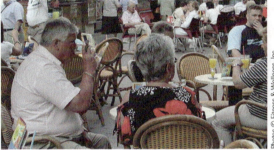

Our environment is not conducive to a healthy, physically active lifestyle.

Community Design

The typical modern lifestyle requires hours spent sitting in cars. Communities are designed around the automobile. City streets make driving convenient and walking or cycling difficult, impossible, or dangerous. For each car in the United States, there are seven parking spaces.[11] Drivers can almost always find a parking spot, but walkers often run out of sidewalks and crosswalks on modern streets.

Streets typically are rated by traffic engineers according to their "level of service"—that is, based on how well they facilitate motorized traffic. A wide, straight street with few barriers to slow motorized traffic gets a high score. According to these guidelines, pedestrians are "obstructions." Only recently have a few local governments and communities started to devise standards to determine how useful streets are for pedestrians and bicyclists and to measure communities by their "walkability score."

Although British street design manuals recommend sidewalks on both sides of the street, American manuals recommend sidewalks on one side of the street only. One measure that encourages activity is the use of "traffic-calming" strategies: intentionally slowing traffic to make the pedestrians' role easier. These strategies were developed and are widely used in Europe. Examples include narrower streets, rougher pavement, pedestrian islands, and raised crosswalks. Neighborhoods where walking is safe, inviting, and a practical means to reach a nearby destination are healthier for their residents. In one large-scale study, the average man in a walkable neighborhood weighed 10 pounds less and the average woman 6 pounds less than their counterparts in less walkable neighborhoods.[12] Many European communities place a high priority on walking and cycling, which make up 40 to 54 percent of all daily trips taken by people in Austria, the Netherlands, Denmark, Italy, and Sweden. By contrast, in the United States, walking and cycling account for 10 percent of daily trips, whereas the automobile accounts for 85 percent.[13]

Many people drive because the distances to cover are on a vast scale. We live in bedroom communities and commute to work. When people live near frequently visited destinations, they are more likely to walk or bike for transportation. In the United States, the automobile is used about half of the time for distances shorter than 500 yards, whereas it is used more than 90 percent of the time for distances greater than two-thirds of a mile. Neighborhoods that mix commercial and residential land use encourage walking over driving because of the short distances among home, shopping, and work. Children also walk or cycle to school less frequently today than in the past.

School and Community Policy

There is tremendous room for growth in the way we encourage and prioritize everyday physical activity and planned exercise. Research shows that physical activity during school and college years is connected not only to better mental and physical health, but also to lifetime adoption of exercise.

GLOSSARY

Anchor points Social norms that individuals use as a reference when considering a new behavior.

Unfortunately, colleges are dropping requirements for physical activity courses to make more time for sit-down courses. Fewer colleges than ever are requiring physical activity courses, with public colleges requiring the courses less often than private colleges.[14] The IRS allows tax deductions for health club memberships only for patients who receive a formal prescription for a specific condition, such as stroke rehabilitation. Health insurance plans cover invasive surgical procedures, including gastric stapling, but will not assist with the cost of a personal fitness trainer. Priorities and incentives ignore prevention and healthy lifestyle factors until an individual is diagnosed with disability or disease.

Environmental Influence on Diet and Nutrition

Our toxic health environment not only decreases opportunities for physical activity but also increases opportunities to overeat. We may begin by considering the amount of calories available to us as a nation.

Food Quality and Abundance

According to the United States Department of Agriculture, the American food supply contains a surplus of 500 calories per day, per person, after wastage. This is a surplus that did not exist in the 1970 food supply. The nutritional quality of the United States food supply does not brighten the outlook. Indeed, if we set about to align the food available in the

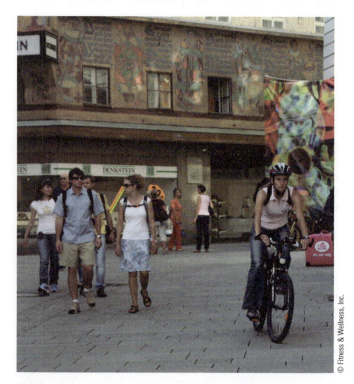

Walking and cycling are priority activities in many European communities.

United States with nutritional guidelines, major changes would be in order. The supply of vegetables would need to rise by 70 percent, the supply of fruit would need to double, and as for the grain supply, four times as much of our grain would need to remain whole instead of being refined.[15] A report on fruit and vegetable consumption by the Centers for Disease Control and Prevention found that fewer than one in ten respondents consumed the recommended 2 to 3 cups per day of vegetables. The study concluded that "substantial new efforts are needed to build consumer demand for fruits and vegetables through competitive pricing, placement and promotion in child care, schools, grocery stores, communities and worksites."[16] Americans who eat the most fruits and vegetables not only have been shown to eat more food by weight each day (because of the higher water and fiber volume of fruits and vegetables), but also have the lowest prevalence of obesity.

The overabundance of food and the need for profits increase pressure on food suppliers to advertise to consumers and lobby to the government to find ways to sell more of their product. As explained by a former executive of a large food company, who left after feeling uncomfortable with industry ethics, "Over the years, relentless efforts were made to increase the number of 'eating occasions' people indulged in and the amount of food they consumed at each."[17]

© Fitness & Wellness, Inc.

> **HOEGER KEY TO WELLNESS**
>
> Increased "eating occasions" are a major contribution to our growing waistlines and have jumped from an average of 3.8 daily occasions 30 years ago to 4.9 daily occasions today.

As Americans, our lives seem to be centered on food, a nonstop string of occasions to eat. We eat during coffee breaks, when we socialize, when we play, when we watch sports, at the movies, and when the clock tells us it's time for a meal. These "eating occasions" are a major contribution to our growing waistlines and have made a notable jump from an average of 3.8 daily occasions in the 1970s to 4.9 daily occasions today.[18] You may take a moment to reflect on your typical day and consider your own average number of eating occasions and how often you allow yourself to begin feeling hungry before you have a meal or snack.

The likelihood of overeating is increased when there is a large variety of food, high visibility of food, food that is physically near, or food that is more convenient. Each of these factors sends an immediate cue to our brain that there is an opportunity to eat. Further, when unhealthy choices outnumber healthy choices, people are less likely to follow their natural cues to choose healthy food. These environmental

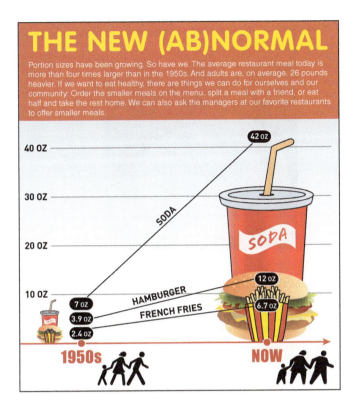

THE NEW (AB)NORMAL

Portion sizes have been growing. So have we. The average restaurant meal today is more than four times larger than in the 1950s. And adults are, on average, 26 pounds heavier. If we want to eat healthy, there are things we can do for ourselves and our community: Order the smaller meals on the menu, split a meal with a friend, or eat half and take the rest home. We can also ask the managers at our favorite restaurants to offer smaller meals.

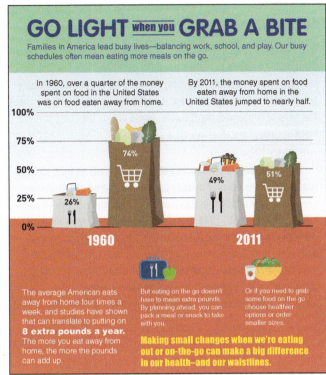

GO LIGHT when you GRAB A BITE

Families in America lead busy lives—balancing work, school, and play. Our busy schedules often mean eating more meals on the go.

In 1960, over a quarter of the money spent on food in the United States was on food eaten away from home.

By 2011, the money spent on food eaten away from home in the United States jumped to nearly half.

The average American eats away from home four times a week, and studies have shown that can translate to putting on **8 extra pounds a year.** The more you eat away from home, the more the pounds can add up.

But eating on the go doesn't have to mean extra pounds. By planning ahead, you can pack a meal or snack to take with you.

Or if you need to grab some food on the go choose healthier options or order smaller sizes.

Making small changes when we're eating out or on-the-go can make a big difference in our health–and our waistlines.

influences that have a negative impact on nutrition can be utilized instead to have a positive impact. For example, having drinkable water physically near has been shown to increase the amount of water an individual drinks in a day. Healthy foods that are convenient and left in highly visible places are more likely to be eaten.

Dining Out

Eating dinner at home around the table accompanied by meaningful conversation (as compared to watching a show) has been linked to a lower body mass index (BMI).[19] Unfortunately, eating out is part of today's lifestyle. In the 1960s, Americans used almost 2 out of 10 dollars from their disposable income on food. About a quarter of that was spent eating away from home. Today, we spend less on food overall, about 1 in 10 dollars, but nearly half of that is on dining out.[20]

Eating out would not be such a problem if portion sizes were reasonable or if restaurant food were similar to food prepared at home. Compared with home-cooked meals, restaurant and fast-food meals are higher in calories, fat, saturated fat, and sodium and lower in vitamins, minerals, and fiber. Today, the average restaurant meal contains more than half of an entire day's caloric and fat allowance and a day and a half's worth of the recommended amount of sodium. Restaurant patrons often underestimate the number of calories they consume during a meal. One study asked trained

dietitians to estimate nutrition information for five restaurant meals. The results showed that the dietitians underestimated the number of calories and amount of fat by 37 and 49 percent, respectively.[21] Findings such as these do not offer much hope for the average consumer who tries to make healthy choices when eating out.

Most restaurants are also pleasurable places to be: colorful, well-lit, and thoughtfully decorated. These intentional features are designed to enhance comfort, appetite, and length of stay. Employees are formally trained in techniques that urge patrons to eat more and spend more. Mention of specific menu items and qualities of taste, texture, and preparation have scientifically been proven to increase a diner's desire for food. Patrons visualizing those items begin to anticipate eating them. Servers, therefore, are prepared to approach the table and suggest specific drinks, appetizers, and daily specials. Following dinner, the server offers desserts and coffee. A person can easily get a full day's worth of calories in one meal.

Even as the awareness of the need for healthful eating habits has grown, few changes have been made in fast food. One recent study found that in a period of 14 years, the nutritional rating of fast-food offerings as measured by the U.S. Department of Agriculture's Healthy Eating Index has improved by only 3 percent.[22] Menu items at many fast-food restaurants frequently are introduced at one size and, over time, popular items are increased in size by two to five times.[23] Large portion sizes are a problem because people

Added Sugar

In our modern food culture, sugar is cheap. Sugar is a low-cost ingredient added to foods to make them more desirable. This has not always been the case. In colonial America, for example, sugar was available only to wealthy households and was kept locked away in a sugar chest. The head of household, not the cook, would unlock the chest to reveal a block or cone of sugar, shave off a small amount of sugar, and deliver it to the kitchen.

Today, the average American gets 350 daily calories from added sugar, or 22 teaspoons of added sugar a day. There has fortunately been some improvement in this number in recent years, down from 16.8 percent in 1988–1994, but our levels of added sugar intake do not begin to approach the American Heart Association's suggested daily limit of six tablespoons for women and nine tablespoons for men. Researchers have recently found that the national rates of not only diabetes, but also heart disease and some cancers move in step with our sugar consumption. Besides being a risk on their own, added

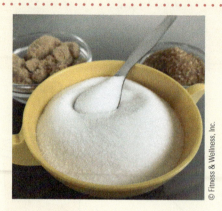

sugar and soft drinks are often the source of calories unaccounted for and increase the likelihood that a person will overeat.

SOURCE: Q. Yang et al., "Added Sugar Intake and Cardiovascular Diseases Mortality Among US Adults," *JAMA Internal Medicine* 174, no. 4 (2014): 516–524.

tend to eat what they are served. A study by the American Institute for Cancer Research found that with bigger portion sizes, 67 percent of Americans ate the larger amount of food they were served.[24] The tendency of most patrons is to clean the plate.

Individuals seem to have the same disregard for hunger cues when snacking. Participants in one study were randomly given an afternoon snack of potato chips in different bag sizes. The participants received bags from 1 to 20 ounces for 5 days. The results showed that the larger the bag, the more the person ate. Of significant interest, the size of the snack did not change the amount of food the person ate during the next meal.[25] Additional research has shown that in our own kitchens, as well as in restaurants, we seem to have taken away from our internal cues the decision of how much to eat. Instead, we have turned that choice over to businesses that profit from overindulgence.

Also working against our hunger cues is our sense of thrift. Restaurants and grocers often appeal to this sense of thrift by using "value marketing," meaning that they offer us a larger portion for only a small price increase. Customers think they are getting a bargain, and the food providers turn a better profit because the cost of additional food is small compared with the cost of marketing, production, and labor. Another example of financial but not nutritional sense is free soft-drink refills. When people choose a high-calorie drink over a lower-calorie drink or water, they do not compensate by eating less food later that day.[26] Liquid calories seem to be difficult for people to account for. People who regularly drink diet sodas tend to gain weight, perhaps because they feel at liberty to eat more. A 2016 study followed the diets of 22,000 adults and found that

regular diet-soda drinkers are also more likely to have treats.[27]

The previously mentioned environmental factors influence our thought processes and hinder our ability to determine what constitutes an appropriate meal based on actual needs. The result: On average, Americans consume 571 more daily calories than they did in the 1970s.[28]

With the information you have been given, you should be able to analyze and identify the environmental influences on your behaviors. Activity 2.1 provides you with the opportunity to determine whether you control your environment or the environment controls you.

2.2 *Keys to Changing Behavior*

Understanding the process of change increases the chances for success for an individual who is motivated and ready to change. In the remainder of the chapter, we will examine what motivates people to change, barriers to change, behavior change theory, the transtheoretical or stages-of-change model, the process of change, and the role of values-based planning and goal setting.

2.3 *Personal Values and Behavior*

To understand human behavior, or why people do what they do, we need to understand values. Values are defined as the core beliefs and ideals that people have. Values govern priorities. Life is full of tradeoffs and values decide

Activity 2.1 **Exercising Control over Your Physical Activity and Nutrition Environment**

Name _____ Date _____

Course _____ Section _____ Gender _____ Age _____

INSTRUCTIONS
Select the appropriate answer to each question and obtain a final score for each section. Then rate yourself according to the guidelines at the end of the lab.

I. Physical Activity

Note: Based on the definitions of *physical activity* and *exercise*, as you take this questionnaire, keep in mind that you can be physically active without exercising, but you cannot exercise without being physically active.

	NEARLY ALWAYS	OFTEN	SELDOM	NEVER
1. Do you identify daily time slots to be *physically active?*	4	3	2	1
2. Do you seek additional opportunities to be active each day (walk, cycle, park farther away, do yard work/gardening)?	4	3	2	1
3. Do you avoid labor-saving devices/activities (escalators, elevators, self-propelled lawn mowers, snow blowers, drive through windows)?	4	3	2	1
4. Does physical activity improve your health and well-being?	4	3	2	1
5. Does physical activity increase your energy level?	4	3	2	1
6. Do you limit your sedentary traveling time on most days to less than one hour?	4	3	2	1
7. Do you take 10-minute activity breaks for every hour you spend sitting, or do you alternate between sitting and standing every 20 minutes?	4	3	2	1
8. Do you seek professional and/or medical (if necessary) advice prior to starting an exercise program or when increasing the intensity, duration, and frequency of exercise?	4	3	2	1
9. Do you identify time slots to *exercise* most days of the week?	4	3	2	1
10. Do you schedule exercise during times of the day when you feel most energetic?	4	3	2	1
11. Do you have an alternative plan to be active or exercise during adverse weather conditions (walk at the mall, swim at the health club, climb stairs, skip rope, dance)?	4	3	2	1
12. Do you cross-train (participate in a variety of activities)?	4	3	2	1
13. Do you surround yourself with people who support your physical activity/exercise goals?	4	3	2	1
14. Do you let family and friends know of your physical activity/exercise interests?	4	3	2	1
15. Do you invite family and friends to exercise with you?	4	3	2	1
16. Do you seek new friendships with people who are physically active?	4	3	2	1
17. Do you select friendships with people whose fitness and skill levels are similar to yours?	4	3	2	1
18. Do you plan social activities that involve physical activity?	4	3	2	1
19. Do you plan activity/exercise when you are away from home (during business and vacation trips)?	4	3	2	1
20. When you have a desire to do so, do you take classes to learn new activity/sport skills?	4	3	2	1
21. Do you limit daily time spent viewing media or using your smartphone?	4	3	2	1
22. Do you spend leisure hours being physically active?	4	3	2	1

Physical Activity Score:_____

© Fitness & Wellness, Inc.

Activity 2.1 Exercising Control over Your Physical Activity and Nutrition Environment *(continued)*

	NEARLY ALWAYS	OFTEN	SELDOM	NEVER

II. Nutrition

1. Do you prepare a shopping list prior to going to the store? — 4 3 2 1

2. Do you select food items primarily from the perimeter of the store (site of most fresh/unprocessed foods)? — 4 3 2 1

3. Do you limit the unhealthy snacks you bring into the home and the workplace? — 4 3 2 1

4. Do you plan your meals and is your pantry well stocked so you can easily prepare a meal without a quick trip to the store? — 4 3 2 1

5. Do you help cook your meals? — 4 3 2 1

6. Do you pay attention to how hungry you are before and during a meal? — 4 3 2 1

7. When reaching for food, do you remind yourself that you have a choice about what and how much you eat? — 4 3 2 1

8. Do you eat your meals at home? — 4 3 2 1

9. Do you eat your meals at the table only? — 4 3 2 1

10. Do you include whole-grain products in your diet each day (whole-grain bread/cereal/crackers/rice/pasta)? — 4 3 2 1

11. Do you make a deliberate effort to include a variety of fruits and vegetables in your diet each day? — 4 3 2 1

12. Do you avoid eating sugary snacks throughout the day and reserve added sugar in your foods for special treats? — 4 3 2 1

13. Do you limit your daily saturated fat and trans fat intake (red meat, whole milk, cheese, butter, hard margarines, luncheon meats, baked goods, processed foods)? — 4 3 2 1

14. Do you avoid unnecessary/unhealthy snacking (at work or play, during TV viewing, at the movies or socials)? — 4 3 2 1

15. Do you plan caloric allowances prior to attending social gatherings that include food and eating? — 4 3 2 1

16. Do you limit alcohol consumption to two drinks a day if you are a man, one drink a day if you are a woman, or none at all if you are a woman with a family history of cancer, especially breast cancer? — 4 3 2 1

17. Are you aware of strategies to decrease caloric intake when dining out (resist the server's offerings for drinks and appetizers, select a low-calorie/nutrient-dense item, drink water, resist cleaning your plate, ask for a doggie bag, share meals, request whole-wheat substitutes, get dressings on the side, avoid cream sauces, skip desserts)? — 4 3 2 1

18. Do you avoid ordering larger meal sizes because you get more food for your money? — 4 3 2 1

19. Do you avoid buying food when you hadn't planned to do so (gas stations, convenience stores, movie theaters)? — 4 3 2 1

20. Do you fill your time with activities that will keep you away from places where you typically consume food (kitchen, coffee room, dining room)? — 4 3 2 1

21. Do you know what situations trigger your desire for unnecessary snacking and overeating (vending machines, TV viewing, food ads, cookbooks, fast-food restaurants, buffet restaurants)? — 4 3 2 1

Nutrition Score: _____

Environmental Control Ratings

≥75	You have good control over your environment
53–74	There is room for improvement
32–52	Your environmental control is poor
≤31	You are controlled by your environment

Total Environmental Score
(add Physical Activity and Nutrition Scores): ☐

Figure 2.2 Values and behavior.

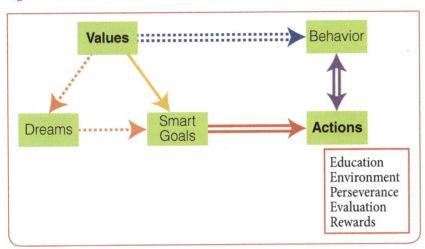

which opportunities will be sacrificed for others that are viewed as more important. Values govern behavior as people look to conduct themselves in a manner that is conducive to living and attaining goals consistent with their beliefs and what is important to them. A person's values reflect who they are.

Values are established through experience and learning, and their development is a lifelong process. Values are first developed within a person's family circles, immediate community, and media and wider culture according to what is acceptable or unacceptable, desirable or undesirable, and rewarded or ignored/punished. Educational experiences play a key role in the establishment of values (see Figure 2.2). Education is power: It provides people with knowledge to form opinions and allows them to better internalize and visualize future outcomes from today's choices. This is especially important because human nature is to focus on the present when making decisions, to give extra weight to immediate benefits and immediate feedback rather than to greater positive impact. Education forces people to question issues and take stands.

Values are also learned through examples and role models. Individuals observe the behaviors of others and choose to emulate the action if they perceive the outcome as positive. According to behavioral scientists, people have a need to maintain a positive view of themselves, which is why it is often helpful and pleasant for people to associate themselves with positive role models. As people look to develop values, they typically search for and emulate people of high ethical values and accomplishments that make them feel positive both about the people whose behaviors they are trying to emulate and themselves.

Core values change throughout life based on education and the environment in which people live. Learning and gaining a belief about a particular issue is most critical in the establishment of values. For example, individuals who lead a sedentary lifestyle and never exercise lack an understanding of and don't experience the myriad benefits and vibrant quality of life obtained through fitness participation. Part of their decision not

to exercise may be due to negative feelings and associations that intuitively arise when they think about exercise. Behavioral scientists refer to these immediate associations as **affect**. Through a book, class, sports participation, or a friend, the person first may be exposed to exercise and an active lifestyle. The individual may then seek an environment wherein he/she can learn and actively participate in a physical activity or exercise program. The feelings of well-being and increased health, functional capacity, and quality of life and the education gained about the benefits of fitness in turn become the reward for program participation. The individual now associates exercise with positive feelings and a positive view of themselves. Their actions and feelings lead to the development of the value that daily activity is vital for health and wellness. Often, deliberate effort is required to be in an environment that rewards the behaviors the individual is trying to live.

2.4 *Your Brain and Your Habits*

Habits are a necessary tool for everyday brain function. Our minds learn to use familiar cues to carry out automatic behavior that has worked successfully in the past. While we carry out these automatic behaviors, we allow our minds to spend energy working on other tasks and puzzling through other problems. If you've ever found yourself driving a familiar route when you had intended to turn off and drive elsewhere, you are performing a habit. Habits happen in familiar environments and not in new environments. Habits, however, can be changed by deliberate choice. During times of stress or when our minds are preoccupied with other problems, we are much more prone to return to and rely on habits, good or bad, and we are less likely to consider deliberate choice, core values, and long-term goals. Members of Alcoholics Anonymous are instructed, for example, that they are less likely to relapse if they can avoid situations where they become hungry, angry, lonely, or tired (H.A.L.T.).

There is a biological explanation for the way habits go from planned to automatic behavior. The area of our brain where habits are formed is known as the basal ganglia. This cluster of nuclei is situated where it can communicate with both the forebrain, involved in decision making, and the midbrain, which controls motor movement. The largest nucleus of the basal ganglia, known as the striatum, plays a key role in habit formation. The striatum is activated by events that are

GLOSSARY

Affect Immediate associations and feelings (either positive or negative) that influence choices.

What Is a Craving?

During a craving, our mind may be experiencing some of the pleasure response it remembers from a specific past experience, like consuming a particular food. Our mind then notices that the act that caused the reward is missing. We are then driven by a desire to eat that food or participate in the desired behavior.

A craving may also be ignited by a perceived opportunity to participate in the desired behavior. An urge to eat a particular food or abuse a desired drug, for example, may be ignited in a setting where a person has encountered that food or drug in the past. A visual cue like an advertisement or a social cue like friends gathering at a bar may also create the perception that there is an opportunity to experience the reward we remember. This is one reason food that is physically near or highly visible is harder to resist. The mind views the accessible food as a perceived opportunity to eat. The same goes for food that is still left on a person's plate after he or she begins to feel full. The food left on the plate represents an opportunity to continue to eat.

Personal cues are the strongest type of cues. A situation that corresponds with an addicted individual's own repeated experiences with a desired substance affects that individual longer than general cues that the substance is available.

Conversely, when a perceived opportunity is eliminated, the craving will often subside, and the individual's attention will naturally go elsewhere. A plate full of brownies on the counter, for example, is a perceived opportunity to eat brownies. A plate of brownies wrapped in freezer paper and stored at the bottom of the freezer is not a strong perceived opportunity.

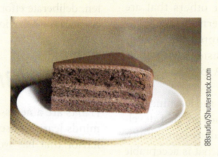

An individual who allows the mind to elaborate on a craving and imagine specific sensory details of the reward may overwhelm the working memory, strengthening the desire to submit to the craving. An individual who is able to consider the craving in abstract terms or in passing, and not dwell on it, is more likely to resist the craving.

Professional behavioral therapists have found that having some kind of preemptive strategy for coping with urges, no matter how simple, greatly improves an individual's chance of success for overcoming and choosing the desired behavior. For example, some studies have shown increased resilience to an urge when subjects responded by taking a 15-minute walk, by using highly visual imagery to picture a favorite place, or by spending 10 minutes on an engaging activity on their smartphones, as long as they can self-regulate their smartphone time.

SOURCE: M. Fatseas, F. Serre, J.-M. Alexandre, R. Debrabant, M. Auriacombe, and J. Swendsen, "Craving and Substance Use among Patients with Alcohol, Tobacco, Cannabis or Heroin Addiction: A Comparison of Substance- and Person-Specific Cues," *Addiction* (2015), doi: 10.1111/add.12882.

88studio/Shutterstock.com

---

rewarding, exciting, unexpected, and intense, as well as by cues from the environment that are associated with those events. The striatum then memorizes events that are pleasurable and rewarding and helps the individual seek opportunities to repeat those events again in the future.

The neurotransmitter dopamine is abundant in the striatum. Dopamine has many functions in the brain, including cognition, learning, behavior, motivation, and reward and punishment. As such, it plays a key role in habit formation. Any activity that links an action to a reward involves dopamine. Following repeated pairings with a reward, the behavior becomes a conditioned response that is now hard-wired in the brain. This behavior is triggered by a familiar environmental cue, upon which the brain automatically responds by performing the habit. As these behaviors become ingrained in the brain, we lose awareness as they are carried out. Once we recognize the familiar trigger, we often follow the habit whether it is helpful or detrimental, and therefore often sabotage the desire for willful change.

Changing Habits through Mindfulness and Repetition

There are likely some habits you would like to break or triggers you would rather not respond to as you usually do.

Perhaps there are positive habits you'd like to create so that in times of pressure and stress you fall into a set of positive behaviors.

There are steps you can take to change unwanted behaviors that have been ingrained in the brain or to create helpful behaviors. First, recognize that there are biological processes that lead to behavioral habits. Take note of the situational cues or stressful experiences that trigger a habit. Researchers have found that 45 percent of our behaviors are conducted in uniform contexts and locations from day to day.[29]

As you are adopting a new habit, repetition is critical. The more you repeat a new behavior under similar circumstances, the more likely you will develop the required circuitry in the striatum to make it a habit. For example, exercising at the same time of day helps develop the exercise habit. In due time, when you fail to exercise, the striatum will let you know that that specific time of the day is exercise time. Or perhaps, when you get in your car, you wait to put on your seatbelt until you are well on your way. Work to use the cue of getting in your car as a signal to immediately strap on your seatbelt and note how long it takes to become a new habit.

You must also consciously prepare to eliminate bad habits, such as not eating while watching television. Instead, use commercial breaks as a cue to stand up and find a quick household task that requires movement. Finally, realize that

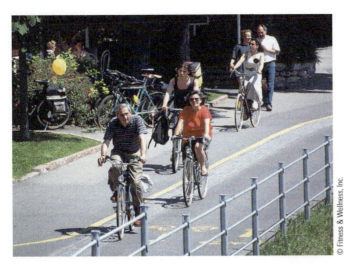

Bicycles are the preferred mode of transportation for local residents in Salzburg, Austria.

© Fitness & Wellness, Inc.

excessive stress (distress—see Chapter 12) often triggers old habits. For example, an argument with a roommate may lead to excessive time watching a TV series while eating unhealthy food. You must prepare for an adequate response in these situations. If you made a mistake and did not adequately respond to that specific situation, chalk it up to experience, use it as a learning tool, and next time come back with the proper response.

Changing Habits by Focusing on Long-Term Values

Understanding how to create and break habits through mindfulness and repetition is a powerful tool. There are greater forces at work in behavioral change than just pathways of automatic behavior, however. Those greater forces are our core values and understanding of who we are and what greater long-term desires we hold. Change in core values often overrules instant rewards as we seek long-term gratification. This ability to change according to values also has a biological explanation.

An entirely separate portion of the brain, the prefrontal cortex, is responsible for reminding us of who we are and of our long-term goals. The prefrontal cortex is also responsible for personality expression; social behavior; and complex thought processing, such as predicting likely outcomes based on prior experience and weighing competing thoughts. When you find yourself leaving your warm, comfortable bed in the morning to go to work or stopping yourself from checking a new text message because you are driving, you are experiencing your prefrontal cortex at work, placing long-term desires ahead of short-term urges.

As you work to change behavior, you will notice competing desires, especially as you begin change. Find ways to guide yourself toward new behaviors by first recognizing that you have two desires, a short-term urge and a long-term desire. Take a few extra minutes to understand and visualize the

reward you are seeking, and to educate yourself about the best way to obtain it. Remind yourself often of your core values, and look for opportunities throughout the day to align your behaviors with those core values. People can improve their chances of overcoming urges for unhealthy behavior by simply being in a frame of mind where they are thinking of the long-term benefits.

2.5 Planning and Willpower

Understanding the concept of willpower, or self-control, is helpful in the process of behavioral change. Many scientists believe that self-restraint against impulses can be built, like a muscle, if built slowly and gradually. Research suggests starting with something small. If you feel you need to read every text message the moment it arrives, you may try to learn to wait a few minutes and finish the activity you are working on and then read your text message. As you do so, you find you are able to carry out your new behavior with positive results, and your ability to exert self-control over that behavior increases.

The most effective use of willpower may be in its use as a planning tool. Individuals who plan ahead, whether it is their weekly schedule or their response in a certain situation, are able to align behavior with their long-term desires. Planning ahead allows individuals to be conscientious about their choices. Individuals who conscientiously plan are likely to be more successful, whether through success in school; having longer marriages; or decreasing their risk of high blood pressure, strokes, and Alzheimer's disease.[30]

Any new behavior you are trying to adopt should be equated with your own personal long-term values (see the section on SMART goals on pages 73–76 of this chapter). One series of studies enlisted participants who were attempting to make healthy lifestyle changes. When participants met with temptation, they were instructed to respond with a phrase: half the participants were instructed to say "I don't" and the other half were instructed to say "I can't." For example, when met with temptation, an individual may say something like "I don't check text messages while driving," versus "I can't check text messages while driving." Or an individual may say "I don't buy food that has trans fat," versus "I can't buy food that has trans fat." The phrase "I don't" was chosen by researchers because it connotes self-driven change while the phrase "I can't" connotes restrictions from an outside source.

The large majority of participants who used the phrase "I don't," which connotes self-driven change, were successful at their chosen behavior change. Those who used the phrase "I can't" were likely to be unsuccessful. The phrase "I don't" helped participants connect the new behavior with their own long-term goals and desires and kept them from feeling that behavior was an imposed restriction.[31]

Willpower is believed by some scientists to be a limited daily resource.[32] Some suggest it is highest in the morning and is depleted as we use it throughout the day, primarily when confronted with difficult challenges and stress. Some behavioral scientists suggest that the simple belief that willpower is limited will make an individual underestimate human resilience and become more tempted to give up on a goal.[33]

Perhaps the best advice is taken from both points of view. When you are planning to take on a significant task, help yourself be successful by choosing a time when you can put aside as many other demands and stressors as possible. And when you meet a failure, do not give up. Instead become a person who pushes past failure and recognizes failure for what it is: a natural process of learning on the way to success.

Studies indicate that willpower reserve can be increased through exercise, balanced nutrition, a good night's sleep, and quality time spent with important people in your life. On the other hand, willpower decreases in times of depression, anxiety, anger, and loneliness.

Researchers have found an actual growth in gray matter in the prefrontal cortex as individuals build self-control. Daily meditation, too, has been proven to develop the self-control "muscle".[34]

Growth versus Fixed Mindset

Behavioral studies have proven the importance of a growth mindset over a fixed mindset. Scientists who warn against viewing willpower as a limited resource do so because they understand the importance of a growth mindset. Individuals are more successful when they are taught that growth is possible for an individual's creativity, work ethic, intelligence, and other changeable traits. They show an increased capacity to learn and improve. Individuals who are taught that changeable traits are fixed at birth do not perform as well and give up more quickly.[35] A growth mindset places value on effort rather than linking an individual's self-valuation to results. This focus on effort has far-reaching effects throughout the individual's life.

Implementation Intentions

Another simple way to keep your values foremost in your mind is by using a research-based strategy that behavior scientists call implementation intentions.[36] The strategy follows what you might expect from the name. You consider a situation in which you are likely to encounter temptation. You then make a plan for the action you will take when faced with that situation. When the situation arises, you are much more likely to succeed with your goal by implementing the planned behavior. For example, if the weather turns bad for your evening walk, you can choose to walk around an indoor track or at the mall, do water aerobics, swim, or play racquetball. If a friend comes into town on a day you plan to exercise, you can opt for a hike together in place of your workout.

2.6 Self-Efficacy

At the heart of behavior modification is the concept of **self-efficacy**, or the belief in one's own ability to perform a given task. Self-efficacy exerts a powerful influence on people's behaviors and touches virtually every aspect of their lives. It affects both motivation for and performance of a specific task. Self-efficacy also influences vulnerability to stress and depression. Furthermore, your confidence in your coping skills determines how resilient you are in the face of adversity. Possessing high self-efficacy enhances wellness in countless ways, including your desire to learn, be productive, and be healthy.

HOEGER KEY TO WELLNESS

People prioritize instant gratification over long-term benefits. This is termed temporal discounting and leads people to choose a benefit that will be felt sooner over one with greater positive impact.

The knowledge and skills you possess, along with the personal support you have from the people around you, further determine what goals you choose to take on or choose not to take on. Mahatma Gandhi once stated: "If I have the belief that I can do it, I shall surely acquire the capacity to do it even if I may not have it at the beginning." Likewise, Teilhard de Chardin, a French paleontologist and philosopher, stated: "It is our duty as human beings to proceed as though the limits of our capabilities do not exist." With this type of attitude, how can you not strive to be the best that you can possibly be?

Sources of Self-Efficacy

The best contributors to self-efficacy are mastery experiences, or personal experiences that one has had with successes and failures. Successful past performances greatly enhance self-efficacy: "Nothing breeds success like success." Persisting through failure in a way an individual feels proud of (personal growth) can also be seen as a success, as the experience brings its own favorable outcomes. Watching consistent efforts add up creates a positive psychological effect as individuals see that, although they may not be able to control everything around them, they can indeed take charge of making positive change in their lives. Too much failure, on the other hand, may undermine confidence—in particular, if it occurs before a sense of efficacy is established.

You should structure your activities in ways that will bring success or that will make you feel good about your effort and feel that you have experienced personal growth. Your success at a particular activity increases your confidence in being able to repeat that activity. Once strong self-efficacy is developed through successful mastery experiences, an occasional setback does not have a significant effect on one's beliefs. Mastery experiences can be made more successful by practicing self-compassion and self-acceptance. By not expecting perfection but rather by being happy to be who you are and learn what you can, you are more likely to feel that your efforts are a success.

Vicarious experiences provided by role models or those one admires also influence personal efficacy. This involves the thought process of your belief that you can also do it. When you observe a peer of similar capabilities master a task, you are more likely to develop a belief that you too can perform that task—"If he can do it, so can I." Here you imitate the model's skill or you follow the same approach that led your model to a successful outcome. You may also visualize success. Visual imagery of successful personal performance—that is, watching yourself perform the skill in your mind—also increases personal efficacy.

Although not as effective as past performances and vicarious experiences, verbal persuasion of one's capabilities to perform a task also contributes to self-efficacy. When you are verbally persuaded that you possess the capabilities, you will be more likely to try the task and believe that you can get it done. The opposite is also true. Negative verbal persuasion has a far greater effect in lowering efficacy than positive messages do to enhance it. If you are verbally persuaded that you lack the skills to master a task, you will tend to avoid the activity and will be more likely to give up without giving yourself a fair chance to succeed.

The least significant source of self-efficacy beliefs are physiological cues that people experience when facing a challenge.

2.7 *Motivation and Locus of Control*

The explanation given for why some people succeed and others give up is often motivation. **Motivation** is the drive that dictates human behavior. Although motivation comes from within, external factors trigger the inner desire to accomplish a given task. These external factors, then, control behavior.

When studying motivation, understanding **locus of control** is helpful. People who believe they have control over events in their lives are said to have an internal locus of control. People with an external locus of control believe that what happens to them is a result of chance or the environment and is unrelated to their behavior. People with an internal locus of control generally are healthier and have an easier time initiating and adhering to a wellness program than those who perceive that they have no control and think of themselves as powerless and vulnerable. People with an external locus of control also are at greater risk for illness. When illness does strike a person, establishing a sense of control is vital to recovery.

Few people have either a completely external or a completely internal locus of control. They fall somewhere along a continuum. The more external one's locus of control is, the greater the challenge to change and adhere to exercise and other healthy lifestyle behaviors. Fortunately, people can develop a more internal locus of control. Understanding that most events in life are not determined genetically or environmentally helps people pursue goals and gain control over their lives. Three impediments, however, can keep people from taking action: lack of competence, lack of confidence, and lack of motivation.[37]

1. *Problems of competence.* Lacking the skills to perform a task leads to reduced competence. If your friends play basketball regularly but you don't know how to play, you might be inclined not to participate. The solution to this problem of competence is to master the skills you require to participate. Most people are not born with all-inclusive natural abilities, including playing sports.

   Another alternative is to select an activity in which you are skilled. It may not be basketball, but it well could be aerobics. Don't be afraid to try new activities. Similarly, if you need to lower your body weight, you could learn to cook healthy, low-calorie meals. Try different recipes until you find foods that you like.

2. *Problems of confidence.* Problems with confidence arise when you have the skill but don't believe you can get it done. Fear and feelings of inadequacy often interfere with the ability to perform the task. You shouldn't talk yourself out of something until you have given it a fair try. Initially, try to visualize yourself doing the task and getting it done. Repeat this several times, then actually try it. You will surprise yourself.

   Sometimes, lack of confidence arises when the task seems insurmountable. In these situations, dividing a goal into smaller, more realistic objectives helps to accomplish the task. You might know how to swim but may need to train for several weeks to swim a continuous mile. Set up your training program so that you swim a little farther each day until you are able to swim the entire mile. If you don't meet your objective on a given day, try it again; reevaluate; cut back a little; and, most important, don't give up.

3. *Problems of motivation.* With problems of motivation, both the competence and the confidence are there, but individuals are unwilling to change because the reasons to change are not important to them. For example, people begin contemplating a smoking-cessation program only when the reasons for quitting outweigh the reasons for smoking. This chapter discusses the causes of feeling unwilling to change and the barriers to change in the following section.

Many people are unaware of the magnitude of benefits of a wellness program. When it comes to a healthy lifestyle, however, you may not get a second chance. A stroke, a heart attack, or cancer can have irreparable or fatal consequences. Greater understanding of what leads to disease can help initiate change. Joy, however, is a greater motivator than fear. Even fear of dying often doesn't instigate change.

---GLOSSARY---

Self-efficacy One's belief in the ability to perform a given task.

Motivation The desire and will to do something.

Locus of control A concept examining the extent to which a person believes he or she can influence the external environment.

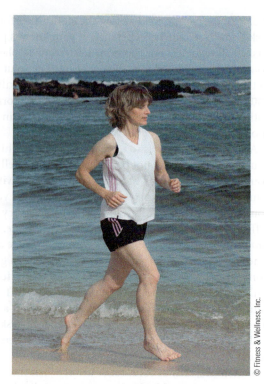

© Fitness & Wellness, Inc.

The higher quality of life experienced by people who are physically fit is hard to explain to someone who has never achieved good fitness.

Two years following coronary bypass surgery (heart disease), most patients' denial returns, and surveys show that they have not done much to alter their unhealthy lifestyle. The motivating factor for the few who do change is the "joy of living." Rather than dwelling on the "fear of dying" and causing patients to live in emotional pain, physicians help patients visualize the way positive changes will help them feel better. They will be able to enhance their quality of life by carrying out activities of daily living without concern for a heart attack, go for a walk without chest pain, play with children, and even resume an intimate relationship.

Also, feeling physically fit is difficult to explain to people unless they have experienced it themselves. Feelings of fitness, self-esteem, confidence, health, and better quality of life cannot be conveyed to someone who is constrained by sedentary living. In a way, wellness is like reaching the top of a mountain. The quiet, the clean air, the lush vegetation, the flowing water in the river, the wildlife, and the majestic valley below are difficult to explain to someone who has spent a lifetime within city limits.

2.8 Barriers to Change

In spite of the best intentions, people make unhealthy choices daily. Some of the most common reasons follow:

1. *Lack of core values.* Many are unwilling to trade convenience (sedentary lifestyle, unhealthy eating, and substance abuse) for health or other benefits.

Tip to initiate change. Subscribe to several reputable health, fitness, and wellness newsletters (see Chapter 15). Visualize positive outcomes to lifestyle change. Seek relationships with others who value healthy choices.

2. *Procrastination.* People seem to think that tomorrow is the best time to start change.

Tip to initiate change. Ask yourself: What simple, achievable step can you take today toward a changed behavior?

3. *Preconditioned cultural beliefs.* If we accept the idea that we are a product of our environment, our cultural beliefs and our physical surroundings pose significant barriers to change.

Tip to initiate change. Find a like-minded partner or search out individuals online or publications that are like-minded.

4. *Gratification.* People often prioritize instant gratification over long-term benefits. This behavior is termed **temporal discounting** and often leads people to choose a benefit that will be felt sooner over a benefit with a far greater positive impact.

Tip to initiate change. When met with temptation, spend more time in a mindset of thinking ahead.

5. *Risk complacency.* Consequences of unhealthy behaviors often don't manifest themselves until years later. People tell themselves, "If I get heart disease, I'll deal with it then. For now, I want to enjoy myself."

Tip to initiate change. Visualize long-term goals that align with your own true core values.

6. *Complexity.* People think the world is too complicated, with too much to think about. If you are living the typical lifestyle, you may feel overwhelmed by everything that seems to be required to lead a healthy lifestyle.

Tip to initiate change. Take it one step at a time. Work on only one or two behaviors at a time so that the task won't seem insurmountable. If you are feeling overwhelmed by a goal, ask yourself, on a scale of 1 to 5: How confident are you that you can make the change now? If you are less than fully confident, consider making your goal simpler and simpler until you have a goal so easy for you to accomplish that you are sure you can be successful. You can then build on your goal as you go.

7. *Indifference and helplessness.* A defeatist thought process often takes over, and we may believe that we have no control over our health (also see discussion of locus of control, pages 59–60).

Tip to initiate change. As author F. Scott Fitzgerald observed, "Trouble has no necessary connection with discouragement. Discouragement has a germ of its own." Ask yourself what small step you can take toward success. Be patient and gentle with yourself as you take further small steps of success and build self-efficacy.

8. *Rationalization.* As noted earlier, humans have a need to maintain a positive view of the person they have chosen to be. One drawback of this need is rationalization. When a person makes a negative choice, which

The Power of Positive Self-Talk

Individuals who are able to reframe problems in a positive way are better able to maintain health and well-being. They can approach imperfect situations productively. They are also able to practice self-compassion and treat themselves with the same kindness they would extend to other people. One way individuals can improve outlook is by fostering the habit of positive self-talk. *Self-talk* is a person's internal dialogue—the continual stream of thoughts an individual thinks during a day, especially in response to one's own behavior. Individuals may not notice whether their self-talk leans positive or negative until they have monitored themselves for a time. For example, after a stressful week when you realize you have eaten poorly you may find yourself saying something negative, like, "Why do I think I can do these things? I can barely keep my life together, let alone eat well." Saying the phrase aloud may help you notice that your thought is destructive to your goal. Or by saying the phrase aloud you may be happy to discover that you are thinking something positive, like "That week was not easy, but I made it through. I certainly learned what does not work for me. I am going to use next week to reset and approach my days in a way that has worked well for me in the past."

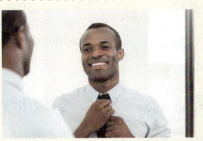

g-stockstudio/Shutterstock.com

Following are suggestions for recognizing self-talk and creating a habit of positive self-talk.

- Learn to identify how you respond to your own behavior. For a few days, take note of self-talk by saying the thought aloud or by writing it down. Or picture the thought as a headline in a magazine.
- Once you have recognized your thought, ask whether a friend would say the same thing to you in the same situation.
- Take a step back. Ask yourself whether there is evidence for what you are thinking. Ask yourself whether you are magnifying the negative side of a situation.
- Consider whether you are filtering out the positive side of a situation.
- Challenge your negative thoughts. Ask yourself if there is a different, more positive, way of viewing the situation. For instance, if you have performed poorly on a school exam, you may notice yourself saying something negative, like "There is no way I am going to get this subject." With some creativity, you may be able to reframe the situation and think something positive, like "The semester isn't over yet. I have always looked for opportunities to talk with my instructors, and this is probably one of those opportunities. I will stop by during office hours today."
- Interrupt your pattern of negative thoughts. Counter with a positive behavior that requires your attention. Or try focusing on positive memories.
- Consider whether you can take any action to change the behavior you are feeling badly about.
- Give yourself permission to find the humor in the situation, to smile and laugh.

---

everyone does occasionally, that person may not choose to change behavior but rather to rationalize behavior in order to maintain a positive self view.

Tip to initiate change. Learn to recognize when you're glossing over or minimizing a problem. Practice a daily habit of looking inward and be honest with yourself. By choosing to be honest and upfront with others, you will be able to recognize more of your own needs. While you are making this change, be kind to yourself and focus on positive self-talk. Let go of preconditioned expectations and focus on self-acceptance. Your health and your life are priceless. Monitoring lifestyle habits through daily logs and then analyzing the results can help you change self-defeating behaviors.

9. *Illusions of invincibility.* At times, people believe that unhealthy behaviors will not harm them. It can be hard to believe that things can go wrong until they do. Young adults often have the attitude that "I can smoke now, and in a few years I'll quit before it causes any damage." Unfortunately, nicotine is one of the most addictive drugs known to us, so quitting smoking is not an easy task. Another example is drinking and driving. The feeling of "I'm in control" or "I can handle it" while under the influence of alcohol is a deadly combination. Others perceive low risk when engaging in negative behaviors with people they like (e.g., sex with someone you've recently met and feel attracted to).

Tip to initiate change. Stay educated about the human body. Take time to feel amazement and awe at its workings and resilience and also to recognize and understand that it can be vulnerable. Viewing or reading the personal story of a victim of unhealthy behavior has been shown to help individuals internalize the true risk of that behavior (see emotional arousal on pages 69–70).

10. *Overplanning.* The human mind is naturally suspicious and fearful of the unknown. We may not always be aware that our hesitation or avoidance of a new behavior stems from this innate tendency. To make

GLOSSARY

Temporal discounting   The human tendency to place more value on immediate feedback and rewards over long-term rewards.

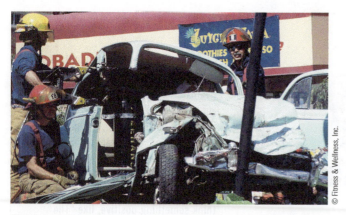

Feelings of invincibility are a strong barrier to change that can bring about life-threatening consequences.

ourselves more comfortable with future change, especially if we fear failure, we may find ourselves researching and planning indefinitely, but never actually starting.

Tip to initiate change. Act now, finish planning later. Try dipping your toe in by taking a small step toward the new behavior before you feel fully prepared. Take action and find out what follows. Once we have tried a new behavior, we naturally feel more courage and confidence, and we gain concrete experience we could not have visualized through planning.

11. *Loss aversion.* In most circumstances, people naturally feel the pain of loss more acutely than they feel the pleasure of gain. This inclination can make harmful behavior harder to give up. It can also make an individual hesitant to make any change that will be followed by tough choices. The individual fears that new choices will mean losing something that is currently part of his or her life.

    Tip to initiate change. If possible, find a way to reframe your choice. For example, financial advisors suggest that investors who need to sell a stock not dwell on selling. Rather investors should imagine that all of their assets are back in their pocket as cash. They can then start with a clear mind to choose investments that are inherently valuable. Sometimes a change of physical setting can help a person think clearly. Focus on the things, people, and behaviors that you hold most dear in your life. Use implementation intentions to plan how you will change behaviors, little by little, to align with those things you value.

HOEGER KEY TO WELLNESS

 Self-efficacy exerts a powerful influence on people's behaviors and touches virtually every aspect of their lives. Possessing high self-efficacy enhances wellness in countless ways.

Critical Thinking

What barriers to exercise do you encounter most frequently? How about barriers that keep you from managing your daily caloric intake?

2.9 Behavior Change Theories

The first step in addressing behavioral change is to recognize that you indeed have a problem. The five general categories of behaviors addressed in the process of willful change are:

1. Stopping a negative behavior
2. Preventing relapse to a negative behavior
3. Developing a positive behavior
4. Strengthening a positive behavior
5. Maintaining a positive behavior

Psychotherapy has been used successfully to help people change their behavior. But most people do not seek professional help. They usually attempt to change by themselves with limited or no knowledge of how to achieve change.

The simplest model of change is the two-stage model of unhealthy behavior and healthy behavior. This model states that

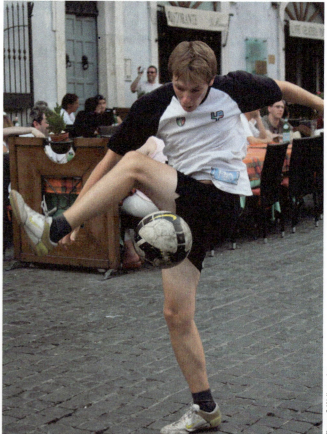

Countering: Substituting healthy behaviors for problem behaviors facilitates change.

either you do it or you don't. Most people who use this model attempt self-change but end up asking themselves why they're unsuccessful. They just can't do it. Their intent to change may be good, but to accomplish it, they need knowledge about how to achieve change. Thus, several theories or models have been developed over the years. Among the most accepted are learning theories, the problem-solving model, social cognitive theory, the relapse prevention model, and the humanistic theory of change. The final theory covered in this chapter, the transtheoretical model of change, has been widely used with much success in helping individuals improve health behaviors and interrupt addictive behavior. The detailed discussion of the transtheoretical model provided later may help you recognize your own readiness for change with a variety of behaviors in your own life.

Learning Theories

Learning theories maintain that most behaviors are learned and maintained under complex schedules of reinforcement and anticipated outcomes. The process involved in learning a new complex behavior requires modifying many smaller, simpler behaviors that shape the new pattern behavior. Reinforcement can be internal or external, positive or negative. External reinforcement can happen to the individual or to someone the individual is observing.

Problem-Solving Model

The **problem-solving model** proposes that many behaviors are the result of making decisions as we seek to solve problems. The decisions are conscious choices and are intended to improve situations we view as problematic. The process of change requires conscious attention, the setting of goals, and a design for a specific plan of action.

Social Cognitive Theory

In **social cognitive theory**,[38] behavior change is influenced by three key factors that also influence one another: the environment, personal factors, and characteristics of the behavior itself. Self-efficacy plays a large role in how the behavior develops.

Relapse Prevention Model

In the **relapse prevention model**, people are taught to anticipate high-risk situations and develop action plans to prevent **lapses** and **relapses**. One way this model is put into practice is through *implementation intentions*, discussed earlier. Examples of factors that disrupt behavior change include negative physiological or psychological states (stress or illness), social pressure, lack of support, limited coping skills, change in work conditions, and lack of motivation.

Humanistic Theory of Change

Humanists believe in the basic goodness of humanity and respect for mankind. At the core of the theory is the belief that people are unique in the development of personal goals—with the ultimate goal being **self-actualization**. Self-actualized people are independent, are creative, set their own goals, and accept themselves. Humanists propose that people are motivated by a hierarchy of needs that begin with basic physical needs like food and sleep, then progress to needs for safety and security, followed by a need for approval and belonging, desires for recognition and achievement, and finally the ultimate desire for self-actualization. In this hierarchy, each need requires fulfillment before the next need becomes relevant. No person will seek recognition and achievements as long as the need for a secure home is not met. Another important belief of this theory is that the present is the most important time for any person, rather than the past or the future. (For example, a person who uses cigarette smoking to maintain weight will not give up smoking unless proper weight management is accomplished by other means like healthy eating habits and increased physical activity. For a full smoking cessation program, see Chapter 13, pages 508–515). The challenge, then, is to identify basic needs at the core of the hierarchy (acceptance, independence, and recognition) before other healthy behaviors (exercise and stress management) are considered.

2.10 The Transtheoretical Model of Change

The **transtheoretical model**, developed by psychologists James Prochaska, John Norcross, and Carlo DiClemente, is based on the theory that change is a gradual process that involves several stages. The model is used most frequently to change

---

GLOSSARY

Learning theories Behavioral modification perspective stating that most behaviors are learned and maintained under complex schedules of reinforcement and anticipated outcomes.

Problem-solving model Behavioral modification model proposing that many behaviors are the result of making decisions as the individual seeks to solve the problem behavior.

Social cognitive theory Behavioral modification model holding that behavior change is influenced by the environment, self-efficacy, and characteristics of the behavior itself.

Relapse prevention model Behavioral modification model based on the principle that high-risk situations can be anticipated through the development of strategies to prevent lapses and relapses.

Lapse (v.) To slip or fall back temporarily into unhealthy behavior(s); (n.) short-term failure to maintain healthy behaviors.

Relapse (v.) To slip or fall back into unhealthy behavior(s) over a longer time; (n.) longer-term failure to maintain healthy behaviors.

Self-actualization The desire that people have to realize their maximum potential and possibilities.

Transtheoretical model Behavioral modification model proposing that change is accomplished through a series of progressive stages in keeping with a person's readiness to change.

Figure 2.3 Stages of change model.

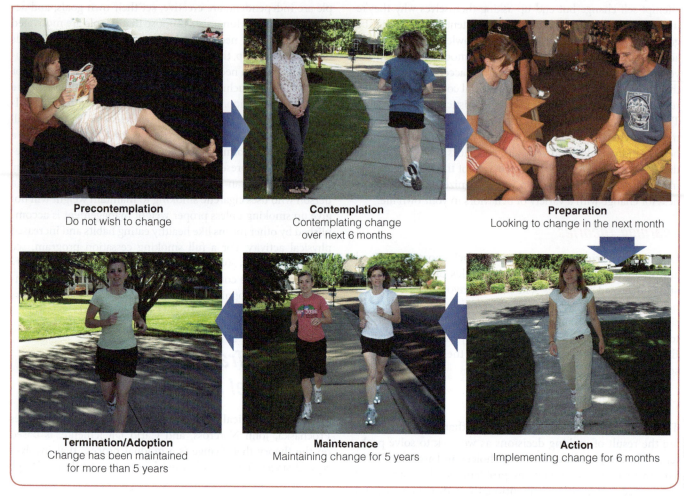

Precontemplation
Do not wish to change

Contemplation
Contemplating change
over next 6 months

Preparation
Looking to change in the next month

Termination/Adoption
Change has been maintained
for more than 5 years

Maintenance
Maintaining change for 5 years

Action
Implementing change for 6 months

© Fitness & Wellness, Inc.

health-related behaviors such as physical inactivity, smoking, poor nutrition, weight problems, stress, and alcohol abuse.

An individual goes through six stages in the process of willful change. The stages describe underlying processes that people go through to change problem behaviors and replace them with healthy behaviors. The six stages of change are precontemplation, contemplation, preparation, action, maintenance, and termination/adoption (see Figure 2.3).

After years of study, researchers indicate that applying specific behavioral-change processes during each stage of the model increases the success rate for change. (The specific processes for each stage are shown in Table 2.1.) Understanding each stage of this model will help you determine where you are in relation to your personal healthy lifestyle behaviors. It also will help you identify processes to make successful changes. The discussion in the remainder of the chapter focuses on the transtheoretical model, with the other models integrated as applicable with each stage of change.

1. *Precontemplation.* Individuals in the **precontemplation stage** are not considering change or do not want to change a given behavior. They typically deny having a problem and have no intention of changing in the immediate future. These people are usually unaware or

underaware of the problem. Other people around them—including family, friends, health care practitioners, and coworkers—however, identify the problem clearly. Precontemplators do not care about the problem behavior and may even avoid information and materials that address the issue. They tend to avoid free screenings and workshops that might help identify and change the problem, even if they receive financial compensation for attending. Often, they actively resist change and seem resigned to accepting the unhealthy behavior as their "fate."

Precontemplators are the most difficult people to inspire toward behavioral change. Many think that change isn't even a possibility. At this stage, knowledge is power. Educating them about the problem behavior is critical to help them start contemplating the process of change. The challenge is to find ways to help them realize that they are ultimately responsible for the consequences of their behavior. Typically, they initiate change only when their values change, their feelings are addressed, or people they respect or job requirements pressure them to do so.

2. *Contemplation.* In the **contemplation stage**, individuals acknowledge that they have a problem and begin to

Table 2.1 Applicable Processes of Change During Each Stage of Change

Precontemplation	Contemplation	Preparation	Action	Maintenance	Termination/Adoption
Consciousness-raising	Consciousness-raising	Consciousness-raising			
Social liberation	Social liberation	Social liberation	Social liberation		
	Self-analysis	Self-analysis			
	Emotional arousal	Emotional arousal			
	Positive outlook	Positive outlook	Positive outlook		
		Commitment	Commitment	Commitment	Commitment
		Behavior analysis	Behavior analysis		
			Mindfulness	Mindfulness	Mindfulness
		Goal setting	Goal setting	Goal setting	
		Self-reevaluation	Self-reevaluation	Self-reevaluation	
			Countering	Countering	
			Monitoring	Monitoring	Monitoring
			Environment control	Environment control	Environment control
			Helping relationships	Helping relationships	Helping relationships
			Rewards	Rewards	Rewards

SOURCE: Adapted from J. O. Prochaska, J. C. Norcross, and C. C. DiClemente, *Changing for Good* (New York: William Morrow, 1994); and W. W. K. Hoeger and S. A. Hoeger, *Principles and Labs for Fitness & Wellness* (Belmont, CA: Wadsworth/Thomson Learning, 2004).

think seriously about overcoming it. Although they are not quite ready for change, they are weighing the pros and cons of changing. Core values are starting to change. Even though they may remain in this stage for years, in their minds they are planning to take some action within the next 6 months. Education and peer support remain valuable during this stage. In Activity 2.2, you will be able to list under the processes of change self-defeating and constructive habits (cons and pros) that work against and for you when attempting to accomplish that specific behavior.

3. *Preparation.* In the **preparation stage**, individuals are seriously considering change and planning to change a behavior within the next month. They are taking initial steps for change and may even try the new behavior for a short while, such as stopping smoking for a day or exercising a few times during the month. During this stage, people define a general goal for behavioral change (e.g., to quit smoking by the last day of the month) and write specific actions (objectives or strategies) to accomplish this goal. It is important to take on goals that are meaningful to you (not to someone else) and that you feel confident you can achieve. To consider whether a goal is right for you, use Figure 2.4: Rate your confidence that you can achieve your goal using a scale of one to ten, with ten being fully confident. Next, rate your motivation on a scale of one to ten, with ten being extremely motivated. If both motivation and confidence rate as a six or higher, the goal is worth pursuing. If not, you are likely still in the contemplation stage for your goal. The discussion on goal setting later in this chapter will help you write SMART goals and specific actions to reach your goal. Continued peer and environmental support is helpful during the preparation stage.

A key concept to keep in mind during the preparation stage is that in addition to being prepared to address the behavioral change or goal you are attempting to reach, you must prepare to address the specific actions (supportive behaviors) required to reach that goal (Figure 2.5). For example, you may be willing to give weight loss a try, but are you prepared to start eating less, eating out less often, eating less calorie-dense foods, shopping and cooking wisely, exercising more, watching television less, and becoming much more active? Achieving goals generally requires changing these supportive behaviors, and you must be prepared to do so.

4. *Action.* The **action stage** requires the greatest commitment of time and energy. Here, the individual is actively doing things to change or modify the problem behavior or to adopt a new, healthy behavior. The action stage requires that the person follow the specific guidelines set forth for that behavior. For example, a person has actually stopped smoking completely, is exercising aerobically three times a week according to exercise prescription guidelines, or is maintaining a healthy diet.

GLOSSARY

Precontemplation stage Stage of change in the transtheoretical model in which an individual is unwilling to change behavior.

Contemplation stage Stage of change in the transtheoretical model in which the individual is considering changing behavior within the next 6 months.

Preparation stage Stage of change in the transtheoretical model in which the individual is getting ready to make a change within the next month.

Action stage Stage of change in the transtheoretical model in which the individual is actively changing a negative behavior or adopting a new, healthy behavior.

Activity 2.2 Behavior Modification Plan

Name _____ Date _____

Course _____ Section _____ Gender _____ Age _____

I. Stages of Change Instructions

Please indicate which response most accurately describes your current _____ and _____ behaviors (in the blank spaces identify the behaviors: smoking, physical activity, stress, nutrition, weight control). Next, select the statement below (select only one) that best represents your current behavior pattern for each. To select the most appropriate statement, fill in the blank for one of the first three statements if your current behavior is a problem behavior. For example, you may say:

"I currently <u>smoke</u>, and I do not intend to change in the foreseeable future" or

"I currently <u>do not exercise</u>, but I am contemplating changing in the next 6 months."

If you have already started to make changes, fill in the blank in one of the last three statements. In this case you may say:

"I currently <u>eat a low-fat diet</u>, but I have only done so within the last 6 months" or

"I currently <u>practice adequate stress management techniques</u>, and I have done so for over 6 months."

You may use this form to identify your stage of change for any health-related behavior. After identifying two problem behaviors, look up your stage of change for each one using Table 2.3 (on page 73).

Behavior #1. Fill in only one blank.

☐ 1. I currently_____, and do not intend to change in the foreseeable future.

☐ 2. I currently_____, but I am contemplating changing in the next 6 months.

☐ 3. I currently_____ regularly, but I intend to change in the next month.

☐ 4. I currently_____, but I have only done so within the last 6 months.

☐ 5. I currently_____, and I have done so for over 6 months.

☐ 6. I currently_____, and I have done so for over 5 years.

Stage of change:_____ (see Table 2.3 on page 73).

Behavior #2. Fill in only one blank.

☐ 1. I currently_____, and do not intend to change in the foreseeable future.

☐ 2. I currently_____, but I am contemplating changing in the next 6 months.

☐ 3. I currently_____ regularly, but I intend to change in the next month.

☐ 4. I currently_____, but I have only done so within the last 6 months.

☐ 5. I currently_____, and I have done so for over 6 months.

☐ 6. I currently_____, and I have done so for over 5 years.

Stage of change: _____ (see Table 2.3 on page 73).

© Fitness & Wellness, Inc.

Activity 2.2 Behavior Modification Plan *(continued)*

II. Processes of Change

According to your stage of change for the two behaviors you have identified, list the processes of change that apply to each behavior (see Table 2.1 on page 65).

Behavior #1: _____

_____

Behavior #2: _____

_____

III. Techniques for Change

List a minimum of three techniques that you will use with each process of change (see Table 2.2 on page 72).

Behavior #1: _____

_____

List:	Self-Destructive Behaviors	Constructive Behaviors
	_____	_____
	_____	_____
	_____	_____
	_____	_____

Behavior #2: _____

_____

List:	Self-Destructive Behaviors	Constructive Behaviors
	_____	_____
	_____	_____
	_____	_____
	_____	_____

Today's date: _____   Completion date: _____   Signature: _____

MINDTAP From Cengage **Complete This Online**
Visit **www.cengagebrain.com** to access MindTap, a complete digital course that includes interactive quizzes, videos, and more.

Figure 2.4 Readiness to change according to confidence and motivation.

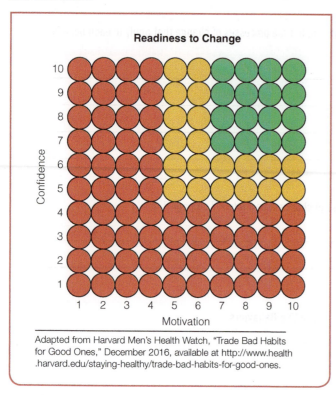

Adapted from Harvard Men's Health Watch, "Trade Bad Habits for Good Ones," December 2016, available at http://www.health .harvard.edu/staying-healthy/trade-bad-habits-for-good-ones.

Figure 2.5 Goal setting and supportive behaviors.

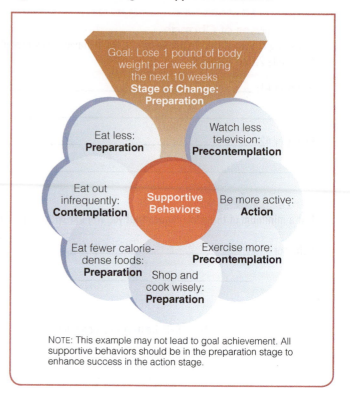

NOTE: This example may not lead to goal achievement. All supportive behaviors should be in the preparation stage to enhance success in the action stage.

Relapse is common during this stage, and the individual may regress to a previous stage. If unsuccessful, a person should reevaluate his or her readiness to change supportive behaviors as required to reach the overall goal. Problem solving that includes identifying barriers to change and specific actions (strategies) to overcome supportive behaviors is useful during relapse. Once people are able to maintain the action stage for 6 consecutive months, they move into the maintenance stage.

5. *Maintenance.* During the **maintenance stage**, the person continues the new behavior for up to 5 years. This stage requires the person to continue to adhere to the specific guidelines that govern the behavior (such as complete smoking cessation, exercising aerobically three times a week, or practicing proper stress management techniques). At this time, the person works to reinforce the gains made through the various stages of change and strives to prevent lapses and relapses.

6. *Termination/adoption.* Once a person has maintained a behavior more than 5 years, he or she is said to be in the **termination or adoption stage** and exits from the cycle of change without fear of relapse. In the case of negative behaviors that are terminated, the stage of change is referred to as termination. If a positive behavior has been adopted successfully for more than 5 years, this stage is designated as adoption.

Many experts believe that once an individual enters the termination/adoption stage, former addictions, problems, or lack of compliance with healthy behaviors no longer present an obstacle in the quest for wellness. The change has become part of one's lifestyle. This phase is the ultimate goal for all people searching for a healthier lifestyle.

HOEGER KEY TO WELLNESS

In the transtheoretical model of change, a person who has maintained a behavior more than 5 years is said to be in the adoption stage and exits from the cycle of change without fear of relapse.

For addictive behaviors such as alcoholism and hard drug use, however, some health care practitioners believe that the individual never enters the termination stage. Chemical dependency is so strong that most former alcoholics and hard-drug users must make a lifetime effort to prevent relapse. Similarly, some behavioral scientists suggest that the adoption stage might not be applicable to health behaviors such as exercise and weight control because the likelihood of relapse is always high.

Use the guidelines provided in Activity 2.2 to determine where you stand in respect to behaviors you want to change or new ones you wish to adopt. As you follow the guidelines, you will realize that you might be at different stages for different behaviors. For instance, you might be in the preparation stage for aerobic exercise and getting regular sleep, in the action stage for strength training, but only in the

Figure 2.6 Model of progression and relapse.

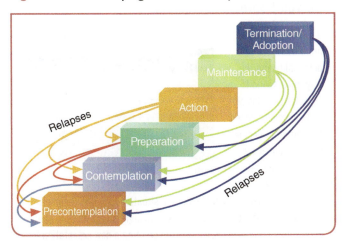

contemplation stage for a healthy diet. Realizing where you are with respect to different behaviors will help you design a better action plan for a healthy lifestyle.

Relapse

After the precontemplation stage, relapse may occur at any level of the model. Even individuals in the maintenance and termination/adoption stages may regress to any of the first three stages of the model (Figure 2.6). Relapse, however, does not mean failure. Failure comes only to those who give up and don't use prior experiences as a building block for future success.

When relapse is viewed as a useful learning experience, the individual should be able to consider the circumstances that led to that relapse and will be better prepared to prevent such in the future. Relapses tend to follow short-term frustrations or underlying difficulties that have been building up to a critical level. A relapse may be a cue that the person should evaluate the stressors they are facing and build the resources and support needed to reach the goal. The chances of moving back up to a higher stage of the model are far better for someone who has previously made it into one of those stages.

2.11 The Process of Change

Using the same plan for everyone who wishes to change a behavior will not work. With exercise, for instance, we provide different prescriptions to people of varying fitness levels Chapter 6). This principle also holds true for individuals who are attempting to change their behaviors.

Timing is important in the process of willful change. People respond more effectively to selected **processes of change** in keeping with the stage of change they have reached at any given time. Thus, applying appropriate processes at each stage of change enhances the likelihood of changing behavior permanently. The following description of 16 of the most common processes of change will help you develop a personal plan for change. The respective stages of change in which each process works best are summarized in Table 2.1.

Consciousness-Raising

The first step in a behavior modification program is consciousness-raising. This step involves obtaining information about the problem so that you can make a better decision about the problem behavior. Possibly, you don't even know that a certain behavior is a problem, such as being unaware of saturated and total fat content in many fast-food items. Consciousness-raising may continue from the precontemplation stage through the preparation stage.

Social Liberation

Social liberation stresses external societal acceptance of and support for positive change. Individuals who receive cues that a new behavior will be accepted and supported in their community will be more likely to succeed at adopting that behavior. Examples of social liberation include pedestrian-only traffic areas, health-oriented cafeterias and restaurants, advocacy groups, civic organizations, policy interventions, and self-help groups.

Self-Analysis

The next process in modifying behavior is developing a decisive desire to do so, called self-analysis. If you have no interest in changing a behavior, you won't do it. You will remain a precontemplator or a contemplator. Take a moment to consider your values. Examine your beliefs and whether they help or hinder you from adopting a healthy lifestyle. Do you value ambition over a healthy lifestyle? Do you admire an artist or celebrity who abuses drugs? Do you value smoking because it has become part of your self-identity and helps you feel like part of your social group? If you have no intention of quitting smoking, you will not quit, regardless of what anyone may say or how strong the evidence in favor of quitting may be. In your self-analysis, you may want to prepare a list of reasons for continuing or discontinuing the behavior. When the reasons for changing outweigh the reasons for not changing, you are ready for the next stage—either the contemplation stage or the preparation stage.

Emotional Arousal

In emotional arousal, a person experiences and expresses feelings about the problem and its solutions. Also referred to as "dramatic release," this process often involves deep emotional experiences. Watching a loved one die from lung cancer caused by cigarette smoking may be all that is needed to make a person quit smoking. As in other examples, emotional arousal might be prompted by a dramatization of the consequences of drug use and abuse, a film about a person

---GLOSSARY---

Maintenance stage Stage of change in the transtheoretical model in which the individual maintains behavioral change for up to 5 years.

Termination/adoption stage Stage of change in the transtheoretical model in which

the individual has eliminated an undesirable behavior or maintained a positive behavior for more than 5 years.

Processes of change Actions that help you achieve change in behavior.

undergoing open-heart surgery, or a book illustrating damage to body systems as a result of unhealthy behaviors.

Positive Outlook

Having a positive outlook means taking an optimistic approach from the beginning and believing in yourself. Behavioral scientists believe that the ability to remain positive is a trait that can be learned.[39] Following the guidelines in this chapter will help you design a plan so that you can work toward change and remain enthused about your progress. Studies of individuals who are trying to quit an addictive behavior have found that asking such persons to reconnect with positive and meaningful goals in their lives greatly improves chances for success. In many cases, goals that will bring the person enjoyment and purpose will be incompatible with the undesired behaviors.

Commitment

Upon making a decision to change, you accept the responsibility to change and believe in your ability to do so. During the commitment process, you engage in preparation and may draw up a specific plan of action. Write down your goals and, preferably, share them with others or announce them! In essence, you are signing a behavioral contract for change. You will be more likely to adhere to your program if others know you are committed to change.

Mindfulness

The simple act of being aware of thoughts and choices is a powerful tool. A person should not feel that having an urge means that they have to act on it. A common technique of mindfulness is referred to as "urge surfing," which directs the person to notice the urge, pay attention to the way the urge feels as it builds, and then simply continue noticing it as the urge subsides.

HOEGER KEY TO WELLNESS

A simple way to keep your values foremost in your mind is to use "implementation intentions." Imagine possible obstacles to your goals, then visualize specifically what you will do to overcome them.

Behavior Analysis

How you determine the frequency, circumstances, and consequences of the behavior to be altered or implemented is known as behavior analysis. If the desired outcome is to consume less trans and saturated fats, you first must find out what foods in your diet are high in these fats, when you eat them, and when you don't eat them—all part of the preparation stage. Knowing when you don't eat them points to circumstances under which you exert control over your diet, which will help as you set goals.

Goals

Goals motivate change in behavior. The stronger the goal or desire, the more motivated you'll be either to change unwanted behaviors or to implement new, healthy behaviors.

Do You Conform or Deviate?

It is important to be mindful of your own personality and the way you respond to expectations. Sociologists have long noted that different people have a tendency to conform or deviate, to fit in or stand out,

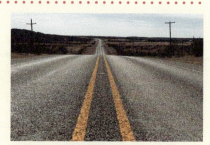

David Dea/Shutterstock.com

according to their personality and the situation they find themselves in. A recent contribution to this body of thought suggests that when people adopt a new behavior, they are creating a new expectation for themselves. Therefore, it is critical for people to understand how they respond to expectations. Some individuals are compelled to follow through with expectations they create for themselves, while others resist expectations they create for themselves. Then, there are those who are compelled to follow through with expectations created for them by others, while some resist expectations created by others. Understanding your own tendencies can help you create the right framework for your own behavioral change.

SOURCE: G. Rubin, *Better Than Before: Mastering the Habits of Our Everyday Lives* (New York: Crown Publishers, 2015).

The discussion on goal setting (beginning on page 73) will help you write goals and prepare an action plan to achieve them. This will aid with behavior modification.

Self-Reevaluation

During the process of self-reevaluation, individuals analyze their feelings about a problem behavior. The pros and cons or advantages and disadvantages of a certain behavior can be reevaluated at this time. For example, you may decide that strength training will help you get stronger and tone up, but implementing this change will require you to wake up earlier three times per week. If you remember a time when you enjoyed feeling fit and capable of meeting daily physical demands with ease, you may feel good about weight loss and enhanced physical capacity as a result of a strength-training program.

Countering

The process whereby you substitute healthy behaviors for a problem behavior, known as countering, is a critical part of the action and maintenance stages of changing behaviors. You need to replace unhealthy behaviors with new, healthy ones. You can use exercise to combat sedentary living, smoking, stress, or overeating. Or you may use exercise, yard work, volunteer work, or reading to prevent overeating and achieve recommended body weight.

Monitoring

During the action and maintenance stages, continuous behavior monitoring increases awareness of the desired outcome.

Sometimes, this process of monitoring is sufficient in itself to cause change. For example, keeping track of daily food intake reveals sources of excessive fat in the diet. This can help you gradually cut down or completely eliminate high-fat foods. If the goal is to increase daily intake of fruits and vegetables, keeping track of the number of servings consumed each day raises awareness and may help increase intake.

Environment Control

In environment control, the person restructures the physical surroundings to avoid problem behaviors and decrease temptations. If you bring baby carrots and nuts to work instead of chips, you are likely to snack better. If you put your favorite workout gear neatly folded at eye level in your closet, you may associate more pleasant feelings with getting ready to exercise.

Similarly, you can create an environment in which exceptions become the norm, and then the norm can flourish. You may leave yourself reminders or prompts that you are likely to see as you are making healthy choices. Such reminders, also referred to as "point-of-decision-prompts," have been used successfully on a public level. For example, reminders on soda machines that "calories count" encourage consumers to look at the calories listed by each soda selection prior to making a choice. Put sugarless gum where you used to put cigarettes. Snap a photo of the schedule for your favorite gym class and set it as the home screen on your phone. Put an electric timer on your computer so it will shut off automatically at 8:00 p.m. All of these tactics will be helpful throughout the action, maintenance, and termination/adoption stages.

Helping Relationships

Surround yourself with people who will work toward a common goal with you or those who care about you and will encourage you along the way. "Helping relationships" will be supportive during the action, maintenance, and termination/adoption stages.

Attempting to quit smoking, for instance, is easier when a person is around others who have already quit or are trying to quit as well. One particular research study examined a social network of 12,000 people to understand the smoking habits of individuals who personally knew someone who had quit. They found that knowing someone who had quit smoking boosted an individual's likelihood to quit or avoid starting in the first place. People were 67 percent less likely to be a smoker than the national average if the person who had quit was their spouse, 36 percent if it was a friend, and 25 percent if it was a sibling.[40] Researchers found that, consistently, it was the closeness of the relationship, and not geographical closeness, that made the difference in health behaviors.

Losing weight is difficult if meal planning and cooking are shared with roommates who enjoy foods that are high in fat and sugar. Peer support is a strong incentive for behavioral change. Thus, the individual should avoid people who will not be supportive and associate with those who will.

In some cases, people who have achieved the same goal already may not be supportive either. For instance, someone may say, "I can do 6 consecutive miles." Your response should be, "I'm proud that I can jog 3 consecutive miles."

Rewards

People tend to repeat behaviors that are rewarded and to disregard those that are not rewarded or are punished. Rewarding oneself or being rewarded by others is a powerful tool during the process of change in all stages. If you have successfully cut down your caloric intake during the week, reward yourself by going to a movie or buying a new pair of shoes. Do not reinforce yourself with destructive behaviors such as eating a calorie-dense dinner. If you fail to change a desired behavior (or to implement a new one), you may want to put off buying those new shoes you had planned for that week. When a positive behavior becomes habitual, give yourself an even better reward. Treat yourself to a weekend away from home or buy a new bicycle.

Behavior Modification Planning

Steps for Successful Behavior Modification

1. Acknowledge that you have a problem.
2. Describe the behavior to change (increase physical activity, stop overeating, quit smoking).
3. List advantages and disadvantages of changing the specified behavior.
4. Decide positively that you will change.
5. Identify your stage of change.
6. Set a realistic goal (SMART goal) and completion date, and sign a behavioral contract.
7. Define your behavioral change plan: List processes of change, techniques of change, and actions that will help you reach your goal.
8. Implement the behavior change plan.
9. Monitor your progress toward the desired goal.
10. Periodically evaluate and reassess your goal.
11. Reward yourself when you achieve your goal.
12. Maintain the successful change for good.

Try It

In your online journal or class notebook, record your answers to the following questions: Have you consciously attempted to incorporate a healthy behavior into or eliminate a negative behavior from your lifestyle? If so, what steps did you follow, and what helped you achieve your goal?

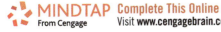

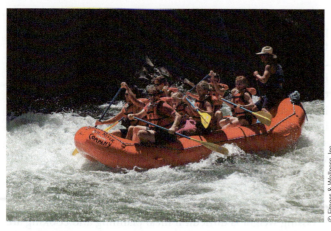

Rewarding oneself when a goal is achieved, such as scheduling a weekend getaway, is a powerful tool during the process of change.

© Fitness & Wellness, Inc.

> ### Critical Thinking
>
> Your friend John is a 20-year-old student who is not physically active. Exercise has never been a part of his life, and it has not been a priority in his family. He has decided to start a jogging and strength-training course in 2 weeks. Can you identify his current stage of change and list processes and techniques of change that will help him maintain a regular exercise behavior?

Techniques of Change

Not to be confused with the processes of change, you can apply any number of **techniques of change** within each process to help you through it (Table 2.2). A technique is simply the specific action you take in your own life to apply a process of change. For example, following dinner, some

Table 2.2 Sample Techniques for Use with Process of Change

Process	Techniques
Consciousness-Raising	Become aware that there is a problem, read educational materials about the problem behavior or about people who have overcome this same problem, find out about the benefits of changing the behavior, watch an instructional program on television, visit a therapist, talk and listen to others, ask questions, or take a class.
Social Liberation	Seek out advocacy groups (Overeaters Anonymous, Alcoholics Anonymous), join a health club, buy a bike, join a neighborhood walking group, and work in nonsmoking areas.
Self-Analysis	Question yourself on the problem behavior, express your feelings about it, become aware that there is a problem, analyze your values, list advantages and disadvantages of continuing (smoking) or not implementing a behavior (exercise), take a fitness test, or do a nutrient analysis.
Emotional Arousal	Practice mental imagery of yourself going through the process of change, visualize yourself overcoming the problem behavior, do some role-playing in overcoming the behavior or practicing a new one, watch dramatizations (a movie) of the consequences or benefits of your actions, or visit an auto salvage yard or a drug rehabilitation center.
Positive Outlook	Believe in yourself, know that you are capable, know that you are special, and draw from previous personal successes.
Commitment	Just do it, set New Year's resolutions, sign a behavioral contract, set start and completion dates, tell others about your goals, and work on your action plan.
Behavior Analysis	Prepare logs of circumstances that trigger or prevent a given behavior and look for patterns that prompt the behavior or cause you to relapse.
Goal Setting	Write goals and actions; design a specific action plan.
Self-Reevaluation	Determine accomplishments and evaluate progress, rewrite goals and actions, list pros and cons, weigh sacrifices (can't eat out with others) versus benefits (weight loss), visualize continued change, think before you act, learn from mistakes, and prepare new action plans accordingly.
Countering	Seek out alternatives: stay busy, walk (don't drive), read a book (instead of snacking), attend alcohol-free social events, carry your own groceries, mow your yard, dance (don't eat), go to a movie (instead of smoking), and practice stress management.
Monitoring	Use exercise logs (days exercised, sets and resistance used in strength training), keep journals, conduct nutrient analyses, count grams of fat, count number of consecutive days without smoking, list days and type of relaxation technique(s) used.
Environment Control	Rearrange your home (no TVs, ashtrays, or large-sized cups), get rid of unhealthy items (cigarettes, junk food, and alcohol), then avoid unhealthy places (bars and happy hour), avoid relationships that encourage problem behaviors, use reminders to control problem behaviors or encourage positive ones (post notes indicating "don't snack after dinner" or "lift weights at 8:00 p.m."). Frequent healthy environments (a clean park, a health club, restaurants with low-fat/low-calorie/nutrient-dense menus, and friends with goals similar to yours).
Helping Relationships	Associate with people who have and want to overcome the same problem, form or join self-help groups, or join community programs specifically designed to deal with your problem.
Rewards	Go to a movie, buy a new outfit or shoes, buy a new bike, go on a weekend getaway, reassess your fitness level, use positive self-talk ("Good job," "That felt good," "I did it," "I knew I'd make it," or "I'm good at this").

Figure 2.7 **Stage of change and behavior modification outline.**

Complete Activity 2.2 to identify your stage of change for two behaviors.
In addition, use this form as a future reference to identify your stage of change for any other behaviors you may like to address.

Please indicate which response most accurately describes your current [ ] behavior. (In the blank space identify the behavior: smoking, physical activity, stress, nutrition, weight control.) Next, select the statement below (select only one) that best represents your current behavior pattern. To select the most appropriate statement, fill in the blank for one of the first three statements if your current behavior is a problem behavior. (For example, you may say, "I currently smoke, and I do *not* intend to change in the foresee- able future," or "I currently *do not exercise,* but I am contemplating changing in the next 6 months.") If you have already started to make changes, fill in the blank in one of the last three statements. (In this case, you may say: "I currently *eat a low-fat diet,* but I have done so only within the past 6 months," or "I currently *practice adequate stress management techniques,* and I have done so for more than 6 months.") As you can see, you may use this form to identify your stage of change for any type of health-related behavior.

1. I currently [ ] , and I do not intend to change in the foreseeable future.

2. I currently [ ] , but I am contemplating changing in the next 6 months.

3. I currently [ ] regularly, but I intend to change in the next month.

4. I currently [ ] , but I have done so only within the past 6 months.

5. I currently [ ] , and I have done so for more than 6 months.

6. I currently [ ] , and I have done so for more than 5 years.

people find it difficult to resist continuous snacking during the rest of the evening until it is time to retire for the night. In the process of countering, for example, an individual can use various techniques to avoid unnecessary snacking. Examples include going for a walk, working on a project, flossing and brushing your teeth immediately after dinner, calling a friend, going out, or going to bed earlier.

As you develop a behavior modification plan, you need to identify specific techniques that may work for you within each process of change. A list of techniques for each process is pro- vided in Table 2.2. This is only a sample list; dozens of other techniques could be used as well. Some of these techniques also can be used with more than one process. Visualization, for example, is helpful in emotional arousal and self-reevaluation.

Now that you are familiar with the stages of change in the process of behavior modification, use Figure 2.7 and Activity 2.2 to identify two problem behaviors in your life. In this activity, you will be asked to determine your stage of change for two behaviors according to six standard statements. Based on your selection, determine the stage of change classification according

to the ratings provided in Table 2.3. Next, develop a behavior modification plan according to the processes and techniques for change that you have learned in this chapter. (Similar exercises to identify stages of change for other fitness and wellness behav- iors are provided in activities for subsequent chapters.)

2.12 *Goal Setting and Evaluation*

To initiate change, **goals** are essential, as goals motivate be- havioral change. Whatever you decide to accomplish, setting goals will provide the road map to help make your dreams a reality. Setting goals, however, is not as simple as it looks. Set- ting goals is more than just deciding what you want to do. A vague statement such as "I will lose weight" is not sufficient to help you achieve this goal.

SMART Goals

Only a well-conceived action plan will help you attain goals. Determining what you want to accomplish is the starting point, but to reach your goal you need to write **SMART goals** (Figure 2.8). These goals are Specific, Measurable, Acceptable, Realistic, and Time specific. In Activity 2.3, you have an

Table 2.3 **Stage of Change Classification**

Selected Statements (see Figure 2.6 and Activity 2.2)	Classification
1	Precontemplation
2	Contemplation
3	Preparation
4	Action
5	Maintenance
6	Termination/Adoption

GLOSSARY

Techniques of change Methods or procedures used during each process of change.

Goals The ultimate aims toward which effort is directed.

SMART (goals) An acronym used in reference to specific, measurable, attainable, realistic, and time-specific goals.

Figure 2.8 SMART goals.

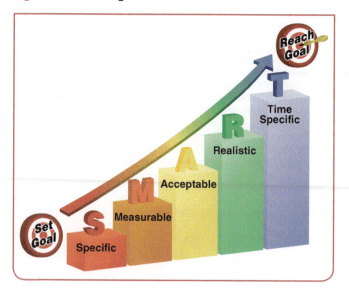

© Fitness & Wellness, Inc.

Avoiding an All-or-Nothing Approach

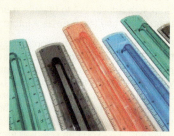

Take the time to evaluate your expectations before setting a goal. What will you expect from yourself? What will you expect from others? The key to setting realistic goals is having healthy, reasonable expectations for yourself, the people in your social circles, and your community. It is important to recognize that life can be a juggling act, and that realistically, you cannot control the outcome of every day. Avoid an all-or-nothing approach to your goals. Expect to be less than perfect and plan to get back on track as soon as you see that you have veered from your goal. Mistakes are learning opportunities and are part of practicing a new behavior.

opportunity to set SMART goals for one behavior (or more) that you wish to change or adopt.

1. *Specific.* When writing goals, state exactly and in a positive manner what you would like to accomplish. For example, if you are overweight at 150 pounds and at 27 percent body fat, to simply state, "I will lose weight" is not a specific goal. Instead, rewrite your goal to state, "I will reduce my body fat to 20 percent (137 pounds) in 12 weeks." This strategy was confirmed by the National Weight Control Registry upon studying people who successfully lost weight and maintained weight loss. These individuals were found to have highly specific goals; they envisioned themselves obtaining a specific percent body fat or fitting into a certain piece of clothing.

   Write down your goals. An unwritten goal is simply a wish. A written goal, in essence, becomes a contract with yourself. Show this goal to a friend or an instructor, and have him or her witness the contract you have made with yourself by signing alongside your signature.

   Once you have identified and written down a specific goal, write the specific **actions** that will help you reach that goal. These actions are necessary steps. For example, a goal might be to achieve recommended body weight. Several specific actions could be to:

   a. Lose an average of 1 pound (or 1 fat percentage point) per week.
   b. Monitor body weight before breakfast every morning.
   c. Assess body composition at 3-week intervals.
   d. Limit fat intake to less than 25 percent of total daily caloric intake.
   e. Eliminate all pastries from the diet during this time.
   f. Walk/jog in the proper target zone for 60 minutes, six times a week.

2. *Measurable.* Whenever possible, goals and actions should be measurable. For example, "I will lose weight" is not measurable, but "to reduce body fat to 20 percent" is measurable. Also note that all of the sample-specific actions (a) through (f) for "Specific" in the previous point are measurable. For instance, you can figure out easily whether you are losing a pound or a percentage point per week; you can conduct a nutrient analysis to assess your average fat intake; or you can monitor your weekly exercise sessions to make sure you are meeting this specific objective.

3. *Acceptable.* Goals that you set for yourself are more motivational than goals that someone else sets for you. These goals will motivate and challenge you and should be consistent with your other goals. As you set an acceptable goal, ask yourself: Do I have the time, commitment, and necessary skills to accomplish this goal? If not, you need to restate your goal so that it is acceptable to you.

   When successful completion of a goal involves others, such as an athletic team or an organization, an acceptable goal must be compatible with those of the other people involved. If a team's practice schedule is set Monday through Friday from 4:00 to 6:00 p.m., it is unacceptable for you to train only three times per week or at a different time of the day.

   Acceptable goals also embrace positive thoughts. Visualize and believe in your success. As difficult as some tasks may seem, where there's a will, there's a way. A plan of action, prepared according to the guidelines in this chapter, will help you achieve your goals.

GLOSSARY

Actions Steps required to reach a goal.

Activity 2.3   **Setting SMART Goals***

Name _____ Date _____

Course _____ Section _____ Gender _____ Age _____

In Activity 2.2, you identified two behaviors that you wish to change. Using SMART goal guidelines, write goals and actions that will provide a road map for behavioral change. In the spaces provided in this lab, indicate how your stated goals meet each one of the SMART goal guidelines.

I. SMART Goals

Goal 1:

_____

_____

Indicate what makes your goal specific.

_____

How is your goal measurable?

_____

_____

Why is this an acceptable goal?

_____

_____

State why you consider this goal realistic.

_____

_____

How is this goal time-specific?

_____

_____

II. Specific Actions
Write a minimum of five specific actions that will help you reach your two SMART goals.

Goal 1: _____

Actions:

1. _____

2. _____

3. _____

4. _____

5. _____

*Make additional copies of this form as needed.

© Fitness & Wellness, Inc.

4. *Realistic.* Goals should be within reach. On the one hand, if you currently weigh 190 pounds and your target weight is 140 pounds, setting a goal to lose 50 pounds in a month would be unsound, if not impossible. Such a goal does not allow you to implement adequate behavior modification techniques or ensure weight maintenance at the target weight. Unattainable goals only set you up for failure, discouragement, and loss of interest. On the other hand, do not write goals that are too easy to achieve and do not challenge you. If a goal is too easy, you may lose interest and stop working toward it.

You can write both short-term and long-term goals. If the long-term goal is to attain recommended body weight and you are 53 pounds overweight, you might set a short-term goal of losing 10 pounds and write specific actions to accomplish this goal. Then the immediate task will not seem as overwhelming and will be easier.

At times, problems arise even with realistic goals. Try to anticipate potential difficulties as much as possible, and plan for ways to deal with them. If your goal is to jog for 30 minutes on 6 consecutive days, what are the alternatives if the weather turns bad? Possible solutions are to jog in the rain, find an indoor track, jog at a different time of day when the weather is better, or participate in a different aerobic activity such as stationary cycling, swimming, Zumba, or step aerobics.

Monitoring your progress as you move toward a goal also reinforces behavior. Keeping an exercise log or doing a body composition assessment periodically enables you to determine your progress at any given time.

5. *Time specific.* A goal should always have a specific date set for completion. The earlier example to reach 20 percent body fat in 12 weeks is time specific. The chosen date should be realistic but not too distant in the future. Allow yourself enough time to achieve the goal, but not too much time, as this could affect your performance. With a deadline, a task is much easier to work toward.

HOEGER KEY TO WELLNESS

Whenever possible, goals and actions should be measurable. Monitoring your progress as you move toward a goal reinforces behavior.

Goal Evaluation

In addition to the SMART guidelines provided, you should conduct periodic evaluations of your goals. Reevaluations are vital to success. You may find that after you have fully committed and put all your effort into a goal, that goal may be unreachable. If so, reassess the goal.

Recognize that you will face obstacles and you will not always meet your goals. Use your setbacks and learn from them. Rewrite your goal and create a plan that will help you get around self-defeating behaviors in the future. Once you achieve a goal, set a new one to improve on or maintain what you have achieved. Goals keep you motivated.

Assess Your Behavior

1. What are your feelings about the science of behavior modification and how its principles may help you on your journey to health and wellness?

2. Can you accept the fact that for various healthy lifestyle factors (e.g., regular exercise, healthy eating, not smoking, stress management, and prevention of sexually transmitted infections), you are either in the precontemplation or contemplation stage of change? As such, are you willing to learn what is required to change and actually eliminate unhealthy behaviors and adopt healthy lifestyle behaviors?

3. Are you now in the action phase (or a later phase) for exercise and healthy eating? If not, what barriers keep you from being so?

Assess Your Knowledge

1. Most of the behaviors that people adopt in life are
   a. a product of their environment.
   b. learned early in childhood.
   c. learned from parents.
   d. genetically determined.
   e. the result of peer pressure.

2. Instant gratification is
   a. a barrier to change.
   b. a factor that motivates change.
   c. one of the six stages of change.
   d. the end result of successful change.
   e. a technique in the process of change.

3. The desire and will to do something are referred to as
   a. invincibility.
   b. confidence.
   c. competence.
   d. external locus of control.
   e. motivation.

4. People who believe they have control over events in their lives
   a. tend to rationalize their negative actions.
   b. exhibit problems of competence.
   c. often feel helpless over illness and disease.
   d. have an internal locus of control.
   e. often engage in risky lifestyle behaviors.

5. Habits are most likely to be repeated
   a. during times of stress.
   b. when an individual is tired.
   c. in familiar environments.
   d. after an action has been repeatedly rewarded.
   e. All of the above.

6. Which of the following is a stage of change in the transtheoretical model?
   a. Recognition
   b. Motivation
   c. Relapse
   d. Preparation
   e. Goal setting

7. A precontemplator is a person who
   a. has no desire to change a behavior.
   b. is looking to make a change in the next 6 months.
   c. is preparing for change in the next 30 days.
   d. willingly adopts healthy behaviors.
   e. is talking to a therapist to overcome a problem behavior.

8. An individual who is trying to stop smoking and has not smoked for 3 months is in the
   a. maintenance stage.
   b. action stage.
   c. termination stage.
   d. adoption stage.
   e. evaluation stage.

9. The process of change in which an individual obtains information to make a better decision about a problem behavior is known as
   a. behavior analysis.
   b. self-reevaluation.
   c. commitment.
   d. positive outlook.
   e. consciousness-raising.

10. A goal is effective when it is
    a. specific.
    b. measurable.
    c. realistic.
    d. time specific.
    e. All of the above.

Correct answers can be found at the back of the book.

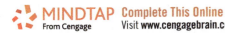

MINDTAP **Complete This Online**
From Cengage   Visit **www.cengagebrain.com** to access MindTap, a complete digital course that includes interactive quizzes, videos, and more.

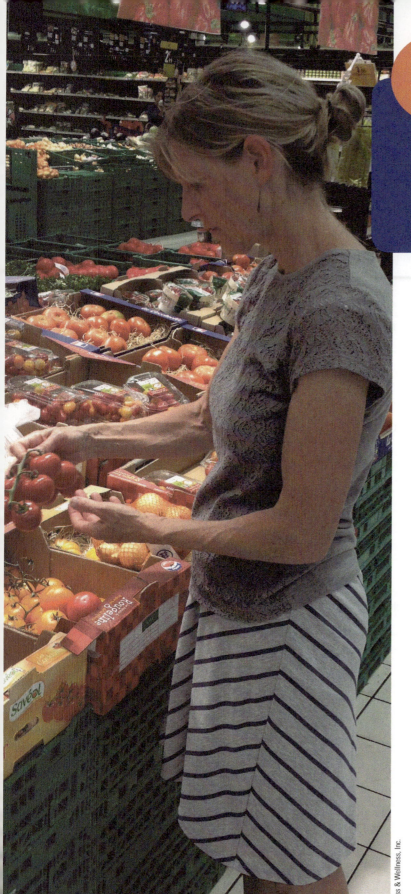

3

Nutrition for Wellness

"Eat to live, don't live to eat."
—Benjamin Franklin

Objectives

3.1 **Define** nutrition and describe its relationship to health and well-being.

3.2 **Learn** to use the U.S. Department of Agriculture MyPlate guidelines for healthier eating.

3.3 **Describe** the functions of the nutrients—carbohydrates, fiber, fats, proteins, vitamins, minerals, and water—in the human body.

3.4 **Conduct** a comprehensive nutrient analysis and implement changes to meet the Dietary Reference Intakes (DRIs).

3.5 **Learn** to balance your diet and achieve a healthy dietary pattern.

3.6 **Identify** myths and fallacies regarding nutrition.

3.7 **Become aware** of guidelines for nutrient supplementation.

3.8 **Learn** the key substrates (energy fuels) for physical activity and dietary recommendations for aerobic and strength-training exercise.

3.9 **Define** osteoporosis and learn recommended guidelines to prevent the disease.

3.10 **Learn** the *2015-2020 Dietary Guidelines for Americans.*

© Fitness & Wellness, Inc.

FAQ

Do I have to follow a diet 24/7 to derive health benefits?

A sound diet is vital for good health and wellness. An extreme approach, however, is not the best advice when it comes to proper nutrition. Health experts believe that such an approach may lead to "orthorexia nervosa," a new category of eating disorder characterized by an unhealthy compulsion over food choices. Moderation and common sense in all things is solid advice when it comes to healthy diet and nutrition. Healthy eating patterns that can be maintained for a lifetime include small and occasional treats.

How much should I worry about sugar in my diet?

Traditionally, the most significant health concerns regarding excessive sugar intake included increased caloric intake, weight gain, obesity, tooth decay, and lower nutrient intake ("empty" or "discretionary" calories with no nutritional benefit whatsoever). In particular, recent studies have determined regular soda consumption is counterproductive to good health.

Data indicate that people who consume 25 percent or more of daily calories from sugar are almost three times more likely to die from cardiovascular disease than those who consume the least. Consumption of two sugar-sweetened beverages per day increases coronary heart disease risk by 35 percent and stroke risk by 20 percent. Excessive added sugar (any sugar removed from its natural product and added to another food) in the diet also raises cholesterol and triglycerides (which clog up the arteries) and increases the risk for pancreatic cancer. Regular soft drink consumers have about an 80 percent greater risk for developing type 2 diabetes. Other data indicate that sugar overconsumption leads to liver cirrhosis and dementia, and individuals who

drink more than five sugary soft drinks per week have reduced bone density in the hips and more than double joint-cushioning cartilage loss in the knees as compared to those who limit daily sugar intake. Excessive consumption of sugary beverages has been linked to more than 180,000 yearly obesity-related deaths worldwide.

The hardest dietary habit for post-heart attack victims to change is drinking sugary drinks, with soft drink consumption being the most difficult habit to kick. In an article published in the *American Journal of Public Health*, scientists established that regardless of weight gain, drinking an 8-ounce daily serving of soda is linked to 1.9 years of additional biological aging and drinking 20 ounces of soda daily is associated with 4.6 years of additional aging.

You do not have to eliminate all sugar from your diet. Data indicate that the typical American consumes about 16 percent of their daily calories from added sugar, or about 350 "empty" calories, the equivalent of 22 teaspoons per day. Most people simply cannot afford all those extra daily empty calories, and the sweet treats often displace more nutritious choices on the plate. People should strive for a "nutrient-rich" diet—that is, a high nutrient-to-calorie ratio. The American Heart Association recommends no more than 6 (100 calories) and 9 (150 calories) daily teaspoons of added sugar for women and men, respectively. And the *2015-2020 Dietary Guidelines* recommend limiting added sugar to 10 percent or less of total daily calories.

Data also indicate that liquid calories (soft drinks) do not result in less food consumption during a meal. Liquid calories are not recognized by the

body as are solid food calories and do little to suppress the body's hunger-stimulating hormone ghrelin; thus, they most often lead to greater caloric consumption per meal. Adults who drink one or more sodas per day are 27 percent more likely to be overweight or obese. Not taking into account the greater caloric intake with meals, even just the one can (12 oz) of soda per day can add 16.5 pounds of body weight per year (160 calories per can × 365 days ÷ 3,500—the equivalent of 1 pound of fat). Thus, for good health and proper weight management, steer clear of liquid calories and hydrate with plain water instead.

Unfortunately, at present, food labels still do not differentiate between natural and added sugars, making it difficult to determine the quantity added to foods and drinks. New food labels requiring added sugar information are not required by the FDA until July 2018; and for smaller manufacturers, not until July 2019. Natural sugars in food (fructose and lactose) are acceptable because these foods contain many other healthful substances. Among others, added sugars listed on food labels include ordinary table sugar (sucrose), raw sugar, cane sugar, brown sugar, invert sugar, high-fructose corn syrup (HFCS), corn syrup, corn sweetener, glucose, dextrose, fructose, lactose, maltose, maltodextrin, molasses, honey, agave syrup, maple syrup, malt syrup, fruit juice concentrate, and sorghum.

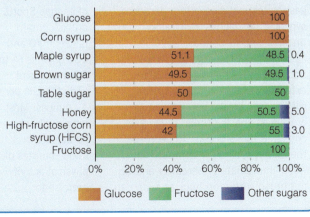

You can estimate the number of teaspoons of sugar in processed food by dividing the total grams of sugar on the label by 4.

Almost half (47 percent) of all the added sugar in our diet comes from beverages. They are the most significant source of added sugars in the American diet. The American Diabetes Association indicates that soft drinks and sweetened drinks are the biggest source of added sugar in the diet, accounting for 38 percent of all added sugar intake. (Each 12-ounce can of soft drink contains about 10 teaspoons of sugar.) Soda consumption in the United States has increased by 500 percent over the past 50 years. The soda industry generates about 47 gallons of soft drink for each American. Other drinks loaded with added sugar include fruit drinks, iced teas, sports drinks, and energy drinks. Plain sugar, candy, and sugar-sweetened baked products account for another 31 percent of the added sugar intake.

Currently, energy drinks are a major health concern in the United States. Besides added sugar or artificial sweeteners, caffeine, and flavorings, they also contain other ingredients like vitamins, ginkgo biloba, and taurine. The caffeine content in these drinks can be five times (250 to 500 mg) what's in a cup of coffee (40 to 90 mg). Several deaths have been attributed to these energy drinks, most likely due to an irregular heartbeat caused by the excess caffeine. Some of the most detrimental health effects of overconsumption of energy drinks include tachycardia (rapid heart rate), chest pain, higher blood pressure, tremors, restlessness, gastrointestinal discomfort, dizziness, syncope, headaches, respiratory distress, and insomnia.

Because of the high acid content, both sports and energy drinks are extremely erosive to tooth enamel, with energy drinks being twice as erosive as sports drinks. If you ever consume these drinks, to decrease the damage, rinse your mouth with water immediately thereafter and do not brush within an hour as such can actually exacerbate the damage on the enamel caused by the acids. The same can be said about soft drinks, but to a lesser damaging extent.

Many researchers have expressed particular concern over HFCS, a liquid sweetener made from cornstarch but greatly enhanced with fructose. HFCS is used in many products, including soft drinks, candies, baked goods, and breakfast cereals. HFCS is thought to be a major contributor to obesity, cardiovascular disease, diabetes, and possibly high blood pressure, liver and kidney disease, and systemic inflammation.

The sugar in HFCS stimulates the brain's reward system by activating the neurotransmitter dopamine, also known as the "craving" hormone. The theory is that consuming HFCS makes you crave even more food and feel hungrier longer.

The advisory committee that developed the *2015–2020 Dietary Guidelines for Americans* also does not recommend the use of sugar substitutes in place of sugar for weight management purposes because long-term effects of their use are still unknown. Furthermore, data indicate that individuals who consume an average of two diet sodas per day actually gain more weight than people who do not consume diet drinks.

Only athletes who participate in vigorous-intensity exercise for longer than 60 minutes at a time benefit from sports drinks as an additional source of energy. Sports drinks contain between 70 and 100 calories (4 to 6 teaspoons of added sugar) per 12 ounces. Most individuals who participate in 30 to 60 minutes of physical activity/ exercise for

health/fitness purposes do not need and will not benefit from sports drinks. For proper weight management and healthy living, moderation is a sound principle regarding added sugar consumption.

What is the difference between antioxidants and phytonutrients?

Antioxidants, comprising vitamins, minerals, and phytonutrients, help prevent damage to cells from highly reactive and unstable molecules known as oxygen free radicals (see page 118). Antioxidants are found both in plant and animal foods, whereas phytonutrients (also known as phytochemicals) are found in plant foods only, including fruits, vegetables, beans, nuts, and seeds. Thousands of these bioactive compounds found in plants offer an array of health benefits ranging from cardiovascular disease and cancer prevention to vision health.

The actions of phytonutrients go beyond those of most antioxidants. In particular, they appear to have powerful anti-cancer properties. For example, at almost every stage of cancer, phytonutrients can block, disrupt, slow, or even reverse the process. In terms of heart disease, they may reduce inflammation, inhibit blood clots, or prevent the oxidation of low-density lipoprotein cholesterol. People should consume ample amounts of plant-based foods to obtain a healthy

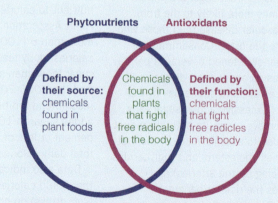

The difference between phytonutrients and antioxidants.

(continued)

supply of antioxidants, including a wide array of phytonutrients.

What is chronic inflammation, and does it relate to diet and nutrition?

Normal body inflammation that develops suddenly is a protective response to injury, infection, or the presence of inflammatory stimulants. Typically it lasts a few days or weeks to help kill or encapsulate microbes, form protective scar tissue, and regenerate damaged tissue. Sudden or acute inflammation as a result of a cold, fever, sprain, strain, bruise, or cut is beneficial because it shows that the immune system is working to respond to invading bacteria and viruses or to repair bodily damage.

Chronic or low-grade inflammation, however, is a persistent condition with tissue destruction and repair taking place at the same time and can last years or decades before damage is apparent. It occurs as a result of the continuous presence of pro-inflammatory stimulants and the body's inability to provide sufficient anti-inflammatory compounds. Chronic inflammation is primarily related to unhealthy lifestyle choices. Most people are unaware of its existence until age-related chronic disease occurs. It is triggered by eating an unhealthy diet, being physically inactive and obese, not getting enough sleep, smoking, drinking too much alcohol, or having an internal injury or infection that produces no outward signs or symptoms.

Chronic inflammation may be the cause of most of the feared chronic diseases of middle and older age. It is a major risk factor in the development of arthritis, metabolic syndrome, heart disease, stroke, diabetes, cancer, chronic obstructive pulmonary disease, Alzheimer's, autoimmune disease, neurological diseases, and asthma. Furthermore, inflammation in one area of the body may not only cause damage in that part of the body but can also cause damage elsewhere. For example, heartburn (gastroesophageal reflux disease or GERD) can lead to esophageal cancer, and gingivitis (inflamed gums) can lead to heart disease, stroke, and diabetes (damage done elsewhere).

Chronic inflammation is definitely related to faulty nutrition. In general, trans fatty acids and partially hydrogenated oils, fried and charred food (high in advanced glycation end products or AGEs—see page 114), sugars and refined grains, and highly processed foods lead to inflammation. Individual food sensitivities can also trigger immune reactions and inflammation. Foods that appear to combat inflammation include omega-3 fatty acids, antioxidant-rich foods, low-glycemic foods, probiotic foods, and spices and herbs (including turmeric, sage, rosemary, thyme, cinnamon, cayenne pepper, clove, ginger, nutmeg, and oregano). Additional information on nutrition and inflammation is provided throughout this chapter.

Should I be concerned about antibiotics in meat?

The use of antibiotics in animals in the United States is a common practice to increase animal growth and prevent chronic livestock illness in overcrowded farms with unsanitary living conditions. Most mass-produced meat in the United States has been injected with antibiotics and hormones. The concern is that overuse may lead to antibiotic resistance in humans, a condition responsible for about 2 million illnesses and 23,000 deaths in the United States each year. The World Health Organization (WHO), the American Medical Association, and the National Resources Defense Council consider nontherapeutic antibiotic use in livestock as a significant public health risk. As a consumer, you are encouraged to minimize the use of meats anyway, for overall health reasons (see page 95), and when you do use meats, search for products from companies that certify antibiotic use in animals for therapeutic purposes only. Imports of United States meats are banned by the European Union, Canada, Japan, Australia, Russia, and Taiwan.

What is gluten sensitivity?

Gluten sensitivity falls under an umbrella of adverse effects on the body caused by gluten, a protein found in wheat, barley, rye, malts, and triticale. Gluten is also used as an additive for flavoring and stabilizing food or as a thickening agent.

About 1 percent of Americans suffer from celiac disease, an autoimmune disorder in genetically predisposed people of all ages that damages the lining of the small intestine and the ability to absorb nutrients. The disease is caused by a reaction to gluten, leading to an inflammatory reaction that induces a series of symptoms, including vomiting, severe abdominal pain, diarrhea, and fatigue. A gluten-free diet is the accepted treatment for individuals with celiac disease.

Many people test negative for celiac disease but appear to be gluten sensitive. They indicate that they feel better when they eliminate gluten from the diet. A gluten-free diet, however, is not completely free of gluten; rather, it contains a low, harmless level. The average consumption of gluten-containing foods has increased significantly in recent years because gluten is now used as a thickener or stabilizing agent added to many processed foods, including processed meats, spice mixes, ketchup, and soy sauce. Switching to a healthy diet often helps gluten-sensitive individuals because highly processed grains and junk foods tend to have high amounts of gluten. Some gluten in the diet may not affect these people much. Whole grains, which may contain some gluten, provide many health benefits and people who are gluten sensitive can still get whole grains by choosing brown and wild rice, quinoa, millet, teff, corn, and buckwheat.

REAL LIFE STORY | Kwame's Experience

Through high school and my first couple years of college, I was in the habit of eating fast food every day. I was usually in a hurry, so going through a drive-through and getting a burger or chicken nuggets was the easiest solution. I pretty much never ate vegetables. I just didn't care for them. The only vegetable I liked was fresh corn the way my mom makes it—with lots of butter. My eating habits caused me to put on some weight over the years, but I still thought I looked okay. It wasn't until I took a Fitness and Wellness class and did a 3-day analysis of my diet that I realized how bad my eating habits really were. Some days I got more than double the amount of saturated fat and sodium that I should be having! I realized that if I went on eating this way, it would catch up with me eventually, and might even take years off my life. So I decided to try to improve my eating habits. I cut way down on the trips to fast food restaurants. It was really hard, because I drive by so many of them, and as soon as I see the sign, I start craving the foods. Sometimes I can almost smell the French fries cooking! At first it took a lot of will-power, but once I got in the habit of driving past without stopping, it got easier and I

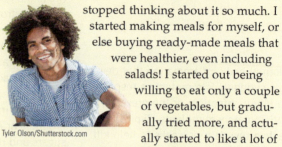

Tyler Olson/Shutterstock.com

stopped thinking about it so much. I started making meals for myself, or else buying ready-made meals that were healthier, even including salads! I started out being willing to eat only a couple of vegetables, but gradually tried more, and actually started to like a lot of them. Now I usually get even more than five servings a day of fruits and vegetables. Since changing my eating habits, I have lost some weight, and I also have more energy. Eating right can still be a challenge, especially when I get stressed and am pressed for time. But I believe that my health is worth the effort.

PERSONAL PROFILE: My Nutrition Habits

I.   Are you aware of the average daily caloric intake and macronutrient content of your diet? ___ Yes ___ No.

II. According to nutritional guidelines, the daily average caloric intake should be distributed so that less than ___ of the calories come from fat.

III. Do you take nutrient supplements to enhance your personal nutrition? ___ Yes ___ No

IV. Are you aware of how much added sugar is in your food, and if so, are you limiting your daily intake of added sugar to no more than 6 teaspoons if you are a woman or 9 teaspoons if you are a man? ___ Yes ___ No

V.   Do you balance daily calories with physical activity to sustain healthy weight and focus on consuming nutrient-dense foods and beverages? ___ Yes ___ No

VI. Do you make an effort to prevent disease and add years to your life by consuming a diet that is primarily based on fruits, vegetables, 100 percent whole grains, lean protein choices, and healthy unsaturated fats? ___ Yes ___ No

MINDTAP From Cengage   **Complete This Online**
Visit **www.cengagebrain.com** to access MindTap, a complete digital course that includes interactive quizzes, videos, and more.

Proper **nutrition** is essential to overall health and wellness. Good nutrition means that a person's diet supplies all the essential nutrients for healthy body functioning, including normal tissue growth, repair, and maintenance. The diet should also provide enough **substrates** to produce the energy necessary for work, physical activity, and relaxation.

Nutrients should be obtained from a wide variety of sources. Figure 3.1 shows U.S. Department of Agriculture (USDA) MyPlate nutrition guidelines and recommended daily food amounts according to various caloric requirements. To lower the risk for chronic disease, an effective wellness program must incorporate healthy eating guidelines. These guidelines will be discussed throughout this chapter and in later chapters.

Too much or too little of any nutrient can precipitate serious health problems. The typical U.S. diet is too high in calories, sugar, saturated fat, and sodium, and not high enough in fiber (whole grains, fruits, and vegetables), vitamin D,

GLOSSARY

Nutrition Science that studies the relationship of foods to optimal health and performance.

Substrates Substances acted on by an enzyme (e.g., carbohydrates, fats).

Nutrients Substances found in food that provide energy, regulate metabolism, and help with growth and repair of body tissues.

Figure 3.1 MyPlate: Steps to a healthier you.

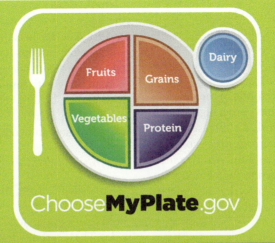

Switch to fat-free or low-fat (1%) milk.

Make at least half your grains whole grains.

Make half your plate fruits and vegetables.

Choose fish and lean or low-fat meat and poultry.

ChooseMyPlate.gov

VEGETABLES	FRUITS	GRAINS	PROTEIN	DAIRY
Any vegetable or 100% vegetable juice counts as a member of the Vegetable Group. Vegetables may be raw or cooked; fresh, frozen, canned, or dried/dehydrated; and may be whole, cut-up, or mashed. Vegetables are organized into 5 subgroups, based on their nutrient content: dark green vegetables, red and orange vegetables, beans and peas, starchy vegetables, and other vegetables.	Any fruit or 100% fruit juice counts as part of the Fruit Group. Fruits may be fresh, canned, frozen, or dried, and may be whole, cut-up, or pureed.	Any food made from wheat, rice, oats, cornmeal, barley, or another cereal grain is a grain product. Bread, pasta, oatmeal, breakfast cereals, tortillas, and grits are examples of grain products. Grains are divided into 2 subgroups: whole grains and refined grains.	All foods made from meat, poultry, seafood, beans, and peas, eggs, processed soy products, nuts, and seeds are considered part of the Protein Foods Group (beans and peas are also part of the Vegetable Group). Select at least 8 ounces of cooked seafood per week. Meat and poultry choices should be lean or low-fat. Young children need less, depending on their age and calories needs. The advice to consume seafood does not apply to vegetarians. Vegetarian options in the Protein Foods Group include beans and peas, processed soy products, and nuts and seeds.	All fluid milk products and many foods made from milk are considered part of this food group. Most Dairy Group choices should be fat-free or low-fat. Foods made from milk that retain their calcium content are part of the group. Foods made from milk that have little to no calcium, such as cream cheese, cream, and butter, are not. Calcium-fortified soymilk (soy beverage) is also part of the Dairy Group.

Recommended Daily Amounts

Women	Vegetables	Fruits	Grains	Protein	Dairy
19–30 years old	2½ cups	2 cups	6 oz equivalents	5½ oz equivalents	3 cups
31–50 years old	2½ cups	1½ cups	6 oz equivalents	5 oz equivalents	3 cups
51+ years old	2 cups	1½ cups	5 oz equivalents	5 oz equivalents	3 cups
Men					
19–30 years old	3 cups	2 cups	8 oz equivalents	6½ oz equivalents	3 cups
31–50 years old	3 cups	2 cups	7 oz equivalents	6 oz equivalents	3 cups
51+ years old	2½ cups	2 cups	6 oz equivalents	6½ oz equivalents	3 cups

Source: http://www.choosemyplate.gov/. Additional information can be obtained on this site, including an online individualized MyPlate eating plan (Plan a Healthy Menu option on the site) based on your age, gender, weight, height, and activity level.

calcium, and potassium—factors that undermine good health. On a given day, nearly half of the people in the United States eat no fruit, and almost one-fourth eat no vegetables.

Food availability is not a problem. The problem is overconsumption of the wrong foods. Diseases of dietary excess and imbalance are among the leading causes of death in many developed countries throughout the world, including the United States.

Diet and nutrition often play a crucial role in the development and progression of chronic diseases. A diet high in saturated fat and trans fat increases the risk for diseases of the cardiovascular system, including atherosclerosis, coronary heart disease (CHD), and strokes. In sodium-sensitive individuals, high salt intake has been linked to high blood pressure. Up to 50 percent of all cancers may be diet related. Obesity, diabetes, and osteoporosis also have been associated with faulty nutrition.

3.1 Nutrients

The essential nutrients that the human body requires are carbohydrates, fat, protein, vitamins, minerals, and water. The first three are called "fuel nutrients" because they are the only substances that the body uses to supply the energy (commonly measured in calories) needed for work and normal body functions. The three others—vitamins, minerals, and water—are regulatory nutrients. They have no caloric value but are still necessary for a person to function normally and maintain good health. Many nutritionists add to this list a seventh nutrient: fiber. This nutrient is vital for good health. Recommended amounts seem to provide protection against several diseases, including cardiovascular disease and some cancers.

Carbohydrates, fats, proteins, and water are termed macronutrients because we need them in proportionately large amounts daily. Vitamins and minerals are required in only small amounts—grams, milligrams, and micrograms instead of, say, ounces—and nutritionists refer to them as micronutrients.

Depending on the amount of nutrients and calories they contain, foods can be classified by their **nutrient density**. Foods that contain few or a moderate number of calories but are packed with nutrients are said to have high nutrient density. Foods that have a lot of calories but few nutrients are of low nutrient density and are commonly called "junk food."

A **calorie** is the unit of measure indicating the energy value of food to the person who consumes it. It also is used to express the amount of energy a person expends in physical activity. Technically, a kilocalorie (kcal), or large calorie, is the amount of heat necessary to raise the temperature of 1 kilogram of water by 1 degree Celsius. For simplicity, people call it a calorie rather than a kcal. For example, if the caloric value of a food is 100 calories (i.e., 100 kcal), the energy in this food would raise the temperature of 100 kilograms of water by 1 degree Celsius. Similarly, walking 1 mile would burn about 100 calories (again, 100 kcal).

3.2 Carbohydrates

Carbohydrates constitute the major source of calories that the body uses to provide energy for work, to maintain cells, and to generate heat. They are necessary for brain, muscle, and nervous system function and help regulate fat and metabolize protein. Each gram of carbohydrate provides the human body with four calories. The major sources of carbohydrates are breads, cereals, fruits, vegetables, and milk and other dairy products. Carbohydrates are classified into simple carbohydrates and complex carbohydrates (Figure 3.2).

Simple Carbohydrates

Often called "sugars," **simple carbohydrates** have little nutritive value. Examples are candy, soda, and cakes. Simple carbohydrates are divided into monosaccharides and disaccharides. These carbohydrates—whose names end in "ose"—often take the place of more nutritive foods in the diet.

Monosaccharides

The simplest sugars are **monosaccharides**. The three most common monosaccharides are glucose, fructose, and galactose.

1. Glucose is a natural sugar found in food and also produced in the body from other simple and complex carbohydrates. It is used as a source of energy, or it may be stored in the muscles and liver in the form of glycogen (a long chain of glucose molecules hooked together). Excess glucose in the blood is converted to fat and stored in **adipose tissue**.
2. Fructose, or fruit sugar, occurs naturally in fruits and honey and is converted to glucose in the body.
3. Galactose is produced from milk sugar in the mammary glands of lactating animals and is converted to glucose in the body.

Figure 3.2 Major types of carbohydrates.

Simple carbohydrates	
Monosaccharides	**Disaccharides**
Glucose	Sucrose (glucose+fructose)
Fructose	Lactose (glucose+galactose)
Galactose	Maltose (glucose+glucose)

Complex carbohydrates	
Polysaccharides	**Fiber**
Starches	Cellulose
Dextrins	Hemicellulose
Glycogen	Pectins
	Gums
	Mucilages

Glycemic Index and Glycemic Load

The glycemic index (GI) provides a numeric value that measures the blood glucose (sugar) response following ingestion of individual carbohydrate foods. Carbohydrates that are quickly absorbed and cause a rapid rise in blood glucose are said to have a high GI. Those that break down slowly and gradually release glucose into the blood have a low GI. Consumption of high-glycemic foods in combination with some fat and protein, nonetheless, brings down the average index. The glycemic load (GL) is calculated by multiplying the GI of a particular food by its carbohydrate content in grams and dividing by 100. The usefulness of the glycemic load is based on the theory that a high-glycemic-index food eaten in small quantities provides a similar effect in blood sugar rise as a consumption of a larger quantity of a low-glycemic food. Research also indicates that a low-GL diet significantly reduces inflammatory conditions that lead to chronic diseases in the human body. The most accurate source of the GI and GL of 750 foods has been published in the *Journal of Clinical Nutrition*. Additional information on the GI is also provided in Chapter 5, pages 169–170.

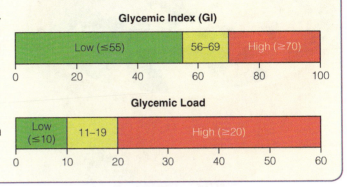

Disaccharides

The three major **disaccharides** are:

1. Sucrose or table sugar (glucose + fructose)
2. Lactose (glucose + galactose)
3. Maltose (glucose + glucose)

These disaccharides are broken down in the body, and the resulting simple sugars (monosaccharides) are used as indicated earlier.

Complex Carbohydrates

Complex carbohydrates are also called polysaccharides. Anywhere from about ten to thousands of monosaccharide molecules can unite to form a single polysaccharide. Examples of complex carbohydrates are starches, dextrins, and **glycogen**.

1. Starch is the storage form of glucose in plants that is needed to promote their earliest growth. Starch is commonly found in grains, seeds, corn, nuts, roots, potatoes, and legumes. In a healthful diet, grains, the richest source of starch, should supply most of the body's energy. Once eaten, starch is converted to glucose for the body's own energy use. High starch consumption, according to some research, has been linked to weight gain and greater risk of developing type 2 diabetes. Although no specific guidelines for daily intake are given, you can compute the starch content in carbohydrate foods by subtracting the fiber and sugar contents from the total carbohydrate in the respective item. For example, a food item with 30 grams of total carbohydrates, 4 grams dietary fiber, and 6 grams of sugars would have a net starch content of 20 grams (30 − 4 − 6).
2. Dextrins are formed from the breakdown of large starch molecules exposed to dry heat, such as in baking bread or producing cold cereals. These complex carbohydrates of plant origin provide many valuable nutrients and can be an excellent source of fiber.
3. Glycogen is the animal polysaccharide synthesized from glucose and is found in only tiny amounts in meats. In essence, we manufacture it; we don't consume it. Glycogen constitutes the body's reservoir of glucose. Thousands of glucose molecules are linked, to be stored as glycogen in the liver and muscle. When a surge of energy is needed, enzymes in the muscle and the liver break down glycogen and thereby make glucose readily available for energy transformation. (This process is discussed under "Nutrition for Athletes," starting on page 126.)

GLOSSARY

Nutrient density A measure of the amount of nutrients and calories in various foods.

Calorie The amount of heat necessary to raise the temperature of 1 gram of water 1 degree Celsius; used to measure the energy value of food and cost (energy expenditure) of physical activity.

Carbohydrates A classification of a dietary nutrient containing carbon, hydrogen, and oxygen; the major source of energy for the human body.

Simple carbohydrates Carbohydrates formed by simple or double sugar units with little nutritive value; divided into monosaccharides and disaccharides.

Monosaccharides The simplest carbohydrates (sugars), formed by five- or six-carbon skeletons. The three most common monosaccharides are glucose, fructose, and galactose.

Adipose tissue Fat cells in the body.

Disaccharides Simple carbohydrates formed by two monosaccharide units linked together, one of which is glucose. The major disaccharides are sucrose, lactose, and maltose.

Complex carbohydrates Carbohydrates formed by three or more simple sugar molecules linked together; also referred to as polysaccharides.

Glycogen Form in which glucose is stored in the body.

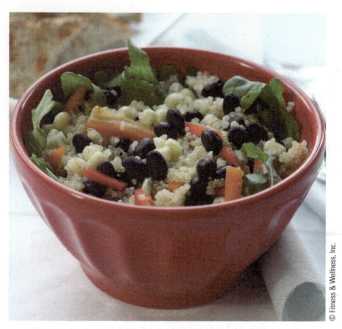

High-fiber foods are essential in a healthy diet.

Fiber

Fiber is a complex non-digestible carbohydrate. A high-fiber diet gives a person a feeling of fullness without adding too many calories to the diet. **Dietary fiber** is present mainly in plant leaves, skins, roots, and seeds. Processing and refining foods removes almost all of their natural fiber. In our diet, the main sources of fiber are whole-grain cereals and breads, fruits, vegetables, and legumes.

Fiber is important in the diet because it is rich in disease-preventing compounds. A fiber-rich diet decreases the risk of inflammation, obesity, diabetes, high blood pressure, and, in particular, the risk for cardiovascular disease (including heart disease and stroke). Increased fiber intake may lower the risk for CHD because saturated fats and trans fats often take the place of fiber in the diet, increasing the formation of cholesterol. Other health disorders that have been tied to low intake of fiber are infections, respiratory diseases, constipation, diverticulitis, hemorrhoids, and gallbladder disease. Data also show that increased fiber intake enhances gastrointestinal health and immune function, promotes the growth of beneficial gut bacteria, and calms inflammation. Individuals who eat the most dietary fiber have a 22 percent lower mortality rate from any cause as compared to those who eat the least amount of fiber.[1] And fiber supplements don't provide the same benefits as high-fiber foods. Other than fiber, whole plant foods contain many nutrients that act in synergy, augmenting the health benefits.

The recommended fiber intake for adults of age 50 years and younger is 25 grams per day for women and 38 grams for men. As a result of decreased food consumption in people older than 50 years of age, an intake of 21 and 30 grams of fiber per day, respectively, is recommended.[2] Most people in the United States eat only 15 grams of fiber per day, putting them at increased risk for disease. You can increase fiber intake by eating more fruits, vegetables, legumes, whole grains, and whole-grain cereals.

Research provides evidence that increasing fiber intake to 30 grams per day leads to a significant reduction in heart attacks, cancer of the colon, breast cancer, diabetes, and diverticulitis. Table 3.1 provides the fiber content of selected foods. A practical guideline to obtain your fiber intake is to eat at least five (preferably nine) daily servings of fruits and vegetables and three servings of whole-grain foods (whole-grain bread, cereal, and rice). Think of your servings of these food items as servings of absolute goodness to your taste and health.

Refined vs. Whole Grains

Whole grains contain the entire (100 percent) grain kernel—that is, the bran, germ, and endosperm. Examples include whole-wheat flour, whole cornmeal, oats and oatmeal, cracked wheat (bulgur), brown rice, quinoa (a grain-like crop), millet, amaranth, barley, corn, rye, buckwheat, and sorghum. **Refined grains** have been milled, a process that removes the bran and germ, the most nutritious parts of wheat grains. They contain vitamin B_1, B_2, B_3, E, folic acid, calcium, phosphorus, zinc, cooper, iron, and dietary fiber. Removal of the bran and germ is done to give *grains* a finer texture and improved shelf life, but it also removes dietary fiber, iron, and some B vitamins. White flour, white bread, degermed cornmeal, and white rice and pasta are examples of refined grain products. Refined grains are often enriched to add back B vitamins and iron. Fiber, however, is not added back.

Whole grains should not be confused with multigrain, which are made out of a variety of grains such as wheat, oat, and barley. Unless the label indicates that the product is made out of whole grain, multigrain products can be made of refined grains and as such are missing the nutrients found in the bran and germ.

Scientists also encourage people to make smart carbohydrate choices. When selecting foods high in carbohydrates, the carb-to-fiber ratio should be 10:1 or less. In the following examples, "cereal A" has a carb-to-fiber ratio of 13:1, whereas "cereal B" has a ratio of 5:1. Thus, cereal B is the much healthier choice.

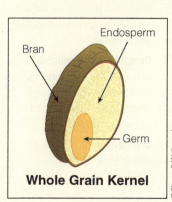

Whole Grain Kernel
(Endosperm, Bran, Germ)

Cereal A
Total Carbohydrate: 26 g
Dietary Fiber: 2 g

Cereal B
Total Carbohydrate: 25 g
Dietary Fiber: 5 g

Table 3.1 Dietary Fiber Content of Selected Foods

Food	Serving Size	Dietary Fiber (gr)
Almonds, shelled	¼ cup	3.9
Apple	1 medium	3.7
Banana	1 small	1.2
Beans (red kidney)	½ cup	8.2
Blackberries	½ cup	4.9
Beets, red, canned (cooked)	½ cup	1.4
Brazil nuts	1 oz	2.5
Broccoli (cooked)	½ cup	3.3
Brown rice (cooked)	½ cup	1.7
Carrots (cooked)	½ cup	3.3
Cauliflower (cooked)	½ cup	5.0
Cereal		
All Bran	1 oz	8.5
Cheerios	1 oz	1.1
Cornflakes	1 oz	0.5
Fruit 'n Fibre	1 oz	4.0
Fruit Wheats	1 oz	2.0
Just Right	1 oz	2.0
Wheaties	1 oz	2.0
Corn (cooked)	½ cup	2.2
Eggplant (cooked)	½ cup	3.0
Lettuce (chopped)	½ cup	0.5
Orange	1 medium	4.3
Parsnips (cooked)	½ cup	2.1
Pear	1 medium	4.5
Peas (cooked)	½ cup	4.4
Popcorn (plain)	1 cup	1.2
Potato (baked)	1 medium	4.9
Strawberries	½ cup	1.6
Summer squash (cooked)	½ cup	1.6
Watermelon	1 cup	0.1

Types of Fiber

Fiber is typically classified according to its solubility in water:

1. Soluble fiber dissolves in water and forms a gel-like substance that encloses food particles. This property allows soluble fiber to bind and excrete fats from the body. This type of fiber has been shown to lower blood cholesterol and blood sugar levels. Soluble fiber is found primarily in oats, fruits, barley, legumes, and psyllium (an ancient Indian grain added to some breakfast cereals).
2. Insoluble fiber is not easily dissolved in water, and the body cannot digest it. This type of fiber is important because it binds water, causing a softer and bulkier stool that increases **peristalsis,** the involuntary muscle contractions of intestinal walls that force the stool through the intestines and enable quicker excretion of food residues. Speeding the passage of food residues through the intestines seems to lower the risk for colon cancer, mainly because it reduces the amount of time that cancer-causing agents are in contact with the intestinal wall. Insoluble fiber is also thought to bind with carcinogens (cancer-producing substances), and more water in the stool may dilute the cancer-causing agents, lessening their potency. Sources of insoluble fiber include wheat, cereals, vegetables, and skins of fruits.

The most common types of fiber are:

1. Cellulose: water-insoluble fiber found in plant cell walls
2. Hemicellulose: water-insoluble fiber found in cereal fibers
3. Pectins: water-soluble fiber found in vegetables and fruits
4. Gums and mucilages: water-soluble fiber also found in small amounts in foods of plant origin

Surprisingly, excessive fiber intake can be detrimental to health. It can produce loss of calcium, phosphorus, and iron, to say nothing of gastrointestinal discomfort. If your fiber intake is less than the recommended amount, increase your intake gradually over several weeks to avoid gastrointestinal disturbances. While increasing your fiber intake, be sure to drink more water to avoid constipation and even dehydration. Excellent complex carbohydrate choices include quinoa (high in protein—a complete protein), beans, and sweet potatoes.

Computing Daily Carbohydrate Requirement

According to the Institute of Medicine, daily carbohydrate intake should be in the range of 45 to 65 percent of the total daily caloric intake (see Table 3.7, page 98). That is, if your total daily intake is 2,000 calories, your carbohydrate intake should be in the range of 900 to 1,300 calories (2,000 × .45 and 2,000 × .65). Because each gram of carbohydrates provides 4 calories (see Figure 3.8), your daily consumption in grams of carbohydrates should be in the range of 225 to 325 grams (900 ÷ 4 and 1,300 ÷ 4). The range is provided to accommodate differences in the amount of daily physical activity and exercise and a few medical conditions that may

GLOSSARY

Dietary fiber A complex carbohydrate in plant foods that is not digested but is essential to digestion.

Whole grains Grains that contain the entire (100 percent) grain kernel—that is, the bran, germ, and endosperm. Examples include whole-wheat flour, whole cornmeal, oats and oatmeal, cracked wheat, brown rice, quinoa (a grain-like crop), millet, amaranth, barley, corn, rye, buckwheat, and sorghum.

Refined grains Grains that have been significantly modified from their natural composition through a process that removes the bran and germ. The process removes dietary fiber, iron, and many B vitamins. White flour, white bread, and white rice and pasta are examples of refined grain products.

Peristalsis Involuntary muscle contractions of intestinal walls that facilitate excretion of wastes.

have specific requirements (e.g., metabolic syndrome; see Chapter 10, page 401). Some athletes may require even more carbohydrates to replace muscle glycogen used during intense training. Elite aerobic endurance athletes training several hours per day actually need up to 70 percent of their daily caloric intake from carbohydrates.

3.3 *Fats (Lipids)*

The human body uses **fats** as a source of energy. Also called lipids, fats are the most concentrated energy source, with each gram of fat supplying 9 calories to the body (in contrast to 4 for carbohydrates). Fats are a part of the human cell structure. Body fat is an endocrine organ (see *Types of Body Fat*, Chapter 4, p. 137) and is used as stored energy and as an insulator to preserve body heat. Fat cells also absorb shock; supply essential fatty acids; and carry the fat-soluble vitamins A, D, E, and K. Fats can be classified into three main groups: simple, compound, and derived (Figure 3.3). The most familiar sources of fat are whole milk and other dairy products, meats, and meat alternatives such as eggs and nuts.

Simple Fats

A simple fat consists of a glyceride molecule linked to one, two, or three units of fatty acids. Depending on the number of fatty acids attached, simple fats are divided into monoglycerides (one fatty acid), diglycerides (two fatty acids), and triglycerides (three fatty acids). More than 90 percent of the weight of fat in foods and more than 95

Figure 3.3 Major types of fats (lipids).

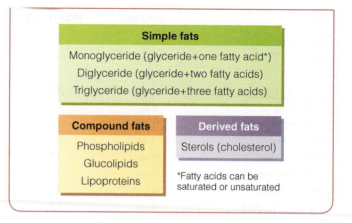

percent of the stored fat in the human body are in the form of triglycerides.

The length of the carbon atom chain and the amount of hydrogen saturation (i.e., the number of hydrogen molecules attached to the carbon chain) in fatty acids vary. Based on the extent of saturation, fatty acids are said to be saturated or unsaturated. Unsaturated fatty acids are classified further into monounsaturated and polyunsaturated fatty acids. Saturated fatty acids are mainly of animal origin, and unsaturated fats are found mostly in plant products.

Saturated Fats

In saturated fatty acids (or "saturated fats"), the carbon atoms are fully saturated with hydrogen atoms; only single bonds link the

---

Behavior Modification Planning

Tips to Increase Fiber in Your Diet

I PLAN TO   **I DID IT**

- ❑ ❑ Eat more vegetables, either raw or steamed.
- ❑ ❑ Eat salads daily that include a wide variety of vegetables.
- ❑ ❑ Eat more fruit, including the skin.
- ❑ ❑ Choose whole-wheat and whole-grain products.
- ❑ ❑ Choose breakfast cereals with more than 5 grams of fiber per serving.
- ❑ ❑ Sprinkle a teaspoon or two of unprocessed bran or 100 percent bran cereal on your favorite breakfast cereal.

- ❑ ❑ Add high-fiber cereals to casseroles and desserts.
- ❑ ❑ Add beans to soups, salads, and stews.
- ❑ ❑ Replace a portion of the meat in dishes such as stews, spaghetti, tacos, enchiladas, and burritos with beans (black, pinto, and kidney beans).
- ❑ ❑ Add vegetables to sandwiches: sprouts, green and red pepper strips, diced carrots, sliced cucumbers, red cabbage, and onions.
- ❑ ❑ Add vegetables to spaghetti: broccoli, cauliflower, sliced carrots, and mushrooms.
- ❑ ❑ Experiment with unfamiliar fruits and vegetables—collards, kale,

broccoflower, asparagus, papaya, mango, kiwi, and starfruit.
- ❑ ❑ Blend fruit juice with small pieces of fruit and crushed ice.
- ❑ ❑ Skip the juice and eat the fruit instead.
- ❑ ❑ When increasing fiber in your diet, drink plenty of fluids.

Try It

Do you know your average daily fiber intake? If you do not know, keep a 3-day record of daily fiber intake. How do you fare against the recommended guidelines? If your intake is low, how can you change your diet to increase your daily fiber intake?

MINDTAP From Cengage   **Complete This Online**
Visit **www.cengagebrain.com** to access MindTap, a complete digital course that includes interactive quizzes, videos, and more.

Figure 3.4 Classification of fats based on the degree of hydrogen saturation.

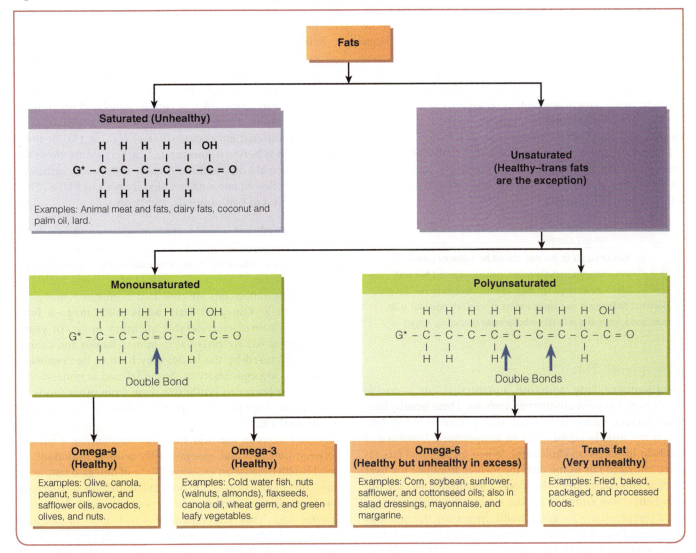

carbon atoms on the chain (Figure 3.4). Foods high in saturated fatty acids are meats, animal fat, lard, whole milk, cream, butter, cheese, ice cream, hydrogenated oils (hydrogenation saturates fat with hydrogens; also known as trans fats), coconut oil, and palm oils. They are also concealed in foods such as cakes, cookies, muffins, biscuits, fried chicken with skin, creamy pasta sauces, mayonnaise, salad dressings, and processed meats.

Saturated fats typically do not melt at room temperature. Coconut and palm oils are exceptions. In general, saturated fats raise the blood cholesterol level. The data on coconut and palm oils are controversial as some research indicates that these oils may be neutral in terms of their effects on cholesterol; that is, they raise both the LDL cholesterol and the HDL cholesterol. The increase in LDL cholesterol, however, may be more damaging than the increase in HDL cholesterol. Some individuals promote the use of coconut oil as a health food, but the scientific evidence to support the claim is not strong. Coconut oil might be better than saturated animal fats, but it is not a good choice as compared to extra virgin olive and canola oils. If you like coconut oil, use it sparingly.

Saturated fats fuel body-wide inflammation, cause heart disease, promote obesity and visceral fat, increase breast cancer risk, and may weaken the immune system. Although saturated fats raise the "bad" low-density lipoprotein (LDL) cholesterol (in particular the less-damaging larger LDL particles) and daily intake should be limited, data indicate that people who replace saturated fat in the diet with refined carbohydrate foods (carbohydrates that have been processed away from their natural state to the point where most of the intact grain has been removed) such as white bread, pasta, sugar, and low-fat sweetened baked goods are at greater risk for heart disease because the latter tend to increase triglycerides (blood fats) and the more dangerous smaller LDL particles.[3]

GLOSSARY

Fats A classification of nutrients containing carbon, hydrogen, some oxygen, and sometimes other chemical elements.

Processed (and packaged) **foods** are often low in fat but high in refined carbohydrates, sugar, and sodium—all three of which, when consumed in large amounts, are worse for the person than moderate consumption of saturated fat. High refined-carbohydrate diets increase palmitoleic acid, a monounsaturated fatty acid (MUFA) that behaves like a saturated fatty acid and causes an increase in LDL cholesterol. Unfortunately, many Americans prefer convenience and taste over health. Surveys tell us that more than 60 percent of the foods we purchase at supermarkets are processed foods.

In terms of fat, to derive significant health benefits, the main focus should be in replacing saturated fat with polyunsaturated fats, as in liquid vegetable oils (see discussion that follows and in Chapter 10 on page 394).

HOEGER KEY TO WELLNESS

 Saturated fat in the diet should be replaced primarily with complex carbohydrates, polyunsaturated fat, and monounsaturated fat. Your risk for cardiovascular disease does not decrease if you replace most of your saturated fat with processed foods and refined carbohydrates (including sugar).

Unsaturated Fats

In unsaturated fatty acids (or "unsaturated fats"), double bonds form between unsaturated carbons. These healthy fatty acids include monounsaturated and polyunsaturated fats, which are usually liquid at room temperature. Unsaturated fats help lower blood cholesterol. When unsaturated fats replace saturated fats in the diet, the former stimulate the liver to clear cholesterol from the blood. Unsaturated fats are not only better than saturated fat, but are also far superior to refined carbohydrates for good health. Increasing the intake of unsaturated fats should be a priority in the American diet.

In monounsaturated fatty acids (MUFA), only one double bond is found along the chain. Monounsaturated fatty acids are found in olive, canola, peanut, and sesame oils. They are also found in avocados and nuts.

Olive oil is considered the healthiest oil because of the nutrients it contains. Extra virgin olive oil contains antioxidants, polyphenols, and omega-3 fatty acids, all of which promote cardiovascular health, improved cognitive function, and a healthier immune system. Olive oil may even help prevent or reverse type 2 diabetes because it helps the body produce adiponectin, a hormone that aids with blood sugar regulation. Olive oil also has anti-inflammatory properties that protect against chronic diseases.

Extra virgin olive oil is produced from the first pressing of the olives and, as such, holds the most nutrients. Virgin olive oil is derived from the second pressing. Juices collected from subsequent pressings are then used to manufacture light and pure olive oils.

Canola oil is also extremely healthy. Its composition is the closest to the optimum requirements of fatty acids by the human body, and it contains a nearly ideal mix of unsaturated fatty acids that promote cardiac health. The omega-3s in canola oil also counteract fibrinogen, a compound in the blood that has been linked to thrombosis (clot formation in the blood vessels) and inflammation.

Extra virgin and virgin olive oils retain the flavor of the olives to a greater extent; thus, they are best used to make tasty dish toppings and salad dressings but may not be the most ideal for cooking or baking. Because olive oil is more expensive than canola oil, you can use canola oil for cooking and reserve olive oil for toppings, dips, and dressings.

Polyunsaturated fatty acids (PUFA) contain two or more double bonds between unsaturated carbon atoms along the chain. Vegetable oils, including corn, cottonseed, safflower, walnut, sunflower, and soybean oils, are high in PUFA. They are also found in fish, almonds, and pecans.

Omega Fatty Acids Unsaturated omega fatty acids have been named based on where the first double bond appears in the carbon chain—starting from the end of the chain; hence, the term "omega" from the end of the Greek alphabet. Accordingly, omega fats are classified as omega-3, omega-6, and omega-9. **Omega-3 fatty acids** and **omega-6 fatty acids** have gained considerable attention in recent years. These fatty acids are essential to human health and cannot be manufactured by the body; they have to be consumed in the diet. Omega-9 fatty acids are defined as nonessential because the body can synthesize them from other foods we eat, and we don't have to depend on direct dietary sources to obtain them.

Some leaders in the field state that maintaining a balance between omega-3 and omega-6 fatty acids is important for good health because an excessive intake of omega-6 fatty acids may contribute to low-grade body inflammation, a risk factor for heart disease, cancer, asthma, arthritis, and depression (Figure 3.5). They recommend a 4-to-1 ratio of omega-6 to omega-3 fatty acids to maintain and improve health. At present, however, there is no solid evidence to substantiate this recommendation. The guideline to maintain healthy weight—a diet high in vegetable polyunsaturated fats, omega-3 fatty acids, slow-digesting carbohydrates (low glycemic loads), antioxidant-rich foods, and probiotic foods, less animal saturated fat and trans fats, and a reduced intake of red meat—is the best advice to prevent low-grade body inflammation.

Most critical in the diet are omega-3 fatty acids, which provide substantial health benefits. Omega-3 fatty acids tend to decrease cholesterol, triglycerides, inflammation, blood clots, abnormal heart rhythms, high blood pressure, and slow growth of plaque in the arteries. They also decrease the risk for heart attack, stroke, Alzheimer's disease, diabetes, dementia, macular degeneration, and joint degeneration and play an important role in fetal brain and eye development.

Unfortunately, only 25 percent of the U.S. population consumes the recommended amount (approximately 500 mg) of omega eicosapentaenoic acid (EPA) and docosahexaenoic acid (DHA) on any given day. These are two of the three major types of omega-3 fatty acids, along with alpha-linolenic acid (ALA). The evidence is strongest for EPA and DHA as being cardioprotective. Once consumed, the body converts ALA to

Figure 3.5 Chronic low-grade inflammation leads to an array of chronic diseases.

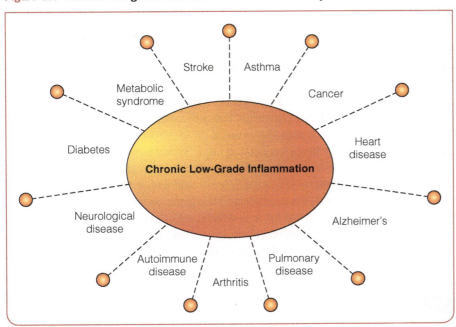

species of fish. Canned fish is best when packed in water. In oil-packed fish, the oil mixes with some of the natural fat in fish. When the oil is drained, some of the omega-3 fatty acids are lost as well. Good sources of omega-3 ALA include flaxseeds, canola oil, walnuts, wheat germ, and green leafy vegetables.

Fish is lower in saturated fat than meat or poultry. Data indicate that eating as little as 6 ounces of fatty fish per week can reduce the risk of premature death from heart disease by one-third and overall death rates by about one-sixth. Fish also appears to have anti-inflammatory properties that can help treat chronic inflammatory kidney disease, osteoarthritis, rheumatoid arthritis, Crohn's disease, and autoimmune disorders like asthma and lupus. Data indicate that consuming fish at least twice per week adds about two years of life to an already 65-year-old person. Thus, fish is one of the healthiest foods we can consume.

EPA and then to DHA, but the process is not very efficient. It is best to increase consumption of EPA and DHA to obtain the greatest health benefit. EPA is also known to inhibit an enzyme that increases the production of inflammatory hormones.

Individuals at risk for heart disease are encouraged to get an average of .5 to 1.8 grams (500 to 1,800 mg) of EPA and DHA per day.[4] These fatty acids protect against irregular heartbeat and blood clots, reduce triglycerides and blood pressure, and defend against inflammation.[5]

Fish—especially fresh or frozen salmon, mackerel, herring, tuna, and rainbow trout—are high in EPA and DHA. Table 3.2 presents a listing of total EPA plus DHA content of selected

The oil in flaxseeds is high in ALA and has been shown to reduce abnormal heart rhythm and prevent blood clots. Flaxseeds are also high in fiber and plant chemicals known as lignans. Studies are being conducted to investigate the potential cancer-fighting ability of lignans. The addition of a daily ounce (3 to 4 tablespoons) of ground flaxseeds to the diet is recommended for a potential decrease in the onset of tumors and may even lead to their shrinkage. Excessive flaxseed in the diet is not recommended. High doses actually may be detrimental to health. Pregnant and lactating women, especially, should not consume large amounts of flaxseed.

Because flaxseeds have a hard outer shell, they should be ground to obtain the nutrients; whole seeds will pass through the body undigested. Grinding the seeds just before use best preserves flavor and nutrients. Pre-ground seeds should be kept sealed and refrigerated. Ground flaxseeds can be mixed with salad dressings, salads, wheat flour, pancakes, muffins, cereals, rice, cottage cheese, and yogurt. Flaxseed oil also may be used, but the oil has little or no fiber and lignans and must be kept refrigerated because it spoils quickly. The oil cannot be used for cooking, either, because it scorches easily.

Table 3.2 Omega-3 Fatty Acid Content (EPA + DHA) per 100 Grams (3.5 oz) of fish

Type of Fish	Total EPA + DHA
Anchovy	1.4 gr
Bluefish	1.2 gr
Halibut	0.4 gr
Herring	1.7 gr
Mackerel	2.4 gr
Sardine	1.4 gr
Salmon, Atlantic	1.0 gr
Salmon, Chinook	1.9 gr
Salmon, Coho	1.2 gr
Salmon, Pink	1.0 gr
Salmon, Sockeye	1.3 gr
Shrimp	0.3 gr
Trout, Rainbow	0.6 gr
Trout, Lake	1.6 gr
Tuna, light (water canned)	0.3 gr
Tuna, white (Albacore)	0.8 gr

GLOSSARY

Processed foods All agricultural commodities that undergo processing (cooking, canning, freezing, dehydration, or milling) or addition of another ingredient.

Omega-3 fatty acids Polyunsaturated fatty acids found primarily in cold-water seafood, flaxseed, and flaxseed oil; thought to lower blood cholesterol and triglycerides.

Omega-6 fatty acids Polyunsaturated fatty acids found primarily in corn and sunflower oils and most oils in processed foods.

Mercury and Fish

Potential contaminants in fish—in particular, mercury—have created concerns among some people. Mercury cannot be removed from food. As it accumulates in the body, it harms the brain and nervous system. Mercury is a naturally occurring trace mineral that can be released into the air from industrial pollution. As mercury falls into streams and oceans, it accumulates in the aquatic food chain. Larger fish accumulate larger amounts of mercury because they eat medium- and small-size fish. Of particular concern are shark, swordfish, king mackerel, pike, bass, and tilefish, which have higher levels. Farm-raised salmon also have slightly higher levels of poly-chlorinated biphenyls (PCBs), which the U.S. Environmental Protection Agency lists as a "probable human carcinogen."

The American Heart Association recommends consuming fish twice a week. Further, the FDA recommends that pregnant women consume at least 8 to 12 ounces of a variety of lower-mercury fish distributed over two to three meals per week. The risk for adverse effects from eating fish is extremely low and primarily theoretical in nature. For most people, eating two servings of fish per week poses no health threat. The best recommendation is to balance the risks against the benefits. If you are still concerned, consume no more than 12 ounces per week of a variety of fish and shellfish that are lower in mercury, including canned light tuna, wild salmon, shrimp, pollock, catfish, and scallops. Twelve ounces per week has been shown to be safe even for pregnant or lactating women without leading to developmental problems in their offspring. And check local advisories about the safety of fish caught by family and friends in local streams, rivers, lakes, and coastal areas. Many preventive medicine experts now believe that fish is most likely the single most important food an individual can consume for good heart health, and that the benefits in terms of reduced heart disease and cancer deaths far outweigh the risks of eating fish.

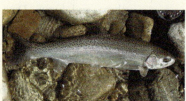
© Fitness & Wellness, Inc.

Low-Mercury Seafood Choices

Anchovy	Oyster	Sole (Pacific)
Catfish	Salmon (wild)	Tilapia
Clam	Sardine	Trout (fresh water)
Crab (domestic)	Scallop	Tuna (canned, light)
Flounder	Shrimp	Whitefish

Most of the PUFA consumption in the United States comes from omega-6, considered healthy fats, but excessive intake may be detrimental to health. Omega-6 fatty acids include linoleic acid (LA), gamma-linolenic acid (GLA), and arachidonic acid (AA). The typical American diet contains 10 to 20 times more omega-6 than omega-3 fatty acids. Most omega-6 fatty acids come in the form of LA from vegetable oils, the primary oil ingredient added to most processed foods, including salad dressing. LA-rich oils include corn, soybean, sunflower, safflower, and cottonseed oils.

Although more research is required, the imbalance between omega-3 and omega-6 fatty acids is thought to be partly responsible for the increased rate of inflammatory conditions seen in the United States today. Furthermore, in terms of heart health, while omega-6 fatty acids lower the "bad" LDL cholesterol, they also lower the "good" HDL cholesterol; thus, their overall effect on cardiac health is neutral. To decrease your intake of LA, watch for corn, soybean, sunflower, and cottonseed oils in salad dressings, mayonnaise, and margarine.

The best source of omega-3 EPA and DHA, the fatty acids that provide the most health benefits, is fish. Data suggest that the amount of fish oil obtained by eating two servings of fish weekly lessens the risk for CHD and may contribute to brain, joint, and vision health. A word of caution: People who have diabetes or a history of hemorrhaging or strokes, are on aspirin or blood-thinning therapy, or are presurgical patients should not consume fish oil except under a physician's instruction.

Omega-9 fatty acids are from a family of polyunsaturated fats generally found in vegetable oils (canola, olive, peanut, safflower, and sunflower oils), but they are also found in avocados, olives, and nuts (almonds, cashews, macadamias, peanuts, pecans, pistachios, and walnuts). These fatty acids are uniquely high in monounsaturated fat, low in saturated fat, and contain zero trans fat. Omega-9 fatty acids are protective against metabolic syndrome and cardiovascular disease because they have been shown to increase HDL cholesterol and decrease LDL cholesterol.

Trans Fatty Acids Hydrogen often is added to monounsaturated and polyunsaturated fats to increase shelf life and to solidify them so that they are more spreadable. During this process, called "partial hydrogenation," the position of hydrogen atoms may be changed along the carbon chain, transforming the fat into a **trans fatty acid**. Some margarine, spreads, shortening, pastries, nut butters, coffee creamers, crackers, cookies, frozen breakfast foods, dairy products, snacks and chips, cake mixes, meats, processed foods, and fast foods contain trans fatty acids.

Trans fatty acids are not essential and provide no known health benefit. In truth, health-conscious people minimize their intake of these types of fats because diets high in trans fatty acids increase LDL cholesterol and decrease HDL cholesterol, increase rigidity of the coronary arteries, contribute to the formation of blood clots that may lead to heart attacks and strokes, and increase visceral fat (fat around the abdomen) by redistributing fat tissue from other parts of the body.

According to research published in the *American Journal of Clinical Nutrition*, high trans fatty acid intake has been associated with an increased risk of all-cause mortality, accounting for an estimated 7 percent of all deaths in the United States in recent years.[6]

Paying attention to food labels is important because the words "partially hydrogenated" and "trans fatty acids" indicate that the product carries a health risk just as high as or higher than that of saturated fat. Since 2006, the U.S. Food and Drug Administration (FDA) requires food labeling of products that contain more than half a gram of trans fats per serving so that consumers can make healthier choices. Subsequently, the Institute of Medicine indicated that there is no safe level of consumption. In 2013, the FDA further proposed regulation to ban trans fats from all products by stating that they are not safe for human health and ordered that they be removed from the "generally recognized as safe" (GRAS) list of food additives.

Compound Fats

Compound fats are a combination of simple fats and other chemicals. Examples are:

1. Phospholipids: similar to triglycerides, except that choline (or another compound) and phosphoric acid take the place of one of the fatty acid units
2. Glucolipids: a combination of carbohydrates, fatty acids, and nitrogen
3. Lipoproteins: water-soluble aggregates of protein and triglycerides, phospholipids, or cholesterol

Lipoproteins (a combination of lipids and proteins) are especially important because they transport fats in the blood. The major forms of lipoproteins are HDL, LDL, and very-low-density lipoprotein (VLDL). Lipoproteins play a large role in developing or in preventing heart disease. High HDL ("good" cholesterol) levels have been associated with lower risk for CHD, whereas high levels of LDL ("bad" cholesterol) have been linked to increased risk for CHD. HDL is more than 50 percent protein and contains little cholesterol. LDL is approximately 25 percent protein and nearly 50 percent cholesterol. VLDL contains about 50 percent triglycerides, only about 10 percent protein, and 20 percent cholesterol.

Derived Fats

Derived fats combine simple and compound fats. **Sterols** are an example. Although sterols contain no fatty acids, they are considered lipids because they do not dissolve in water. The sterol mentioned most often is cholesterol, which is found in many foods or can be manufactured in the body—primarily from saturated fats, trans fats, and refined carbohydrates.

In the 1980s and 1990s, people were concerned with overall fat intake. As a result, they cut back on fats and started to overconsume refined carbohydrates. Nowadays, people understand that healthy unsaturated fats and caloric balance are essential to good health. The latter is important because overconsumption of even healthy fats leads to weight gain. Keep in mind that as you add something healthy to your diet, you need to remove an equal amount of calories from a different food item, preferably a less healthy item.

HOEGER KEY TO WELLNESS

The healthiest diets are rich in vegetables, fruits, whole grains, fish, vegetable oils, beans, yogurt, and nuts and low in red and processed meats, saturated fat, trans fat, sodium, refined grains, and sugar.

3.4 *Proteins*

Proteins are the main substances the body uses to build and repair tissues such as muscles, blood, internal organs, skin, hair, nails, and bones. They form a part of hormone, antibody, and enzyme molecules. **Enzymes** play a key role in all of the body's processes. Because proteins form all enzymes, these nutrients are necessary for normal functioning. Proteins also help maintain the normal balance of body fluids.

Proteins can be used as a source of energy, too, but only if sufficient carbohydrates are not available. Each gram of protein yields four calories of energy (the same as carbohydrates). The main sources of protein are meats and meat alternatives, milk, and other dairy products. Excess proteins may be converted to glucose or fat, or even excreted in the urine.

The human body uses 20 **amino acids** to form various types of protein. Amino acids contain nitrogen, carbon, hydrogen, and oxygen. Of the 20 amino acids, 9 are called essential amino acids because the body cannot produce them. The other 11, termed nonessential amino acids, can be manufactured in the body if food proteins in the diet provide enough nitrogen (see Table 3.3). For the body to function normally, all amino acids must be present in the diet.

GLOSSARY

Trans fatty acid Solidified fat formed by adding hydrogen to monounsaturated and polyunsaturated fats to increase shelf life.

Lipoproteins Lipids covered by proteins; these transport fats in the blood. Types are LDL, HDL, and VLDL.

Sterols Derived fats, of which cholesterol is the best-known example.

Proteins A classification of nutrients consisting of complex organic compounds containing nitrogen and formed by combinations of amino acids; the main substances used in the body to build and repair tissues.

Enzymes Catalysts that facilitate chemical reactions in the body.

Amino acids Chemical compounds that contain nitrogen, carbon, hydrogen, and oxygen; the basic building blocks the body uses to build different types of protein.

Importance of Adequate Daily Protein Intake

Adequate protein intake with each meal is crucial for satiety and weight management and to help build, repair, and maintain lean tissue. The latter has even greater relevance for people who are physically active. Loss of lean tissue with sedentary living, aging, exhaustive exercise training, and while dieting (negative caloric balance) without proper energy and protein intake is inevitable. Loss of lean tissue is never desirable because of the decrease in functional physical capacity (the ability to perform ordinary and unusual tasks of daily living), as well as in the resting metabolic rate.

Protein is also important for bone health. About 50 percent of bone volume and 30 percent of bone mass are protein. Contrary to previous beliefs, data indicate that when consumed during the same meal,

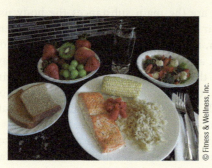

© Fitness & Wellness, Inc.

protein and calcium interact and actually help improve bone health. Furthermore, an intake above the recommended RDA of 0.8 g/day can improve health by helping prevent obesity, osteoporosis, and metabolic syndrome. The current RDA, nonetheless, is the same for people of all ages. During growth in youth, body hormones help the body use proteins quite efficiently. Such is not the case as people age. In fact, adults have greater protein needs to help maintain lean tissue (muscles and bones) necessary for a healthy metabolic rate, blood sugar regulation, and bone health. The protein requirement is actually higher in older adults because caloric intake typically decreases as people age, yet the protein need does not.

As an individual, you can prevent or even completely reverse such a loss. The recommendation is that we distribute our protein intake in equal parts throughout the day. To do so, determine your daily intake in grams (see Table 3.4) and divide by three (meals per day). For example, if you are young, weigh 141 pounds (64 kg), and you are physically active, your total protein intake should be between 64 and 77 grams per day (64 × 1.0 and 64 × 1.2, or the equivalent of 256 to 308 calories derived from protein each day—each gram of protein supplies the body with 4 calories) or 21 to 26 grams of protein per meal. The range of protein intake for most healthy adults is between 25 and 40 grams of high-quality protein at breakfast, lunch, and dinner.

Table 3.3 Amino Acids

Essential Amino Acids*	Nonessential Amino Acids
Histidine	Alanine
Isoleucine	Arginine
Leucine	Asparagine
Lysine	Aspartic acid
Methionine	Cysteine
Phenylalanine	Glutamic acid
Threonine	Glutamine
Tryptophan	Glycine
Valine	Proline
	Serine
	Tyrosine

*NOTE: Must be provided in the diet because the body cannot manufacture them.

Proteins that contain all the essential amino acids, known as "complete" or "higher-quality" proteins, are usually of animal origin. If one or more of the essential amino acids are missing, the proteins are termed incomplete or lower-quality proteins. The essential amino acid that is missing in an incomplete protein is called the limiting amino acid. All plant products, including grains, fruits, vegetables, beans, nuts, and seeds, are incomplete proteins. The only exceptions of complete proteins found in plant products are soy and quinoa.

Individuals have to take in enough protein to ensure nitrogen for adequate production of all amino acids. On a vegetarian diet, consumption of a variety of food sources is required

so that the diet supplies all the essential amino acids within a meal or a given day. When different foods are consumed, the limiting amino acid in one food can be obtained from another food source. This principle is referred to as complementing proteins. For example, grains and legumes complement each other when they are consumed together. Legumes and nuts also complement each other. Nuts and grains, however, are not complementary proteins. Soy and quinoa can also be used to complement the limiting amino acids in grains, legumes, nuts, and seeds.

Protein deficiency is not a problem in the typical United States diet. Two glasses of skim milk combined with about 4 ounces of poultry or fish meet the daily protein requirement. High intake of protein foods from animal sources, however, can be a concern because they are often high in saturated fat, which leads to cardiovascular disease. You can determine your recommended daily protein intake using the guidelines provided in Table 3.4. To obtain your body weight in kilograms, divide your weight in pounds by 2.2046.

Table 3.4 Recommended Daily Protein Intake

Category	Grams/kg of Body Weight
Sedentary	0.8 g/kg
Healthy older adult (65+)	1.0–1.2 g/kg
Physically active	1.0–1.2 g/kg
Athlete	1.2–2.0 g/kg
Weight gain/loss	1.5–2.0 g/kg

Limit Red Meat Consumption

Several recent research articles provide strong evidence that excessive red meat consumption increases the risk of premature death, primarily from heart disease, stroke, some cancers, and type 2 diabetes. Consumption of both unprocessed red meat (beef, pork, and lamb) and processed red meat (cold cuts, ham, bacon, bologna, sausage, and hot dogs) leads to this outcome.

Researchers believe that it is not just the saturated fat that is the culprit. L-carnitine, a compound abundant in red meat, feeds intestinal bacteria. These bacteria digest *L-carnitine* and turn it into a compound called trimethylamine-N-oxide (TMAO) that is believed to cause atherosclerosis (obstruction of the arteries) that increases the risk for heart attack, stroke, and memory loss. Red-meat eaters also have a higher incidence of pancreatic, prostate, and esophageal cancers. Nitrites, chemical compounds used to cure (preserve) meats, are believed to increase the risk. Processed meats labeled as "no nitrite added" most likely are not nitrite-free because nitrite and nitrate (which the body can convert to nitrite) occur naturally in meats.

Eating less red meat also protects the environment by requiring less cattle feed and water, decreasing the production of methane gas and solid waste by the animals, reducing the requirement of nitrous oxide used in fertilizers to grow the feed, and leading to less deforestation to make pasture and farmland.

The most compelling evidence comes from a study of more than 120,000 people at the Harvard School of Public Health showing a 30 percent increased risk of premature death among people who eat the most red meat as compared to those who eat the least (about half a

serving per day). In the study, 3 ounces of unprocessed red meat were considered as one serving, but only 1 ounce of processed red meat was viewed as a serving. The mortality rate was highest among processed red-meat eaters. Eating just one serving per day increased the risk between 13 (unprocessed) and 20 percent (processed).

The data also indicated that replacing one serving a day of red meat with fish, poultry, nuts, beans, low-fat dairy, or whole grains decreased the chances of premature death in the range of 7 to 19 percent. The researchers concluded that, *"The message we want to communicate is it would be great if you could reduce your intake of red meat consumption to half a serving a day or two to three servings a week, and severely limit processed red meat intake."*

A study involving almost half a million people from ten European countries found that individuals eating 5.7 ounces of processed meats (the equivalent of two daily sausages and a slice of bacon) had a 44 percent greater risk of dying during the 13-year study. One in every 17 people followed during this time died, and almost twice as many from cancer as from heart disease. A subsequent study that included almost 150,000 health professionals found that people who increase red meat consumption by more than half a serving per day have a 48 percent greater risk of developing type 2 diabetes over the next 4 years. In contrast, people who cut their daily intake in half had a 14 percent lower risk of type 2 diabetes.

As mentioned earlier, a well-balanced diet contains a variety of foods from all five basic food groups, including a wise selection of foods from animal sources (see also "Balancing the Diet" in this chapter). Based on current nutrition data, meat (particularly red meat or excessive poultry and fish) should be replaced by grains, legumes, vegetables, and fruits as main courses. Meats should be used more for flavoring than for volume. Daily consumption of beef, poultry, or fish should be limited to 3 ounces (smaller than a deck of cards) or less.

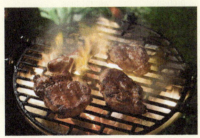

Viktor1/Shutterstock.com

SOURCES: A. Pan et al., "Red Meat Consumption and Mortality: Results from 2 Prospective Cohort Studies," *Archives of Internal Medicine* 172 (2012): 555–563; S. Rohrmann et al., "Meat Consumption and Mortality—Results from the European Prospective Investigation into Cancer and Nutrition," *BMC Medicine 2013*, 11: 63 doi:10.1186/1741-7015-11-63; A. Pan et al., "Changes in Red Meat Consumption and Subsequent Risk of Type 2 Diabetes Mellitus," *Journal of the American Medical Association Internal Medicine* 173 (2013): 1328–1335.

3.5 *Vitamins*

Vitamins are necessary for normal bodily metabolism, growth, and development. Vitamins are classified into two types based on their solubility:

1. Fat soluble (A, D, E, and K)
2. Water soluble (B complex and C)

The body does not manufacture most vitamins, so they can be obtained only through a well-balanced diet. To decrease loss of vitamins during cooking, natural foods should be microwaved or steamed rather than boiled in water that is thrown out later.

A few exceptions, such as vitamins A, D, and K, are formed in the body. Vitamin A is produced from beta-carotene,

found mainly in yellow/orange foods such as carrots, pumpkin, and sweet potatoes. Vitamin D is found in certain foods and is created when ultraviolet light from the sun transforms 7-dehydrocholesterol, a compound in human skin. Vitamin K is created in the body by intestinal bacteria. The major functions of vitamins are outlined in Table 3.5.

Vitamins C, E, and beta-carotene also function as antioxidants, which are thought to play a key role in preventing chronic diseases. (The specific functions of these antioxidant nutrients and of the mineral selenium, also an antioxidant, are discussed under "Antioxidants," page 118.)

GLOSSARY

Vitamins Organic nutrients essential for normal metabolism, growth, and development of the body.

Table 3.5 Major Functions of Vitamins

Nutrient	Good Sources	Major Functions	Deficiency Symptoms
Vitamin A	Milk, cheese, eggs, liver, yellow and dark green fruits and vegetables	Required for healthy bones, teeth, skin, gums, and hair; maintenance of inner mucous membranes, thereby increasing resistance to infection; adequate vision in dim light.	Night blindness; decreased growth; decreased resistance to infection; rough, dry skin
Vitamin D	Fortified milk, cod liver oil, salmon, tuna, egg yolk	Necessary for bones and teeth; needed for calcium and phosphorus absorption.	Rickets (bone softening), fractures, muscle spasms
Vitamin E	Vegetable oils, yellow and green leafy vegetables, margarine, wheat germ, whole-grain breads and cereals	Related to oxidation and normal muscle and red blood cell chemistry.	Leg cramps, red blood cell breakdown
Vitamin K	Green leafy vegetables, cauliflower, cabbage, eggs, peas, potatoes	Essential for normal blood clotting.	Hemorrhaging
Vitamin B$_1$ (Thiamine)	Whole-grain or enriched bread, lean meats and poultry, fish, liver, pork, poultry, organ meats, legumes, nuts, dried yeast	Assists in proper use of carbohydrates, normal functioning of nervous system, maintaining good appetite.	Loss of appetite, nausea, confusion, cardiac abnormalities, muscle spasms
Vitamin B$_2$ (Riboflavin)	Eggs, milk, leafy green vegetables, whole grains, lean meats, dried beans and peas	Contributes to energy release from carbohydrates, fats, and proteins; needed for normal growth and development, good vision, and healthy skin.	Cracking of the corners of the mouth, inflammation of the skin, impaired vision
Vitamin B$_6$ (Pyridoxine)	Vegetables, meats, whole grain cereals, soybeans, peanuts, potatoes	Necessary for protein and fatty acids metabolism and for normal red blood cell formation.	Depression, irritability, muscle spasms, nausea
Vitamin B$_{12}$	Meat, poultry, fish, liver, organ meats, eggs, shellfish, milk, cheese	Required for normal growth, red blood cell formation, and nervous system and digestive tract functioning.	Impaired balance, weakness, drop in red blood cell count
Niacin	Liver and organ meats, meat, fish, poultry, whole grains, enriched breads, nuts, green leafy vegetables, and dried beans and peas	Contributes to energy release from carbohydrates, fats, and proteins; normal growth and development; and formation of hormones and nerve-regulating substances.	Confusion, depression, weakness, weight loss
Biotin	Liver, kidney, eggs, yeast, legumes, milk, nuts, dark green vegetables	Essential for carbohydrate metabolism and fatty acid synthesis.	Inflamed skin, muscle pain, depression, weight loss
Folic Acid	Leafy green vegetables, organ meats, whole grains and cereals, dried beans	Needed for cell growth and reproduction and for red blood cell formation.	Decreased resistance to infection
Pantothenic Acid	All natural foods, especially liver, kidney, eggs, nuts, yeast, milk, dried peas and beans, green leafy vegetables	Related to carbohydrate and fat metabolism.	Depression, low blood sugar, leg cramps, nausea, headaches
Vitamin C (Ascorbic acid)	Fruits, vegetables	Helps protect against infection; required for formation of collagenous tissue, normal blood vessels, teeth, and bones.	Slow-healing wounds, loose teeth, hemorrhaging, rough scaly skin, irritability

3.6 *Minerals*

Approximately 25 minerals have important roles in body functioning. **Minerals** are inorganic substances contained in all cells, especially those in hard parts of the body (bones, nails, and teeth). Minerals are crucial to maintaining water balance and the acid-base balance. They are essential components of respiratory pigments, enzymes, and enzyme systems, and they regulate muscular and nervous tissue impulses, blood clotting, and normal heart rhythm. The four minerals mentioned most often are calcium, iron, sodium, and selenium. Calcium deficiency may result in osteoporosis, and low iron intake can induce iron-deficiency anemia (see page 131). High sodium intake may contribute to high blood pressure. Selenium seems to be important in preventing certain types of cancer. Specific functions of some of the most important minerals are given in Table 3.6.

Table 3.6 Major Functions of Minerals

Nutrient	Good Sources	Major Functions	Deficiency Symptoms
Calcium	Milk, yogurt, cheese, green leafy vegetables, dried beans, sardines, salmon	Required for strong teeth and bone formation; maintenance of good muscle tone, heartbeat, and nerve function.	Bone pain and fractures, periodontal disease, muscle cramps
Copper	Seafood, meats, beans, nuts, whole grains	Helps with iron absorption and hemoglobin formation; required to synthesize the enzyme cytochrome oxidase.	Anemia (although deficiency is rare in humans)
Iron	Organ meats, lean meats, seafood, eggs, dried peas and beans, nuts, whole and enriched grains, green leafy vegetables	Major component of hemoglobin; aids in energy utilization.	Nutritional anemia, overall weakness
Phosphorus	Meats, fish, milk, eggs, dried beans and peas, whole grains, processed foods	Required for bone and teeth formation and for energy release regulation.	Bone pain and fracture, weight loss, weakness
Zinc	Milk, meat, seafood, whole grains, nuts, eggs, dried beans	Essential component of hormones, insulin, and enzymes; used in normal growth and development.	Loss of appetite, slow-healing wounds, skin problems
Magnesium	Green leafy vegetables, whole grains, nuts, soybeans, seafood, legumes	Needed for bone growth and maintenance, carbohydrate and protein utilization, nerve function, temperature regulation.	Irregular heartbeat, weakness, muscle spasms, sleeplessness
Sodium	Table salt, processed foods, meat	Needed for body fluid regulation, transmission of nerve impulses, heart action.	Rarely seen
Potassium	Legumes, whole grains, bananas, orange juice, dried fruits, potatoes	Required for heart action, bone formation and maintenance, regulation of energy release, acid-base regulation.	Irregular heartbeat, nausea, weakness
Selenium	Seafood, meat, whole grains	Component of enzymes; functions in close association with vitamin E.	Muscle pain, possible deterioration of heart muscle, possible hair loss and nail loss

3.7 *Water*

The most important nutrient is **water** because it is involved in almost every vital body process: in digesting and absorbing food, in producing energy, in the circulatory process, in regulating body heat and electrolyte balance, in removing waste products, in building and rebuilding cells, in transporting essential nutrients, and in cushioning joints and organs. In men, about 61 percent of total body weight is water. The proportion of water in body weight in women is 56 percent (Figure 3.6). The difference is due primarily to the higher amount of muscle mass in men.

Inadequate fluid intake results in body dehydration and can lead to decreased mental and physical performance, cardiovascular strain, and heat illness (see Chapter 9, page 357). On average, adequate daily fluid intake is about 13 cups for men and 9 for women. People with increased perspiration due to work, athletic participation, or warm environmental conditions require additional fluid intake.

Almost all foods contain water, but it is found primarily in liquid foods, fruits, and vegetables. People obtain about 80 percent of the daily water needs from beverages and the remaining 20 percent from foods. A panel of scientists at the Institute of Medicine of the National Academy of Sciences (NAS) indicated that most people are getting enough water from the liquids (milk, juices, sodas, coffee) and the moisture content of solid foods. Most Americans and Canadians remain well hydrated simply by using thirst as their guide. Caffeine-containing drinks also are acceptable as a water source because data indicate that people who regularly consume such beverages do not have more 24-hour urine output than those who don't.

An exception to not waiting for the thirst signal to replenish water loss is when an individual exercises in the heat, or does so for an extended time (see Chapter 9, page 357). Water lost under these conditions must be replenished regularly. If you wait for the thirst signal, you may have lost too much water already. At 2 percent of body weight lost, a person is dehydrated. At 5 percent, one may become dizzy and disoriented, have trouble with cognitive skills and heart function, and even lose consciousness.

GLOSSARY

Minerals Inorganic nutrients essential for normal body functions; found in the body and in food.

Water The most important classification of essential body nutrients, involved in almost every vital body process.

Figure 3.6 Approximate proportions of nutrients in the human body.

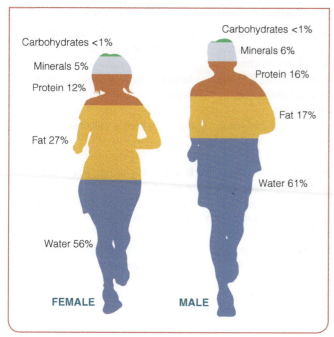

Carbohydrates <1%
Minerals 5%
Protein 12%
Fat 27%
Water 56%
FEMALE

Carbohydrates <1%
Minerals 6%
Protein 16%
Fat 17%
Water 61%
MALE

Table 3.7 The American Diet: Current and Recommended Carbohydrate, Fat, and Protein Intake Expressed as a Percentage of Total Calories

	Current Percentage	Recommended Percentage*
Carbohydrates:	50%	45–65%
Simple	26%	Less than 25%
Complex	24%	20–40%
Fat:	34%	20–35%**
Monounsaturated:	11%	Up to 20%
Polyunsaturated:	10%	Up to 10%
Saturated:	13%	Less than 6%
Protein:	16%	10–35%

*SOURCE: Adapted from the National Academy of Sciences, Institute of Medicine. *Dietary Reference Intakes for Energy Carbohydrates, Fiber, Fat, Protein and Amino Acids (macronutrients).* Washington DC: National Academy Press, 2002.

**Less than 30% is recommended by most major national health organizations. Up to 35% is allowed for individuals with metabolic syndrome who may need additional fat in the diet.

3.8 *A Healthy Diet*

One of the fundamental ways to enjoy good health and live life to its fullest is through a well-balanced diet. Several guidelines have been published to help you accomplish this. As illustrated in Table 3.7, the most recent recommended guidelines by the NAS state that daily caloric intake should be distributed so that 45 to 65 percent of total calories come from carbohydrates (mostly complex carbohydrates and less than 25 percent from sugar), 20 to 35 percent from fat, and 10 to 35 percent from protein.[7] The recommended ranges allow for flexibility in planning diets according to individual health and physical activity needs. The fat percentage is up to 35 percent to accommodate individuals with metabolic syndrome (see Chapter 10, page 401), who have an abnormal insulin response to carbohydrates and may need additional fat in the diet. For all other individuals, daily fat intake should not exceed 30 percent of total caloric intake.

In addition to the macronutrients, the diet must include all of the essential vitamins, minerals, and water. The source of fat calories is also critical. In late 2013, the American Heart Association (AHA) and the American College of Cardiology released a new recommendation that saturated fat should constitute less than 5 to 6 percent, whereas polyunsaturated fat can be up to 10 percent and monounsaturated fat up to 20 percent of total daily calories. The *2015-2020 Dietary Guidelines for Americans* allow up to 10 percent of the total daily caloric intake from saturated fat, an amount that many preventive medicine specialists consider too high. Rating a particular diet accurately is difficult without a complete nutrient analysis. To determine your caloric distribution from the various nutrients, you have an opportunity to perform a complete nutrient analysis in Activity 3.1 and Activity 3.2.

The NAS recommendations will be effective only if people consistently replace saturated and trans fatty acids with unsaturated fatty acids. The latter will require changes in the typical "unhealthy" American diet, which is generally high in red meat, whole dairy products, and fast foods—all of which are high in saturated and/or trans fatty acids.

Diets in most developed countries changed significantly in the early 20th century. Today, people eat more calories and fat, fewer complex carbohydrates, and about the same amount of protein. People also weigh more than they did in 1900, an indication that we are eating more calories and are not as physically active as our forebears.

Surveys indicate that, on average, people now eat out one meal per day compared to only two per week in the 1970s. Not only do Americans eat more when they eat out, but they also eat far fewer healthy foods than at home. Data indicate that people who cook and eat at home consume about 200 fewer calories per day and have a lower intake of saturated fat, refined carbohydrates, sugar, and salt. Among the most popular foods ordered at restaurants and fast-food places today are French fries, hamburgers, and pizza. About one-fifth of all restaurant meals are purchased at drive-throughs, with almost one-half of young people and a third of baby boomers indicating that they eat full meals in the car. In contrast, whenever possible, healthy eating implies consuming primarily whole, fresh, or locally grown food items made with few ingredients and minimal processing and packaging.

3.9 *Nutrition Standards*

Nutritionists use a variety of nutrient standards. Each standard has a different purpose and utilization in dietary planning and assessment. The most widely known are the Dietary Reference Intakes and the Daily Values.

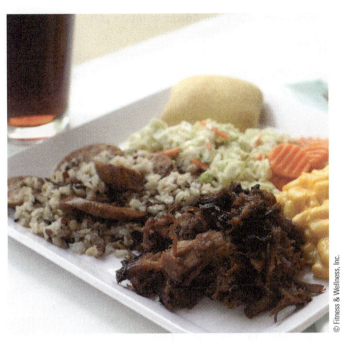

© Fitness & Wellness, Inc.

The typical American diet is too high in calories, sugar, sodium (salt), and unhealthy fats.

Dietary Reference Intakes

To help people meet dietary guidelines, the NAS developed the **Dietary Reference Intakes (DRIs)** for healthy people in the United States and Canada. The DRIs are based on a review of the most current research on nutrient needs of healthy people. The DRI reports are written by the Food and Nutrition Board of the Institute of Medicine in cooperation with scientists from Canada.

The DRI encompass four types of reference values for planning and assessing diets and for establishing adequate amounts and maximum safe nutrient intakes in the diet. These four reference values are the **Recommended Dietary Allowance (RDA), Estimated Average Requirement (EAR), Adequate Intake (AI),** and **Tolerable Upper Intake Levels (UL)**. The type of reference value used for a given nutrient and a specific age/gender group is determined according to available scientific information and the intended use of the dietary standard. Nutrients for which a daily DRI has been set are given in Table 3.8.

Estimated Average Requirement

The EAR is the amount of a nutrient that is estimated to meet the nutrient requirement of half the healthy people in specific age and gender groups. At this nutrient intake level, the nutritional requirements of 50 percent of the people are not met. For example, looking at 300 healthy women at age 26, the EAR would meet the nutritional requirement for only half of these women.

Recommended Dietary Allowance

The RDA is the daily amount of a nutrient that is considered adequate to meet the known nutrient needs of nearly all healthy people in the United States. A committee of the Food and Nutrition Board of the NAS determines RDAs of nutrients. Because the committee must decide what level of intake to recommend for everybody, the RDA is set well above the EAR and covers about 98 percent of the population. Stated another way, the RDA recommendation for any nutrient is well above almost everyone's actual requirement. The RDA could be considered a goal for adequate intake. The process for determining the RDA depends on being able to set an EAR because RDAs are determined statistically from the EAR values. If an EAR cannot be set, no RDA can be established.

Adequate Intake

When data are insufficient or inadequate to set an EAR, an AI value is determined instead of the RDA. The AI value is derived from approximations of observed nutrient intakes among a group or groups of healthy people. The AI value for children and adults is expected to meet or exceed the nutritional requirements of a corresponding healthy population.

Tolerable Upper Intake Level

The UL establishes the highest level of nutrient intake that seems to be safe for most healthy people, beyond which exists an increased risk for adverse effects. As intakes increase above the UL, so does the risk for adverse effects. Established UL values are presented in Table 3.9.

Daily Values

The **Daily Values (DV)** are reference values for nutrients and food components listed on food-packaging labels. The DVs include measures of fat, saturated fat, and carbohydrates (as

GLOSSARY

Dietary Reference Intake (DRI) A general term that describes four types of nutrient standards that establish adequate amounts and maximum safe nutrient intakes in the diet: Estimated Average Requirements (EAR), Recommended Dietary Allowances (RDA), Adequate Intakes (AI), and Tolerable Upper Intake Levels (UL).

Recommended Dietary Allowance (RDA) The daily amount of a nutrient (statistically determined from the EARs) that is considered adequate to meet the known nutrient needs of almost 98 percent of all healthy people in the United States.

Daily Values (DV) Reference values for nutrients and food components used in food labels.

Estimated Average Requirement (EAR) The amount of a nutrient that meets the dietary needs of half the people.

Adequate Intake (AI) The recommended amount of a nutrient intake when sufficient evidence is not available to calculate the EAR and subsequent RDA.

Tolerable Upper Intake Level (UL) The highest level of nutrient intake that seems safe for most healthy people, beyond which exists an increased risk of adverse effects.

Table 3.8 Dietary Reference Intakes (DRIs): Recommended Dietary Allowances (RDA) and Adequate Intake (AI) for Selected Nutrients

	Recommended Dietary Allowances (RDA)															Adequate Intakes (AI)			
	Thiamin (mg)	Riboflavin (mg)	Niacin (mg NE)	Vitamin B6 (mg)	Folate (µg)	Vitamin B12 (µg)	Phosphorus (mg)	Magnesium (mg)	Vitamin A (µg)	Vitamin C (mg)	Vitamin D (IU)	Vitamin E (mg)	Selenium (mcg)	Iron (mg)	Calcium (mg)	Fluoride (mg)	Pantothenic acid (mg)	Biotin (mg)	Choline (mg)
Males																			
14–18	1.2	1.3	16	1.3	400	2.4	1,250	410	900	75	600	15	55	11	1,300	3	5.0	25	550
19–30	1.2	1.3	16	1.3	400	2.4	700	400	900	90	600	15	55	8	1,000	4	5.0	30	550
31–50	1.2	1.3	16	1.3	400	2.4	700	420	900	90	600	15	55	8	1,000	4	5.0	30	550
51–70	1.2	1.3	16	1.7	400	2.4	700	420	900	90	600	15	55	8	1,000	4	5.0	30	550
>70	1.2	1.3	16	1.7	400	2.4	700	420	900	90	800	15	55	8	1,200	4	5.0	30	550
Females																			
14–18	1.0	1.0	14	1.2	400	2.4	1,250	360	700	65	600	15	55	15	1,300	3	5.0	25	400
19–30	1.1	1.1	14	1.3	400	2.4	700	310	700	75	600	15	55	18	1,000	3	5.0	30	425
31–50	1.1	1.1	14	1.3	400	2.4	700	320	700	75	600	15	55	18	1,000	3	5.0	30	425
51–70	1.1	1.1	14	1.5	400	2.4	700	320	700	75	600	15	55	8	1,200	3	5.0	30	425
>70	1.1	1.1	14	1.5	400	2.4	700	320	700	75	800	15	55	8	1,200	3	5.0	30	425
Pregnant (19–30)	1.4	1.4	18	1.9	600	2.6	700	350	770	85	600	15	60	27	1,000	3	6.0	30	450
Lactating (19–30)	1.4	1.6	17	2.0	500	2.8	700	310	1,300	120	600	19	70	9	1,000	3	7.0	35	550

SOURCE: Reprinted with permission from "Dietary Reference Intakes: Recommended Dietary Allowances and Adequate Intakes, Elements," and "Dietary Reference Intakes for Calcium and Vitamin D," 2011 by the National Academy of Sciences, Courtesy of the National Academics Press, Washington D.C.

Table 3.9 Tolerable Upper Intake Levels (UI) of Selected Nutrients for Adults (19–70 years)

Nutrient	UL per Day
Calcium	2.5 g
Phosphorus	4.0 g*
Magnesium	350 mg
Vitamin D	50 mcg
Fluoride	10 mg
Niacin	35 mg
Iron	45 mg
Vitamin B6	100 mg
Folate	1,000 mcg
Choline	3.5 g
Vitamin A	3,000 mcg
Vitamin C	2,000 mg
Vitamin E	1,000 mg
Selenium	400 mcg

*3.5 g per day for pregnant women.

SOURCE: Adapted from the National Academy of Sciences, Institute of Medicine. *Dietary Reference Intakes for Tolerable Upper Intake Levels, Vitamins.* Washington, DC: National Academy Press, 2011.

expressed as percentages for a 2,000-calorie diet and therefore may require adjustments depending on an individual's daily **estimated energy requirement (EER)** in calories. For example, for a 2,000-calorie diet (the EER), the recommended carbohydrate intake is about 300 grams (about 60 percent of the EER), and the recommendation for fat is 65 grams (about 30 percent of EER). The vitamin, mineral, and protein DVs were adapted from the RDA. The DVs also are not as specific for age and gender groups as are the DRI. Both the DRI and the DV apply to only healthy adults. They are not intended for people who are ill, who may require additional nutrients. Figure 3.7 shows a food label with U.S. Recommended Daily Values.

The FDA is now recommending the first major food label change since 1994. The proposed revision includes a major update to present caloric value per serving bigger and bolder and make the serving size more realistic to

a percent of total calories); cholesterol, sodium, and potassium (in milligrams); and fiber and protein (in grams). The DVs for total fat, saturated fat, and carbohydrates are

GLOSSARY

Estimated energy requirement (EER) The average dietary energy (caloric) intake that is predicted to maintain energy balance in a healthy adult of defined age, gender, weight, height, and level of physical activity, consistent with good health.

Figure 3.7 Food label with U.S. recommended Daily Values.

1 Design
Nutrition Facts
The food label provides information on the macronutrients and other food components important to decrease the risk of developing chronic diseases.

2 Serving size
Check here first
Serving sizes typically are unrealistic. Most people consume more than the small portion sizes listed. If you eat more, you need to adjust all nutrients, including the increase in calories consumed.

3 Percent Daily Value (% DV)
How much are you really getting?
The % DV are based on a 2,000 calories/day diet. You will need to adjust your values based on how much you eat in a serving. This listing can help you choose foods rich in nutrients deficient in your diet (choose items with at least 20% DV) or decrease food items you need to limit for health reasons.

4 Limit these nutrients
Know what you want to minimize
These are nutrients that most people need to limit on a daily basis: Trans fat, saturated fat, sodium, and cholesterol. Be on the lookout for hydrogenated and partially-hydrogenated oils. For poly-unsaturated and monounsaturated fats, you may consume up to 10 percent and 20 percent, respectively, of your total daily calories. For better health, make sure to choose items with less than 5% DV for foods you wish to avoid. Note also that if there is less than .5 g or less of trans fat per serving, manufacturers do not have to list it here and it may simply state 0%. 20% DV is high in sodium.

5 Know your nutrients
Know the nutrients to increase
For good health, consume sufficient beneficial nutrients like dietary fiber, protein, calcium, vitamins, and nutrients needed every day. Be sure, however, to consume primarily complex carbohydrates and limit the intake of food items with a close ratio of total carbohydrates to sugars. Limit foods with more than 5 g of sugar per serving. Check the protein content to make sure you meet the recommended daily requirement, particularly if you are highly active, on a weight loss program, or if you are an older adult.

6 Ingredient list
Always read the list
The ingredients are listed in descending order of predominance (the ingredient that weighs the most is listed first and the ingredient that weighs the least is listed last). Choose whole, minimally processed foods with ingredients that you are familiar with in your kitchen. Foods with a shorter ingredient list indicates that the foods are less processed. A good guideline is to choose items with 5 or fewer ingredients. In particular pay attention to and minimize the use of foods with the following ingredients on the list: trans fats, saturated fat, hydrogenated and partially-hydrogenated oils, grains that are not 100 percent whole grain, added sugars, high fructose corn syrup (and other sugars), artificial ingredients, nitrates, and nitrites in the ingredient list.

7 Other facts
Descriptors, health claims, and allergies
Certain terms such as "good source of fiber," "low-fat," "fat-free," as well as selected health claims are allowed on food labels. Laws require that such descriptors and claims meet legal definitions. Food labels must also list major food allergens (milk, eggs, fish, crustacean shellfish, tree nuts, wheat, peanuts, and soybeans).

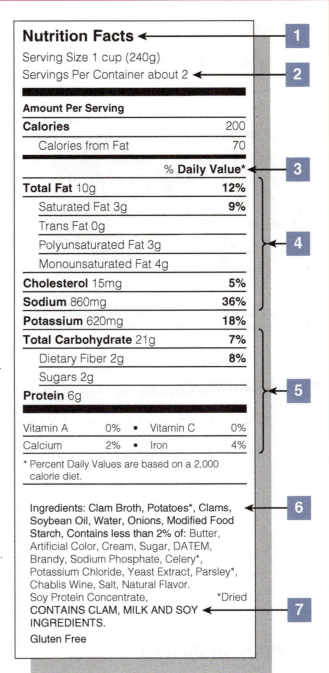

Reprinted with permission from the American Institute for Cancer Research.

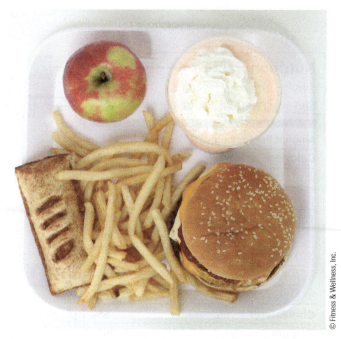

© Fitness & Wellness, Inc.

An apple a day will not keep the doctor away if most meals are high in calories, saturated fat, and trans fat content.

reflect the amount people typically eat. These changes are proposed to emphasize the need for adequate daily caloric balance. Added sugar information along with DV information for sodium, potassium, fiber, and vitamin D are also recommended. The listing of calories from fat on the label is to be removed because the emphasis needs to be on the type of fat consumed (unsaturated) rather than the total amount.

> **!** **Critical Thinking**
>
> What do the nutrition standards mean to you? How much of a challenge would it be to apply those standards in your daily life?

3.10 *Nutrient Analysis*

The first step in evaluating your diet is to conduct a nutrient analysis. This can be quite educational because most people do not realize how harmful and nonnutritious many common foods are. The top sources of calories in the American diet are soft drinks, sweet rolls, pastries, doughnuts, cakes, hamburgers, cheeseburgers, meatloaf, pizza, potato and corn chips, and buttered popcorn—all of which are low in essential nutrients and high in fat and/or sugar and calories.

Most nutrient analyses cover calories, carbohydrates, fats, cholesterol, and sodium, as well as eight essential nutrients: protein, calcium, iron, vitamin A, thiamine, riboflavin, niacin, and vitamin C. If the diet has enough of these eight nutrients,

the foods consumed in natural form to provide these nutrients typically contain all the other nutrients the human body needs.

To do your own nutrient analysis, keep a three-day record of everything you eat using Activity 3.1 (make additional copies of this form as needed). At the end of each day, look up the nutrient content for those foods in the list of Nutritive Values of Selected Foods (in Appendix B, available in MindTap at www.cengagebrain.com). Record this information on the form in Activity 3.1. If you do not find a food in Appendix B, the information may be on the food container itself.

When you have recorded the nutritive values for each day, add up each column and write the totals at the bottom of the chart. After the third day, fill in your totals in Activity 3.2 and compute an average for the three days. To rate your diet, compare your figures with those in the RDA (see Table 3.8). The results will give a good indication of areas of strength and deficiency in your current diet.

Some of the most revealing information learned in a nutrient analysis is the source of excessive fat and saturated fat intake in the diet. The average daily fat consumption in the United States diet is about 34 percent of the total caloric intake, much of it from saturated fats, which increases the risk for chronic diseases such as cardiovascular disease, cancer, diabetes, and obesity. Although fat provides a smaller percentage of our total daily caloric intake compared with two decades ago (37 percent), the decrease in percentage is simply because Americans now eat more calories than 20 years ago (335 additional daily calories for women and 170 for men).

As illustrated in Figure 3.8, 1 gram of carbohydrates or protein supplies the body with 4 calories, and fat provides 9 calories per gram consumed (alcohol yields 7 calories per gram). Therefore, looking at only the total grams consumed for each type of food can be misleading.

For example, a person who eats 160 grams of carbohydrates, 100 grams of fat, and 70 grams of protein has a total intake of 330 grams of food. This indicates that 30 percent of

Figure 3.8 **Caloric value of food (fuel nutrients).**

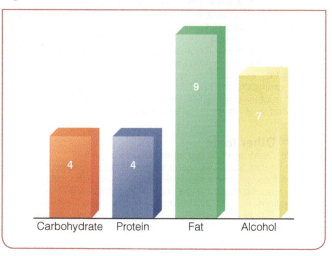

Carbohydrate 4   Protein 4   Fat 9   Alcohol 7

Activity 3.1   **Daily Nutrient Intake***

Date:

Foods	Amount	Calories	Protein (g)	Fat (total g)	Sat. Fat (g)	Cho-lesterol (mg)	Carbo-hydrates (g)	Dietary Fiber (g)	Calcium (mg)	Iron (mg)	Sodium (mg)	Vit. E (mg)	Folate (mcg)	Vit. C (mg)	Selenium (mcg)
Totals															

*Make additional copies of this form as needed.

MINDTAP **Complete This Online**
From Cengage
Visit **www.cengagebrain.com** to access MindTap, a complete digital course that includes interactive quizzes, videos, and more.

Activity 3.2   Analysis of Daily Nutrient Intake

Name: _____

Day	Calories	Protein (g)	Fat (g)	Sat. Fat (g)	Cholesterol (mg)	Carbohydrates (g)	Dietary Fiber (g)	Calcium (mg)	Iron (mg)	Sodium (mg)	Vit. E (mg)	Folate (mcg)	Vit. C (mg)	Selenium (mcg)	
One															
Two															
Three															
Totals															
Average[a]															
Percentages[b]															
Recommended Dietary Allowances*															
Men															
14–18 yrs	See below[c]	See below[d]	20–30%[e]	7%	<300	45–65%	38	1,300	12	2,300	15	400	75	55	
19–30 yrs			20–30%[e]	7%	<300	45–65%	38	1,000	10	2,300	15	400	90	55	
31–50 yrs			20–30%[e]	7%	<300	45–65%	38	1,000	10	2,300	15	400	90	55	
51+ yrs			20–30%[e]	7%	<300	45–65%	30	1,000	10	2,300	15	400	90	55	
Women															
14–18 yrs			20–30%[e]	7%	<300	45–65%	25	1,300	15	2,300	15	400	65	55	
19–30 yrs			20–30%[e]	7%	<300	45–65%	25	1,000	15	2,300	15	400	75	55	
31–50 yrs			20–30%[e]	7%	<300	45–65%	25	1,000	15	2,300	15	400	75	55	
51+ yrs			20–30%[e]	7%	<300	45–65%	21	1,200	15	2,300	15	400	75	55	
Pregnant			20–30%[e]	7%	<300	45–65%	25	1,200	30	2,300	15	600	85	60	
Lactating			20–30%[e]	7%	<300	45–65%	25	1,200	15	2,300	15	500	120	70	

[a] Divide totals by 3 or number of days assessed.

[b] Percentages: Protein and carbohydrates = multiply average by 4, divide by average calories, and multiply by 100.
Fat and saturated fat = multiply average by 9, divide by average calories, and multiply by 100.

[c] Use Table 5.2 (page 187) for all categories.

[d] Protein intake should be between .8 and 2.0 grams per kilogram of body weight (see Table 3.4, page 94). Pregnant women should consume an additional 15 grams of daily protein, and lactating women should have an extra 20 grams.

[e] Based on recommendations by nutrition experts. Up to 35% is allowed for individuals who suffer from metabolic syndrome.

* Adapted from *Recommended Dietary Allowances*, 10th Edition, and the Dietary Reference Intakes series, National Academy of Sciences 1989, 1997, 1998, 2000, 2001, Washington, DC.

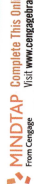

MINDTAP From Cengage   **Complete This Online**
Visit **www.cengagebrain.com** to access MindTap, a complete digital course that includes interactive quizzes, videos, and more.

Behavior Modification Planning

Caloric and Fat Content of Selected Fast Food Items

	Calories	Total Fat (grams)	Saturated Fat (grams)	Percent Fat Calories
Burgers				
McDonald's Big Mac	590	34	11	52
McDonald's Big N' Tasty with Cheese	590	37	12	56
McDonald's Quarter Pounder with Cheese	530	30	13	51
Burger King Whopper	760	46	15	54
Burger King Bacon Double Cheeseburger	580	34	18	53
Burger King BK Smokehouse Cheddar Griller	720	48	19	60
Burger King Whopper with Cheese	850	53	22	56
Burger King Double Whopper	1,060	69	27	59
Burger King Double Whopper with Cheese	1,150	76	33	59
Wendy's Baconator	830	51	22	55
Sandwiches				
Arby's Regular Roast Beef	350	16	6	41
Arby's Super Roast Beef	470	23	7	44
Arby's Roast Chicken Club	520	28	7	48
Arby's Market Fresh Roast Beef & Swiss	810	42	13	47
McDonald's Crispy Chicken	430	21	8	43
McDonald's Filet-O-Fish	470	26	5	50
McDonald's Chicken McGrill	400	17	3	38
Wendy's Chicken Club	470	19	4	36
Wendy's Breast Fillet	430	16	3	34
Wendy's Grilled Chicken	300	7	2	21
Burger King Specialty Chicken	560	28	6	45
Subway Veggie Delight*	226	3	1	12
Subway Turkey Breast	281	5	2	16
Subway Sweet Onion Chicken Teriyaki	374	5	2	12
Subway Steak & Cheese	390	14	5	32
Subway Cold Cut Trio	440	21	7	43
Subway Tuna	450	22	6	44
Mexican				
Taco Bell Crunchy Taco	170	10	4	53
Taco Bell Taco Supreme	220	14	6	57
Taco Bell Soft Chicken Taco	190	7	3	33
Taco Bell Bean Burrito	370	12	4	29
Taco Bell Fiesta Steak Burrito	370	12	4	29
Taco Bell Grilled Steak Soft Taco	290	17	4	53
Taco Bell Double Decker Taco	340	14	5	37
French Fries				
Wendy's, biggie (5½ oz)	440	19	7	39
McDonald's, large (6 oz)	540	26	9	43
Burger King, large (5½ oz)	500	25	13	45
Shakes				
Wendy's Frosty, medium (16 oz)	440	11	7	23
McDonald's McFlurry, small (12 oz)	610	22	14	32
Burger King, Old Fashioned Ice Cream Shake, medium (22 oz)	760	41	29	49
Hash Browns				
McDonald's Hash Browns (2 oz)	130	8	4	55
Burger King, Hash Browns, small (2½ oz)	230	15	9	59

*6-inch sandwich with no mayo

Try It

Using the information in the table, record in your online journal or class notebook ways you can restructure fast-food consumption to decrease caloric value and saturated fat content in your diet.

SOURCE: Adapted from *Restaurant Confidential*. Copyright © 2002 by the Center for Science in the Public Interest. Used by permission of Workman Publishing Co., Inc., New York. All rights reserved.

the total grams of food is in the form of fat (100 grams of fat ÷ 330 grams of total food = 0.30; 0.30 × 100 = 30 percent)—and, in reality, almost half of that diet is in the form of fat calories. In the sample diet, 640 calories are derived from carbohydrates (160 grams × 4 calories per gram), 280 calories from protein (70 grams × 4 calories per gram), and 900 calories from fat (100 grams × 9 calories per gram), for a total of 1,820 calories. If 900 calories are derived from fat, almost half of the total caloric intake is in the form of fat (900 ÷ 1,820 × 100 = 49.5 percent).

Each gram of fat provides 9 calories—more than twice the calories of a gram of carbohydrate or protein. The fat content of selected foods, given in grams and as a percent of total calories, is presented in Figure 3.9. The percentage of fat is further subdivided into saturated, monounsaturated, polyunsaturated, and other fatty acids.

3.11 *Achieving a Balanced Diet*

Anyone who has completed a nutrient analysis and has given careful attention to Table 3.5 (vitamins) and Table 3.6 (minerals) probably will realize that a well-balanced diet entails eating a variety of nutrient-dense foods and monitoring total daily caloric intake. The MyPlate healthy food plan in Figure 3.1 (page 83) contains five major food groups. The food groups are fruits, vegetables, grains, protein, and dairy. A Healthy Eating Plate, based on the MyPlate guidelines, is provided in Figure 3.10 to offer specific recommendations for healthier food choices within the various food groups.

For most meals, three quarters of the plate should be taken up by fruits, vegetables, and grains because they provide the nutritional base for a healthy diet. When increasing the intake of these food groups, it is important to decrease the

Figure 3.9 Fat content of selected foods.

Food	Calories	Total fat (grams)	% fat calories
Avocado/Florida (1)	340	27	71.5
Bacon (3 pieces)	109	9	74.3
Beef/ground/lean/broiled (4 oz)	318	20	56.6
Beef/sirloin (4 oz)	320	21	59.1
Beef/T-bone (4 oz)	338	24	63.9
Butter (1 tbs)	102	11	97.1
Cheese/American (1 oz)	93	7	67.7
Cheese/cheddar (1 oz)	114	9	71.1
Cheese/cottage 4% (1 cup)	216	9	37.5
Cheese/cream (1 oz)	99	10	90.9
Cheese/Parmesan (1 oz)	129	9	62.8
Cheese/Swiss (1 oz)	106	8	67.9
Cheeseburger (1)	305	13	38.4
Chicken/breast/no skin (4 oz)	188	4	19.1
Chicken/thigh/no skin (4 oz)	232	13	50.4
Egg/hard-cooked (1)	77	5	58.4
Frankfurter/beef & pork (1)	182	17	84.1
Halibut/baked (4 oz)	159	3	17.0
Hamburger (1)	255	9	31.8
Ice cream/vanilla (1 cup)	267	15	50.6
Ice milk/vanilla (1 cup)	182	6	29.7
Lamb/lean & fat (4 oz)	293	19	58.4
Margarine (1 tbs)	101	11	98.0
Mayonnaise (1 tbs)	99	11	100.0
Milk/2% (1 cup)	121	5	37.2
Milk/skim (1 cup)	85	.5	5.3
Milk/whole (1 cup)	149	8	48.3
Nuts/cashew/oil roasted (1 oz)	163	14	77.3
Nuts/peanuts/oil roasted (1 oz)	165	14	76.4
Oil/canola (1 tbs)	126	14	100.0
Oil/coconut (1 tbs)	120	13.5	100.0
Oil/flaxssed (1 tbs)	120	13.5	100.0
Oil/olive (1 tbs)	124	14	100.0
Oil/palm (1 tbs)	120	13.5	100.0
Oil/peanut (1 tbs)	120	13.5	100.0
Salmon/baked (4 oz)	245	12	44.1
Sherbet (1 cup)	266	4	13.5
Shrimp/boiled (3 oz)	85	1	10.6
Tuna/oil/drained (3 oz)	167	7	37.7
Tuna/water/drained (3 oz)	99	1	9.1
Turkey/dark meat/no skin (4 oz)	212	8	34.0
Turkey/light meat/no skin (4 oz)	117	4	30.8

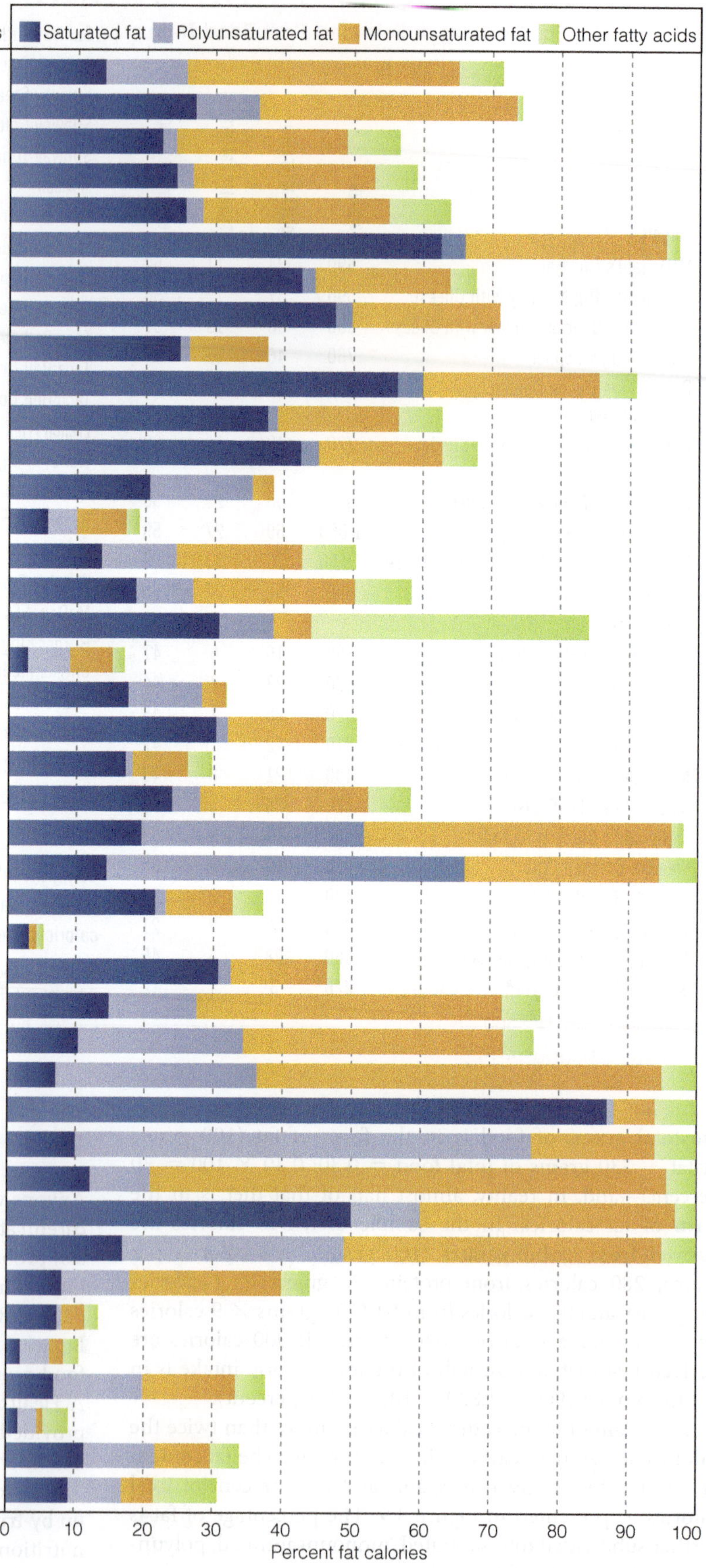

Legend: ■ Saturated fat ■ Polyunsaturated fat ■ Monounsaturated fat ■ Other fatty acids

Percent fat calories

Figure 3.10 Healthy eating plate.

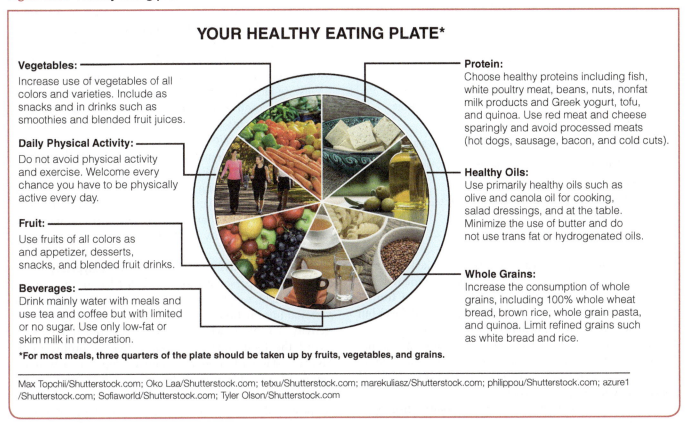

YOUR HEALTHY EATING PLATE*

Vegetables:
Increase use of vegetables of all colors and varieties. Include as snacks and in drinks such as smoothies and blended fruit juices.

Daily Physical Activity:
Do not avoid physical activity and exercise. Welcome every chance you have to be physically active every day.

Fruit:
Use fruits of all colors as and appetizer, desserts, snacks, and blended fruit drinks.

Beverages:
Drink mainly water with meals and use tea and coffee but with limited or no sugar. Use only low-fat or skim milk in moderation.

Protein:
Choose healthy proteins including fish, white poultry meat, beans, nuts, nonfat milk products and Greek yogurt, tofu, and quinoa. Use red meat and cheese sparingly and avoid processed meats (hot dogs, sausage, bacon, and cold cuts).

Healthy Oils:
Use primarily healthy oils such as olive and canola oil for cooking, salad dressings, and at the table. Minimize the use of butter and do not use trans fat or hydrogenated oils.

Whole Grains:
Increase the consumption of whole grains, including 100% whole wheat bread, brown rice, whole grain pasta, and quinoa. Limit refined grains such as white bread and rice.

*For most meals, three quarters of the plate should be taken up by fruits, vegetables, and grains.

Max Topchii/Shutterstock.com; Oko Laa/Shutterstock.com; tetxu/Shutterstock.com; marekuliasz/Shutterstock.com; philippou/Shutterstock.com; azure1/Shutterstock.com; Sofiaworld/Shutterstock.com; Tyler Olson/Shutterstock.com

intake of low-nutrient foods to effectively balance caloric intake with energy needs. These foods should be complemented with low-fat milk/dairy products and small amounts of lean sources of protein.

In addition to providing nutrients crucial to health, fruits and vegetables are the sole source of **phytonutrients** ("phyto" comes from the Greek word for plant). These compounds show promising results in the fight against cancer and heart disease. More than 4,000 phytonutrients have been identified. The main function of phytonutrients in plants is to protect them from sunlight. In humans, phytonutrients seem to have a powerful ability to block the formation of cancerous tumors. Their actions are so diverse that at almost every stage of cancer, phytonutrients have the ability to block, disrupt, slow, or even reverse the process. In terms of heart disease, they may reduce inflammation, inhibit blood clots, or prevent the oxidation of LDL cholesterol. For many phytonutrients, it's not the phytonutrient itself that provides the benefits, but rather the end product of its absorption and metabolism by the gut flora, the liver, the lungs, and other tissues that is used by the human body to prevent and fight disease.

The consistent message is to eat a diet with ample fruits and vegetables. The daily recommended amount of fruits and vegetables has absolutely no substitute. Unfortunately, based on the most recent data from the Centers for Disease Control and Prevention, only 13 percent of Americans eat the recommended two servings of fruit per day and 9 percent the recommended three daily servings of vegetables.

Many scientific studies have linked fruit and vegetable consumption with many health benefits, including a substantial decrease in the risk for cardiovascular disease, cancer, diabetes mellitus, obesity, high blood pressure, metabolic syndrome, and osteoporosis and increased cognitive function, among many others. And research states that, on average, people who consume five servings per day live 3 years longer than people who seldom or ever eat fruits and vegetables. Science has not yet found a way to allow people to eat a poor diet, pop a few pills, and derive the same benefits. For individuals who feel that fruits and vegetables are too expensive (as compared to what?), they are certainly much cheaper than eating out. The most valuable possession that you have is your health. Ask yourself: What is it worth to you? For health and wellness, fruits and vegetables (fresh, frozen, canned, dried, or juiced) should be included at each meal and snack.

Whole grains are a major source of fiber as well B vitamins and iron. The amount of flavorful whole-grain products in supermarkets today has substantially increased. Ten to 20 years ago, most whole-grain products were not very flavorful. Nowadays, excellent choices of whole-grain breads, flour, rice, pasta, crackers, and pancake and waffle mixes are available. Many of these products, such as brown,

GLOSSARY

Phytonutrients Compounds thought to prevent and fight cancer; found in large quantities in fruits and vegetables.

Preserving Produce Nutrients at Home

- Freeze produce immediately after harvesting. It helps retain most vitamins and minerals.

- Avoid cooking produce in water. Up to 50 percent of vitamins can be lost in the process. Steaming, stir-frying, and micro-waving are better options. If you do boil produce, reuse the cooking water in soups and sauces.

- Peel less. Nutrient content is often higher near the surface.

- Refrigerate produce. Fewer nutrients are lost in cooler temperatures.

- Chop less. The greater the surface area that is exposed to heat, light, and water, the greater the nutrient loss.

multi-grain, and wild rice, can now also be cooked in micro-waves in less than 2 minutes. Available also are many products made with whole-wheat white flour (derived from a different strain of wheat) that is lighter in color and flavor but still provides the nutrient benefits of whole grains.

Milk and milk products (select low-fat or nonfat) can decrease the risk of low bone mass (osteoporosis) throughout life. Besides calcium, other nutrients derived from milk are potassium, vitamin D, and protein.

Foods in the protein group consist of poultry, fish, eggs, nuts, legumes, and seeds. Nutrients in this group include protein, B vitamins, vitamin E, iron, zinc, and magnesium. Choose low-fat or lean meats and poultry and bake, grill, or broil them at low temperature (to prevent the formation of advanced glycation end products, see page 114). Most

Americans eat sufficient foods from this group but need to choose leaner foods and a greater variety of fish, dry beans, nuts, and seeds. In terms of meat, poultry, and fish, the rec-ommendation is to consume about 3 ounces and not to ex-ceed 6 ounces daily. All visible fat and skin should be trimmed off meats and poultry before cooking.

Oils are fats that come from different plants and fish and are liquid at room temperature. Choose carefully and avoid oils that have trans fats (check the food label) or saturated fats. Fats that are solid at room temperature come from ani-mal sources or can be made from vegetable oils through the process of hydrogenation.

As an aid to balancing your diet, the form in Activity 3.3 enables you to record your daily food intake. This record is much easier to keep than the complete nutrient analysis in Activity 3.1 and Activity 3.2. Make one copy for each day you wish to record.

To start the activity, go to www.choosemyplate.gov and establish your personal Daily Checklist based on your age, gender, height, weight, and physical activity level. Fill in your personal information and record it on the form provided in Activity 3.3. Next, whenever you have something to eat, record the food and the amount eaten according to the MyPlate standard amounts (ounce, cup, or teaspoon—Figure 3.1). Do this immediately after each meal so you will be able to keep track of your actual food intake more easily. At the end of the day, evaluate your diet by checking whether you ate the minimum required amounts for each food group. If you meet the minimum required servings at the end of each day and your caloric intake is in balance with the recommended amount, you are taking good steps to a healthier you.

Behavior Modification Planning

"Super" Foods

The following "super" foods that fight disease and promote health should be included often in the diet.

I PLAN TO / **I DID IT**

- ☐ ☐ Acai berries
- ☐ ☐ Avocados
- ☐ ☐ Bananas
- ☐ ☐ Barley
- ☐ ☐ Beans
- ☐ ☐ Beets
- ☐ ☐ Blueberries
- ☐ ☐ Broccoli

- ☐ ☐ Butternut squash
- ☐ ☐ Carrots
- ☐ ☐ Goji berries
- ☐ ☐ Grapes
- ☐ ☐ Kale
- ☐ ☐ Kiwifruit
- ☐ ☐ Flaxseeds
- ☐ ☐ Lentils
- ☐ ☐ Nuts (Brazil, walnuts)
- ☐ ☐ Salmon (wild)
- ☐ ☐ Soy
- ☐ ☐ Oats and oatmeal
- ☐ ☐ Olives and olive oil
- ☐ ☐ Onions
- ☐ ☐ Oranges

- ☐ ☐ Peppers
- ☐ ☐ Pomegranates
- ☐ ☐ Quinoa
- ☐ ☐ Strawberries
- ☐ ☐ Spinach
- ☐ ☐ Sweet potatoes
- ☐ ☐ Tea (green, black, red)
- ☐ ☐ Tomatoes
- ☐ ☐ Walnuts
- ☐ ☐ Watermelon
- ☐ ☐ Yogurt

Try It

Using this list, make a list of super foods you can add to your diet and when you can eat them (snacks/meals). List meals that you can add these foods to.

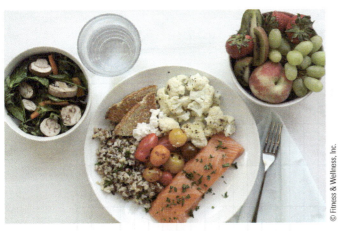

You can restructure your meals so that whole grains and vegetables constitute the major portion of the meal; meats or fish are on the side and added primarily for flavoring; fruits are used for desserts; and low-fat or nonfat milk products are used.

3.12 *Choosing Healthy Foods*

Once you have completed the nutrient analysis and the My-Plate record form (Activity 3.1, Activity 3.2, and Activity 3.3), you may conduct a self-evaluation of your current nutritional habits. In Activity 3.4, you can also assess your current stage of change regarding healthy nutrition and list strategies to help you improve your diet.

Initially, developing healthy eating habits requires a conscious effort to select nutritious foods (see box on page 112). You must learn the nutritive value of typical foods that you eat. You can do so by reading food labels and looking up the nutritive values using listings such as that provided in Appendix B or by using computer software available for such purposes.

Although not a major concern, be aware that in a few cases there is label misinformation. Whether it is a simple mistake or outright deception is difficult to determine because there is little testing of food products and there are limited risks (penalties) if label misrepresentation occurs. The FDA simply does not have adequate staffing to regularly check food labels.

A limited number of organizations are trying to help. For example, the Florida Department of Agriculture and Consumer Services has found a 10 percent violation rate in food products tested. As a consumer, you may never know which products are mislabeled, although in a few cases you may be able to discern the truth by yourself. If a product claims to be low in calories and fat but tastes "too good to be true," that may indeed be the case. For example, an independent analysis of Rising Dough Bakery cookies found that the oatmeal cranberry cookie (the size of a compact disk) had more than twice as many calories as those listed on the label.

HOEGER KEY TO WELLNESS

Preparing most meals at home is one of the surest ways to eat healthier and enjoy a longer, more productive, and better life. If you feel that you don't have time to cook, or don't care to cook, sooner or later you will have to make time to treat and care for illness and disease.

In most cases, when monitoring caloric intake, doing your own food preparation using healthy cooking methods is a better option than eating out or purchasing processed foods. The American Society for Nutrition indicates that processed foods account for approximately 50 percent of the saturated fat, 57 percent of the sodium, and 75 percent of the sugars in the American diet. Healthy eating requires proper meal planning and adequate coping strategies when confronted with situations that encourage unhealthy eating and overindulgence. Additional information on these topics is provided in the weight management chapter (Chapter 5).

3.13 *Vegetarianism*

About 7.5 million people in the United States are vegetarians and another 23 million people follow a vegetarian-inclined diet. **Vegetarians** rely primarily on foods from the bread, cereal, rice, pasta, and fruit and vegetable groups and avoid most foods from animal sources in the dairy and protein groups. The basic types of vegetarians are as follows:

1. **Vegans** eat no animal products at all.
2. **Ovovegetarians** allow eggs in the diet.
3. **Lactovegetarians** allow foods from the milk group.
4. **Ovolactovegetarians** include egg and milk products in the diet.
5. **Semivegetarians** do not eat red meat, but do include fish (pescovegetarian) and poultry in addition to milk products and eggs in their diet.

Vegetarian diets can be healthful and consistent with the Dietary Guidelines for Americans and can meet the DRIs for nutrients. Vegetarians who do not select their food combinations properly, however, can develop nutritional deficiencies of protein, vitamins, minerals, and even calories. Even greater attention should be paid when planning vegetarian diets for infants and children. Unless carefully planned, a strict plant-based diet will prevent proper growth and development.

Nutrient Concerns

In some vegetarian diets, protein deficiency can be a concern. Vegans in particular must be careful to eat foods that provide a balanced distribution of essential amino acids, such as grain

---

GLOSSARY

Vegetarians Individuals whose diet is of vegetable or plant origin.

Vegans Vegetarians who eat no animal products at all.

Ovovegetarians Vegetarians who allow eggs in their diet.

Lactovegetarians Vegetarians who eat foods from the milk group.

Ovolactovegetarians Vegetarians who include eggs and milk products in their diet.

Semivegetarians Vegetarians who include milk products, eggs, and fish and poultry in the diet.

Activity 3.3 MyPlate Record Form

Name: _____ Gender: _____ Date: _____

Course: _____ Section: _____ Age: _____

No.	Food*	Calories	Fat (gr)	Food Groups Daily Goals (see Figure 3.1) Grains (oz.)	Vegetables (cups)	Fruits (cups)	Dairy (cups)	Protein Foods (oz.)	Oils (tsp.)
1									
2									
3									
4									
5									
6									
7									
8									
9									
10									
11									
12									
13									
14									
15									
16									
17									
18									
19									
20									
21									
22									
23									
24									
25									
26									
27									
28									
29									
30									
Totals									
Recommended Amount: Obtain online at www.choosemyplate.gov based on age, gender, weight, height, and activity level		**							
Deficiencies/Excesses									

*See "List of Nutritive Value of Selected Foods" in Appendix B, available in MindTap at www.cengagebrain.com

**Multiply the recommended amount of calories by .30 (30%) and divide by 9 to obtain the daily recommended amount of grams of fat.

MINDTAP Complete This Online
From Cengage Visit **www.cengagebrain.com** to access MindTap, a complete digital course that includes interactive quizzes, videos, and more.

Activity 3.4	**Nutrition Behavior Modification Plan**

Name _____ Date _____

Course _____ Section _____ Gender _____ Age _____

Nutrition Stage of Change

Using Figure 2.7 and Table 2.3 (page 73) identify your current stage of change for nutrition (healthy diet):

[   ]

What I Learned and What I Can Do to Improve My Nutrition:

Based on the nutrient analysis and your healthy diet plan, explain what these experiences have taught you, and list specific changes and strategies that you can use to improve your present nutrition habits. Use an extra blank sheet of paper as needed.

Briefly state what you learned from the online MyPlate experience at www.choosemyplate.gov/: _____

_____

_____

_____

_____

Specific changes I plan to make: _____

_____

_____

_____

_____

Strategies I will use: _____

_____

_____

_____

_____

_____

Current number of daily steps: [   ]   **Category** (Use Table 1.4, page 25): _____

MINDTAP From Cengage   **Complete This Online**
Visit **www.cengagebrain.com** to access MindTap, a complete digital course that includes interactive quizzes, videos, and more.

Behavior Modification Planning

Selecting Nutritious Foods

To select nutritious foods:

I PLAN TO
I DID IT

1. Given the choice between whole foods and refined, processed foods, choose the former (apples rather than apple pie, potatoes rather than potato chips). No nutrients have been refined out of the whole foods, and they contain less fat, salt, and sugar.

2. Choose the leaner cuts of meat. Select fish or poultry often, beef seldom. Ask for broiled, not fried, to control your fat intake.

3. Use both raw and cooked vegetables and fruits. Raw foods offer more fiber and vitamins, such as folate and thiamine, which are destroyed by cooking. Cooking foods frees other vitamins and minerals for absorption.

4. Include milk, milk products, or other calcium sources for the calcium you need. Use low-fat or nonfat items to reduce fat and calories.

5. Learn to use margarine, butter, and oils sparingly. A little gives flavor; a lot overloads you with fat and calories.

6. Vary your choices. Eat broccoli today, carrots tomorrow, and corn the next day. Eat Chinese today, Italian tomorrow, and broiled fish with brown rice and steamed vegetables the third day.

7. Load your plate with vegetables and unrefined starchy foods. A small portion of meat or cheese is all you need for protein.

8. When choosing breads and cereals, choose the 100% whole-grain varieties.

To select nutritious fast foods:

9. Choose the broiled or grilled sandwich with lots of vegetables—and hold the mayo—rather than the crispy, crunchy, breaded, battered, or tempura fish or chicken patties.

10. Select a healthy salad—and use more plain vegetables than those mixed with oily or mayonnaise-based dressings.

11. Order chili with more beans than meat. Choose a soft bean burrito over tacos with fried shells.

12. Drink water or low-fat milk rather than a cola beverage.

When choosing from a vending machine:

13. Choose cracker sandwiches over chips and pork rinds (virtually pure fat). Choose peanuts, pretzels, and popcorn over cookies and candy.

14. Choose low-fat milk and fruit juices over cola beverages. Better yet, drink water and save your calories for actual fruits.

15. Forgo the low-nutrient density food items such as chips, pretzels, and cookies. Instead, look for fresh fruits and vegetables, hummus, 100% whole wheat crackers, and nuts.

Try It

Based on what you have learned, list strategies you can use to increase food variety, enhance the nutritive value of your diet, and decrease fat and caloric content in your meals.

Adapted from W. W. K. Hoeger, L. W. Turner, and B. Q. Hafen, *Wellness: Guidelines for a Healthy Lifestyle* Belmont, CA: (Wadsworth Cengage Learning, 2007).

---

products and legumes. Strict vegans also need a supplement of vitamin B$_{12}$. This vitamin is not found in plant foods; its only source is animal foods. Deficiency of this vitamin can lead to anemia and nerve damage.

The key to a healthful vegetarian diet is to eat foods that possess complementary proteins because most plant-based products lack one or more essential amino acids in adequate amounts. For example, both grains and legumes are good protein sources, but neither provides all the essential amino acids. Grains and cereals are low in the amino acid lysine, and legumes lack methionine. Foods from these two groups—such as combinations of tortillas and beans, rice and beans, rice and soybeans, or wheat bread and peanuts—complement each other and provide all required protein nutrients. Complementing protein foods include grains with legumes; legumes with nuts and seeds; or soy and quinoa with grains, legumes, or nuts and seeds (see

Figure 3.11). These complementary proteins may be consumed over the course of 1 day, but it is best if they are consumed during the same meal (also see discussion under Proteins on pages 93–94).

Other nutrients likely to be deficient in vegetarian diets—and ways to compensate—are as follows:

- Vitamin D can be obtained from moderate exposure to the sun or by taking a supplement.
- Riboflavin can be found in green leafy vegetables, whole grains, and legumes.
- Calcium can be obtained from fortified soybean milk or fortified orange juice, calcium-rich tofu, and selected cereals. A calcium supplement is also an option.
- Iron can be found in whole grains, dried fruits and nuts, and legumes. To enhance iron absorption, a good source of vitamin C should be consumed with these foods. (Calcium and iron are the most difficult

Figure 3.11 Complementing proteins for vegetarians.

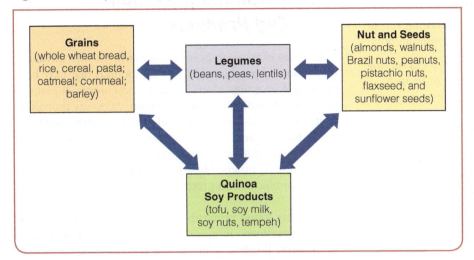

nutrients to consume in sufficient amounts in a strict vegan diet.)

- Zinc can be obtained from whole grains, wheat germ, beans, nuts, and seeds.

MyPlate also can be used as a guide for vegetarians. The key is food variety. Most vegetarians today eat dairy products and eggs. They can replace meat with legumes, nuts, seeds, eggs, and meat substitutes (tofu, tempeh, soy milk, and commercial meat replacers such as veggie burgers and soy hot dogs). For additional MyPlate healthy eating tips for vegetarians and how to get enough of the previously mentioned nutrients, go to www.choosemyplate.gov. Those who are interested in vegetarian diets are encouraged to consult additional resources because special vegetarian diet planning cannot be covered adequately in a few paragraphs.

3.14 *Nuts*

Consumption of nuts has received considerable attention in recent years. Although nuts are 70 to 90 percent fat, most of this is healthy unsaturated fats. Nuts are known to be nutrient

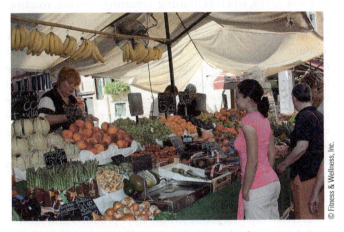

Most fruits and vegetables contain large amounts of cancer-preventing phytonutrients.

powerhouses. They are an excellent source of vitamin E and magnesium, and provide selenium, folate, vitamin K, beta-carotene, phosphorus, copper, potassium, zinc, and many phytonutrients. A combined analysis of several studies with a total of almost 355,000 participants showed that eating about a daily ounce of nuts (a medium handful) resulted in a 27 percent lower risk of all-cause mortality and a 39 percent reduced risk of cardiovascular mortality.[8] Cancer mortality also decreased when comparing the highest group of consumers with the lowest group. Previous research had already shown that people who eat nuts several times a week have a lower risk of early mortality and heart disease, and enjoy beneficial effects on cholesterol, blood pressure, respiratory disease, insulin regulation (type 2 diabetes), and blood glucose control; nuts also help decrease inflammation and the risk for dementia. Walnuts have also been shown to trigger a series of cancer-blocking changes in the body.

Nuts do have a drawback: They are high in calories. One ounce, less than a handful of nuts, provides 160 to 200 calories and a cup of mixed nuts packs 800 calories. People who snack on *modest* amounts of nuts, however, do not gain weight and nut consumption may even aid with weight loss. Because of their protein, fiber, and high unsaturated fat content, nuts are known to be satiating, leading to less snacking and eating in subsequent meals. Furthermore, due to the hard walls on their cells, nuts are resistant to digestion. About one-fifth of the fat content in nuts does not get absorbed by the body. Nuts are particularly recommended for use in place of high-protein foods such as meats, bacon, and eggs or as part of a meal in fruit or vegetable salads, homemade bread, pancakes, casseroles, yogurt, and oatmeal. Peanut butter is also healthier than cheese or some cold cuts in sandwiches.

3.15 *Soy Products*

The popularity of soy foods, including use in vegetarian diets, is attributed primarily to Asian research that points to less heart disease and fewer hormone-related cancers in people who regularly consume soy foods. A benefit of eating soy is that it replaces unhealthy animal products high in saturated fat. Soy is rich in plant protein, unsaturated fat, and fiber, and some soy is high in calcium.

The benefits of soy lie in its high protein content and plant chemicals, known as isoflavones, which act as antioxidants and are thought to protect against estrogen-related cancers (breast, ovarian, and endometrial). The compound genistein, one of many phytonutrients in soy, may reduce the risk for breast cancer, and soy consumption also may lower the risk for prostate cancer. Limited animal studies have suggested an actual increase in breast cancer risk. Human studies are still inconclusive but tend to favor a slight protective effect in premenopausal women.

Until more data become available, the following recommendations have been issued regarding soy consumption[9]:

1. Do not exceed three servings of soy per day (a serving constitutes half a cup of tofu, edamame, or tempeh; one-fourth cup of roasted soy nuts; or one cup of soy yogurt or soy milk).
2. Limit soy intake to just a few servings per week if you now have or have had breast cancer.
3. Avoid soy supplements because they may contain higher levels of isoflavones than those found in soy foods. Individuals with a history of breast cancer and women who are pregnant or lactating should especially avoid them altogether.

3.16 Probiotics

Yogurt is rated in the "super-foods" category because, in addition to being a good source of calcium, potassium, riboflavin, and protein, it contains **probiotics**. The latter are friendly "for life" microbes that are thought to rebalance the naturally present intestinal bacteria. These microorganisms help break down foods and are thought to prevent disease-causing organisms from settling in. Although low-fat or nonfat yogurt is an excellent choice, you should not consume yogurt expecting miraculous medical benefits. Probiotics have been found to offer protection against gastrointestinal infections and boost immune activity. Additional research, nonetheless, is needed to further investigate probiotic benefits.

Yogurts are cultured with *Lactobacillus bulgaricus* and *Streptococcus thermophilus* probiotics. When selecting yogurt, preferably look for low-fat or nonfat products that also contain L-acidophilus, Bifidus, and the prebiotic (substances on which probiotics feed) inulin. The latter, a soluble fiber, appears to enhance calcium absorption. Avoid yogurt with added fruit jam, sugar, and candy. Most yogurts have lots of added sugar and limited fruit. Thus, it is best to buy plain yogurt and add fresh fruit.

A fast-growing trend in nutrition is the relationship between a healthy diet and *gut microbes*. These microorganisms have a remarkable impact on the immune system and disease prevention. They feed primarily on complex/fiber-rich carbohydrates and introduce additional live bacteria to the gut. Thus, a diet high in whole plant foods, including whole grains, legumes, fruit, vegetables, seeds, nuts, and fermented foods, results in increased microbial diversity and positive health outcomes.

3.17 Advanced Glycation End Products

A new area of research in nutrition has to do with **advanced glycation end products (AGEs)**, compounds that have been implicated in aging, adverse effects, and chronic diseases by increasing oxidation and inflammation. AGEs are thought to contribute to the development of atherosclerosis, heart disease, diabetes and diabetes-related complications, kidney disease, osteoarthritis, rheumatoid arthritis, and Alzheimer's disease, among others. These compounds are produced when glucose combines with proteins, lipids, and other ingredients in foods.

AGEs are found primarily in foods cooked in dry heat, at high temperatures, in processed foods, and in foods high in fat content. Broiling, grilling, and frying create the highest levels of AGEs, whereas braising, steaming, stewing, roasting, boiling, and poaching decrease the levels. French-fried potatoes have about eight times the amount of AGEs in the same amount of a baked potato. Fast-food restaurants take advantage of the flavor-enhancing effects of AGEs by adding these toxic compounds to their foods to increase the foods' appeal to the consumer. The take-home message to the consumer here is once again moderation. You do not have to completely eliminate grilling, frying, and fast foods, but common sense is vital to maintain good health.

The following guidelines can help you decrease AGEs in your diet:

1. Limit cooking meats at high temperatures.
2. Avoid high-fat foods (whole-milk products and meats).
3. Increase intake of fruits, vegetables, grains, fish, and low-fat milk products.
4. Choose unprocessed rather than processed foods by cooking fresh foods from scratch.
5. Eat at home most of the time and avoid prepackaged and fast foods as much as possible.
6. Avoid browning. (The process of browning sugars and proteins on food surfaces increases the formation of AGEs.)

3.18 Diets From Other Cultures

Increasingly, Americans are eating foods reflecting the ethnic composition of people from other countries. Learning how to wisely select from the wide range of options is the task of those who seek a healthy diet.

Mediterranean Diet

The **Mediterranean diet** receives much attention because people in that region have notably lower rates of diet-linked diseases and a longer life expectancy. The diet focuses on minimally processed (whole) foods. It features an abundance of fresh fruits and vegetables, olive oil, whole grains, and legumes; features, in moderation, fish, red wine, nuts, and

HOEGER KEY TO WELLNESS

Decrease your risk for chronic diseases and accelerated aging by limiting red meat consumption and processed meats to less than 3.0 ounces and 1.0 ounce, respectively, two times per week or less. To minimize the consumption of advanced glycation end products (AGEs), do not cook meats at high temperatures, reduce high-fat foods, and avoid browning sugars and proteins.

Figure 3.12 Mediterranean diet pyramid.

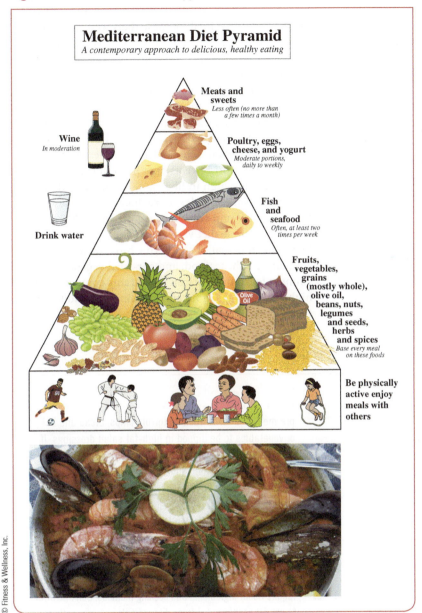

a lower incidence of heart disease (33 percent) and deaths from cancer (24 percent). Another study involving more than 120,000 men and women reported an increase in life expectancy of 15.1 and 8.4 years in women and men, respectively, who followed a combined healthy lifestyle approach: (1) regular physical activity, (2) eating a Mediterranean diet, (3) not smoking, and (4) maintaining healthy body weight.[11]

A subsequent study published in 2013, the first randomized **clinical study** on the diet, was terminated early because individuals on a Mediterranean diet had an almost 30 percent decreased risk of heart disease.[12] The Mediterranean diet has also been linked to lower risk for metabolic syndrome and stroke, improved brain health and cognitive function, lower risk for Alzheimer's disease, and better weight management. Although most people in the United States focus on the olive oil component of the diet, olive oil is used mainly as a means to increase consumption of vegetables because vegetables sautéed in oil taste better than steamed vegetables.

Ethnic Diets

As people migrate, they take their dietary practices with them. Many ethnic diets are healthier than the typical American diet because they emphasize consumption of complex carbohydrates and limit fat intake. The predominant minority ethnic groups in the United States are African American, Hispanic American, and Asian American. Unfortunately, the generally healthier ethnic diets quickly become Americanized when these groups adapt to the United

dairy products (mostly yogurt and cheese); and limits sweets, refined carbohydrates, sodium, and red and processed meats. Although it is a semivegetarian diet, up to 40 percent of the total daily caloric intake may come from fat—mostly monounsaturated fat from olive oil. Moderate intake of red wine is included with meals. The dietary plan also encourages regular physical activity (Figure 3.12).

More than a "diet," the Mediterranean diet is a dietary pattern that has existed for centuries. According to the largest and most comprehensive **observational study** on this dietary pattern, the health benefits and decreased mortality are not linked to any specific component of the diet (such as olive oil or red wine) but are achieved through the interaction of all the components of the pattern.[10] Those who adhere most closely to the dietary pattern have

© Fitness & Wellness, Inc.

---GLOSSARY---

Probiotics Healthy microbes (bacteria) that help break down foods and prevent disease-causing organisms from settling in the intestines.

Advanced glycation end products (AGEs) Derivatives of glucose-protein and glucose-lipid interactions that are linked to aging and chronic diseases.

Mediterranean diet Typical diet of people around the Mediterranean region, focusing on olive oil, red wine, fish, grains, legumes, vegetables, and fruits, with limited amounts of red meat, fish, milk, and cheese.

Observational study A research study in which the investigator does not intervene to make changes but only observes the outcomes based on a particular lifestyle pattern.

Clinical study A research study in which the investigator intervenes (makes certain changes or uses certain interventions or programs) to prevent or treat a disease.

States. Often, they cut back on vegetables and add meats and salt to the diet in conformity with the American consumer.

Ethnic dishes can be prepared at home. They are easy to make and much healthier when one uses the typical (original) variety of vegetables, corn, rice, spices, and condiments. Ethnic health recommendations also encourage daily physical activity and suggest no more than two alcoholic drinks per day. Three typical ethnic diets are as follows:

- The African American diet ("soul food") is based on the regional cuisine of the American South. Soul food includes yams, black-eyed peas, okra, and peanuts. The latter have been combined with American foods such as corn products and pork. Today, most people think of soul food as meat, fried chicken, sweet potatoes, and chitterlings.
- Many ethnic foods in the United States arrived with the conquistadores and evolved through combinations with other ethnic diets and local foods available in Latin America.

    For example, Cuban cuisine combined Spanish, Chinese, and native foods; Puerto Rican cuisine

developed from Spanish, African, and native products; and Mexican diets evolved from Spanish and native foods. Prominent in all of these diets were corn, beans, squash, chili peppers, avocados, papayas, and fish. The colonists later added rice and citrus foods. Today, the Hispanic diet incorporates a wide variety of foods, including red meat and cheese, but the staple still consists of rice, corn, and beans.

- Asian American diets are characteristically rich in vegetables and use minimal meat and fat. The Okinawan diet in Japan, where some of the healthiest and oldest people in the world live, is high in fresh (versus pickled) vegetables, high in fiber, and low in fat and salt. Chinese cuisine includes more than 200 vegetables, and fat-free sauces and seasoning are used to enhance flavor. The Chinese diet varies by region in China. The lowest in fat is that of southern China, with most meals containing fish, seafood, and stir-fried vegetables. Chinese food in American restaurants contains a much higher percentage of fat and protein than traditional Chinese cuisine.

Behavior Modification Planning

Strategies for Healthier Restaurant Eating

On average, Americans eat out six times per week. Research indicates that when dining out, most people consume too many calories and too much fat. Such practice is contributing to the growing obesity epidemic and chronic conditions afflicting most Americans in the 21st century. The following are strategies that you can implement to eat healthier when dining out.

I PLAN TO **I DID IT**

❏ ❏ Plan ahead. Decide before you get to the restaurant that you will select a healthy meal. Then stick to your decision. If you are unfamiliar with the menu, you may be able to access the menu at the restaurant's website beforehand or you can obtain valuable nutrition information at HealthyDiningFinder.com. This website is maintained by registered dietitians and provides information on many restaurant chains located in your area.

❏ ❏ Be aware of calories in drinks. You can gulp down several hundred extra calories through drinks alone. Restaurants and beverage industries are eager to get your money, and servers wouldn't mind a larger tip by having you consume additional items on the menu. Water, sparkling soda water, or unsweetened teas are good choices.

❏ ❏ Avoid or limit appetizers, regardless of how tempting they might be. Ask your server not to bring to the table high-fat

pre-meal free foods such as tortilla chips, bread and butter, or vegetables to be dipped in high-fat salad dressings. If you munch on food freebies or appetizers (or make a meal out of them), have your server box up half or the entire meal for you to take home. If you box up an entire meal, you now have two additional meals that you can consume at home; most restaurant meals can be split into two meals.

❏ ❏ Request a half-size or a child's portion. If you are unable to do so, split the meal with your dining partner or box up half the meal before you start to eat.

❏ ❏ Inquire about ingredients and cooking methods. Don't be afraid to ask for healthy substitutes. For example, you may request that meat be sautéed instead of deep fried or that canola or olive oil be used instead of other oil choices. You can also request a baked potato or brown rice instead of French fries or white rice. Ask for dressing, butter, or sour cream on the side. Request 100% whole-wheat bread for sandwiches. Furthermore, avoid high-fat foods or ingredients such as creamy or cheese sauces, butter, oils, and fatty/fried/crispy meats. When in doubt, ask the server for additional information. If the server can't answer your questions, select a different meal.

Try It

Implement as many of these strategies as possible every time you dine out. Take pride in your healthy choices. Your long-term health and well-being are at stake. You will feel much better about yourself following a healthy meal than you would otherwise.

Table 3.10 Ethnic Eating Guide

	Choose Often	Choose Less Often
Chinese	Beef with broccoli	Crispy duck
	Chinese greens	Egg rolls
	Steamed rice, brown or white	Fried rice
	Steamed beef with pea pods	Kung pao chicken (fried)
	Stir-fry dishes	Peking duck
	Teriyaki beef or chicken	Pork spareribs
	Wonton soup	
Japanese	Chiri nabe (fish stew)	Tempura (fried
	Grilled scallops	chicken, shrimp, or
	Sushi, sashimi (raw fish)	vegetables)
	Teriyaki	Tonkatsu (fried pork)
	Yakitori (grilled chicken)	
Italian	Cioppino (seafood stew)	Antipasto
	Minestrone (vegetarian soup)	Cannelloni, ravioli
	Pasta with marinara sauce	Fettuccini alfredo
	Pasta primavera (pasta with	Garlic bread
	vegetables)	White clam sauce
	Steamed clams	
Mexican	Beans and rice	Chili rellenos
	Black bean/vegetable soup	Chimichangas
	Burritos, bean	Enchiladas, beef or
	Chili	cheese
	Enchiladas, bean	Flautas
	Fajitas	Guacamole
	Gazpacho	Nachos
	Taco salad	Quesadillas
	Tamales	Tostadas
	Tortillas, steamed	Sour cream (as topping)
Middle Eastern	Tandoori chicken	Falafel
	Curry (yogurt-based)	
	Rice pilaf	
	Lentil soup	
	Shish kebab	
French	Poached salmon	Beef Wellington
	Spinach salad	Escargot
	Consommé	French onion soup
	Salad niçoise	Sauces in general
Soul Food	Baked chicken	Fried chicken
	Baked fish	Fried fish
	Roasted pork (not smothered	Smothered pork
	or "etouffe")	tenderloin
	Sautéed okra	Okra in gumbo
	Baked sweet potato	Sweet potato casserole
		or pie
Greek	Gyros	Baklava
	Pita	Moussaka
	Lentil soup	

SOURCE: Adapted from P. A. Floyd, S. E. Mimms, and C. Yelding-Howard, *Personal Health: Perspectives & Lifestyles* (Belmont, CA: Wadsworth/Cengage Learning, 1998).

All healthy diets have similar characteristics: They are high in fruits, vegetables, and grains and low in saturated fat. Healthy diets also use low-fat or fat-free dairy products, and they emphasize portion control—essential in a healthy diet plan.

Some people think that if a food item is labeled "low fat" or "fat free," they can consume it in large quantities. "Low fat" or "fat free" does not imply "calorie free." Many people who consume low-fat diets eat more (and thus increase their caloric intake), which in the long term leads to obesity and its associated health problems.

3.19 *Nutrient Supplementation*

The Academy of Nutrition and Dietetics states that consuming a wide variety of nutrient-dense foods is more effective for good health and chronic disease prevention than taking vitamin and mineral supplements. Approximately half of all adults in the United States, nonetheless, take daily nutrient **supplements**. Americans spend an estimated $32 billion on dietary supplements each year, leading to about 23,000 emergency-room visits and more than 2,000 hospitalizations per year. Weight-loss and energy-boosting supplements account for most of these ER visits, including chest pain problems and irregular and rapid heartbeat.

A significant area of concern is the safety of these products, including adulteration or ingredients not listed or present in greater or lesser quantities than indicated. In one particular case, testing vitamin D pills from one manufacturer, but different batches, yielded a range of 9 percent to 140 percent of the listed amount. The FDA estimates that 70 percent of the dietary-supplement companies fail to adhere to basic quality-control standards. The best recommendation is to look for supplements with the U.S. Pharmacopeia (USP) stamp on them. This stamp requires the supplements to contain no less than 90 percent and no more than 110 percent of the listed dose. Compliance with this standard, however, is voluntary. If the container has the USP stamp on it, you can be pretty confident that the listed potency is found in the supplement.

Nutrient requirements for the body normally can be met by consuming as few as 1,500 calories per day, as long as the diet contains the recommended amounts of food from the different food groups. Many supplements are promoted for disease prevention, yet science does not support this statement. Still, many people consider it necessary to take vitamin supplements.

It's true that the body cannot retain water-soluble vitamins as long as fat-soluble vitamins. The body excretes excessive

Table 3.10 provides a list of healthier foods to choose from when dining at selected ethnic restaurants. Additionally, you can consult the box on the previous page for strategies that you can use for healthy dining out.

GLOSSARY

Supplements Tablets, pills, capsules, liquids, or powders that contain vitamins, minerals, antioxidants, amino acids, herbs, or fiber that individuals take to increase their intake of these nutrients.

intakes readily, although it can retain small amounts for weeks or months in various organs and tissues. Fat-soluble vitamins, by contrast, are stored in fatty tissue. Therefore, daily intake of these vitamins is not as crucial.

People should not take **megadoses** of vitamins and minerals. For some nutrients, a dose of five times the RDA taken over several months may create problems. For other nutrients, it may not pose a threat to human health. Vitamin and mineral doses should not exceed the UL (with the possible exception of vitamin D; see pages 120–121). For nutrients that do not have an established UL, one day's dose should be no more than three times the RDA.

Iron deficiency (determined through blood testing) is more common in women than men. Iron supplementation is frequently recommended for women who have a heavy menstrual flow. Pregnant and lactating women also may require supplements. The average pregnant woman who eats an adequate amount of a variety of foods should take a low dose of an iron supplement daily. Women who are pregnant with more than one baby may need additional supplements. Folate supplements also are encouraged prior to and during pregnancy to prevent certain birth defects (see the following discussions of antioxidants and folate). In the previously listed instances, individuals should take supplements under a physician's supervision.

Adults older than the age of 60 may need to supplement with a daily multivitamin. Aging may decrease the body's ability to absorb and utilize certain nutrients. Nutrient deficiencies in older adults include vitamins C, D, B_6, B_{12}, folate, and the minerals calcium, zinc, and magnesium. Iron needs, however, decrease with age; thus a supplement with lower levels of iron is recommended.

Other people who may benefit from supplementation are those with nutrient deficiencies, alcoholics and street-drug users who do not have a balanced diet, smokers, vegans (strict vegetarians), individuals on low-calorie diets (fewer than 1,500 calories per day), and people with disease-related disorders or who are taking medications that interfere with proper nutrient absorption.

Although supplements may help a small group of individuals, most supplements do not provide clear benefits to healthy people who eat a balanced diet. A supplement cannot replace the array of nutrients found in whole foods. These nutrients often work in synergy; that is, the interaction of the nutrients when combined is greater than the sum of their individual effects. The synergy between nutrients in one particular food item or among fruits, vegetables, and whole grains explains why people do not derive the same benefits when taking isolated supplements as compared to eating whole foods. Studies published show that there is no clear health benefit to most vitamin and mineral supplements.

A multivitamin supplement will not act as an "insurance policy" for people with unhealthy diets because it is quite clear that it will never replace the vitamins, minerals, antioxidants, phytonutrients, anti-inflammatory properties, and additional benefits obtained by consuming fruits, vegetables, whole grains, and fiber as a part of a well-balanced diet. If you still choose to take a multivitamin, pick one that does not exceed 100 percent of the DVs for most vitamins and minerals (men and postmenopausal women are advised to select one without iron, as such is not necessary).

Understand that supplements do not prevent chronic diseases (including heart disease and cancer) or help people run faster, jump higher, relieve stress, improve sexual prowess, cure a common cold, or boost energy levels. Before deciding to take a supplement, you are encouraged to consult a reputable source, such as the National Institutes of Health (NIH) Office of Dietary Supplements (ods.od.nih.gov) or ConsumerLab.com. Also, consult with your health care provider, especially if you are pregnant, nursing, or have a medical condition such as heart disease, diabetes, or hypertension because some supplements interfere with both prescribed and over-the-counter medications.

Antioxidants

Much research and discussion are taking place regarding the effectiveness of **antioxidants** in thwarting several chronic diseases. Although foods probably contain more than 4,000 antioxidants, the four most studied antioxidants are vitamins E and C, beta-carotene (a precursor to vitamin A), and the mineral selenium (technically not an antioxidant but a component of antioxidant enzymes).

Oxygen is used during metabolism to change carbohydrates and fats into energy. During this process, oxygen is transformed into stable forms of water and carbon dioxide. A small amount of oxygen, however, ends up in an unstable form, referred to as **oxygen free radicals**. A free radical molecule has a normal proton nucleus with a single unpaired electron. Having only one electron makes the free radical extremely reactive, and it looks constantly to pair its electron with one from another molecule. When a free radical steals a second electron from another molecule, that other molecule in turn becomes a free radical. This chain reaction goes on until two free radicals meet to form a stable molecule.

Free radicals attack and damage proteins and lipids—in particular, cell membranes and DNA. This damage is thought to contribute to the development of conditions such as cardiovascular disease, cancer, emphysema, cataracts, Parkinson's disease, and premature aging. Solar radiation, cigarette smoke, air pollution, radiation, some drugs, injury, infection, chemicals (such as pesticides), and other environmental factors also seem to encourage the formation of free radicals. Antioxidants are thought to offer protection by absorbing free radicals before they can cause damage and also by interrupting the sequence of reactions once damage has begun, thwarting certain chronic diseases (Figure 3.13).

The body's own antioxidant defense systems typically neutralize free radicals so they don't cause any damage.

Figure 3.13 Antioxidant protection: blocking and absorbing oxygen free radicals to prevent chronic disease.

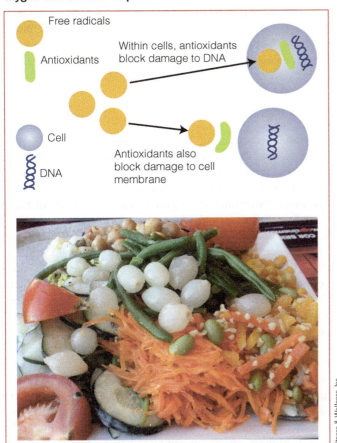

© Fitness & Wellness, Inc.

This system includes a complex network of compounds that includes enzymes and proteins. When free radicals are produced faster than the body can neutralize them, they can damage the cells; foster inflammation; and interfere with blood glucose control, blood vessel function, and normal cell growth. Research also indicates that the body's antioxidant defense system improves as fitness improves.[13] That is, physically fit people have greater protection against free radicals.

Antioxidants are found abundantly in food, especially in fruits and vegetables. Unfortunately, most Americans do not eat the minimum recommended amounts of fruits and vegetables. Plant foods enhance the body's defense system to help combat oxidative stress and its damaging effects.

Antioxidants work best in the prevention and progression of disease, but they cannot repair damage that has already occurred or cure people who have disease. The benefits are obtained primarily from food sources themselves, and controversy surrounds the benefits of antioxidants taken in supplement form.

For a few years, people believed that taking antioxidant supplements could further prevent free radical damage, but a report published in the *Journal of the American Medical Association* indicated that antioxidant supplements actually increase the risk of death.[14] Vitamin E, beta-carotene, and vitamin A increased the risk for mortality by 4 percent, 7 percent, and 16 percent, respectively. Vitamin C had no effect on mortality, while selenium decreased risk by 9 percent. Some researchers, however, have questioned the design and conclusions of this report. More research is definitely required to settle the controversy.

Vitamin E

The RDA for vitamin E is 15 mg or 22 **international units (IU).** Although no evidence indicates that vitamin E supplementation less than the upper limit of 1,000 mg per day is harmful, little or no clinical research supports any health benefits. Vitamin E is found primarily in oil-rich seeds and vegetable oils. Foods high in vitamin E include almonds, hazelnuts, peanuts, canola oil, safflower oil, cottonseed oil, kale, sunflower seeds, shrimp, wheat germ, sweet potato, avocado, and tomato sauce. You should incorporate some of these foods regularly in the diet to obtain the RDA.

Vitamin C

Studies have shown that vitamin C may offer benefits against heart disease, cancer, and cataracts. People who consume the recommended amounts of daily fruits and vegetables, nonetheless, need no supplementation because they obtain their daily vitamin C requirements through the diet alone.

Vitamin C is water soluble, and the body eliminates it in about 12 hours. For best results, consume food rich in vitamin C twice a day. High intake of a vitamin C supplement, above 500 mg per day, is not recommended. The body absorbs very little vitamin C beyond the first 200 mg per serving or dose. Foods high in vitamin C include oranges and other citrus fruit, kiwi fruit, cantaloupe, guava, bell peppers, strawberries, broccoli, kale, cauliflower, and tomatoes.

Beta-Carotene

Obtaining the daily recommended dose of beta-carotene (20,000 IU) from food sources rather than supplements is preferable. Clinical trials have found that beta-carotene supplements do not offer protection against heart disease or

---

GLOSSARY

Megadoses For most vitamins, 10 times the RDA or more; for vitamin A, 5 times the RDA.

Antioxidants Compounds such as vitamins C and E, beta-carotene, and selenium that prevent oxygen from combining with other substances in the body to form harmful compounds.

Oxygen free radicals Substances formed during metabolism that attack and damage proteins and lipids, in particular the cell membrane and DNA, leading to diseases such as heart disease, cancer, and emphysema.

International unit (IU) Measure of nutrients in foods.

cancer or provide any other health benefits. Therefore, the recommendation is to "skip the pill and eat the carrot." One medium raw carrot contains about 20,000 IU of beta-carotene. Other foods high in beta-carotene include sweet potatoes, pumpkin, cantaloupe, squash, kale, broccoli, tomatoes, peaches, apricots, mangoes, papaya, turnip greens, and spinach.

Selenium

Early research on individuals who took 200 micrograms (mcg) of selenium daily indicates that it decreased the risk for prostate, colorectal, and lung cancers and may have decreased the risk for cancers of the breast, liver, and digestive tract. More recent research, however, has failed to confirm such benefits, and experts recommend caution with selenium supplements, as such may increase the risk for diabetes.

At present, the best recommendation available is not to exceed a daily supplement of 100 mcg of selenium. Based on the current body of research, 100 to 200 mcg of selenium per day seems to provide the necessary amount of antioxidant for this nutrient. Although the UL for selenium has been set at 400 mcg, a person has no reason to take more than 200 mcg daily. Too much selenium can damage cells rather than protect them.

One Brazil nut that you crack yourself provides about 100 mcg of selenium. Shelled nuts found in supermarkets average only about 20 mcg each. Other foods high in selenium include red snapper, salmon, cod, tuna, noodles, whole grains, and meats.

Multivitamins

Although much interest has been generated in the previously mentioned individual supplements, the American people still prefer multivitamins as supplements. One-third of all Americans take a multivitamin supplement. At present, several large-scale, well-designed studies have provided no evidence that multivitamins decrease the risk for either cardiovascular disease or cancer, but they cause no harm either. The most convincing data came from a study on more than 161,000 postmenopausal women taking multivitamin pills.[15] The results showed no benefits in terms of cardiovascular, cancer, or premature mortality risk reduction in women taking a multivitamin complex for an average of 8 years compared with those who did not. A panel of experts from the NIH has indicated that there aren't enough data to support the use of multivitamins.

If you take a multivitamin for general health reasons, it doesn't grant you a license to eat carelessly. Multivitamins are not magic pills. They don't provide energy, fiber, or phytonutrients. People who eat a healthy diet, with ample amounts of fruits, vegetables, and grains, have a low risk of cardiovascular disease and cancer compared with people with deficient diets who take a multivitamin complex.

HOEGER KEY TO WELLNESS

There is no solid scientific evidence that multivitamin supplementation provides any significant health benefits. Your best choice to prevent disease and increase physical capacity is through a nutrient-rich diet.

Vitamin D

Vitamin D is attracting a lot of attention because research suggests that the vitamin possesses anticancer properties, especially against breast, colon, and prostate cancers and, possibly, lung and digestive cancers. It is also believed that it decreases inflammation, fighting cardiovascular disease, periodontal disease, and atherosclerosis. Furthermore, other scientists believe that vitamin D strengthens the immune system, controls blood pressure, helps maintain muscle strength, decreases the risk for arthritis and dementia, prevents birth defects, and may help deter diabetes and fight depression. Vitamin D is necessary for absorption of calcium, a nutrient critical for building and maintaining bones to prevent osteoporosis and for dental health.

The theory that vitamin D protects against cancer is based on studies showing that people who live farther north (who have less sun exposure during the winter months) have a higher incidence of cancer. Furthermore, people diagnosed with breast, colon, or prostate cancer during the summer months, when vitamin D production by the body is at its highest, are 30 percent less likely to die from cancer, even 10 years following the initial diagnosis. Researchers think that vitamin D level at the time of cancer onset affects survival rates.

Technically, vitamin D is a prohormone. Its metabolic product, calcitriol, is a secosteroid hormone that influences more than 2,000 genes affecting health and well-being. During the winter months, most people in the United States living north of a 35-degree latitude (above the states of Georgia and Texas) and in Canada are not getting enough vitamin D. The body uses ultraviolet B (UVB) rays to generate vitamin D. UVB rays are shorter than ultraviolet A rays, so they penetrate the atmosphere at higher angles. During the winter season, the sun is too far south for the UVB rays to get through.

In 2010, the Institute of Medicine of the NAS increased the DRI of vitamin D to 600 IU (15 mcg) for children and adults up to 70 years of age. Older adults should get 800 IU (20 mcg) per day. Vitamin D experts had hoped for higher levels, considering these amounts to be too low for most individuals, especially during the winter months. Preliminary evidence suggests that people should get between 1,000 and 2,000 IU (25 to 50 mcg) of vitamin D per day. For now, the UL has been set at 2,000 IU (50 mcg).

The most accurate test to measure how much vitamin D is in the body is the 25-hydroxyvitamin D test. Currently, there is no consensus as to the optimal blood level of vitamin D. Most leaders in the field recommend a blood level of at least

30 nanograms per milliliter (ng/mL) throughout the year, while some recommend a level between 40 and 50 ng/mL. The majority of laboratories classify a range of 30 to 100 ng/ml as optimal and between 12 and 29 ng/mL as moderately deficient. Toxicity, although rare, may occur at blood levels above 150 ng/mL. If you are deficient, the Vitamin D Council recommends that all adults supplement their diets with 5,000 IU of vitamin D daily for 3 months and then take a 25-hydroxyvitamin D test.[16] You may then adjust your supplement dosage based on your test results, daily sun exposure, and the season of the year.

Depending on skin tone and sun intensity, about 15 minutes of unprotected sun exposure (without sunscreen) of the face, arms, hands, and lower legs during peak daylight hours (10:00 a.m. and 4:00 p.m.—when your shadow is shorter than your actual height) generates between 2,000 and 5,000 IU of vitamin D. Thus, it makes no sense that the UL is set at 2,000 when the human body manufactures more than that in just 15 minutes of unprotected sun exposure. The UL of 2,000 IU will most likely be revised in the next update of the DRI.

Good sources of vitamin D in the diet include salmon, mackerel, tuna, and sardines. Fortified milk, yogurt, orange juice, margarines, and cereals are also good sources. To obtain up to 2,000 IU per day from food sources alone, however, is difficult (see Table 3.11). Thus, daily safe sun exposure and supplementation (especially during the winter months) are highly recommended.

The best source of vitamin D is sunshine. UVB rays lead to the production on the surface of the skin of inactive oil-soluble vitamin D_3. The inactive form is then transformed by the liver, and subsequently the kidneys, into the active form of vitamin D. Sun-generated vitamin D is better than that obtained from foods or supplements.

Vitamin D_3 generated on the surface of the skin, however, doesn't immediately penetrate into the blood. It takes up to 48 hours to absorb most of the vitamin. Because it is an oil-soluble compound, experts recommend that you avoid using soap following safe sun exposure, as it would wash off most of the vitamin. You may use soap for your armpits, groin area, and feet, but avoid using soap on the newly sun-exposed skin.

Excessive sun exposure can lead to skin damage and skin cancer. It is best to strive for daily *safe sun* exposure, that is, 10 to 20 minutes (based on skin tone and sun intensity) of unprotected sun exposure during peak hours of the day a few times a week. Generating too much vitamin D from the sun is impossible because the body generates only what it needs. If you have sensitive skin, you may start with 5 minutes and progressively increase sun exposure by 1 minute per day. If your skin turns a slight pink following exposure, you have overdone it and need to cut back on the time that you are out in the sun.

People at the highest risk for low vitamin D levels are older adults, those with dark skin (they make less vitamin D), and individuals who spend most of their time indoors and get little sun exposure. On average, a 65-year-old person synthesizes only about 25 percent as much vitamin D as a 20-year-old from similar sun exposure. Over a span of 6 to 7 years, individuals 65 and older with low blood levels of vitamin D are two-and-a-half times more likely to die in that time frame than those with high levels, two studies have found. People with darker skin also need 5 to 10 times the sun exposure of lighter-skinned people to generate the same amount of vitamin D. The skin's dark pigment reduces the ability of the body to synthesize vitamin D from the sun by up to 95 percent.

In the United States and Canada, most of the population does not make vitamin D from the sun during the winter months when UVB rays do not get through; most people's time is spent indoors, and extra clothing is worn to protect against the cold. According to data, about 40 percent of the United States population doesn't have a 25-hydroxyvitamin D level of even 20 ng/mL. The highest deficiency rate is seen in Blacks and Hispanics, with about 80 percent and 70 percent deficiency rates, respectively. During periods of limited sun exposure, you should consider a daily vitamin D_3 supplement of up to 2,000 IU per day. Some vitamins contain vitamin D_2, which is a less potent form of the vitamin. In addition to the previously discussed conditions, vitamin D production also decreases during cloudy weather conditions, with the use of sunscreen or protective clothing, and at lower altitudes because the sun's rays travel through more atmosphere prior to reaching the earth's surface.

Folate

Although it is not an antioxidant, 400 mcg of **folate** (a B vitamin) is recommended for all premenopausal women. Folate helps prevent some birth defects and seems to offer protection against colon and cervical cancers. Women who might become pregnant should plan to take a folate

Table 3.11 Good Sources of Vitamin D

Food	Amount	IU*
Multivitamins (most brands)	Daily dose	400
Salmon	3.5 oz	360
Mackerel	3.5 oz	345
Sardines (oil/drained)	3.5 oz	250
Shrimp	3.5 oz	200
Orange juice (D-fortified)	8 oz	100
Milk (any type/D-fortified)	8 oz	100
Margarine (D-fortified)	1 tbsp	60
Yogurt (D-fortified)	6-8 oz	60
Cereal (D-fortified)	¾-1 C	40
Egg	1	20

*IU = International units

GLOSSARY

Folate One of the B vitamins.

Sun Exposure

Managing sun exposure is critical to optimal health and disease prevention. Use the following information to help you gauge how to achieve sufficient vitamin D levels through sunlight exposure while avoiding overexposure and risk for skin cancer. To reach adequate vitamin D levels throughout the year, you either need to take a vitamin D supplement or expose your face, arms, and lower legs to the sun several times a week for a short amount of time: Roughly half the time it takes your skin to begin to turn pink. Overexposure to sun is a major risk factor for skin cancer and should be completely avoided (one or two sunburns in youth alone can cause skin cancer later in life). Once you have been exposed to sunlight for a few minutes on a near-daily basis, find shade or cover up.

Sun exposure changes with

- *Weather conditions.* Direct sunlight hastens exposure while cloudy conditions subdue it.

- *Skin color.* Lighter skin takes less time than darker skin to obtain sufficient levels of sunlight for vitamin D generation. Lighter skin also takes less time for skin damage to occur.

- *Sunscreen, protective clothing, and amount of skin you exposed.* The more skin that is exposed to the sun the more vitamin D your body will produce. To avoid cancer risk, sunscreen needs to be reapplied continuously, or protective clothing must be worn.

- *Altitude.* At high altitudes the sun travels through less atmosphere so exposure happens more rapidly.

- *Reflection.* Reflection from sand, water, or snow increases both vitamin D production and the risk for skin damage.

- *Glass.* UVB rays are blocked by glass, making sunlight exposure through glass not viable for vitamin D production. Glass lets UVA rays through, allowing for skin tanning but at a slower rate.

- *Soap.* Skin sun-exposed areas should not be washed with soap for up to 48 hours following exposure if the skin is to produce vitamin D.

- *Time of day.* Sun exposure is greatest at midday, generally between the hours of 10 a.m. and 4 p.m. Use the shadow test to gauge sun exposure. If your shadow is shorter than your height, sun exposure is at its strongest and is sufficient for optimal vitamin D production (but you also are more apt to suffer skin damage if overexposed).

- *Time of year.* Summer sun exposure is more direct than winter sun exposure.

- *Latitude.* The closer you are to the equator the more direct the sun's rays. Higher latitudes require the sun to travel through more atmosphere because it travels at an angle. This is one reason vacationers to tropical locations often underestimate the direct angle of the sun and their need for sun protection. High latitudes during winter months do not have any time of day when sunlight is direct enough to cause vitamin D production.

---

supplement because studies have shown that folate before and during pregnancy can prevent serious birth defects (in particular, spina bifida). Some of these defects occur during the first few days and weeks of pregnancy. Adequate folate intake can also prevent congenital heart defects, early miscarriages, and premature birth. Thus, women who may become pregnant need to have adequate folate levels before conception and throughout pregnancy.

Some evidence also indicates that adequate intake of folate along with vitamins B_6 and B_{12} prevents heart attacks by reducing homocysteine levels in the blood (see Chapter 10). High concentrations of homocysteine accelerate the process of plaque formation (atherosclerosis) in the arteries. Five servings of fruits and vegetables per day usually meet the needs for these nutrients. Almost nine of ten adults in the United States do not obtain the recommended 400 mcg of folate per day, and less than 8 percent eat the recommended daily servings of fruits and vegetables.

With the possible exception of women of childbearing age, obtaining your daily folate RDA from natural foods is preferable to getting it from supplements. The UL for folate has been set at 1,000 mcg/day. Evidence suggests that exceeding 1,000 mcg through a combination of diet and supplements may actually fuel the progression of precancerous growths

and cancer.[17] A daily multivitamin or a serving of a highly fortified cereal each provide 400 mcg of folate. In combination with a supplement, one can easily exceed the UL of 1,000 mcg/day. To date, no data have linked folate obtained from natural foods to increased cancer risk. On the contrary, natural foods have been found to have a cancer-protective effect.

In an updated recommendation released in 2014, the U.S. Preventive Services Task Force concludes that, "the current evidence is insufficient to assess the balance of benefits and harms of the use of multivitamins for the prevention of cardiovascular disease or cancer." Many nutrition supplements are promoted to prevent disease, yet the scientific evidence does not support this notion.

A further word of caution when taking supplements: The quality and safety of dietary supplements in today's market is questionable. Supplements are exempt from the strict regulatory oversight applied to prescription drugs, and often, they do not contain the ingredient(s) or nutrient(s) listed on the label. According to the American College of Gastroenterology, some of these supplements taken over a long term or in high doses can be toxic to the human body. There is no shortcut to healthy nutrition: You are better off eating right and not relying on supplements for health and wellness.

3.20 *Benefits of Foods*

In its latest position statement on nutrient supplements, the Academy of Nutrition and Dietetics indicates that the best nutrition-based strategy for promoting optimal health and reducing the risk of chronic disease is to wisely choose a wide variety of foods. Additional nutrients from supplements can help some people meet their nutrient needs, as specified by science-based nutrition standards such as the DRIs.[18]

Fruits and vegetables are the richest sources of antioxidants and phytonutrients. For example, researchers at the USDA compared the antioxidant effects of vitamins C and E with those of various common fruits and vegetables. The results indicated that three-fourths of a cup of cooked kale (which contains only 11 IU of vitamin E and 76 mg of vitamin C) neutralized as many free radicals as did approximately 800 IU of vitamin E or 600 mg of vitamin C. A list of top antioxidant foods is presented in Table 3.12.

Many people who eat unhealthily think that they need supplementation to balance their diets. This is a fallacy about nutrition. The problem here is not necessarily a lack of vitamins and minerals, but rather a diet too high in calories, saturated fat, trans fats, and sodium. Vitamin, mineral, and fiber supplements do not supply all of the nutrients and other beneficial substances present in food and needed for good health.

Wholesome foods contain vitamins, minerals, carbohydrates, fiber, proteins, fats, and phytonutrients, along with other substances not yet discovered. Researchers do not know whether the protective effects are caused by the antioxidants alone, by a combination of antioxidants with other nutrients, or by some other nutrients in food that have not been investigated yet. Many nutrients work in **synergy**, enhancing chemical processes in the body.

As stated previously, supplementation will not offset poor eating habits. Pills are no substitute for common sense. If you think your diet is not balanced, you first need to conduct a nutrient analysis (see Activity 3.1 and Activity 3.2) to determine which nutrients you lack in sufficient amounts. Eat more of them, as well as foods that are high in antioxidants and phytonutrients. Following a nutrient assessment, a **registered dietitian (RD)** can help you decide what supplement(s), if any, might be necessary.

Furthermore, the AHA does not recommend antioxidant supplements either, until more definite research is available. If you take any supplements in pill form, however, look for products that meet the disintegration standards of the USP on the bottle. The USP standard suggests that the supplement should completely dissolve in 45 minutes or less. Supplements that do not dissolve, of course, cannot get into the bloodstream.

Critical Thinking

Do you take supplements? If so, for what purposes are you taking them—and do you think you could restructure your diet so that you could do without them?

3.21 *Functional Foods*

Functional foods are foods or food ingredients that offer specific health benefits beyond those supplied by the traditional nutrients they contain. Many functional foods come in their natural forms. A tomato, for example, is a functional food because it contains the phytonutrient lycopene, thought to reduce the risk for prostate cancer. Other examples of functional foods are kale, broccoli, blueberries, red grapes, and green tea.

The term "functional food," however, has been used primarily as a marketing tool by the food industry to attract consumers. Unlike **fortified foods,** which have been modified to help prevent nutrient deficiencies, functional

Table 3.12 Top Antioxidant Foods

Food
Red beans
Wild blueberries
Red kidney beans
Pinto beans
Blueberries
Cranberries
Artichokes
Blackberries
Kale
Prunes
Raspberries

SOURCE: U.S. Department of Agriculture.

GLOSSARY

Synergy A reaction in which the result is greater than the sum of its two parts.

Registered dietitian (RD) A person with a college degree in dietetics who meets all certification and continuing education requirements of the Academy of Nutrition and Dietetics or Dietitians of Canada.

Functional foods Foods or food ingredients containing physiologically active substances that provide specific health benefits beyond those supplied by basic nutrition.

Fortified foods Foods that have been modified by the addition or increase of nutrients that either were not present or were present in insignificant amounts with the intent of preventing nutrient deficiencies.

Behavior Modification Planning

Guidelines for a Healthy Diet

I PLAN TO	I DID IT	
❏	❏	Use portion control by keeping them small to moderate.
❏	❏	Base your diet on a large variety of foods and focus on high-fiber foods.
❏	❏	Consume a rainbow of colors, including ample amounts of green, yellow, red, blue/purple, and orange fruits and vegetables.
❏	❏	Eat more whole grains, foods high in complex carbohydrates, including at least three 1-ounce servings of whole-grain foods per day. Limit refined carbohydrates.
❏	❏	Eat foods rich in vitamin D.
❏	❏	Maintain adequate daily calcium intake from food sources and consider a supplement with vitamin D_3.
❏	❏	Consume protein in moderation and spread it out throughout the day.
❏	❏	Limit meat consumption to three ounces per day and minimize the use of red and processed meats.
❏	❏	Emphasize healthy unsaturated fats and limit trans fat and saturated fat intake.
❏	❏	Limit sodium intake to 2,300 mg per day.
❏	❏	Limit sugar intake.
❏	❏	Limit liquid calories, especially those with added sugar.
❏	❏	If you drink alcohol, do so in moderation (one daily drink for women and two for men).
❏	❏	Obtain most vitamins and minerals from food sources. If deficient, consider taking a daily multivitamin (preferably one that includes vitamin D_3).

Try It

Carefully analyze these guidelines and note the areas where you can improve your diet. Work on one guideline each week until you are able to adhere to all of the guidelines.

MINDTAP From Cengage **Complete This Online**
Visit **www.cengagebrain.com** to access MindTap, a complete digital course that includes interactive quizzes, videos, and more.

foods are created by the food industry by the addition of ingredients aimed at treating or preventing symptoms or disease. In functional foods, the added ingredients are typically not found in the food item in its natural form but are added to allow manufacturers to make appealing health claims.

In most cases, only one extra ingredient is added (a vitamin, mineral, phytonutrient, or herb). An example is calcium added to orange juice to make the claim that a brand offers protection against osteoporosis. Food manufacturers now offer cholesterol-lowering margarines (enhanced with plant stanol), cancer-protective ketchup (fortified with lycopene), memory-boosting candy (with ginkgo added), calcium-fortified chips, and corn chips containing kava kava (to enhance relaxation).

The use of some functional foods, however, may undermine good nutrition. Margarines still may contain saturated fats or partially hydrogenated oils. Regularly consuming ketchup on top of large orders of fries adds many calories and fat to the diet. Sweets are also high in calories and sugar. Chips are high in calories, salt, and fat. In all of these cases, the consumer would be better off taking the specific ingredient in a supplement form rather than consuming the functional food with its extra calories, sugar, salt, and/or fat.

Functional foods can provide added benefits if used in conjunction with a healthful diet. You may use nutrient-dense functional foods in your overall wellness plan as an adjunct to health-promoting strategies and treatments.

3.22 *Organic Foods*

Concerns over food safety have led many people to turn to organic foods. Currently, there is no solid evidence that organic food is more nutritious than conventional food, but pesticide residues in organic foods are substantially lower than in conventionally grown foods. Health risks from pesticide exposure from foods are relatively small for healthy adults. The health benefits of produce far outweigh the risks. Children, older adults, pregnant and lactating women, and people with weak immune systems, however, may be vulnerable to some types of pesticides.

Organic foods, including crops, meat, poultry, eggs, and dairy products, are produced under strict government regulations in the way they are grown, handled, and processed. Organic crops have to be grown without the use of conventional pesticides, artificial fertilizers, human waste, or sewage sludge and have to be processed without ionizing radiation or food additives. Harmful microbes in manure must also be destroyed prior to use, and genetically modified organisms may not be used. Organic livestock are raised under certain grazing conditions, use organic feed, and are raised without the use of antibiotics and growth hormones.

Organic foods can just as easily be contaminated with bacteria, pathogens, and heavy metals that pose major health risks. The soil itself may become contaminated, or if the produce comes in contact with feces of grazing cattle, wild animals/birds, farm workers, or any other source, potentially harmful microorganisms can contaminate the produce. The

Behavior Modification Planning

Minimizing the Risk of Food Contamination and Pesticide Residues

Most food is safe to eat, but there is no 100 percent guarantee that all produce is free of contamination.

I PLAN TO **I DID IT**

❑ ❑ Wash your hands thoroughly before and after touching raw produce.

❑ ❑ Do not place raw fruits and vegetables next to uncooked meat, poultry, or fish.

❑ ❑ Trim all visible fat from meat and remove the skin from poultry and fish prior to cooking (pesticides concentrate in animal fat).

❑ ❑ Rinse, scrub, and peel. Use a scrub brush to wash fresh produce under running water. Pay particular attention to crevices in the produce. Washing fresh produce reduces pesticide levels but does not completely eliminate them. Eat a variety of foods to decrease exposure to any given pesticide.

❑ ❑ Select produce that is free of dirt and does not have holes or cuts or other signs of spoilage.

❑ ❑ Discard the outermost leaves of leafy vegetables such as lettuce and cabbage.

❑ ❑ Cut your own fruits and vegetables instead of getting them precut. Wash all produce thoroughly before cutting, even melons and avocados. Cutting into potentially contaminated (unwashed) inedible rinds of fruit can contaminate the inside of the fruit. Always use a knife to remove orange peels instead of biting into them. Peel waxed fruits and vegetables and other produce as necessary (cucumbers, carrots, peaches, and apples).

❑ ❑ Store produce in the refrigerator in clean containers or clean plastic bags. (Previously used bags that are not kept cold can grow harmful bacteria.)

❑ ❑ For some produce, consider buying certified organic foods. Look for the "USDA Organic" seal. According to data from the Environmental Working Group, a nonprofit consumer activist organization, conventional produce with the most pesticide residue includes peaches, apples, sweet bell peppers, celery, nectarines, strawberries, grapes, lettuce, imported grapes, pears, spinach, and potatoes. Among the least contaminated are onions, avocados, sweet corn, pineapples, mangos, sweet peas, asparagus, kiwifruit, bananas, cabbage, broccoli, and eggplant (list of foods downloaded from https://www.ewg.org/foodnews/).

Try It

Lifestyle behavior patterns are difficult to change. These recommendations can minimize your risk of food contamination and ingestion of pesticide residues. Make a copy of the recommendations and determine how many of these suggestions you are able to include in daily life over the course of the next 7 days.

---

best safeguard to protect yourself is to follow the food safety guidelines provided on the previous page.

3.23 *Genetically Modified Crops*

In a genetically modified organism (GMO), the DNA (or basic genetic material) is genetically engineered (manipulated or modified) to obtain certain results. This is done by inserting genes with desirable traits from one plant, animal, or microorganism into another one to either introduce new traits or enhance existing traits.

Crops are genetically modified to make them better resist disease and extreme environmental conditions (such as heat and frost), require fewer fertilizers and pesticides, last longer, and improve their nutrient content and taste. GMOs could help save billions of dollars by producing more crops and helping to feed the hungry in developing countries around the world.

Concern over the safety of **genetically engineered (GE) foods** has led to heated public debates in Europe and, to a lesser extent, in the United States. The concern is that genetic modifications create "transgenic" organisms that have not previously existed and that have potentially unpredictable effects on the environment and on humans. Also, there is some concern that GE foods may cause illness or allergies in humans and that cross-pollination may destroy other plants or create "superweeds" with herbicide-resistant genes. Some researchers believe that GE crops have increased usage of harmful herbicides, causing an overall negative impact on the environment.

GE crops were first introduced into the United States in 1996. This technology is moving forward so rapidly that the USDA already has approved more than 60 GE crops. Avoiding GE foods is difficult because more than 75 percent of processed foods on the market today contain GMOs. Currently, the FDA does not mandate labels for foods

GLOSSARY

Genetically engineered (GE) foods Foods whose basic genetic material (DNA) is manipulated by inserting genes with desirable traits from one plant, animal, or microorganism into another one either to introduce new traits or to enhance existing ones.

containing GE ingredients. At least 64 other countries are currently requiring labeling of GE foods.

Americans have been consuming GE foods for two decades now with no apparent detrimental health consequences. If people do not wish to consume GE foods, organic foods are an option because organic trade organizations do not certify foods with genetic modifications. Produce bought at the local farmers' market also may be an option because small farmers are less likely to use this technology.

At this point, the World Health Organization, the American Medical Association, and the National Academy of Sciences have indicated that there is no evidence of any hazards from GE foods. Many questions remain, and much research is required in this field. As a consumer, you must continue educating yourself as more evidence becomes available in the next few years.

3.24 Energy Substrates for Physical Activity

The two main fuels that supply energy for physical activity are glucose (sugar) and fat (fatty acids). The body uses amino acids, derived from proteins, as an energy substrate when glucose is low, such as during fasting, prolonged aerobic exercise, or a low-carbohydrate diet.

Glucose is derived from foods that are high in carbohydrates, such as breads, cereals, grains, pasta, beans, fruits, vegetables, and sweets in general. Glucose is stored as glycogen in muscles and the liver. Fatty acids (discussed on pages 88–93) are the product of the breakdown of fats. Unlike glucose, an almost unlimited supply of fatty acids, stored as fat in the body, can be used during exercise.

Energy (ATP) Production

The energy derived from food is not used directly by the cells. It is first transformed into **adenosine triphosphate (ATP)**. The subsequent breakdown of this compound provides the energy used by all energy-requiring processes of the body (Figure 3.14).

ATP must be recycled continually to sustain life and work. ATP can be resynthesized in three ways:

1. *ATP-CP system.* The body stores small amounts of ATP and creatine phosphate (CP). These stores are used during all-out activities such as sprinting, long jumping, and weight lifting. The amount of stored ATP provides energy for just 1 or 2 seconds. During brief all-out efforts, ATP is resynthesized from CP, another high-energy phosphate compound. This is the ATP-CP, or phosphagen, system. Depending on the amount of physical training, the concentration of CP stored in cells is sufficient to allow maximum exertion for up to 10 seconds. Once the CP stores are depleted, the person is forced to slow down or rest to allow ATP to form through anaerobic and aerobic pathways.

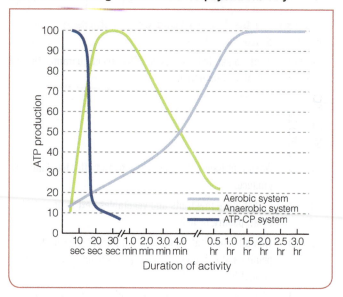

Figure 3.14 Contributions of the energy formation mechanisms during various forms of physical activity.

2. *Anaerobic or lactic acid system.* During maximal-intensity exercise that is sustained for 10 to 180 seconds, ATP is replenished primarily from the breakdown of glucose through a series of chemical reactions that do not require oxygen (hence, "anaerobic"). In the process, though, **lactic acid** is produced. As lactic acid accumulates, it leads to muscle fatigue.

   Because of the accumulation of lactic acid with high-intensity exercise, the formation of ATP during anaerobic activities is limited to about 3 minutes. A recovery period of several minutes then is necessary to allow for the removal of lactic acid. Formation of ATP through the anaerobic system requires glucose (carbohydrates).

3. *Aerobic system.* The production of energy during slow-sustained exercise is derived primarily through aerobic metabolism. Glucose (carbohydrates), fatty acids (fat), and oxygen (hence "aerobic") are required to form ATP using this process; and under steady-state exercise conditions, lactic acid accumulation is minimal or nonexistent.

Because oxygen is required, a person's capacity to utilize oxygen is crucial for successful athletic performance in aerobic events. The higher one's maximal oxygen uptake (VO_{2max}) (see pages 224–225), the greater one's capacity to generate ATP through the aerobic system—and the better one's athletic performance in long-distance events. From the previous discussion, it becomes evident that for optimal performance, both recreational and highly competitive athletes must make the required nutrients a part of their diet.

3.25 Nutrition for Athletes

During resting conditions, fat supplies about two-thirds of the energy to sustain the body's vital processes. During exercise, the body uses both glucose (glycogen) and fat in combination to supply the energy demands. The proportion of fat to glucose changes with the intensity of exercise. When a person is exercising below 60 percent of his or her maximal work capacity (VO$_{2max}$), fat is used as the primary energy substrate. As the intensity of exercise increases, so does the percentage of glucose utilization—up to 100 percent during maximal work that can be sustained for only 2 to 3 minutes. In general, athletes do not require special supplementation or any other special type of diet. Unless the diet is deficient in basic nutrients, no special secret or magic diet will help people perform better or develop faster as a result of what they eat. As long as they eat a balanced diet—that is, based on a large variety of nutrients from all basic food groups—athletes do not require additional supplements. Even in strength-training and bodybuilding, protein in excess of 20 percent of total daily caloric intake is not necessary. The recommended daily protein intake ranges from 0.8 gram per kilogram of body weight for sedentary people to 2.0 grams per kilogram for extremely active individuals (Table 3.4).

The main difference between a sensible diet for a sedentary person and a sensible diet for a highly active individual is the total number of calories required daily and the amount of carbohydrate intake needed during prolonged physical activity. People in training consume more calories because of their greater energy expenditure—which is required as a result of intense physical training.

Carbohydrate Loading

On a regular diet, the body is able to store between 1,500 and 2,000 calories in the form of glycogen. About 75 percent of this glycogen is stored in muscle tissue. This amount, however, can be increased greatly through **carbohydrate loading**.

A regular diet should be altered during several days of heavy aerobic training or when a person is going to participate in a long-distance event of more than 90 minutes (e.g., marathon, triathlon, road cycling). For events shorter than 90 minutes, carbohydrate loading does not seem to enhance performance.

During prolonged exercise, glycogen is broken down into glucose, which then is readily available to the muscles for energy production. In comparison with fat, glucose frequently is referred to as the "high-octane fuel" because it provides about 6 percent more energy per unit of oxygen consumed.

Heavy training over several consecutive days leads to depletion of glycogen faster than it can be replaced through the diet. Glycogen depletion with heavy training is common in athletes. Signs of depletion include chronic fatigue, difficulty in maintaining accustomed exercise intensity, and lower performance.

On consecutive days of exhaustive physical training (this means several hours daily), a carbohydrate-rich diet—70 percent of total daily caloric intake or 8 grams of carbohydrate per kilogram (2.2 pounds) of body weight—is recommended. This diet often restores glycogen levels in 24 hours. Along with the high-carbohydrate diet, a day of rest or a day

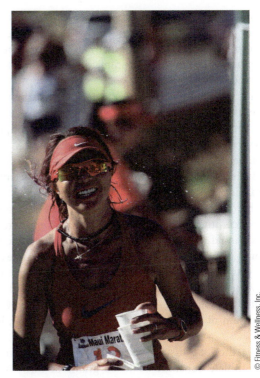

Fluid and carbohydrate replenishment during exercise is essential when participating in long-distance aerobic endurance events, such as a marathon or a triathlon.

© Fitness & Wellness, Inc.

with decreased training intensity is needed to allow the muscles to recover from glycogen depletion following days of intense training. For people who exercise less than an hour a day, a 60 percent carbohydrate diet, or 6 grams of carbohydrate per kilogram of body weight, is enough to replenish glycogen stores.

Following an exhaustive workout, eating a combination of carbohydrates and protein (such as a tuna sandwich) within 30 minutes of exercise seems to speed up glycogen storage even more. Protein intake increases insulin activity, thereby enhancing glycogen replenishment. A 70 percent carbohydrate intake then should be maintained throughout the rest of the day.

By following a special diet and exercise regimen 5 days before a long-distance event, highly (aerobically) trained individuals are capable of storing two to three times the amount of glycogen found in the average person. Athletic performance may be enhanced for long-distance events of more than 90 minutes by eating a regular balanced diet

GLOSSARY

Adenosine triphosphate (ATP) A high-energy chemical compound that the body uses for immediate energy.

Lactic acid End product of anaerobic glycolysis (metabolism).

Carbohydrate loading Increasing intake of carbohydrates during heavy aerobic training or prior to aerobic endurance events that last longer than 90 minutes.

(50 to 60 percent carbohydrates), along with intensive physical training on the fifth and fourth days before the event, followed by a diet high in carbohydrates (about 70 percent) and a gradual decrease in training intensity over the last 3 days before the event.

The amount of glycogen stored as a result of a carbohydrate-rich diet does not seem to be affected by the proportion of complex and simple carbohydrates. The intake of simple carbohydrates (sugars) can be raised while on a 70 percent carbohydrate diet, as long as it doesn't exceed 25 percent of the total calories. Complex carbohydrates provide more nutrients and fiber, making them a better choice for a healthier diet.

On the day of the long-distance event, carbohydrates are still the recommended choice of substrate. As a general rule, athletes should consume 1 gram of carbohydrates for each kilogram (2.2 pounds) of body weight 1 hour prior to exercise (i.e., if you weigh 160 pounds, you should consume 160 ÷ 2.2 = 72 grams). If the pre-event meal is eaten earlier, the amount of carbohydrates can be increased to 2, 3, or 4 grams per kilogram of weight 2, 3, or 4 hours, respectively, before exercise.

During the long-distance event, researchers recommend that the athlete consume 30 to 60 grams of carbohydrates (120 to 240 calories) every hour. This is best accomplished by drinking 8 ounces of a 6 to 8 percent carbohydrate sports drink every 15 minutes (check labels to ensure proper carbohydrate concentration). This also lessens the chance of dehydration during exercise, which hinders performance and endangers health. The percentage of the carbohydrate drink is determined by dividing the amount of carbohydrate (in grams) by the amount of fluid (in milliliters) and then multiplying by 100. For example, 18 grams of carbohydrate in 240 milliliters (8 ounces) of fluid yields a drink that is 7.5 percent (18 ÷ 240 × 100) carbohydrate.

Strenuous Exercise and Strength Training

Meeting your protein needs close to your training time is critical during high-intensity aerobic workouts and in strength training. Minute tears in muscle tissue occur during intense training. The availability of protein to the muscles promotes faster repair and development and may even prevent damage from taking place in the first place. Thus, consuming a light carbohydrate/protein snack 30 to 60 minutes prior to intense exercise and immediately following exercise (10 to 20 g of protein) is beneficial to repair and maintain muscle and further promote muscle growth. Additional protein taken with meals throughout the day is needed for optimal development. More information on this topic is provided in Chapter 7 under "Dietary Guidelines for Strength and Muscular Development" (page 274).

Hyponatremia

In some cases, athletes participating in long- or ultra-long-distance races may suffer from **hyponatremia**, or low sodium concentration in the blood. The longer the race, the greater the risk of hyponatremia. This condition occurs as lost sweat, which contains salt and water, is replaced by only water (no salt) during a very long-distance race. Although the athlete is overhydrated, blood sodium is diluted and hyponatremia occurs. Typical symptoms are similar to those of heat illness and include fatigue, weakness, disorientation, muscle cramps, bloating, nausea, dizziness, confusion, slurred speech, fainting, and even seizures and coma in severe cases.

Based on estimates, about 30 percent of the participants in the Hawaii Ironman Triathlon suffer from hyponatremia. The condition, however, is rare in the everyday exerciser. To help prevent hyponatremia, athletes should ingest extra sodium prior to the event and then adequately monitor fluid intake during the race to prevent overhydration. Sports drinks that contain sodium (ingest about 1 gram of sodium per hour) should be used during the race to replace **electrolytes** lost in sweat and to prevent blood sodium dilution.

Creatine Supplementation

Creatine is an organic compound obtained in the diet primarily from meat and fish. In the human body, creatine combines with inorganic phosphate and forms **creatine phosphate (CP)**, a high-energy compound. CP then is used to resynthesize ATP during short bursts of all-out physical activity. Individuals on a normal mixed diet consume an average of 1 gram of creatine per day. Each day, 1 additional gram is synthesized from various amino acids. One pound of meat or fish provides approximately 2 grams of creatine.

Creatine supplementation is popular among individuals who want to increase muscle mass and improve athletic performance. Creatine monohydrate—a white, tasteless powder that is mixed with fluids prior to ingestion—is the form most popular among people who use the supplement. Supplementation can result in an approximate 20 percent increase in the amount of creatine that is stored in muscles. Most of this creatine binds to phosphate to form CP, and 30 to 40 percent remains as free creatine in the muscle. Increased creatine storage is believed to enable individuals to train more intensely—thereby building more muscle mass and enhancing performance in all-out activities of very short duration (less than 30 seconds).

Creatine supplementation has two phases: the loading phase and the maintenance phase. During the loading phase, the person consumes between 20 and 25 grams (1 teaspoonful is about 5 grams) of creatine per day for 5 to 6 days, divided into four or five dosages of 5 grams each throughout the day. (This amount represents the equivalent of consuming 10 or more pounds of meat per day.) Research also suggests that the amount of creatine stored in muscle is enhanced by taking creatine in combination with a high-carbohydrate food. Once the loading phase is complete, taking 2 grams per day seems to be sufficient to maintain the increased muscle stores.

To date, no serious side effects have been documented in people who take up to 25 grams of creatine per day for 5 days. Stomach distress and cramping have been reported only in rare instances. The 2 grams taken per day during the maintenance phase is just slightly above the average intake in our daily diet. Long-term effects of creatine supplementation on health, however, have not been established.

A frequently documented result following 5 to 6 days of creatine loading is an increase of 2 to 3 pounds in body weight. This increase appears to be related to the increased water retention necessary to maintain the additional creatine stored in muscles. Some data, however, suggest that the increase in stored water and CP stimulates protein synthesis, leading to an increase in lean body mass.

The benefits of elevated creatine stores may be limited to high-intensity/short-duration activities such as sprinting, strength training (weight lifting), and sprint cycling. Supplementation is most beneficial during exercise training itself, rather than as an aid to enhance athletic performance a few days before competition.

Enhanced creatine stores do not benefit athletes competing in aerobic endurance events because CP is not used in energy production for long-distance events. Actually, the additional weight can be detrimental in long-distance running and swimming events because the athlete must expend more energy to carry the extra weight during competition.

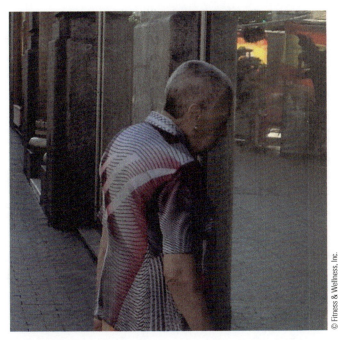

© Fitness & Wellness, Inc.

Osteoporosis is a leading cause of serious morbidity and functional loss in the elderly.

3.26 *Bone Health and Osteoporosis*

Osteoporosis, literally meaning "porous bones," is a condition in which bones lack the minerals required to keep them strong. In osteoporosis, bones—primarily of the hip, wrist, and spine—become so weak and brittle that they fracture readily. The process begins slowly in the third and fourth decades of life. Women are especially susceptible after menopause because of the accompanying loss of **estrogen**, which increases the rate at which bone mass is broken down.

According to the National Osteoporosis Foundation, 54 million Americans have osteoporosis and low bone density. Based on estimates, one in two women and one in four men over the age of 50 will suffer a bone fracture due to osteoporosis.

Osteoporosis is the leading cause of serious morbidity and functional loss in the elderly population. One of every two women and up to one in four men over age 50 will have an osteoporotic-related fracture at some point in their lives. The chances of a postmenopausal woman developing osteoporosis are much greater than her chances of developing breast cancer or incurring a heart attack or stroke. Up to 20 percent of people who have a hip fracture die within a year because of complications related to the fracture. As alarming as these figures are, they do not convey the pain and loss of quality of life in people who suffer the crippling effects of osteoporotic fractures.

Although osteoporosis is viewed primarily as a woman's disease, more than 30 percent of all men will be affected by age 75. About 100,000 of the yearly 300,000 hip fractures in the United States occur in men.

Despite the strong genetic component, osteoporosis is preventable. Maximizing bone density at a young age and subsequently decreasing the rate of bone loss later in life are critical factors in preventing osteoporosis.

Normal hormone levels prior to menopause and adequate calcium intake and physical activity throughout life cannot be overemphasized. These factors are all crucial in preventing osteoporosis. The absence of any one of these three factors leads to bone loss for which the other two factors never completely compensate. Smoking and excessive use of alcohol and corticosteroid drugs also accelerate the rate of bone loss in women and men alike. And osteoporosis is more common in whites, Asians, and people with small frames. Figure 3.15 depicts these variables.

GLOSSARY

Hyponatremia A low sodium concentration in the blood caused by overhydration with water.

Electrolytes Substances that become ions in solution and are critical for proper muscle and neuron activation (include sodium, potassium, chloride, calcium, magnesium, phosphate, and bicarbonate, among others).

Creatine An organic compound derived from meat, fish, and amino acids that combines with inorganic phosphate to form creatine phosphate.

Creatine phosphate (CP) A high-energy compound that the cells use to resynthesize ATP during all-out activities of very short duration.

Osteoporosis A condition of softening, deterioration, or loss of bone mineral density that leads to disability, bone fractures, and even death from medical complications.

Estrogen Female sex hormone essential for bone formation and conservation of bone density.

Figure 3.15 Threats to bone health (osteoporosis).

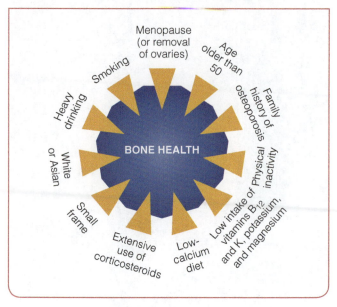

Table 3.14 Calcium-Rich Foods

Food	Amount	Calcium (mg)	Calories
Beans, red kidney, cooked	1 cup	70	218
Beet, greens, cooked	½ cup	82	19
Bok choy (Chinese cabbage)	1 cup	158	20
Broccoli, cooked, drained	1 cup	72	44
Burrito, bean (no cheese)	1	57	225
Cottage cheese, 2% low-fat	½ cup	78	103
Ice milk (vanilla)	½ cup	102	100
Instant Breakfast, nonfat milk	1 cup	407	216
Kale, cooked, drained	1 cup	94	36
Milk, nonfat, powdered	1 tbsp	52	15
Milk, skim	1 cup	296	88
Oatmeal, instant, fortified, plain	½ cup	109	70
Okra, cooked, drained	½ cup	74	23
Orange juice, fortified	1 cup	300	110
Soy milk, fortified, fat free	1 cup	400	110
Spinach, raw	1 cup	56	12
Turnip greens, cooked	1 cup	197	29
Tofu (some types)	½ cup	138	76
Yogurt, fruit	1 cup	372	250
Yogurt, low-fat, plain	1 cup	448	155

Bone health begins at a young age. Some experts have called osteoporosis a "pediatric disease." Bone density can be promoted early in life by making sure the diet has sufficient calcium and participating in weight-bearing activities. Adequate calcium intake in women and men alike is also associated with a reduced risk for colon cancer. The RDA for calcium is between 1,000 and 1,300 mg per day (see Table 3.13).

To obtain your daily calcium requirement, get as much calcium as possible from calcium-rich foods, including calcium-fortified foods. If you don't get enough, you need to make a conscious and deliberate effort to reach the RDA through foods in the diet. Calcium supplements are no longer recommended because they may cause more harm than good, including a modest increase in risk of heart attacks, kidney stones in both men and women, and possibly an increased risk of prostate cancer in men. Calcium obtained from food has not been linked to these negative health risks. Supplements are only warranted in extreme cases, when dietary intake from food absolutely does not supply the need.

Table 3.14 provides a list of selected foods and their calcium content. Along with having an adequate calcium intake, taking a minimum of 400 to 800 IU of vitamin D daily is

recommended for optimal calcium absorption (for overall health benefits, 1,000 to 2,000 IU of vitamin D is preferable). Close to half of people older than 50 are also vitamin D deficient. Without vitamin D, it is practically impossible for the body to absorb sufficient calcium to protect the bones.

Protein is also necessary for the continuous rebuilding of bones. Excessive protein, however, is detrimental to bone health because it makes the blood more acidic. To neutralize the acid, calcium is taken from the bones and released into the bloodstream. The more protein we eat, the higher the calcium content in the urine (i.e., the more calcium excreted). This might be the reason that countries with a high protein intake, including the United States, also have the highest rates of osteoporosis. Individuals should aim to achieve the RDA for protein, nonetheless, because people who consume too little protein (less than 35 grams per day) lose more bone mass than those who eat too much (more than 100 grams per day).

Vitamin B_{12} may also be a key nutrient in the prevention of osteoporosis. Several reports have shown an association between low vitamin B_{12} and lower bone mineral density in both men and women. Vitamin B_{12} is found primarily in dairy products, meats, poultry, fish, and some fortified cereals. Other nutrients vital for bone health are potassium (also neutralizes acid), vitamin K (works with bone-building proteins), and magnesium (also keeps bone from becoming too brittle).

Soft drinks and alcoholic beverages also can contribute to a loss in bone density if consumed in large quantities. Although they may not cause the damage directly, they often take the place of dairy products in the diet.

Table 3.13 Recommended Daily Calcium Intake

Age	Amount (mg)
9–18	1,300
19–50	1,000
51–70 Men	1,000
51–70 Women	1,200
>70	1,200

Pregnant and lactating women should follow the recommendation for their respective age group.

Exercise plays a key role in preventing osteoporosis by decreasing the rate of bone loss following the onset of menopause. Active people are able to maintain bone density much more effectively than their inactive counterparts. A combination of weight-bearing exercises, such as walking or jogging and strength training, is especially helpful.

The benefits of exercise go beyond maintaining bone density. Exercise strengthens muscles, ligaments, and tendons—all of which provide support to the bones (skeleton). Exercise also improves balance and coordination, which can help prevent falls and injuries.

People who are active have higher bone mineral density than inactive people do. Similar to other benefits of participating in exercise, there is no such thing as "bone in the bank." To have good bone health, people need to participate in a regular lifetime exercise program.

Prevailing research also tells us that estrogen is the most important factor in preventing bone loss. Lumbar bone density in women who have always had regular menstrual cycles exceeds that of women with a history of **oligomenorrhea** and **amenorrhea** interspersed with regular cycles. Furthermore, the lumbar density of these two groups of women is higher than that of women who have never had regular menstrual cycles.

For instance, athletes with amenorrhea (who have lower estrogen levels) have lower bone mineral density than even non-athletes with normal estrogen levels. Studies have shown that amenorrheic athletes at age 25 have the bones of women older than 50. It has become clear that sedentary women with normal estrogen levels have better bone mineral density than active amenorrheic athletes. Many experts believe the best predictor of bone mineral content is the history of menstrual regularity.

As a baseline, women age 65 and older should have a bone density test to establish the risk for osteoporosis. Younger women who are at risk for osteoporosis should discuss a bone density test with their physician at menopause. The test also can be used to monitor changes in bone mass over time and to predict the risk of future fractures. The bone density test is a painless scan requiring only a small amount of radiation to determine bone mass of the spine, hip, wrist, heel, or fingers. The amount of radiation is so low that technicians administering the test can sit next to the person receiving it. The procedure often takes less than 15 minutes.

Various therapy modalities available to prevent and/or treat osteoporosis should be discussed with a physician. If you have osteoporosis, lifestyle changes may be required, and you may also need medication to prevent future fractures. A calcium-rich diet, adequate vitamin D, daily exercise, and drug therapy are all treatment options.

New medical treatments have been developed and continue to evolve to prevent and treat bone loss. The newer medications can be classified into two categories: antiresorptive and anabolic. Antiresorptive medications slow bone loss, but the body still makes new bone at the same rate, so bone density may increase. The drugs that fall into this category include bisphosphonates, calcitonin, denosumab, estrogen agonists/antagonists (also referred to as selective estrogen receptor modulators, or SERMs), and menopausal hormone therapy (MHT). Anabolic medications increase the rate of bone formation. The only FDA approved drug in this category is teriparatide, a form of parathyroid hormone.

MHT may be the most effective treatment to relieve acute (short-term) symptoms of menopause, such as hot flashes, mood swings, sleep difficulties, and vaginal dryness. Due to potential health risks, experts recommend that women on MHT use the lowest dose that still provides benefits and use it for the shortest time needed. Regardless of the treatment modality, women should always work with a physician to determine the best course of action.

3.27 *Iron Deficiency*

Iron is a key element of **hemoglobin** in blood. The RDA for iron for adult women is between 15 and 18 mg per day (8 to 11 mg for men). Inadequate iron intake is often seen in children, teenagers, women of childbearing age, and endurance athletes. If iron absorption does not compensate for losses or if dietary intake is low, iron deficiency develops. As many as half of American women have an iron deficiency. Over time, excessive depletion of iron stores in the body leads to iron-deficiency anemia, a condition in which the concentration of hemoglobin in the red blood cells is lower than it should be.

Physically active individuals—in particular, women—have a greater than average need for iron. Heavy training creates a demand for iron that is higher than the recommended intake because small amounts of iron are lost through sweat, urine, and stools. Mechanical trauma, caused by the pounding of the feet on the pavement during extensive jogging, may also lead to destruction of iron-containing red blood cells.

A large percentage of female endurance athletes are reported to have iron deficiency. The blood **ferritin** levels of women who participate in intense physical training should be checked frequently.

The rates of iron absorption and iron loss vary from person to person. In most cases, though, people can get enough iron by eating more iron-rich foods such as beans, peas, green leafy vegetables, enriched grain products, egg yolk, fish, and lean meats. A list of foods high in iron is given in Table 3.15.

If you are iron-deficient, be aware that calcium interferes with iron absorption. Thus, try not to include dietary sources of calcium with your main iron-rich meal. The intake of these

---

GLOSSARY

Oligomenorrhea Irregular menstrual cycles.

Amenorrhea Cessation of regular menstrual flow.

Hemoglobin Protein-iron compound in red blood cells that transports oxygen in the blood.

Ferritin A blood cell protein that contains iron (a ferritin test helps determine how much iron the body is storing).

Table 3.15 Iron-Rich Foods

Food	Amount	Iron (mg)	Calories
Beans, red kidney, cooked	1 cup	3.2	218
Beef, ground lean (21% fat)	3 oz	2.1	237
Beef, sirloin, lean only	3 oz	2.9	171
Beef, liver, fried	3 oz	5.3	184
Beet, greens, cooked	½ cup	1.4	19
Broccoli, cooked, drained	1 cup	1.3	44
Burrito, bean (no cheese)	1	2.3	225
Egg, hard-cooked	1	.7	77
Farina (Cream of Wheat), cooked	½ cup	5.2	65
Instant Breakfast, nonfat milk	1 cup	4.8	216
Peas, frozen, cooked, drained	½ cup	1.3	62
Shrimp, boiled	3 oz	2.7	87
Spinach, raw	1 cup	1.5	12
Vegetables, mixed, cooked	1 cup	1.5	108

two minerals should be separated as much as possible. This is particularly critical in young menstruating women who need the iron.

3.28 *2015–2020 Dietary Guidelines for Americans*

The secretaries of the Department of Health and Human Services (DHHS) and the USDA appoint an expert Dietary Guidelines advisory committee every 5 years to issue a report and make recommendations concerning dietary guidelines for Americans. The guidelines are intended for healthy people 2 years and older and provide guidance to help people achieve a healthy eating pattern, improve diet quality, and shape nutrition education programs. You can access the complete guidelines at http://health.gov/dietaryguidelines/2015/guidelines/. The recommendations encourage people to:[19]

1. Follow a healthy eating pattern across the lifespan. All food and beverage choices matter. Choose a healthy eating pattern at an appropriate calorie level to help achieve and maintain a healthy body weight, support nutrient adequacy, and reduce the risk of chronic disease.
2. Focus on variety, nutrient density, and amount. To meet nutrient needs within calorie limits, choose a va-

riety of nutrient-dense foods across and within all food groups in recommended amounts.
3. Limit calories from added sugars and saturated fats and reduce sodium intake. Consume an eating pattern low in added sugars, saturated fats, and sodium. Cut back on foods and beverages higher in these components to amounts that fit within healthy eating patterns.
4. Shift to healthier food and beverage choices. Choose nutrient-dense foods and beverages across and within all food groups in place of less healthy choices. Consider cultural and personal preferences to make these shifts easier to accomplish and maintain.
5. Support healthy eating patterns for all. Everyone has a role in helping to create and support healthy eating patterns in multiple settings nationwide, from home to school to work to communities.

The Dietary Guidelines website also provides examples of healthy eating patterns, including the Healthy US-Style Eating Pattern, Healthy Mediterranean-Style Eating Pattern, Healthy Vegetarian Eating Pattern, and the DASH Eating Plan.

Key Recommendations

The Dietary Guidelines for healthy eating patterns should be applied in their entirety, given the interconnected relationship that each dietary component can have with others. **Consume a healthy eating pattern that accounts for all foods and beverages within an appropriate calorie level.**
A healthy eating pattern includes:

- A variety of vegetables from all of the subgroups—dark green, red and orange, legumes (beans and peas), starchy, and other

---

Changing Genetic Destiny with Nutrition

Although you may have inherited a genetic predisposition to a certain disease(s), genes can be switched on and off. Emerging research tells us that DNA and some proteins have molecular "tags" that can activate or inactivate a gene. Our environment and lifestyle can cause these tags to be added or removed. The field of nutrigenomics (science that studies how foods affect our genes) tells us that nutritious foods have many bioactive ingredients that trigger genes to express health—essentially turning the disease predisposition off.

For example, people with a diet rich in fruits, vegetables, and nuts who also have a genetic variant that may lead to heart disease have as low a risk for heart disease as those individuals who do not have this genetic variant. Antioxidants, found abundantly in fruits and vegetables, cause changes in gene expression that fortify the body's defense processes. A healthy diet pattern has also been found to alter your genetic expression toward cancer protection. In essence, we can directly influence our genetic destiny toward health. *It's truly up to us to make the environment work for us and not against us!*

- Fruits, especially whole fruits
- Grains, at least half of which are whole grains
- Fat-free or low-fat dairy, including milk, yogurt, cheese, and/or fortified soy beverages
- A variety of protein foods, including seafood, lean meats and poultry, eggs, legumes (beans and peas), and nuts, seeds, and soy products
- Oils

A healthy eating pattern limits:

- Saturated fats and *trans* fats, added sugars, and sodium
    Key recommendations that are quantitative are provided for several components of the diet that should be limited. These components are of particular public health concern in the United States, and the specified limits can help individuals achieve healthy eating patterns within calorie limits:
- Consume less than 10 percent of calories per day from added sugars.
- Consume less than 10 percent of calories per day from saturated fats.
- Consume less than 2,300 milligrams (mg) per day of sodium.
- If alcohol is consumed, it should be consumed in moderation—up to one drink per day for women and up to two drinks per day for men—and only by adults of legal drinking age.

Physical Activity Recommendation

In tandem with the preceding recommendations, Americans of all ages—children, adolescents, adults, and older adults—should meet the *Physical Activity Guidelines for Americans* to help promote health and reduce the risk of chronic disease. Americans should aim to achieve and maintain a healthy body weight. The relationship between diet and physical activity contributes to calorie balance and managing body weight. As such, the *Dietary Guidelines* includes a key recommendation to meet the *Physical Activity Guidelines for Americans.*

3.29 Proper Nutrition: A Lifetime Prescription for Healthy Living

The three factors that do the most for health, longevity, and quality of life are proper nutrition, a sound exercise program, and quitting (or never starting) smoking. Achieving and maintaining a balanced diet is not as difficult as most people think. If everyone were more educated about their own nutrition habits and the nutrition habits of their children, the current magnitude of nutrition-related health problems would be much smaller. Although treatment of obesity is important, we should place far greater emphasis on preventing obesity in youth and adults in the first place.

Specific Nutrition Recommendations for Americans

A healthy dietary pattern includes:

- Whole fruits and a variety of vegetables
- Grains, at least half as whole grains
- Low-fat dairy products
- A variety of lean protein choices, including seafood, legumes, nuts, seeds, and soy products
- Healthy oils

A healthy dietary pattern also limits:

- Processed foods
- Saturated fat
- Trans fats
- Added sugar
- Sodium
- Alcohol

Children tend to eat the way their parents do. If parents adopt a healthy diet, children most likely will follow. The difficult part for most people is to retrain themselves—to closely examine the eating habits they learned from their parents—to follow a lifetime healthy nutrition plan that includes grains, legumes, fruits, vegetables, nuts, seeds, and low-fat dairy products, with moderate use of animal protein, junk food, sodium, and alcohol.

Critical Thinking

What factors in your life and the environment have contributed to your current dietary habits? Do you need to make changes? What may prevent you from doing so?

In spite of the ample scientific evidence linking poor dietary habits to early disease and mortality rates, many people remain precontemplators: They are not willing to change their eating patterns. Even when faced with obesity, elevated blood lipids, hypertension, and other nutrition-related conditions, people do not change. The motivating factor to change one's eating habits seems to be a major health breakdown, such as a heart attack, a stroke, or cancer—by which time the damage has been done already. In many cases, it is irreversible and, for some, fatal.

An ounce of prevention is worth a pound of cure. The sooner you implement the dietary guidelines presented in this chapter, the better your chances of preventing chronic diseases and reaching a higher state of wellness.

Assess Your Behavior

1. Are whole grains, fruits, vegetables, legumes, and nuts the staples of your diet?

2. Are you meeting your personal MyPlate recommendations for daily fruits, vegetables, grains, protein, and dairy?

3. Will the information presented in this chapter change in any manner the way you eat?

4. Are there dietary changes that you need to implement to meet energy, nutrition, and disease risk-reduction guidelines and improve health and wellness? If so, list these changes and indicate what you will do to make it happen.

Assess Your Knowledge

1. The science of nutrition studies the relationship of
   a. vitamins to minerals.
   b. foods to optimal health and performance.
   c. carbohydrates, fats, and proteins to the development and maintenance of good health.
   d. the macronutrients and micronutrients to physical performance.
   e. kilocalories to calories in food items.

2. Faulty nutrition often plays a crucial role in the development and progression of which disease?
   a. Cardiovascular disease
   b. Cancer
   c. Osteoporosis
   d. Diabetes
   e. All are correct choices.

3. According to MyPlate guidelines,
   a. about 50 percent of the daily caloric intake should come from protein.
   b. dairy products are not required in the daily diet.
   c. approximately three quarters of the plate should be taken up by fruits, vegetables, and grains.
   d. most daily fat intake should come from saturated fat.
   e. all of the above.

4. The recommended amount of fiber intake for adults 50 years and younger is
   a. 10 grams per day for women and 12 grams for men.
   b. 21 grams per day for women and 30 grams for men.
   c. 28 grams per day for women and 35 grams for men.
   d. 25 grams per day for women and 38 grams for men.
   e. 45 grams per day for women and 50 grams for men.

5. Unhealthy fats include
   a. unsaturated fatty acids.
   b. monounsaturated fats.
   c. polyunsaturated fatty acids.
   d. saturated fats.
   e. all of the above.

6. Which of the following is classified as an unsaturated fatty acid?
   a. Omega-9
   b. Trans fat
   c. Omega-3
   d. Omega-6
   e. All of the above are unsaturated fatty acids.

7. The amount of a nutrient that is estimated to meet the nutrient requirement of half the healthy people in specific age and gender groups is known as the
   a. Estimated Average Requirement.
   b. Recommended Dietary Allowance.
   c. Daily Values.
   d. Adequate Intake.
   e. Dietary Reference Intake.

8. Regular consumption of red meat is detrimental to health because it
   a. increases the intake of L-carnitine.
   b. leads to the production of TMAO.
   c. increases the consumption of saturated fat.
   d. promotes atherosclerosis.
   e. All are correct choices.

9. Probiotics are
   a. healthy microbes that help break down food and help prevent disease.
   b. a specialized type of antibiotics prescribed to cure chronic diseases.
   c. also known as advanced glycation end products.
   d. found in abundance in fruits and vegetables.
   e. All are correct choices.

10. Antioxidant and multivitamin supplements are encouraged to
    a. prevent illness.
    b. cure several chronic diseases.
    c. increase the amount of disease-fighting oxygen free radicals.
    d. promote the inflammatory response to fight chronic diseases.
    e. All are incorrect choices.

Correct answers can be found at the back of the book.

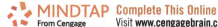

MINDTAP From Cengage **Complete This Online**
Visit **www.cengagebrain.com** to access MindTap, a complete digital course that includes interactive quizzes, videos, and more.

4

Body Composition

Achieving recommended body weight improves health parameters, but most importantly, it improves quality of life by allowing you to pursue tasks of daily living, along with leisure and recreational activities, without functional limitations. You will also rejoice in the way you feel if you follow a healthy diet, remain physically active, and maintain a lifetime exercise program.

Objectives

4.1 **Define** body composition and understand how it relates to recommended body weight.

4.2 **Explain** the difference between essential fat and storage fat.

4.3 **Differentiate** between types of body fat and describe their effects on disease risk.

4.4 **Describe** various techniques used to assess body composition.

4.5 **Assess** body composition using skinfold thickness and girth measurements.

4.6 **Understand** the importance of body mass index (BMI) and waist circumference (WC) in the assessment of risk for disease.

4.7 **Determine** recommended weight according to recommended percent body fat values and BMI.

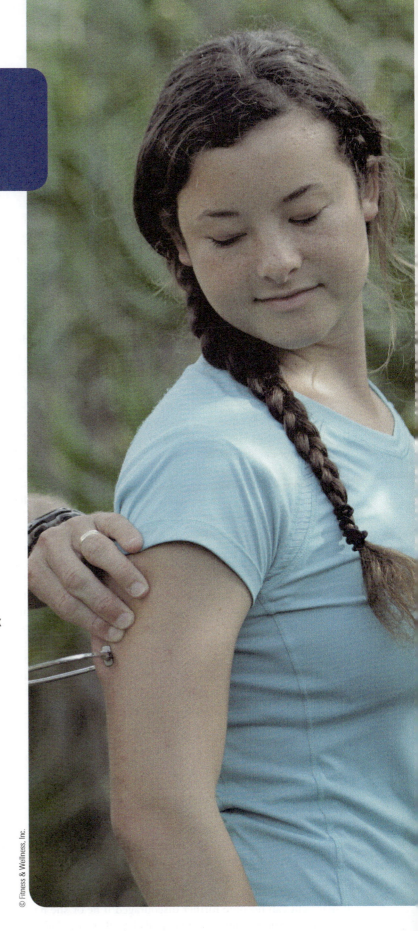

© Fitness & Wellness, Inc.

135

FAQ

What constitutes ideal body weight?

There is no such thing as ideal body weight. Health and fitness professionals prefer to use the terms "recommended" or "healthy" body weight. Let's examine the question by considering an individual example. For a 40-year-old man, 25 percent body fat is the recommended health fitness standard. For the average, apparently healthy individual, this body fat percentage does not constitute a threat to good health. Due to genetic and lifestyle conditions, however, if a 40-year-old man at 25 percent body fat is prediabetic, prehypertensive, and has abnormal blood lipids (see Chapter 10 to read about cholesterol and triglycerides), that individual may be recommended to reduce his percent body fat. Thus, what will work as recommended weight for most individuals may not be the best standard for individuals with disease risk factors. The current recommended or healthy weight standards (based on percent body fat, BMI, or waist-to-height ratio) are established at the point where there appears to be a lower incidence for overweight-related conditions for most people. Individual differences have to be taken into consideration when making a final recommendation, especially in people with risk factors or a personal and family history of chronic conditions.

How accurate are body composition assessments?

Most of the techniques to determine body composition require proper training on the part of the technician administering the test (skinfolds, hydrostatic weighing, DXA, Bod Pod) and, in the case of hydrostatic weighing, proper performance on the part of the person being tested. As detailed in this chapter, body composition assessment is not a precise science. Some of the procedures are more accurate than others. Before undergoing body composition testing, make sure that you understand the accuracy of the technique (see standard error of estimates [SEEs] included under the description of each technique); and even more important, inquire about the training and experience of the person administering the test. We often encounter individuals who have been tested elsewhere by any number of assessments, particularly skinfolds, who come to our laboratory in disbelief and rightfully so because of the results that were given to them. To obtain the best possible results, look for trained and experienced technicians.

Is there a future trend in body composition assessment?

The area of the body where a person stores fat directly affects that individual's chance of developing disease. Individuals with fat stored around internal organs (known as visceral fat) are at greater risk for chronic disease than individuals with the same amount of fat stored just beneath the skin (known as subcutaneous fat). A person with a large abdominal girth certainly has visceral fat. Visceral fat cells (around internal organs) are biologically active in different ways than subcutaneous fat cells (just beneath the skin) and contribute to a higher risk for chronic diseases. Thus, future body composition tests will be designed to get a clearer view of where the abdominal fat lies.

Currently, scans to detect the location of fat are costly and are not widely available. In contrast, metrics such as body mass index (BMI) and waist-to-height ratio (WHtR) are simple, free, and are an excellent starting point for detecting disease risk. Researchers suggest that physicians record abdominal girth along with height and weight as a routine part of every health care visit.

Most people manage their weight by using two sources of feedback—the numbers on the scale and the way their clothing fits. As you will read in this chapter, these evaluations do not tell the full story and can sometimes be misleading. A person may feel discouraged when he or she is, in fact, making progress in losing body fat and gaining muscle mass or may feel optimistic when he or she is, in fact, losing critical lean body mass. A person who is attempting to lose weight can become further discouraged if he or she has unrealistic expectations or vague goals based on the "ideal body" that is portrayed in media. Understanding personal recommended body weight and body composition is vital to setting clear and realistic weight loss goals.

4.1 What Is Body Composition?

To understand the concept of **body composition**, we must recognize that the human body consists of fat and nonfat components. The fat component is called fat mass or **percent body fat**. The nonfat component is termed **lean body mass**.

To determine **recommended body weight**, we need to find out what percent of total body weight is fat and what amount is lean tissue—in other words, assess body composition. Body composition should be assessed by a well-trained technician who understands the procedure being used.

Once the fat percentage is known, recommended body weight can be calculated from recommended body fat.

REAL LIFE STORY | Shondra's Experience

I was surprised at my results of the body composition assessments that we did in our lab. The BMI calculation told me I was at a healthy weight (about 24). But when we did the skinfold test, I found out that I was almost 29 percent body fat, which is considered overweight. I talked about it with my instructor, and I told her that for the first 2 years after starting college I had yo-yo dieted. I would eat a lot less, lose weight, and then get sick of dieting,

eat what I wanted, and gain it all back, plus more. Also, I hated to exercise, so I didn't do anything other than just walking from class to class. My instructor said she felt that my higher percent body fat might be due to my weight loss history. Each time I dieted, I probably lost lean body mass along with fat, and then when I gained weight back, I mainly gained fat, so over time my percent body fat went up. The good news is that over the course of the year,

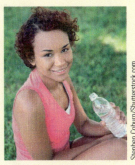
Stephen Coburn/Shutterstock.com

I became much more active and even started doing some basic strength training. Even though I didn't lose any weight, my percent body fat went down to 23 percent, which is a lot healthier.

PERSONAL PROFILE: My Body Composition

Please answer the following questions to the best of your ability. If you cannot answer all of them at this time, you will be able to do so as you work through the chapter contents.

I.   Can you relate to Shondra's experience, and what can you do in your life to avoid the same pitfalls? _____

_____

II. Do you understand the concept of body composition and its relationship to recommended body weight, proper weight management, and good health?   ____ Yes ____ No

III. What better motivates you to keep a healthy body weight: the way you look or the knowledge that you are taking care of your body and avoiding disease risk? Do you believe that the body weight you desire is a healthy weight for you? _____

_____

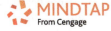 **Complete This Online**
Visit **www.cengagebrain.com** to access MindTap, a complete digital course that includes interactive quizzes, videos, and more.

Guidelines for recommended body weight, also called "healthy weight," have been set at values where there are no medical conditions that would improve with weight loss. The guidelines take into consideration body shape (or fat distribution pattern) that is not associated with higher risk for illness.

Types of Body Fat

Our understanding of human body fat and its functions has only just begun. Over the past decade research has uncovered ways that body fat interacts with other body systems that we never before imagined as possible. Body fat is an endocrine organ—it responds to stimuli and releases hormones to communicate with the brain and body. Our new understanding has the power to prevent disease. In this chapter you will gain that understanding as you read about essential versus storage fat, subcutaneous versus visceral fat, abdominal versus hip and thigh fat, and brown and beige versus white fat. You will come to understand how these types of body fat affect you every day, and you will see the real control you gain over your own heath by monitoring and maintaining your body composition properly.

Essential and Storage Fat

Total fat in the human body is classified into essential fat and storage fat. **Essential fat** is needed for normal physiological function. Without it, human health and physical performance deteriorate. This type of fat is found within tissues such as muscles, nerve cells, bone marrow, intestines, heart, liver, and lungs. Essential fat constitutes about 3 percent of

> **GLOSSARY**
>
> **Body composition** The fat and nonfat components of the human body; important in assessing recommended body weight.
>
> **Percent body fat** Proportional amount of fat in the body based on the person's total weight; includes both essential fat and storage fat; also termed fat mass.
>
> **Lean body mass** Body weight without body fat.
>
> **Recommended body weight** Body weight at which there seems to be no harm to human health; healthy weight.
>
> **Essential fat** Minimal amount of body fat needed for normal physiological functions; constitutes about 3 percent of total weight in men and 12 percent in women.

Figure 4.1 **Typical body composition of an adult man and an adult woman.**

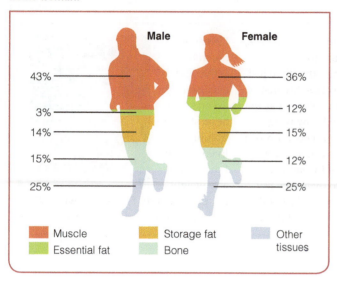

Figure 4.2 **Mortality risk versus body mass index.**

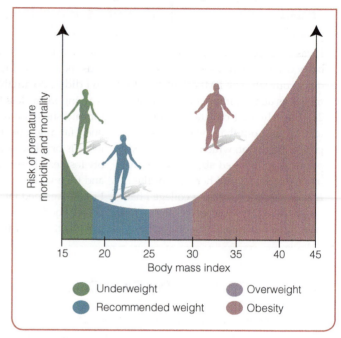

the total weight in men and 12 percent in women (see Figure 4.1). The percentage is higher in women because it includes gender-specific fat, such as that found in the breast tissue, the uterus, and other related fat deposits.

HOEGER KEY TO WELLNESS

Essential fat constitutes about 3 percent of the total weight in men and 12 percent in women.

Storage fat is the fat stored in adipose tissue, mostly just beneath the skin (subcutaneous fat) and around major organs in the body (visceral fat). This fat performs four basic functions: it stores calories to be mobilized when a person gets hungry, it releases hormones that control metabolism, it insulates the body to retain heat, and it acts as padding against physical trauma to the body.

The amount of storage fat does not differ between men and women, except that men tend to store fat around the waist and women around the hips and thighs.

4.2 Why Does Body Composition Matter?

When studying large populations, simple height/weight measurements provide important feedback. By averaging data across large groups of individuals, scientists have been able to establish that the risk for premature illness and death is greater for those who are overweight and that the risk is also increased for individuals who are underweight[1] (see Figure 4.2). When it comes to understanding personal risk,

however, simply finding the point where height and weight intersect on a graph does not provide sufficient information about how your body weight may affect your health.

Formerly, people relied on simple height/weight charts to determine their recommended body weight, but these tables can be highly inaccurate and can fail to identify critical fat values associated with higher risk for disease. Standard height/weight tables, first published in 1912, were based on average weights (while wearing shoes and clothing) for men and women who obtained life insurance policies between 1888 and 1905—a notably unrepresentative population. The recommended body weight on these tables was obtained according to gender, height, and frame size. Because no scientific guidelines were given to determine frame size, most people chose their frame size based on the column in which the weight came closest to their own!

High Body Weight Does Not Always Mean High Body Fat

The best way to determine whether people are truly **overweight** or falsely at recommended body weight is through assessment of body composition. **Obesity** is an excess of body fat. If body weight is the only criterion, an individual might easily appear to be overweight according to height/weight charts yet have a healthy amount of body fat. Typical examples are football players, body builders, weight lifters, and other athletes with large muscle size. Some athletes who appear to be 20 or 30 pounds overweight really have little body fat.

The importance of body composition was clearly demonstrated when a young man who weighed about 225 pounds applied to join a city police force but was turned down without having been granted an interview. The reason? He was "too fat." When this young man's body composition was assessed at a preventive medicine clinic, it was determined that only 5 percent of his total body weight was in the form of fat— considerably less than the recommended standard. In the words of the director of the clinic, "The only way this fellow could come down to the chart's target weight would have been through surgical removal of a large amount of his muscle tissue."

Low Body Weight Does Not Always Mean Low Body Fat

At the other end of the spectrum, some people who weigh very little (and may be viewed as skinny or underweight) actually can be classified as overweight because of their high body fat content. People who weigh as little as 120 pounds but are more than 30 percent fat (about one-third of their total body weight) are not rare. These cases are found more readily in the sedentary population and among people who are always dieting.

Weight Loss versus Fat Loss

Loss in overall body weight can include a combination of loss in water weight, lean body mass, muscle mass, and body fat. Although individuals may lose overall body weight when dieting, the weight loss may not always include the desired loss of body fat, but rather the loss of lean body mass and muscle mass. As discussed in Chapter 5, both physical inactivity and an ongoing negative caloric balance due to dieting can lead to a loss in lean body mass. A loss in lean body mass results in a decrease in calories burned each day through the basal metabolic rate (see Chapter 5), among other adverse effects. This loss of lean body mass can be offset or eliminated, however, by combining a sensible diet with exercise. By tracking body composition, dieters can identify fad diets that promote the loss of water and lean body mass, especially muscle mass. They can opt instead for lifestyle changes that decrease body fat while maintaining or increasing lean body mass.

As you begin to increase exercise and adopt a healthy nutrition plan, your body responds with the beneficial change of increasing muscle mass. Muscle is heavier than fat and, although fat is being lost, little or no weight change is noticeable if you are simply monitoring weight changes on the scale. Do not let this lack of weight change discourage you. Fat loss typically increases after this initial period.

Avoiding Creeping Changes in Body Composition

Knowing your body composition will be an advantage to you not only during your efforts to lose weight but also throughout life. Consider the following pattern that is common in the United States and the developed world. The majority of

Figure 4.3 Typical body composition changes for adults in the United States.

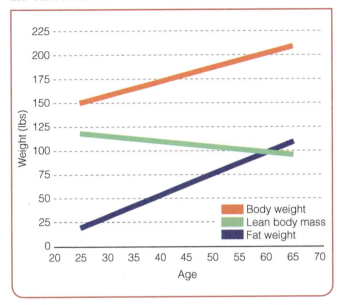

children do not start life with a weight problem. Although a few struggle with weight throughout life, most are not overweight in the early years of life.

> **HOEGER KEY TO WELLNESS**
>
> On average, adults in the United States gain one to two pounds per year. They also lose half a pound of lean tissue each year due to low physical activity. A span of 40 years produces a fat gain of 60 to 100 pounds accompanied by a 20-pound loss of lean body mass.

Trends indicate that adults in the United States gain one to two pounds per year. Over a span of 40 years, the average American will have gained 40 to 80 pounds. Because of the typical reduction in physical activity in our society, however, the average person also loses half a pound of lean tissue each year. Therefore, this span of 40 years has produced an actual fat gain of 60 to 100 pounds accompanied by a 20-pound loss of lean body mass (Figure 4.3). These changes can be better detected by routinely assessing body composition.

GLOSSARY

Storage fat Body fat in excess of essential fat; stored in adipose tissue.

Overweight An excess amount of weight against a given standard, such as height or recommended percent body fat.

Obesity An excessive accumulation of body fat, usually at least 30 percent greater than recommended body weight.

Can I Influence My Body Shape?

Be aware that spot reducing of body fat is a myth (for more information see Chapter 5, page 172). Individuals are not able to reduce body fat in one isolated region of the body by simply working the muscles specific to that area of the body. Abdominal crunches by themselves, for example, will not get rid of excess abdominal fat. Rather, an individual can use diet, exercise, and physical activity to control lean body mass and overall percent body fat. When it comes to the areas where that individual stores body fat (apples vs. pears), gender and genetics are in control. Women also have an increased tendency to store fat in the abdominal area following menopause. When it comes to fat being stored as subcutaneous fat or visceral fat, however, an individual does have some control. An active individual who remains overweight will tend to store body fat as subcutaneous fat, whereas an inactive individual will tend to store it as the more risky visceral fat.

When it comes to diet and disease risk, studies indicate that not all excess calories appear to end up in the same place. To a certain extent, food selections help determine where the fat ends up. Saturated and

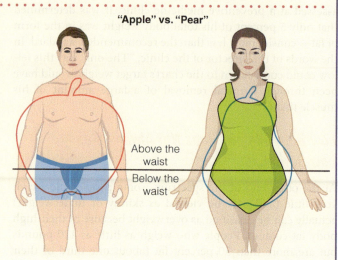

"Apple" vs. "Pear"

Above the waist

Below the waist

trans fats, excessive calories from alcohol, and added sugars (such as sucrose, fructose, and high-fructose corn syrup), all tend to end up as visceral fat.

4.3 Body Shape and Health Risk

As you have seen, body weight affects more than just physical appearance. Excessive body weight and lower health have been linked by research for decades. There is, however, another critical element at work. A person's total amount of body fat by itself is not the best predictor of increased risk for disease but, rather, the location of the fat. Scientific evidence suggests that the way people store fat affects their risk for disease.

- **Android obesity** is seen in individuals who tend to store fat in the trunk or abdominal area (which produces the "apple" shape).
- **Gynoid obesity** is seen in people who store fat primarily around the hips and thighs (which creates the "pear" shape).

Compared with people whose body fat is stored primarily in the hips and thighs, obese individuals with abdominal fat are at higher risk for heart disease, hypertension, type 2

White, Beige, and Brown Fat

Scientists have known for decades about a type of fat called brown fat that helps small mammals like mice, hibernating mammals like bears, and even human infants stay warm in cold conditions. While the purpose of regular fat cells is to store fat, the purpose of brown fat cells is to burn fat and thereby generate body heat. In 2009 scientists discovered that some human adults have a few ounces of brown fat around the collarbone, neck, upper back, and spine. Brown fat burns energy for heat similar to the way muscle burns energy to provide fuel for movement. Brown fat cells contain many more mitochondria (the "powerhouses" of the cell—see Chapter 6, page 221) than regular "white" fat cells do. Scientists have found brown fat in some adults only. Subjects who are overweight and older are less likely to have brown fat. Even more recently, in 2015, scientists discovered another type of energy-burning fat cell referred to as beige fat or brite (brown in white) fat. While brown fat cells are related to muscle cells, beige fat cells seem to be related to regular white fat cells. Both brown and beige fat cells are activated in cold conditions and with exercise. When beige fat cells are activated to their full potential, they may burn 300 to

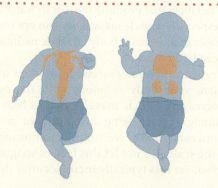

Human infants keep warm with the help of brown fat stores around their neck and shoulders.

500 calories per day from energy stored in regular white fat cells. Beige fat cells may also help prevent insulin resistance.[2] Scientists are now working to understand how big a role brown and beige fat have in regulating body weight.

diabetes ("non–insulin-dependent" diabetes), stroke, some types of cancer, kidney disease, migraines, and diminished lung function. Abdominal fat has also been shown to triple the risk of dementia in older adults[3]. One poignant study followed more than 350,000 people for almost 10 years and concluded that even when body weight is viewed as "normal," individuals with a large waist circumference are at nearly double the risk for premature death.

Subcutaneous and Visceral Fat

Large abdominal girth is a risk factor all its own. Evidence indicates, however, that among individuals with a lot of abdominal fat, two different internal locations of abdominal fat have different effects on disease risk (see Figure 4.4).

- **Subcutaneous fat** is the fat you can grasp just beneath the skin. *Sub-* means "beneath" and *-cutaneous* comes from the original Latin word *cutis* meaning "skin" (as also used in the word *cuticle*). Individuals with fat stored primarily as subcutaneous fat have a better metabolic profile than those with fat stored primarily as visceral fat (see below). Subcutaneous fat cells release more beneficial hormones,[4] communicating with the brain to suppress appetite and burn stored fat and with the liver and muscles to increase sensitivity to insulin. When a person gains fat weight, however, the hormone that increases sensitivity to insulin slows down or stops entirely.

- **Visceral fat** is located around the liver, intestines, and other abdominal organs and in an apron of tissue[5] that lies under the abdominal muscles. It is also known as intra-abdominal fat. *Visceral* means "deep and inward"; you may have heard this term used in the phrase "visceral feelings." Visceral fat poses a much greater risk for disease than subcutaneous fat.[6] Visceral fat creates proteins that

encourage low-level inflammation, proteins that encourage blood vessels to constrict, and proteins that increase insulin resistance.[7] Another type of fat, **retroperitoneal fat,** is located behind (retro) the abdominal cavity (see Figure 4.4) and is often measured as part of visceral fat.

Our new understanding of the dangers of visceral fat comes with a silver lining: Visceral fat metabolizes into fatty acids more readily than subcutaneous fat, and therefore responds more efficiently to diet and especially to exercise. A healthy diet alone will begin to reduce visceral fat stores, but exercise appears to be especially effective for burning away visceral fat from around your waistline (see Figure 4.5). A person who exercises regularly will reduce visceral fat and increase lean body mass even if weight is not lost (for more information on exercise and loss of visceral fat, see the box in Chapter 5 titled "Diet, Exercise, and Visceral Fat" on p. 196). Further, the same positive lifestyle changes that improve other aspects of health have been directly tied to avoiding abdominal adiposity. Individuals who do not smoke, have healthy sleep patterns, are less prone to hostility or depression, and avoid fructose-sweetened foods and hydrogenated vegetable oils are less likely to have their adipose tissue stored as visceral fat.

GLOSSARY

Android obesity Obesity pattern seen in individuals who tend to store fat in the trunk or abdominal area.

Gynoid obesity Obesity pattern seen in people who store fat primarily around the hips and thighs.

Subcutaneous fat Fat deposits directly under the skin.

Visceral fat Fat deposits located around internal organs linked with greater risk for disease; also called intra-abdominal fat.

Retroperitoneal fat Fat deposits in the abdominal cavity behind (retro) the peritoneum.

Figure 4.4 Visceral (VSC) fat is a greater risk factor for heart disease, stroke, hypertension, diabetes, and cancer than subcutaneous (SBC) or retroperitoneal (RTP) fat.

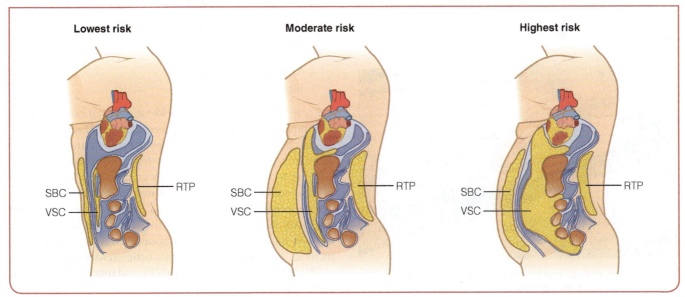

Lowest risk   Moderate risk   Highest risk

Figure 4.5 Body fat in physically active individuals is less likely to be stored as visceral fat, whereas inactive individuals store a greater amount of visceral fat.

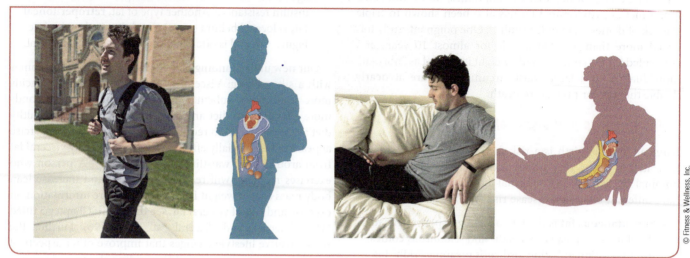

© Fitness & Wellness, Inc.

4.4 *Techniques to Assess Body Composition*

Body composition can be estimated using several methods. There is no method that can determine a person's exact amount of body fat. Some techniques, however, are more accurate than others. The following pages describe the most commonly used procedures for estimating body composition, along with a standard error of estimate (SEE) for each procedure. The SEE is a measure of the accuracy of the prediction for each specific technique, determining how many percentage points a result may deviate from the true percentage. For example, if the SEE for a given technique is 3.0 and the individual tests at a fat percentage of 18.0, the actual fat percentage may range from 15 to 21 percent.

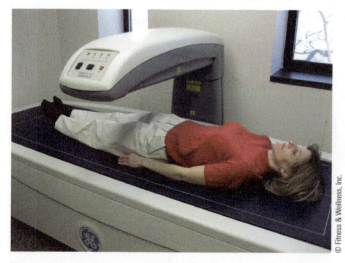

The dual energy x-ray absorptiometry (DXA) technique to assess body composition and bone density.

© Fitness & Wellness, Inc.

Dual Energy X-ray Absorptiometry

Dual energy x-ray absorptiometry (DXA) is a method to assess body composition that is used most frequently in research and by medical facilities. A radiographic technique, DXA uses very low-dose beams of x-ray energy (hundreds of times lower than a typical body x-ray) to measure total body fat mass, fat distribution pattern, and bone density. Bone density is measured to assess the risk for osteoporosis. The procedure itself is simple and takes less than 15 minutes to administer. Many exercise scientists consider DXA to be the standard technique to assess body composition. The SEE for this technique is ±1.8 percent.

Because of its accuracy, DXA is used as a standard of comparison for all other body composition tests. Due to costs, however, DXA is not readily available to most fitness participants. Thus, other methods to estimate body composition are used. The most common of these are:

1. Hydrostatic or underwater weighing
2. Air displacement
3. Skinfold thickness
4. Girth measurements
5. Bioelectrical impedance

Because these procedures yield estimates of body fat, each technique may yield slightly different values. Therefore, when assessing changes in body composition, be sure to use the same technique for pre- and post-test comparisons.

Other techniques to assess body composition are available, but the equipment is costly and not easily accessible to the general population. In addition to percentages of lean tissue and body fat, some of these methods also provide information on total body water and bone mass. These techniques include air displacement, magnetic resonance imaging (MRI), computed tomography (CT), and total body electrical conductivity (TOBEC).

Hydrostatic Weighing

Until the advent of DXA, **hydrostatic weighing** had been the most common technique used in determining body composition in exercise physiology laboratories. With hydrostatic weighing, a person's "regular" weight is compared with a weight taken underwater. Because fat is more buoyant than lean tissue, comparing the two weights can determine a person's percentage of fat. The procedure requires a considerable amount of time, skill, space, and equipment and must be administered by a well-trained technician. The SEE for hydrostatic weighing is ±2.5 percent.

This technique has several drawbacks. First, because each individual assessment can take as long as 30 minutes, hydrostatic weighing is not feasible when testing a lot of people. Furthermore, the person's residual lung volume (amount of air left in the lungs following complete forceful exhalation) should be measured before testing. If residual volume cannot be measured, as is the case in some laboratories and health/fitness centers, it is estimated using the predicting equations, which may decrease the accuracy of hydrostatic weighing. Also, the requirement of being completely underwater makes hydrostatic weighing difficult to administer to **aquaphobic** people. For accurate results, the individual must be able to perform the test properly. Forcing all of the air out of the lungs is not easy for everyone but is important to obtain an accurate reading. Leaving additional air (beyond residual volume) in the lungs makes a person more buoyant. Because fat is less dense than water, overweight individuals weigh less in water. Additional air in the lungs makes a person lighter in water, yielding a false, higher body fat percentage.

For each underwater weighing trial, the person has to (a) force out all of the air in the lungs, (b) lean forward and completely submerge underwater for about 5 to 10 seconds (long enough to get the underwater weight), and (c)

remain as calm as possible (chair movement makes reading the scale difficult). This procedure is repeated eight to ten times.

Air Displacement

When using **air displacement** (also known as air displacement plethysmography), an individual sits inside a small chamber, commercially known as the **Bod Pod**. Computerized pressure sensors determine the amount of air displaced by the person inside the chamber. Body volume is calculated by subtracting the air volume with the person inside the chamber from the volume of the empty chamber. The amount of air in the person's lungs also is taken into consideration when determining actual body volume. Body density and percent body fat then are calculated from the obtained body volume.

The procedure to assess body composition according to air displacement takes only about 15 minutes. Initial research showed that this technique compared favorably with hydrostatic weighing while being less cumbersome to administer. The published SEE for air displacement was originally ±2.2 percent; however, the SEE may actually be higher. Subsequent research determined that percent body fat is about 5 percentage points higher with air displacement than with hydrostatic weighing.[8] Researchers have concluded that further technical work is required to make air displacement an acceptable technique to determine body composition. Furthermore, research is required to determine its accuracy among different age groups, ethnic backgrounds, and athletic populations.

HOEGER KEY TO WELLNESS

Before undergoing body composition testing, make sure you understand the accuracy of the technique and inquire about the experience of the person administering the test.

Hydrostatic or underwater weighing technique.

Bod Pod, used for assessment of body composition.

© Fitness & Wellness, Inc.

GLOSSARY

Dual energy x-ray absorptiometry (DXA) Method to assess body composition that uses very low-dose beams of x-ray energy to measure total body fat mass, fat distribution pattern, and bone density; considered the most accurate of the body composition assessment techniques.

Hydrostatic weighing Underwater technique to assess body composition.

Aquaphobic Having a fear of water.

Air displacement Technique to assess body composition by calculating the body volume from the air replaced by an individual sitting inside a small chamber.

Bod Pod Commercial name of the equipment used to assess body composition through the air displacement technique.

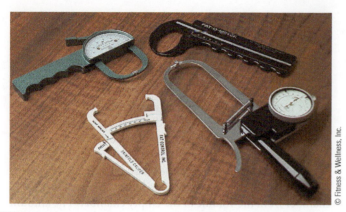

Various types of calipers used to assess skinfold thickness.

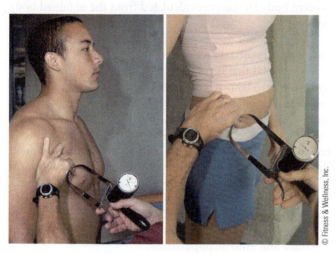

Chest and suprailium skinfold assessments.

Skinfold Thickness

Because of the cost, time, and complexity of hydrostatic weighing and the expense of Bod Pod equipment, most health and fitness programs use **anthropometric measurement** techniques. These techniques, primarily skinfold thickness and girth measurements, allow quick, simple, and inexpensive estimates of body composition.

Assessing body composition using **skinfold thickness** is based on the principle that the amount of subcutaneous fat is proportional to total body fat. Valid and reliable measurements of this tissue give a good indication of percent body fat. The SEE for skinfold analysis is ±3.5 percent.

The skinfold test is done with the aid of pressure calipers. Several techniques requiring measurement of three to seven sites have been developed. The following three-site procedure is the most commonly used technique. The sites measured are as follows (also see Figure 4.6). All measurements should be taken on the right side of the body.

Women: triceps, suprailium, and thigh skinfolds
Men: chest, abdomen, and thigh

With the skinfold technique, training is necessary to obtain accurate measurements. In addition, different technicians may produce slightly different measurements of the same person. Therefore, the same technician should take pre- and post-test measurements.

Measurements should be done at the same time of the day—preferably in the morning—because changes in water hydration from activity and exercise can affect skinfold girth. The procedure is given in Figure 4.6. If skinfold calipers are available, you may assess your percent body fat

Figure 4.6 Procedure and anatomical landmarks for skinfold measurements.

Skinfold Measurement

1. Select the proper anatomical sites. For men, use chest, abdomen, and thigh skinfolds. For women, use triceps, suprailium, and thigh skinfolds. Take all measurements on the right side of the body with the person standing.

2. Measure each site by grasping a double thickness of skin firmly with the thumb and forefinger, pulling the fold slightly away from the muscular tissue. Hold the caliper perpendicular to the fold and take the measurement 1/2″ below the finger hold. Measure each site three times and read the values to the nearest .1 to .5 mm. Record the average of the two closest readings as the final value for that site. Take the readings without delay to avoid excessive compression of the skinfold. Release and refold the skinfold between readings.

3. When doing pre- and post-assessments, conduct the measurement at the same time of day. The best time is early in the morning to avoid water hydration changes resulting from activity or exercise.

4. Obtain percent fat by adding the skinfold measurements from all three sites and looking up the respective values in Tables 4.1, 4.2, or 4.3.

For example, if the skinfold measurements for an 18-year-old female are (a) triceps = 16, (b) suprailium = 4, and (c) thigh = 30 (total = 50), the percent body fat is 20.6%.

Chest (diagonal fold halfway between shoulder crease and nipple)

Abdomen (vertical fold taken about 1/2″ to 1″ to the right of umbilicus)

Triceps (vertical fold on back of upper arm, halfway between shoulder and elbow)

Suprailium (diagonal fold above crest of ilium, on the side of the hip)

Thigh (vertical fold on front of thigh, midway between knee and hip)

Table 4.1 Skinfold Thickness Technique: Percent Fat Estimates for Women Calculated from Triceps, Suprailium, and Thigh

Sum of 3 Skinfolds	Age at Last Birthday								
	22 or Under	23 to 27	28 to 32	33 to 37	38 to 42	43 to 47	48 to 52	53 to 57	58 and Over
23–25	9.7	9.9	10.2	10.4	10.7	10.9	11.2	11.4	11.7
26–28	11.0	11.2	11.5	11.7	12.0	12.3	12.5	12.7	13.0
29–31	12.3	12.5	12.8	13.0	13.3	13.5	13.8	14.0	14.3
32–34	13.6	13.8	14.0	14.3	14.5	14.8	15.0	15.3	15.5
35–37	14.8	15.0	15.3	15.5	15.8	16.0	16.3	16.5	16.8
38–40	16.0	16.3	16.5	16.7	17.0	17.2	17.5	17.7	18.0
41–43	17.2	17.4	17.7	17.9	18.2	18.4	18.7	18.9	19.2
44–46	18.3	18.6	18.8	19.1	19.3	19.6	19.8	20.1	20.3
47–49	19.5	19.7	20.0	20.2	20.5	20.7	21.0	21.2	21.5
50–52	20.6	20.8	21.1	21.3	21.6	21.8	22.1	22.3	22.6
53–55	21.7	21.9	22.1	22.4	22.6	22.9	23.1	23.4	23.6
56–58	22.7	23.0	23.2	23.4	23.7	23.9	24.2	24.4	24.7
59–61	23.7	24.0	24.2	24.5	24.7	25.0	25.2	25.5	25.7
62–64	24.7	25.0	25.2	25.5	25.7	26.0	26.2	26.4	26.7
65–67	25.7	25.9	26.2	26.4	26.7	26.9	27.2	27.4	27.7
68–70	26.6	26.9	27.1	27.4	27.6	27.9	28.1	28.4	28.6
71–73	27.5	27.8	28.0	28.3	28.5	28.8	29.0	29.3	29.5
74–76	28.4	28.7	28.9	29.2	29.4	29.7	29.9	30.2	30.4
77–79	29.3	29.5	29.8	30.0	30.3	30.5	30.8	31.0	31.3
80–82	30.1	30.4	30.6	30.9	31.1	31.4	31.6	31.9	32.1
83–85	30.9	31.2	31.4	31.7	31.9	32.2	32.4	32.7	32.9
86–88	31.7	32.0	32.2	32.5	32.7	32.9	33.2	33.4	33.7
89–91	32.5	32.7	33.0	33.2	33.5	33.7	33.9	34.2	34.4
92–94	33.2	33.4	33.7	33.9	34.2	34.4	34.7	34.9	35.2
95–97	33.9	34.1	34.4	34.6	34.9	35.1	35.4	35.6	35.9
98–100	34.6	34.8	35.1	35.3	35.5	35.8	36.0	36.3	36.5
101–103	35.2	35.4	35.7	35.9	36.2	36.4	36.7	36.9	37.2
104–106	35.8	36.1	36.3	36.6	36.8	37.1	37.3	37.5	37.8
107–109	36.4	36.7	36.9	37.1	37.4	37.6	37.9	38.1	38.4
110–112	37.0	37.2	37.5	37.7	38.0	38.2	38.5	38.7	38.9
113–115	37.5	37.8	38.0	38.2	38.5	38.7	39.0	39.2	39.5
116–118	38.0	38.3	38.5	38.8	39.0	39.3	39.5	39.7	40.0
119–121	38.5	38.7	39.0	39.2	39.5	39.7	40.0	40.2	40.5
122–124	39.0	39.2	39.4	39.7	39.9	40.2	40.4	40.7	40.9
125–127	39.4	39.6	39.9	40.1	40.4	40.6	40.9	41.1	41.4
128–130	39.8	40.0	40.3	40.5	40.8	41.0	41.3	41.5	41.8

Body density is calculated based on the generalized equation for predicting body density of women developed by A. S. Jackson, M. L. Pollock, and A. Ward and published in *Medicine and Science in Sports and Exercise* 12 (1980): 175–182. Percent body fat is determined from the calculated body density using the Siri formula.

with the help of your instructor or an experienced technician (also see Activity 4.1). Then locate the percent fat estimates in Table 4.1, Table 4.2, or Table 4.3, as appropriate.

Girth Measurements

Another method that is frequently used to estimate body fat is to measure circumferences, or **girth measurements**, at various body sites. This technique requires only a standard measuring tape. The limitation is that it may not be valid for

GLOSSARY

Anthropometric measurement Techniques to measure body girths at different sites.

Skinfold thickness Technique to assess body composition by measuring a double thickness of skin at specific body sites.

Girth measurements Technique to assess body composition by measuring circumferences at specific body sites.

Table 4.2 Skinfold Thickness Technique: Percent Fat Estimates for Men Younger Than 40 Calculated from Chest, Abdomen, and Thigh

Sum of 3 Skinfolds	Age at Last Birthday							
	19 or Under	20 to 22	23 to 25	26 to 28	29 to 31	32 to 34	35 to 37	38 to 40
8–10	.9	1.3	1.6	2.0	2.3	2.7	3.0	3.3
11–13	1.9	2.3	2.6	3.0	3.3	3.7	4.0	4.3
14–16	2.9	3.3	3.6	3.9	4.3	4.6	5.0	5.3
17–19	3.9	4.2	4.6	4.9	5.3	5.6	6.0	6.3
20–22	4.8	5.2	5.5	5.9	6.2	6.6	6.9	7.3
23–25	5.8	6.2	6.5	6.8	7.2	7.5	7.9	8.2
26–28	6.8	7.1	7.5	7.8	8.1	8.5	8.8	9.2
29–31	7.7	8.0	8.4	8.7	9.1	9.4	9.8	10.1
32–34	8.6	9.0	9.3	9.7	10.0	10.4	10.7	11.1
35–37	9.5	9.9	10.2	10.6	10.9	11.3	11.6	12.0
38–40	10.5	10.8	11.2	11.5	11.8	12.2	12.5	12.9
41–43	11.4	11.7	12.1	12.4	12.7	13.1	13.4	13.8
44–46	12.2	12.6	12.9	13.3	13.6	14.0	14.3	14.7
47–49	13.1	13.5	13.8	14.2	14.5	14.9	15.2	15.5
50–52	14.0	14.3	14.7	15.0	15.4	15.7	16.1	16.4
53–55	14.8	15.2	15.5	15.9	16.2	16.6	16.9	17.3
56–58	15.7	16.0	16.4	16.7	17.1	17.4	17.8	18.1
59–61	16.5	16.9	17.2	17.6	17.9	18.3	18.6	19.0
62–64	17.4	17.7	18.1	18.4	18.8	19.1	19.4	19.8
65–67	18.2	18.5	18.9	19.2	19.6	19.9	20.3	20.6
68–70	19.0	19.3	19.7	20.0	20.4	20.7	21.1	21.4
71–73	19.8	20.1	20.5	20.8	21.2	21.5	21.9	22.2
74–76	20.6	20.9	21.3	21.6	22.0	22.2	22.7	23.0
77–79	21.4	21.7	22.1	22.4	22.8	23.1	23.4	23.8
80–82	22.1	22.5	22.8	23.2	23.5	23.9	24.2	24.6
83–85	22.9	23.2	23.6	23.9	24.3	24.6	25.0	25.3
86–88	23.6	24.0	24.3	24.7	25.0	25.4	25.7	26.1
89–91	24.4	24.7	25.1	25.4	25.8	26.1	26.5	26.8
92–94	25.1	25.5	25.8	26.2	26.5	26.9	27.2	27.5
95–97	25.8	26.2	26.5	26.9	27.2	27.6	27.9	28.3
98–100	26.6	26.9	27.3	27.6	27.9	28.3	28.6	29.0
101–103	27.3	27.6	28.0	28.3	28.6	29.0	29.3	29.7
104–106	27.9	28.3	28.6	29.0	29.3	29.7	30.0	30.4
107–109	28.6	29.0	29.3	29.7	30.0	30.4	30.7	31.1
110–112	29.3	29.6	30.0	30.3	30.7	31.0	31.4	31.7
113–115	30.0	30.3	30.7	31.0	31.3	31.7	32.0	32.4
116–118	30.6	31.0	31.3	31.6	32.0	32.3	32.7	33.0
119–121	31.3	31.6	32.0	32.3	32.6	33.0	33.3	33.7
122–124	31.9	32.2	32.6	32.9	33.3	33.6	34.0	34.3
125–127	32.5	32.9	33.2	33.5	33.9	34.2	34.6	34.9
128–130	33.1	33.5	33.8	34.2	34.5	34.9	35.2	35.5

Body density is calculated based on the generalized equation for predicting body density of men developed by A. S. Jackson, M. L. Pollock, and A. Ward and published in *Medicine and Science in Sports and Exercise* 40 (1978): 497–504. Percent body fat is determined from the calculated body density using the Siri formula.

athletic individuals (men or women) who participate actively in strenuous physical activity or for people who can be classified visually as thin or obese. The SEE for girth measurements is approximately ±4 percent.

The required procedure for girth measurements is given in Figure 4.7; conversion factors are in Table 4.4 and Table 4.5. Measurements for women are the upper arm, hip, and wrist; for men, the waist and wrist.

Table 4.3 Skinfold Thickness Technique: Percent Fat Estimates for Men Older Than 40 Calculated from Chest, Abdomen, and Thigh

Sum of 3 Skinfolds	Age at Last Birthday							
	41 to 43	44 to 46	47 to 49	50 to 52	53 to 55	56 to 58	59 to 61	62 and Over
8–10	3.7	4.0	4.4	4.7	5.1	5.4	5.8	6.1
11–13	4.7	5.0	5.4	5.7	6.1	6.4	6.8	7.1
14–16	5.7	6.0	6.4	6.7	7.1	7.4	7.8	8.1
17–19	6.7	7.0	7.4	7.7	8.1	8.4	8.7	9.1
20–22	7.6	8.0	8.3	8.7	9.0	9.4	9.7	10.1
23–25	8.6	8.9	9.3	9.6	10.0	10.3	10.7	11.0
26–28	9.5	9.9	10.2	10.6	10.9	11.3	11.6	12.0
29–31	10.5	10.8	11.2	11.5	11.9	12.2	12.6	12.9
32–34	11.4	11.8	12.1	12.4	12.8	13.1	13.5	13.8
35–37	12.3	12.7	13.0	13.4	13.7	14.1	14.4	14.8
38–40	13.2	13.6	13.9	14.3	14.6	15.0	15.3	15.7
41–43	14.1	14.5	14.8	15.2	15.5	15.9	16.2	16.6
44–46	15.0	15.4	15.7	16.1	16.4	16.8	17.1	17.5
47–49	15.9	16.2	16.6	16.9	17.3	17.6	18.0	18.3
50–52	16.8	17.1	17.5	17.8	18.2	18.5	18.8	19.2
53–55	17.6	18.0	18.3	18.7	19.0	19.4	19.7	20.1
56–58	18.5	18.8	19.2	19.5	19.9	20.2	20.6	20.9
59–61	19.3	19.7	20.0	20.4	20.7	21.0	21.4	21.7
62–64	20.1	20.5	20.8	21.2	21.5	21.9	22.2	22.6
65–67	21.0	21.3	21.7	22.0	22.4	22.7	23.0	23.4
68–70	21.8	22.1	22.5	22.8	23.2	23.5	23.9	24.2
71–73	22.6	22.9	23.3	23.6	24.0	24.3	24.7	25.0
74–76	23.4	23.7	24.1	24.4	24.8	25.1	25.4	25.8
77–79	24.1	24.5	24.8	25.2	25.5	25.9	26.2	26.6
80–82	24.9	25.3	25.6	26.0	26.3	26.6	27.0	27.3
83–85	25.7	26.0	26.4	26.7	27.1	27.4	27.8	28.1
86–88	26.4	26.8	27.1	27.5	27.8	28.2	28.5	28.9
89–91	27.2	27.5	27.9	28.2	28.6	28.9	29.2	29.6
92–94	27.9	28.2	28.6	28.9	29.3	29.6	30.0	30.3
95–97	28.6	29.0	29.3	29.7	30.0	30.4	30.7	31.1
98–100	29.3	29.7	30.0	30.4	30.7	31.1	31.4	31.8
101–103	30.0	30.4	30.7	31.1	31.4	31.8	32.1	32.5
104–106	30.7	31.1	31.4	31.8	32.1	32.5	32.8	33.2
107–109	31.4	31.8	32.1	32.4	32.8	33.1	33.5	33.8
110–112	32.1	32.4	32.8	33.1	33.5	33.8	34.2	34.5
113–115	32.7	33.1	33.4	33.8	34.1	34.5	34.8	35.2
116–118	33.4	33.7	34.1	34.4	34.8	35.1	35.5	35.8
119–121	34.0	34.4	34.7	35.1	35.4	35.8	36.1	36.5
122–124	34.7	35.0	35.4	35.7	36.1	36.4	36.7	37.1
125–127	35.3	35.6	36.0	36.3	36.7	37.0	37.4	37.7
128–130	35.9	36.2	36.6	36.9	37.3	37.6	38.0	38.5

Body density is calculated based on the generalized equation for predicting body density of men developed by A. S. Jackson and M. L. Pollock and published in the *British Journal of Nutrition* 40 (1978): 497–504. Percent body fat is determined from the calculated body density using the Siri formula.

Bioelectrical Impedance

The **bioelectrical impedance** technique is much simpler to administer, but its accuracy is questionable. In this technique, sensors are applied to the skin and a weak (totally painless) electrical current is run through the body to measure its

GLOSSARY

Bioelectrical impedance Technique to assess body composition by running a weak electrical current through the body.

Table 4.4 Girth Measurement Technique: Conversion Constants to Calculate Body Density for Women

Upper Arm (cm)	Constant A	Age	Constant B	Hip (cm)	Constant C	Hip (cm)	Constant C	Wrist (cm)	Constant D
20.5	1.0966	17	.0086	79	.0957	114.5	.1388	13.0	.0819
21	1.0954	18	.0091	79.5	.0963	115	.1394	13.2	.0832
21.5	1.0942	19	.0096	80	.0970	115.5	.1400	13.4	.0845
22	1.0930	20	.0102	80.5	.0976	116	.1406	13.6	.0857
22.5	1.0919	21	.0107	81	.0982	116.5	.1412	13.8	.0870
23	1.0907	22	.0112	81.5	.0988	117	.1418	14.0	.0882
23.5	1.0895	23	.0117	82	.0994	117.5	.1424	14.2	.0895
24	1.0883	24	.0122	82.5	.1000	118	.1430	14.4	.0908
24.5	1.0871	25	.0127	83	.1006	118.5	.1436	14.6	.0920
25	1.0860	26	.0132	83.5	.1012	119	.1442	14.8	.0933
25.5	1.0848	27	.0137	84	.1018	119.5	.1448	15.0	.0946
26	1.0836	28	.0142	84.5	.1024	120	.1454	15.2	.0958
26.5	1.0824	29	.0147	85	.1030	120.5	.1460	15.4	.0971
27	1.0813	30	.0152	85.5	.1036	121	.1466	15.6	.0983
27.5	1.0801	31	.0157	86	.1042	121.5	.1472	15.8	.0996
28	1.0789	32	.0162	86.5	.1048	122	.1479	16.0	.1009
28.5	1.0777	33	.0168	87	.1054	122.5	.1485	16.2	.1021
29	1.0775	34	.0173	87.5	.1060	123	.1491	16.4	.1034
29.5	1.0754	35	.0178	88	.1066	123.5	.1497	16.6	.1046
30	1.0742	36	.0183	88.5	.1072	124	.1503	16.8	.1059
30.5	1.0730	37	.0188	89	.1079	124.5	.1509	17.0	.1072
31	1.0718	38	.0193	89.5	.1085	125	.1515	17.2	.1084
31.5	1.0707	39	.0198	90	.1091	125.5	.1521	17.4	.1097
32	1.0695	40	.0203	90.5	.1097	126	.1527	17.6	.1109
32.5	1.0683	41	.0208	91	.1103	126.5	.1533	17.8	.1122
33	1.0671	42	.0213	91.5	.1109	127	.1539	18.0	.1135
33.5	1.0666	43	.0218	92	.1115	127.5	.1545	18.2	.1147
34	1.0648	44	.0223	92.5	.1121	128	.1551	18.4	.1160
34.5	1.0636	45	.0228	93	.1127	128.5	.1558	18.6	.1172
35	1.0624	46	.0234	93.5	.1133	129	.1563		
35.5	1.0612	47	.0239	94	.1139	129.5	.1569		
36	1.0601	48	.0244	94.5	.1145	130	.1575		
36.5	1.0589	49	.0249	95	.1151	130.5	.1581		
37	1.0577	50	.0254	95.5	.1157	131	.1587		
37.5	1.0565	51	.0259	96	.1163	131.5	.1593		
38	1.0554	52	.0264	96.5	.1169	132	.1600		
38.5	1.0542	53	.0269	97	.1176	132.5	.1606		
39	1.0530	54	.0274	97.5	.1182	133	.1612		
39.5	1.0518	55	.0279	98	.1188	133.5	.1618		
40	1.0506	56	.0284	98.5	.1194	134	.1624		
40.5	1.0495	57	.0289	99	.1200	134.5	.1630		
41	1.0483	58	.0294	99.5	.1206	135	.1636		
41.5	1.0471	59	.0300	100	.1212	135.5	.1642		
42	1.0459	60	.0305	100.5	.1218	136	.1648		
42.5	1.0448	61	.0310	101	.1224	136.5	.1654		
43	1.0434	62	.0315	101.5	.1230	137	.1660		
43.5	1.0424	63	.0320	102	.1236	137.5	.1666		
44	1.0412	64	.0325	102.5	.1242	138	.1672		
		65	.0330	103	.1248	138.5	.1678		
		66	.0335	103.5	.1254	139	.1685		
		67	.0340	104	.1260	139.5	.1691		

(continued)

Upper Arm (cm)	Constant A	Age	Constant B	Hip (cm)	Constant C	Hip (cm)	Constant C	Wrist (cm)	Constant D
		68	.0345	104.5	.1266	140	.1697		
		69	.0350	105	.1272	140.5	.1703		
		70	.0355	105.5	.1278	141	.1709		
		71	.0360	106	.1285	141.5	.1715		
		72	.0366	106.5	.1291	142	.1721		
		73	.0371	107	.1297	142.5	.1728		
		74	.0376	107.5	.1303	143	.1733		
		75	.0381	108	.1309	143.5	.1739		
				108.5	.1315	144	.1745		
				109	.1321	144.5	.1751		
				109.5	.1327	145	.1757		
				110	.1333	145.5	.1763		
				110.5	.1339	146	.1769		
				111	.1345	146.5	.1775		
				111.5	.1351	147	.1781		
				112	.1357	147.5	.1787		
				112.5	.1363	148	.1794		
				113	.1369	148.5	.1800		
				113.5	.1375	149	.1806		
				114	.1382	149.5	.1812		
						150	.1818		

electrical resistance, which is then used to estimate body fat, lean body mass, and body water.

The technique is based on the principle that fat tissue is a less efficient conductor of electrical current than is lean tissue. The easier the conductance is, the leaner the individual. Specialized equipment or simple body weight scales with sensors on the surface can be used to perform this procedure.

The accuracy of equations used to estimate percent body fat with this technique may not be reliable. A single equation cannot be used for everyone, but rather valid and accurate equations to estimate body fat for the specific population (age, gender, and ethnicity) are required. Several factors can affect the results, including the individual's water intake and body temperature. Following all manufacturers' instructions will ensure the most accurate result, but even then percent body fat may be off—typically on the higher end, by as much as 10 percentage points (or even more on some scales).

4.5 *Metrics Used to Assess Body Size and Shape*

As you evaluate your body weight and the weight you would like to reach and maintain throughout life, there are a few metrics that will be helpful to know in addition to knowing your body composition. They are body mass index (BMI), waist-to-height ratio (WHtR), and waist circumference (WC). Assessments for these metrics require only a scale and a measuring tape, are quick and easy to obtain, and offer a realistic way for you to track your body weight and shape throughout the years.

Body Mass Index

The technique most widely used over recent decades to determine thinness and excessive fatness is the **body mass index (BMI)**. BMI incorporates height and weight to estimate critical fat values at which the risk for disease increases. BMI is calculated by one of two methods:

1. Dividing the weight in kilograms by the square of the height in meters.
2. Multiplying body weight in pounds by 703 and dividing this figure by the square of the height in inches.

For example, the BMI for an individual who weighs 172 pounds (78 kg) and is 67 inches (1.7 m) tall would be 27: [$78 \div (1.7)^2$] or [$172 \times 703 \div (67)^2$]. You also can look up your BMI in Table 4.6 using your height and weight.

The math for BMI originally came from Lambert Adolphe Jacques Quetelet, a Belgian mathematician in the 1830s. He sought equations to define several features of the average man, including the average build. He surveyed several hundred individuals and settled on the equation of dividing weight by the square of the person's height, which generally followed the average results for the builds of the men measured. This equation was not connected to obesity until the 1970s, when a large-scale study made the equation popular as a way to combine

GLOSSARY

Body mass index (BMI) Technique to determine thinness and excessive fatness that incorporates height and weight to estimate critical fat values at which the risk for disease increases.

Figure 4.7 **Procedure for body fat assessment according to girth measurements.**

Girth Measurements for Women*

1. Using a regular tape measure, determine the following girth measurements in centimeters (cm):

   Upper arm: Take the measure halfway between the shoulder and the elbow.

   Hip: Measure at the point of largest circumference.

   Wrist: Take the girth in front of the bones where the wrist bends.

2. Obtain the person's age.

3. Using Table 4.4, find the subject's age and girth measurement for each site, then look up the respective constant value for each. These values will allow you to derive body density (BD) by substituting the constants in the following formula:

   $$BD = A - B - C + D$$

4. Using the derived body density, calculate percent body fat (%F) according to the following equation:

   $$\%F = (495 \div BD) - 450**$$

Example: Jane is 20 years old, and the following girth measurements were taken: biceps = 27 cm, hip = 99.5 cm, wrist = 15.4 cm

Data	Constant
Upper arm = 27 cm	A = 1.0813
Age = 20	B = .0102
Hip = 99.5 cm	C = .1206
Wrist = 15.4 cm	D = .0971

$$BD = A - B - C + D$$
$$BD = 1.0813 - .0102 - .1206 + .0971 = 1.0476$$
$$\%F = (495 \div BD) - 450$$
$$\%F = (495 \div 1.0476) - 450 = 22.5$$

Girth Measurements for Men***

1. Using a regular tape measure, determine the following girth measurements in inches (the men's measurements are taken in inches, as opposed to centimeters for women):

   Waist: Measure at the umbilicus (belly button).

   Wrist: Measure in front of the bones where the wrist bends.

2. Subtract the wrist from the waist measurement.

3. Obtain the weight of the subject in pounds.

4. Look up the percent body fat (%F) in Table 4.5 by using the difference obtained in number 2 above and the person's body weight.

Example: John weighs 160 pounds, and his waist and wrist girth measurements are 36.5 and 7.5 inches, respectively.

Waist girth = 36.5 inches
Wrist girth = 7.5 inches
Difference = 29.0 inches
Body weight = 160.0 lbs.
%F = 22

*From R. B. Lambson, "Generalized body density prediction equations for women using simple anthropometric measurements." Unpublished doctoral dissertation, Brigham Young University, Provo, UT, August 1987. Reproduced by permission.
**From W. E. Siri, *Body Composition from Fluid Spaces and Density* (Berkeley: University of California, Donner Laboratory of Medical Physics, March 19, 1956.)
***K. W. Penrouse, A. G. Nelson, and A. G. Fisher, "Generalized body composition equation for men using simple measurement techniques," *Medicine and Science in Sports and Exercise* 17, no. 2 (1985): 189. © American College of Sports Medicine, 1985.

height and weight into a single number. The equation was coined BMI and was immediately adopted by researchers studying large populations as a simple way to sift through massive amounts of data, allowing them to connect general trends in height and weight to health outcomes. Some modern researchers contend that a proper equation for BMI should be more complex, as short and tall individuals may receive an inaccurate prediction of health risk. Regardless of its accuracy for large populations, BMI was not initially created to be used as a predictor of health outcomes for individuals.

BMI is important to understand, however, because it is the most widely used method to determine overweight and obesity across the world. Due to the various limitations of previously mentioned body composition techniques—including cost, availability, and lack of consistency—BMI is used almost exclusively in place of body composition tests to determine health risks and mortality rates associated with excessive body weight. As long as its limitations are kept in mind, BMI can add to our general knowledge of the relationship between body size and disease risk, especially when used in conjunction with waist circumference.

BMI and disease risk

Scientific evidence indicates that the risk for disease starts to increase when BMI exceeds 25.[9] Although a BMI between 18.5 and 25 is considered normal (see Table 4.7 and Table 4.9), the lowest risk for chronic disease is in the 22 to 25 range.[10] Individuals are classified as overweight if their index lies between 25 and 30. A BMI of 30 or greater is defined as obese, and one less than 18.5 is considered **underweight**.

GLOSSARY

Underweight Extremely low body weight.

Table 4.5 Girth Measurement Technique: Estimated Percent Body Fat for Men

Waist Minus Wrist Girth Measurement (inches)

Body Weight (pounds)	22	22.5	23	23.5	24	24.5	25	25.5	26	26.5	27	27.5	28	28.5	29	29.5	30	30.5	31	31.5	32	32.5	33	33.5	34	34.5	35	35.5	36	36.5	37	37.5	38	38.5	39	39.5	40	40.5	41	41.5	42	42.5	43	43.5	44	44.5	45	45.5	46	46.5	47	47.5	48	48.5	49	49.5	50
120	4	6	8	10	12	14	16	18	20	21	23	25	27	29	31	33	35	37	39	41	43	45	47	49	50	52	54	56	58																											
125	4	6	7	9	11	13	15	17	18	20	22	24	26	28	30	32	33	35	37	39	41	43	45	46	48	50	52	54	56	58																										
130	3	5	7	9	11	12	14	16	18	20	21	23	25	27	28	30	32	34	36	37	39	41	43	44	46	48	50	52	53	55	57																								
135	3	5	7	8	10	12	14	15	17	19	20	22	24	26	27	29	31	32	34	36	38	39	41	43	44	46	48	50	51	53	55	56																							
140	3	5	6	8	10	11	13	15	16	18	20	22	23	25	27	28	30	31	33	35	36	38	40	41	43	44	46	48	49	51	53	54	56																						
145	3	4	6	8	9	11	13	14	16	17	19	21	22	24	26	27	29	30	32	34	35	37	38	40	42	43	45	46	48	50	51	53	54	55																					
150	2	4	6	7	9	11	12	14	15	17	18	20	22	23	25	26	28	29	31	33	34	36	38	39	41	42	44	45	47	49	50	52	53	55	55																				
155	2	4	5	7	8	10	12	13	15	16	18	19	21	23	24	26	27	29	30	32	34	35	37	38	40	42	43	45	46	48	50	51	53	54	55	55																			
160	2	4	5	6	8	9	11	12	14	15	17	18	20	22	23	25	26	28	29	31	33	34	36	37	39	40	42	44	45	47	48	50	52	53	54	54	54																		
165	2	4	5	6	7	9	11	12	13	15	16	18	19	21	22	24	25	27	28	30	31	33	35	36	38	39	41	43	44	46	47	49	51	52	53	54	54	54																	
170	2	3	5	6	7	9	10	12	13	14	16	17	19	20	22	23	25	26	28	29	31	32	34	36	37	39	40	42	44	45	47	48	50	52	53	54	54	53	53																
175	2	3	4	6	7	8	10	11	13	14	15	17	18	20	21	23	24	26	27	29	30	32	33	35	36	38	40	41	43	44	46	48	49	51	52	53	54	53	52	53															
180	3	4	5	6	8	9	10	12	13	15	16	17	19	20	22	23	25	26	28	29	30	32	33	35	37	38	40	41	43	44	46	47	49	50	52	53	54	52	52	52	53														
185	3	4	5	6	7	9	10	11	13	14	15	17	18	20	21	22	24	25	27	28	30	31	32	34	35	37	38	40	42	43	45	46	48	49	51	53	53	51	51	52	53	53													
190	2	4	5	6	7	8	10	11	12	14	15	16	18	19	21	22	23	25	26	28	29	30	32	33	35	36	38	39	41	42	44	45	47	48	50	51	52	50	51	51	52	52	52												
195	2	3	4	5	7	8	9	10	12	13	14	16	17	18	20	21	22	24	25	27	28	29	31	32	34	35	36	38	39	41	42	44	45	47	48	50	51	49	50	50	51	51	52	52											
200	2	3	4	5	6	8	9	10	11	13	14	15	17	18	19	21	22	23	25	26	27	29	30	32	33	34	36	37	39	40	41	43	44	46	47	49	50	48	49	49	50	51	51	51	52										
205	2	3	4	5	6	7	9	10	11	12	14	15	16	18	19	20	22	23	24	26	27	28	30	31	32	34	35	36	38	39	41	42	43	45	46	48	49	47	48	48	49	50	50	51	51	51									
210	2	3	4	5	6	7	8	10	11	12	13	15	16	17	19	20	21	23	24	25	27	28	29	31	32	33	35	36	38	39	40	42	43	44	46	47	48	46	47	48	48	49	50	50	51	51	51								
215	2	3	4	5	6	7	8	9	11	12	13	14	16	17	18	19	21	22	23	25	26	27	29	30	31	33	34	35	37	38	39	41	42	43	45	46	47	45	46	47	48	48	49	50	50	51	51	51							
220	2	3	4	5	6	7	8	9	10	12	13	14	15	17	18	19	20	22	23	24	26	27	28	29	31	32	33	35	36	37	39	40	41	42	44	45	46	44	45	46	47	48	48	49	50	50	51	51	51						
225	2	3	4	5	6	7	8	9	10	11	13	14	15	16	17	19	20	21	22	24	25	26	28	29	30	31	33	34	35	37	38	39	40	42	43	44	46	43	44	45	46	47	48	49	49	50	50	51	51	51					
230	2	3	4	5	6	7	8	9	10	11	12	14	15	16	17	18	20	21	22	23	25	26	27	28	30	31	32	34	35	36	37	39	40	41	42	44	45	42	43	44	45	46	47	48	48	49	50	50	51	51	51				
235	2	3	4	5	6	7	8	9	10	11	12	13	15	16	17	18	19	21	22	23	24	26	27	28	29	30	32	33	34	36	37	38	39	41	42	43	44	41	42	43	44	45	46	47	48	48	49	49	50	51	51	51		
240	2	3	4	5	6	7	8	9	9	11	12	13	14	15	16	18	19	20	21	22	24	25	26	27	29	30	31	32	33	35	36	37	38	40	41	42	43	40	41	42	43	44	45	46	47	48	49	49	50	50	51	50	50	
245	2	3	4	5	6	6	7	8	9	10	11	13	14	15	16	17	18	20	21	22	23	24	26	27	28	29	30	32	33	34	35	37	38	39	40	41	43	39	40	41	42	43	44	45	46	47	48	49	49	50	51	49	49	49
250	2	3	3	4	5	6	7	8	9	10	11	12	14	15	16	17	18	19	20	22	23	24	25	26	28	29	30	31	32	34	35	36	37	38	40	41	42	38	39	40	41	42	43	44	45	46	47	48	49	50	51	48	49	49
255	2	2	3	4	5	6	7	8	9	10	11	12	13	14	16	17	18	19	20	21	22	24	25	26	27	28	29	31	32	33	34	35	37	38	39	40	41	37	38	39	40	42	43	44	45	46	47	48	49	50	51	52	48	48
260	2	2	3	4	5	6	7	8	8	9	10	12	13	14	15	16	17	18	19	21	22	23	24	25	26	28	29	30	31	32	33	35	36	37	38	39	40	36	37	38	39	40	41	42	44	45	46	47	48	49	50	51	52	50
265	2	2	3	4	5	6	6	7	8	9	10	11	12	14	15	16	17	18	19	20	21	22	24	25	26	27	28	29	30	32	33	34	35	36	37	38	40	35	36	37	38	39	40	41	42	43	44	45	46	47	48	49	51	49
270	2	2	3	4	4	5	6	7	8	9	10	11	12	13	14	16	17	18	19	20	21	22	23	24	26	27	28	29	30	31	32	34	35	36	37	38	39	34	35	36	37	38	39	40	41	43	44	45	46	47	48	49	50	49
275	2	2	3	3	4	5	6	7	8	9	9	11	12	13	14	15	16	17	18	19	21	22	23	24	25	26	27	28	29	31	32	33	34	35	36	37	39	34	35	36	37	38	39	40	41	42	43	44	45	46	47	48	50	49
280	2	2	3	3	4	5	6	7	7	8	9	10	11	12	14	15	16	17	18	19	20	21	22	23	24	26	27	28	29	30	31	32	33	34	36	37	38	33	34	35	36	37	38	39	40	41	42	43	44	45	46	47	49	48
285	2	2	3	3	4	5	6	6	7	8	9	10	11	12	13	14	15	17	18	19	20	21	22	23	24	25	26	27	28	30	31	32	33	34	35	36	37	32	33	34	35	36	37	38	39	40	41	42	43	45	46	47	48	48
290	2	2	2	3	4	5	5	6	7	8	9	10	11	12	13	14	15	16	17	18	19	21	22	23	24	25	26	27	28	29	30	31	32	33	34	36	37	32	33	34	35	36	37	38	39	40	41	42	43	44	45	46	47	47
295	2	2	2	3	4	4	5	6	7	8	8	10	11	12	13	14	15	16	17	18	19	20	21	22	23	24	25	26	27	28	29	31	32	33	34	35	36	31	32	33	34	35	36	37	38	39	40	41	42	43	44	45	46	46
300	2	2	2	3	3	4	5	6	7	7	8	9	10	11	12	13	14	15	16	17	18	19	20	21	22	23	24	25	26	27	28	29	30	31	32	34	35	30	31	32	33	34	35	36	37	38	39	40	41	42	43	44	45	43

Table 4.6 Determination of Body Mass Index (BMI)

Determine your BMI by looking up the number where your weight and height intersect on the table. According to the results, look up your disease risk in Tables 4.7 and 4.9.

Height	Weight																												
	110	115	120	125	130	135	140	145	150	155	160	165	170	175	180	185	190	195	200	205	210	215	220	225	230	235	240	245	250
5'0"	21	22	23	24	25	26	27	28	29	30	31	32	33	34	35	36	37	38	39	40	41	42	43	44	45	46	47	48	49
5'1"	21	22	23	24	25	26	26	27	28	29	30	31	32	33	34	35	36	37	38	39	40	41	42	43	43	44	45	46	47
5'2"	20	21	22	23	24	25	26	27	27	28	29	30	31	32	33	34	35	36	37	37	38	39	40	41	42	43	44	45	46
5'3"	19	20	21	22	23	24	25	26	27	27	28	29	30	31	32	33	34	35	35	36	37	38	39	40	41	42	43	43	44
5'4"	19	20	21	21	22	23	24	25	26	27	27	28	29	30	31	32	33	33	34	35	36	37	38	39	39	40	41	42	43
5'5"	18	19	20	21	22	22	23	24	25	26	27	27	28	29	30	31	32	32	33	34	35	36	37	37	38	39	40	41	42
5'6"	18	19	19	20	21	22	23	23	24	25	26	27	27	28	29	30	31	31	32	33	34	35	36	36	37	38	39	40	40
5'7"	17	18	19	20	20	21	22	23	23	24	25	26	27	27	28	29	30	31	31	32	33	34	34	35	36	37	38	38	39
5'8"	17	17	18	19	20	21	21	22	23	24	24	25	26	27	27	28	29	30	30	31	32	33	33	34	35	36	36	37	38
5'9"	16	17	18	18	19	20	21	21	22	23	24	24	25	26	27	27	28	29	30	30	31	32	32	33	34	35	35	36	37
5'10"	16	17	17	18	19	19	20	21	22	22	23	24	24	25	26	27	27	28	29	29	30	31	32	32	33	34	34	35	36
5'11"	15	16	17	17	18	19	20	20	21	22	22	23	24	24	25	26	26	27	28	29	29	30	31	31	32	33	33	34	35
6'0"	15	16	16	17	18	18	19	20	20	21	22	22	23	24	24	25	26	26	27	28	28	29	30	31	31	32	33	33	34
6'1"	15	15	16	16	17	18	18	19	20	20	21	22	22	23	24	24	25	26	26	27	28	28	29	30	30	31	32	32	33
6'2"	14	15	15	16	17	17	18	19	19	20	21	21	22	22	23	24	24	25	26	26	27	28	28	29	30	30	31	31	32
6'3"	14	14	15	16	16	17	17	18	19	19	20	21	21	22	22	23	24	24	25	26	26	27	27	28	29	29	30	31	31
6'4"	13	14	15	15	16	16	17	18	18	19	19	20	21	21	22	23	23	24	24	25	26	26	27	27	28	29	29	30	30

Compared with individuals who have a BMI of 22 to less than 25, people with a BMI of 25 to less than 30 (overweight) exhibit a mortality rate up to 25 percent higher; the rate for those with a BMI of 30 or greater (obese) is 50 to 100 percent higher.[11] Table 4.7 provides disease risk categories when BMI is used as the sole criterion to identify people at risk. Currently, more than one-third of the U.S. adult population has a BMI of 30 or more. Overweight and obesity trends starting in 1960 according to BMI are shown in Figure 4.8. In addition, the prevalence of obesity by classification (obesity I, II, and III) is provided in Figure 4.9.

Figure 4.8 Overweight and obesity trends in the United States, 1960–2010.

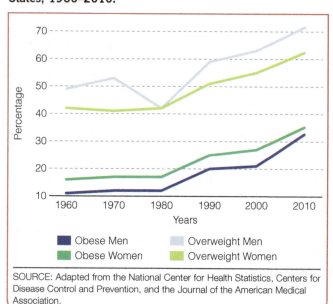

SOURCE: Adapted from the National Center for Health Statistics, Centers for Disease Control and Prevention, and the Journal of the American Medical Association.

Figure 4.9 Obesity prevalence by classification in U.S. adults (>20 years of age), 2011–2012.

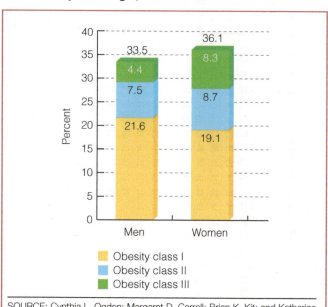

SOURCE: Cynthia L. Ogden; Margaret D. Carroll; Brian K. Kit; and Katherine M. Flegal, "Prevalence of Childhood and Adult Obesity in the United States, 2011–2012" *The Journal of the American Medical Association*, 2014; 311(8): 806–814.

Table 4.7 Disease Risk according to Body Mass Index (BMI)

BMI	Disease Risk	Classification
<18.5	Increased	Underweight
18.5–21.99	Low	Acceptable
22.0–24.99	Very low	Acceptable
25.0–29.99	Increased	Overweight
30.0–34.99	High	Obesity I
35.0–39.99	Very high	Obesity II
≥40.0	Extremely high	Obesity III

Table 4.8 Disease Risk according to Waist Circumference (WC)

Men	Women	Disease Risk
<35.5	32.5	Low
35.5–40.0	32.5–35.0	Moderate
>40.0	>35.0	High

Table 4.9 Disease Risk according to Body Mass Index (BMI) and Waist Circumference (WC)

Classification	BMI (kg/m²)	Disease Risk Relative to Normal Weight and WC		
		Men ≤40″ (102 cm) Women ≤35″ (88 cm)	Men >40″ (102 cm) Women >35″ (88 cm)
Underweight	<18.5	Increased	Low
Normal	18.5–24.9	Very low	Increased
Overweight	25.0–29.9	Increased	High
Obesity Class I	30.0–34.9	High	Very high
Obesity Class II	35.0–39.9	Very high	Very high
Obesity Class III	40.0	Extremely high	Extremely high

Adapted from Expert Panel, Executive Summary of the Clinical Guidelines on the Identification, Evaluation, and Treatment of Overweight and Obesity in Adults, *Archives of Internal Medicine* 158:1855-1867, 1998.

Waist Circumference

Researchers have firmly established that one of the most helpful ways to connect a person's fat distribution pattern to their disease risk is also the simplest: measuring the waistline. Other methods of determining abdominal obesity are available. Complex scanning techniques can identify high intra-abdominal fatness, but these methods are costly, while a simple **waist circumference (WC)** measure has proven to be a reliable way to assess risk. WC seems to predict abdominal visceral fat as accurately as the DXA technique. [12]

WC and disease risk

A waist circumference of more than 40 inches in men and 35 inches in women indicates a higher risk for cardiovascular disease, hypertension, and type 2 diabetes (Table 4.8). Weight loss is encouraged when individuals exceed these measurements.

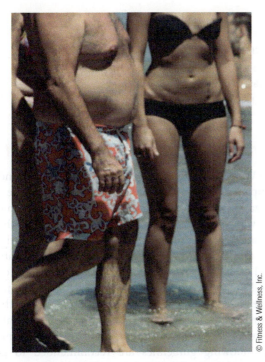

Individuals who accumulate body fat around the midsection ("apple" shape) are at greater risk for disease than those who accumulate body fat in the hips and thighs ("pear" shape).

Research indicates that as independent metrics, WC is a better predictor than BMI of the risk for disease, with waist-to-height ratio (WHtR, see discussion that follows) being perhaps the best predictor. Combining these measurements, however, helps better identify individuals at higher risk resulting from excessive body fat. Table 4.9 provides guidelines to identify people at risk according to BMI and WC.

Waist-to-Height Ratio: "Keep your waist circumference to less than half your height."

The **waist-to-height ratio (WHtR)** is the newest of these metrics to assess health risk. Research indicates that it is a better predictor of health outcomes, including cardiac and metabolic complications, than BMI or WC, even across multiple ethnic groups. [13] While WC is superior to BMI, two individuals with a similar WC (e.g., 43) but of different heights may not be at the same risk for disease, whereas the new WHtR method discriminates between individuals of different heights.

GLOSSARY

Waist circumference (WC) A waist girth measurement to assess potential risk for disease based on intra-abdominal fat content.

Waist-to-Height Ratio (WHtR) A waist-to-height ratio assessment equally applicable to tall and short persons used to determine potential risk for disease based on excessive body weight.

Figure 4.10 **The Ashwell® Shape Chart (waist-to-height ratio).**

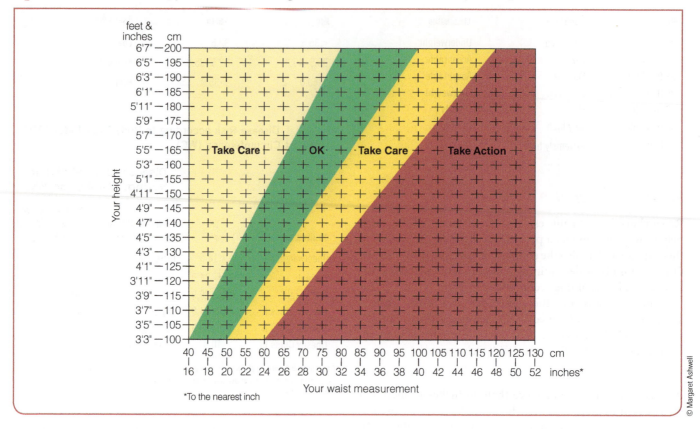

WHtR and disease risk

WHtR is determined simply by dividing the waist circumference in inches by the height in inches. As illustrated in Figure 4.10, a ratio of .4 to .5 indicates the lowest risk for disease, whereas less than .4 or between .5 and .7 requires "care" to decrease health risks, and a ratio of .7 or greater requires "action" to conform to the lowest health risk category of .4 to .5. An example of the WHtR for a person with a WC of 32 inches and a height of 68 inches (5'8") would be .47 (32 ÷ 68).

Researchers have begun promoting a public health message indicating that you should "keep your waist circumference to less than half your height." The simplicity of the message, and the fact that WHtR can be easily determined and used with any other assessment, makes it all the more plausible that it may become a standard worldwide health index. This metric can be implemented anywhere with just a measuring tape or a piece of string. It can empower health care practitioners to intervene before the onset of disease and slow or even reverse the trend of growing mortality rates from preventable chronic disease.

Table 4.10 lists the various risk categories according to WHtR.

Table 4.10 **Health Categories according to Waist-to-Height Ratio (WHtR)**

Category	WHtR (Waist/Height)	Disease Risk
Take Care	<.4	Increased
Acceptable (OK)	.4–.5	Very low
Take Care	.5–.7	Increased
Take Action	>.7	Highest

Obtaining an Accurate Waist Measurement

Before WHtR can be implemented on a global scale and used to compare risk factors across populations, worldwide health organizations will need to agree on precisely how high or low on the waist the measurement should be taken. An abdominal measurement could be taken at the navel or at the narrowest point of the waist; however, the best estimation of visceral fat is likely provided by locating the bottom of your ribs and the top of your hip bone and wrapping the measuring tape around your waist at the mid-point between the two. It is important when recording your own abdominal measurements to be consistent about the site of measurement.

The following guidelines are recommended to get an accurate and repeatable waist measurement:

1. Stand in front of a mirror while taking the measurement to ensure the measuring tape is horizontal.

HOEGER KEY TO WELLNESS

Keep your waist circumference to less than half your height. Intra-abdominal or visceral fat, seen in people with a large waist circumference, secretes harmful inflammatory substances that contribute to chronic disease.

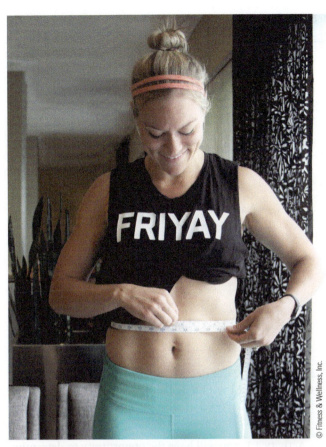

When taking your own abdominal measurement, be sure to stay consistent about the site of measurement.

2. Use a measuring tape that is not elastic, and hold it snug against the skin, but do not compress the waist.
3. Choose a site on the waist and be sure to consistently measure at the same site.
4. When the tape is in place, relax, exhale, and then take the reading.

4.6 Determining Recommended Body Weight

Calculating recommended body weight is not only a scientific process, it is also a personal one. You will need to consider your lifestyle and the benefits that are important to you as you decide whether to target health or high fitness standards.

Begin with Your Current Body Composition

Once you know your percent body fat, you can determine your current body composition classification by consulting Table 4.11, which presents percentages of fat according to both the health fitness standard and the high physical fitness standard (see discussion in Chapter 1).

For example, the recommended health fitness fat percentage for a 20-year-old female is 28 percent or less. Although there are no clearly identified percent body fat levels at which

the risk for disease definitely increases, the health fitness standard in Table 4.11 is currently the best estimate of the point at which there seems to be no harm to health.

According to Table 4.11, the high physical fitness range for this same 20-year-old woman would be between 18 and 23 percent. The high physical fitness standard does not mean that you cannot be somewhat less than this number. Many highly trained male athletes are as low as 3 percent, and some female distance runners have been measured at 6 percent body fat (which may not be healthy).

Not only obese people but also underweight people are at risk for higher mortality. "Underweight" and "thin" do not necessarily mean the same thing. The body fat of a healthy thin person is near the high physical fitness standard, whereas an underweight person has extremely low body fat, even to the point of compromising the essential fat.

The 3 percent essential fat for men and 12 percent for women seem to be the lower limits for people to maintain good health. Below these percentages, normal physiological functions can be seriously impaired. Some experts point out that a little storage fat (in addition to the essential fat) is better than no storage fat at all. As a result, the health and high fitness standards for percent fat in Table 4.11 are set higher than the minimum essential fat requirements, at a point beneficial to optimal health and well-being. Finally, because lean tissue decreases with age, one extra percentage point is allowed for every additional decade of life.

> **!** **Critical Thinking**
>
> Do you think you have a weight problem? Do your body composition results make you feel any different about the way you perceive your current body weight and image?

Calculate Your Recommended Body Weight

Your recommended body weight is computed based on the selected health or high fitness fat percentage for your age and gender. Your decision to select a "desired" fat percentage should be based on your current percent body fat and your personal health/fitness objectives. Following are steps to compute your own recommended body weight:

1. Determine the pounds of body weight that are fat (FW) by multiplying your body weight (BW) by the current percent fat (%F) expressed in decimal form (FW = BW × %F).
2. Determine lean body mass (LBM) by subtracting the weight in fat from the total body weight (LBM = BW − FW). (Anything that is not fat must be part of the lean component.)
3. Select a desired body fat percentage (DFP) based on the health or high fitness standards given in Table 4.11.
4. Compute recommended body weight (RBW) according to the formula RBW = LBM ÷ (1.0 − DFP).

Table 4.11 Body Composition Classification according to Percent Body Fat

		MEN				
Age	Underweight	Excellent	Good	Moderate	Overweight	Obese
19	<3	12.0	12.1–17.0	17.1–22.0	22.1–27.0	≥27.1
20–29	<3	13.0	13.1–18.0	18.1–23.0	23.1–28.0	≥28.1
30–39	<3	14.0	14.1–19.0	19.1–24.0	24.1–29.0	≥29.1
40–49	<3	15.0	15.1–20.0	20.1–25.0	25.1–30.0	≥30.1
50	<3	16.0	16.1–21.0	21.1–26.0	26.1–31.0	≥31.1
		WOMEN				
Age	Underweight	Excellent	Good	Moderate	Overweight	Obese
≤19	<12	17.0	17.1–22.0	22.1–27.0	27.1–32.0	≥32.1
20–29	<12	18.0	18.1–23.0	23.1–28.0	28.1–33.0	≥33.1
30–39	<12	19.0	19.1–24.0	24.1–29.0	29.1–34.0	≥34.1
40–49	<12	20.0	20.1–25.0	25.1–30.0	30.1–35.0	≥35.1
≥50	<12	21.0	21.1–26.0	26.1–31.0	31.1–36.0	≥36.1

High physical fitness standard

Health fitness standard

As an example of these computations, a 19-year-old female who weighs 160 pounds and is 30 percent fat would like to know what her recommended body weight would be at 22 percent:

Sex: female
Age: 19
BW: 160 lb
%F: 30% (.30 in decimal form)

1. FW = BW × %F
   FW = 160 × .30 = 48 lb
2. LBM = BW − FW
   LBM = 160 − 48 = 112 lb

3. DFP: 22% (.22 in decimal form)
4. RBW = LBM ÷ (1.0 − DFP)
   RBW = 112 ÷ (1.0 − .22)
   RBW = 112 ÷ .78 = 143.6 lb

In Activity 4.1, you will have the opportunity to determine your own body composition and recommended body weight. A second column is provided in the activity for a follow-up assessment at a future date. The disease risk according to BMI and WC and recommended body weight according to BMI also are determined in Activity 4.2. You can also set goals to accomplish by the end of the term.

Behavior Modification Planning

Tips for Lifetime Weight Management

Maintenance of recommended body composition is one of the most significant health issues of the 21st century. If you are committed to lifetime weight management, the following strategies will help:

I PLAN TO **I DID IT**

❑ ❑ Accumulate 60 to 90 minutes of physical activity daily.

❑ ❑ Exercise at a brisk aerobic pace for a minimum of 20 minutes three times per week.

❑ ❑ Strength train two to three times per week.

❑ ❑ Manage daily caloric intake by keeping in mind long-term benefits (recommended body weight) instead of instant gratification (overeating).

❑ ❑ "Junior-size" instead of "super-size."

❑ ❑ Regularly monitor body weight, body composition, body mass index, and waist circumference.

❑ ❑ Do not allow increases in body weight (percent fat) to accumulate; deal immediately with the problem through moderate reductions in caloric intake and maintenance of physical activity and exercise habits.

Try It

In your online journal or your class notebook, note which of these tips you are already using and which ones you can incorporate into your daily habits right away.

Other than DXA and hydrostatic weighing, skinfold thickness seems to be the most practical and valid technique to estimate body fat, unless the person is significantly overweight and an accurate skinfold cannot be measured. If skinfold calipers are available, use this technique to assess your percent body fat. If none of these techniques is available to you, estimate your percent fat according to girth measurements (or another technique available to you). You also may wish to use several techniques and compare the results.

> **!** **Critical Thinking**
>
> What influence does society have on the way you perceive yourself in terms of your weight? Does knowing your body composition help give you a more realistic picture of what the recommended weight may be for you?

4.7 Importance of Regularly Assessing Body Composition

If you are on a diet/exercise program, you should repeat your percent body fat assessment and recommended weight computations about once a month. This is important because lean body mass is affected by weight-reduction programs and amount of physical activity. As lean body mass changes, so will your recommended body weight. To make valid comparisons, use the same technique for both pre- and post-program assessments.

Changes in body composition resulting from a weight control/exercise program were illustrated in a co-ed aerobic dance course taught during a brief 6-week summer term. Students participated in a 60-minute aerobics routine four times a week. On the first and last days of class, several

Figure 4.11 Effects of a 6-week aerobics exercise program on body composition.

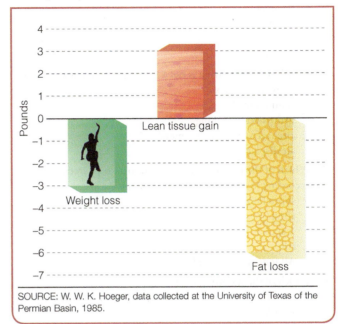

SOURCE: W. W. K. Hoeger, data collected at the University of Texas of the Permian Basin, 1985.

physiological parameters, including body composition, were assessed. Students also were given information on diet and nutrition, but they followed their own dietary program.

At the end of the 6 weeks, the average weight loss for the entire class was three pounds (Figure 4.11). But, because body composition was assessed, class members were surprised to find that the average fat loss was actually six pounds, accompanied by a three-pound increase in lean body mass.

Assessing body composition offers real-time feedback on your efforts to improve nutrition and physical activity. Learning to track it periodically will be an advantage to you during a weight loss program and throughout life. It will help you avoid creeping increases in body fat and will go a long way to demystify the connection between your efforts and results.

Assess Your Behavior

1. Do you know what your percent body fat is according to a reliable body composition assessment technique administered by a qualified technician?
2. Do you know your disease risk according to BMI and WC parameters?
3. Do you know your WHtR category?
4. Have you been able to maintain your body weight at a stable level during the past 12 months?

Assess Your Knowledge

1. Body composition incorporates
   a. a fat component.
   b. a nonfat component.
   c. percent body fat.
   d. lean body mass.
   e. all of the above.

2. Recommended body weight can be determined through
   a. body mass index.
   b. body composition analysis.
   c. BMI and waist circumference.
   d. waist circumference.
   e. all of the above.

3. Essential fat in women is
    a. 3 percent.
    b. 5 percent.
    c. 8 percent.
    d. 12 percent.
    e. 17 percent.

4. Which of the following is *not* a technique to assess body fat?
    a. body mass index
    b. skinfold thickness
    c. hydrostatic weighing
    d. circumference measurements
    e. air displacement

5. Which of the following sites is used to assess percent body fat according to skinfold thickness in men?
    a. suprailium
    b. chest
    c. scapular
    d. triceps
    e. All four sites are used.

6. Which of the following is true?
    a. Visceral fat stores are *less* dangerous than subcutaneous fat stores.
    b. Visceral fat stores do not respond to exercise.
    c. Visceral fat stores are *more* dangerous than subcutaneous fat stores.
    d. Visceral fat is the fat you can grasp just beneath the skin.
    e. none of the above

7. Waist circumference can be used to
    a. determine percent body fat.
    b. assess risk for disease.
    c. measure lean body mass.
    d. identify underweight people.
    e. All of the above are correct.

8. An acceptable BMI is between
    a. 15 and 18.49.
    b. 18.5 and 24.99.
    c. 25 and 29.99.
    d. 30 and 34.99.
    e. 35 and 39.99.

9. The health fitness percent body fat for women of various ages is in the range of
    a. 3 to 7 percent.
    b. 7 to 12 percent.
    c. 12 to 20 percent.
    d. 20 to 27 percent.
    e. 27 to 31 percent.

10. When a previously inactive individual starts an exercise program, the person may
    a. lose weight.
    b. gain weight.
    c. improve body composition.
    d. lose more fat pounds than total weight pounds.
    e. do all of the above.

Correct answers can be found at the back of the book.

MINDTAP **Complete This Online**
From Cengage   Visit **www.cengagebrain.com** to access MindTap, a complete digital course that includes interactive quizzes, videos, and more.

Activity 4.1   **Body Composition Assessment and Recommended Body Weight Determination**

Name _____   Date _____

Course _____   Section _____   Gender _____   Age _____

I. Percent Body Fat according to Skinfold Thickness

Men

Chest (mm):   _____

Abdomen (mm):   _____

Thigh (mm):   _____

Total (mm):   _____

% Fat: _____

Women

Triceps (mm):   _____

Suprailium (mm):   _____

Thigh (mm):   _____

Total (mm):   _____

% Fat: _____

Follow Up

Date _____

% Fat _____ %

II. Percent Fat according to Girth Measurements (use inches for men and centimeters for women.)

Men   Waist (inches): [   ]   Wrist (inches): [   ]   Difference: [   ]   Body weight: [   ]   lbs.   % Fat: [   ]

Women   Upperarm (cm): [   ]   Age: [   ]   Hip (cm): [   ]   Wrist (cm): [   ]

Constants: A = Upperarm [   ]   B = Age [   ]   C = Hip [   ]   D = Wrist [   ]

BD* = A − B − C + D = [   ] − [   ] − [   ] + [   ] = [   ]

% Fat = (495/BD) − 450 = (495/_____) − 450 = [   ]

*BD = body density, carry the computation out to at least four decimal places.

III. Recommended Body Weight Determination

A. Body weight (BW): [   ] lbs.

B. Current %F*: [   ] %

C. Fat weight (FW) = BW × %F

FW = [   ] × [   ] = [   ] lbs.

D. Lean body mass (LBM) = BW − FW = [   ] − [   ] = [   ] lbs.

E. Age: [   ]

F. Desired fat percent (DFP − see Table 4.11, page 156): [   ] %

G. Recommended body weight (RBW) = LBM ÷ (1.0 − DFP*)

RBW = [   ] ÷ (1.0 − [   ]) = [   ] lbs.

_____

*Express percentages in decimal form (for example, 25% = .25).

Follow Up

Date: [   ]

A. BW: [   ] lbs.

B. %F: [   ] %

C. FW: [   ] lbs.

D. LBM: [   ] lbs.

E. Age: [   ]

F. DFP: [   ] %

G. RBW: [   ] lbs.

© Fitness & Wellness, Inc.

MINDTAP From Cengage   **Complete This Online**
Visit **www.cengagebrain.com** to access MindTap, a complete digital course that includes interactive quizzes, videos, and more.

Activity 4.2 **Disease Risk Using Waist Circumference and Body Mass Index**

I. Body Mass Index

Weight: ☐ lb ☐ kg

Height: ☐ in ☐ m

BMI = Weight (lb) × 703 ÷ Height (in) ÷ Height (in)

BMI = ☐ (lb) × 703 ÷ ☐ (in) ÷ ☐ (in)

BMI = ☐ Disease Risk: (use Table 4.7, page 153): ☐

Follow Up Date ☐ BMI = ☐ Disease Risk (use Table 4.7, page 153): ☐

II. Waist Circumference

Follow Up

Waist (in): ☐

Disease Risk (use Table 4.8, page 153): ☐

Date: ☐

Waist: ☐

Disease Risk: ☐

III. Disease Risk according to BMI and WC (use Table 4.9, page 153): ☐

IV. Target Body Weight (TBW) according to BMI

TBW based on BMI = Desired BMI × height (in) × height (in) ÷ 703

TBW at BMI of 25 = 25 × ☐ × ☐ ÷ 703 = ☐ lbs.

TBW at BMI of 22 = 22 × ☐ × ☐ ÷ 703 = ☐ lbs.

V. Waist-to-Height Ratio (WHtR)

WHtR = ☐ (Waist, in) ÷ ☐ (Height, in) = ☐

Health Category (use Table 4.10, page 154): ☐

VI. Determining Body Composition Results and Goals

Briefly state your feelings about your body composition results and your recommended body weight using both percent body fat and BMI. Do you plan to reduce your percent body fat and increase your lean body mass? Write the goal(s) you want to achieve by the end of the term and indicate how you plan to achieve them.

_____

_____

_____

_____

_____

_____

© Fitness & Wellness, Inc.

5

Weight Management

Physical activity is the cornerstone of any sound weight management program. If you are unwilling to increase daily physical activity, you might as well not even attempt to lose weight because, in all likelihood you won't be able to keep it off.

Objectives

5.1 **Describe** the health consequences of obesity.

5.2 **Expose** some popular fad diets and myths and fallacies regarding weight control.

5.3 **Understand** the mental and emotional aspects of proper weight management.

5.4 **Describe** eating disorders and their associated medical problems and behavior patterns and outline the need for professional help in treating these conditions.

5.5 **Explain** the physiology of weight loss, including the effects of diet on basal metabolic rate.

5.6 **Explain** the key role of a lifetime exercise program in a successful weight loss and weight maintenance program.

5.7 **Understand** the roles of strength-training and moderate- versus vigorous-intensity aerobic exercise in weight management.

5.8 **Implement** a physiologically sound weight reduction and weight maintenance program.

5.9 **Describe** behavior modification techniques that help support adherence to a lifetime weight maintenance program.

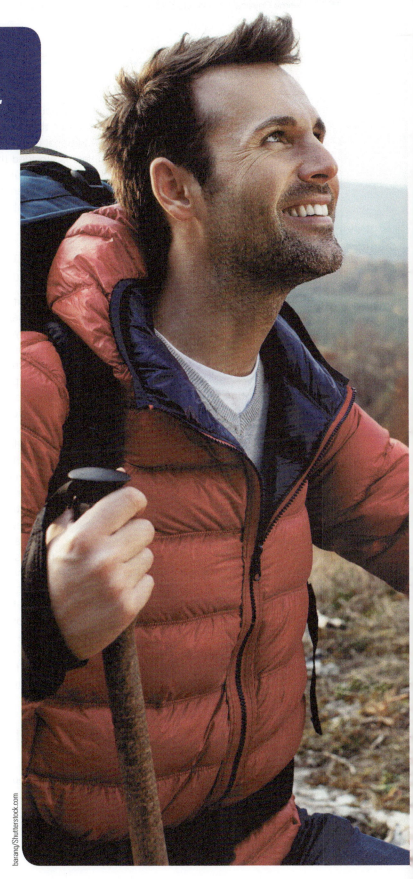

barang/Shutterstock.com

FAQ

Why can't I lose weight with exercise?

During the past few years, there has been a fair amount of media distortion stating "exercise makes a person fat." There is ample scientific evidence that exercise is an important component of a successful weight-loss program. The problem is that following exercise, many people eat more (particularly more junk food). They feel justified in doing so because they exercised. It is clear that weight loss is more effective when you cut back on calories (dieting), as opposed to only increasing physical activity or exercise.

When attempting to lose weight, initial lengthy exercise sessions (longer than 60 minutes) by unfit people may not be the best approach to weight loss—unless they carefully monitor daily caloric intake and avoid caloric compensation for the energy expended during exercise. In active or fit individuals, lengthy exercise sessions are not counterproductive.

Body composition changes are also more effective when dieting and exercise are combined while attempting to lose body weight. Most weight loss when dieting with exercise comes in the form of body fat and not lean body tissue, a desirable outcome. Weight loss maintenance, however, in most cases is possible only with 60 to 90 minutes of sustained daily physical activity and exercise.

If you are still not convinced that exercise is the best approach to weight management, take a look around the gym or the jogging trail. If this were the case, wouldn't those who regularly exercise be the fattest?

Additional information on this subject is provided throughout this chapter, in particular in the section "The Roles of Exercise Intensity and Duration in Weight Management" on page 198.

Are some diet plans more effective than others?

The term "diet" implies a negative caloric balance. A negative caloric balance means that you are consuming fewer calories than those required to maintain your current weight. When energy output surpasses energy intake, weight loss occurs. Popular diets differ widely in the food choices that you are allowed to have, but regardless of which diet you follow, as long as there is a negative caloric balance, you will lose weight. The more limited the choices, the lower the chances to overeat and thus the lower the caloric intake. And the fewer calories you consume, the greater the weight loss. For health reasons, to obtain the variety of nutrients the body needs, even during weight loss periods, you should not consume less than 1,500 calories per day (unless you are a very small individual). These calories should be distributed over a range of foods, emphasizing grains, fruits, vegetables, and small amounts of low-fat animal products or fish.

Why is it so difficult to change dietary habits?

In most developed countries, there is an overabundance of food and practically an unlimited number of food choices. With unlimited supply and choices, most people do not have the willpower, stemming from their core values, to avoid overconsumption.

Our bodies were not created to go hungry or to overeat. We are uncomfortable overeating, and we feel even worse when we have to go hungry. Our health values, however, are not strong enough to prevent overconsumption. The end result: weight gain. Next, we restrict calories (go on a diet), we feel hungry, and we have a difficult time adhering to the diet. Stated quite simply, going hungry is an uncomfortable and unpleasant experience.

To avoid this vicious cycle, our dietary habits (and most likely physical activity habits) must change. A question you need to ask yourself is: Do I value health and quality of life more than food overindulgence? If you do not, then the achievement and maintenance of recommended body weight and good health is a moot point. If you desire to avoid disease and increase quality of life, you have to value health more than food overconsumption. If you have spent the past 20 years tasting and "devouring" every food item in sight, it is time to make healthy choices and consume only moderate amounts of food at a time (portion control). You do not have to taste and eat everything that is placed before your eyes. If you can make such a change in your eating habits, you may not have to worry about another diet for the rest of your life.

REAL LIFE STORY | Sam's Experience

A couple of times over the last few years, I tried to diet. It would usually start around New Year's, when I would make a resolution to lose the extra weight I was carrying. For a few weeks I would try to cut out desserts, avoid second helpings, and eat lower fat foods. At times when I would weigh myself, even if I thought I had really followed my diet well, the scale still wouldn't show any difference, which was really discouraging. Sometimes when I lost a few pounds, I would look in the mirror, but I still looked flabby. I didn't consider adding any exercise to my routine because I hate to sweat, I hate being out of breath, and I hate feeling bad because I'm not able to keep up with other, more fit people. Besides,

after a long day of classes and homework, I would rather spend my free time updating Facebook, playing video games, or watching TV. But when I took a health and fitness class as a general elective, I learned about how important exercise was for proper weight management. It turns out that even if you are successful at losing weight through diet alone, you probably lose muscle along with the fat, so that even if your weight goes down, your body stays flabby. Also, your metabolism slows down, so it is easy to gain back all the weight. While taking the class, I got motivated

Arek_malang/Shutterstock.com

and started exercising while also changing my diet. I started lifting weights and walking and jogging on the treadmill at the student fitness center. I tried not to pay attention to how other people could lift more or run so much faster than me, and gradually my fitness improved. Now, several months later, my efforts have really paid off. So far I have lost more than 30 pounds. And what's more, getting regular exercise has helped me be more positive and feel stronger and more energetic. I am pretty sure that exercise is going to be a lifetime habit and that I will never want to go back to my couch potato ways.

PERSONAL PROFILE: Personal Weight Management Program

To the best of your ability, answer the following questions. If you do not know the answer(s), this chapter will guide you through them.

I. Do you understand the concept of recommended body weight? ____ Yes ____ No Do you consider yourself to be at this weight? ____ Yes ____ No

II. What type of exercise program do you consider most effective for weight management (mark one): ____ aerobic exercise or ____ strength-training?

III. Have you gained weight since you started college? ____ Yes ____ No

IV. Do you understand the concept of long-term gratification derived through a lifetime exercise program and the required process to do so? ____ Yes ____ No

MINDTAP From Cengage **Complete This Online**
Visit www.cengagebrain.com to access MindTap, a complete digital course that includes interactive quizzes, videos, and more.

Obesity is a health hazard of epidemic proportions in most developed countries around the world. According to the World Health Organization, an estimated 35 percent of the adult population in industrialized nations is obese. Obesity has been defined as a body mass index (BMI) of 30 or higher. The obesity level has been set at this number because this is the tipping point at which excess body fat can lead to significant health problems. This means that more than one in three people in industrialized nations are at greater risk for developing major chronic illness.

5.1 Weight Management in the Modern Environment

The current 21st-century environment in which we live is rich in cues to overeat high-calorie, high-fat, sugary foods 24/7. Food overconsumption coupled with advances in modern technology

that minimize the need for daily physical activity have led to the current obesogenic culture that promotes weight gain and the array of chronic conditions caused by excessive weight.

As for the United States, the problem is not improving. Data indicate that almost 71 percent of U.S. adults age 20 and older are overweight (have a BMI ≥25), and 36.5 percent are obese (Figure 5.1).[1] Between 1960 and 2015, the overall (men and women combined) prevalence of adult obesity increased from about 13 to 36.5 percent. This change is primarily attributed to a lack of physical activity and poor dietary habits by the American people. The average weight of American adults between the ages of 20 and 74 has increased 25 pounds or more since 1965, most of the weight gain (15 pounds) coming since 1990. Nearly half of all adults in the United States do not achieve the minimum recommended amount of physical activity (see Figure 1.12, page 24). On average, Americans are consuming approximately 250 additional calories per day as compared to 1970.

Figure 5.1 Percentage of the adult population (≥20 years) that is normal weight (BMI <25), overweight (BMI ≥ 25–29.99), or obese (BMI ≥30) in the United States.

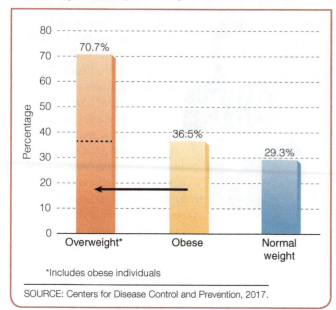

*Includes obese individuals

SOURCE: Centers for Disease Control and Prevention, 2017.

poll, men indicate their "ideal" body weight is 185 pounds, the highest ever, and 14 pounds above the 1990 weight as determined by this same poll. Women indicate their "ideal" weight to be 11 pounds heavier than in 1990, at 140 pounds.

The prevalence of obesity increases with age and is higher in certain ethnic groups, especially African Americans and Hispanic Americans (see Figure 5.3). Furthermore, as the nation continues to evolve into a more mechanized and automated society (relying on escalators, elevators, remote controls, computers, e-mail, cell phones, and automatic-sensor doors),

Figure 5.3 Obesity rates (BMI ≥30) by age and ethnicity, 2015.

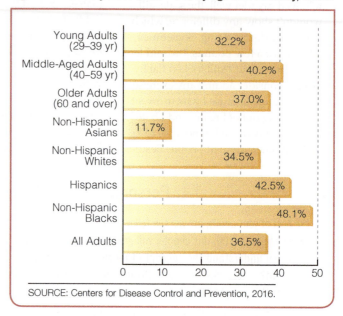

SOURCE: Centers for Disease Control and Prevention, 2016.

Prior to 1985, no single state reported an obesity rate above 15 percent of the state's total population (which includes both adults and children). By 2015 (see Figure 5.2), no state had a prevalence of obesity less than 20 percent.

As of the end of 2012, the average man weighed 196 pounds and the average woman 156 pounds. As pointed out in Chapter 2, the human mind has a tremendous capability to adapt and accept change, even if such is detrimental to one's health. And so it is with body weight. According to a Gallup

Figure 5.2 Percent of the adult population based on BMI ≥30 or 30 pounds overweight, by state, which is obese in the United States, 2015.

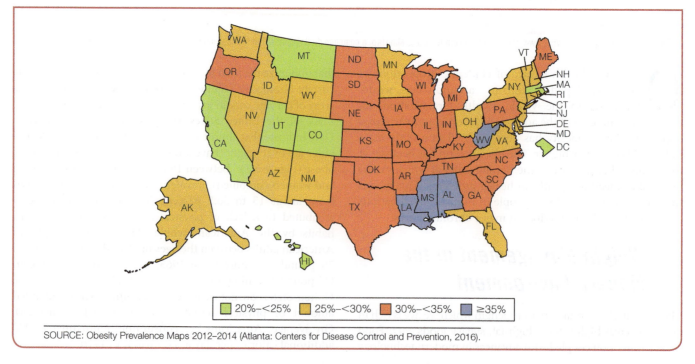

SOURCE: Obesity Prevalence Maps 2012–2014 (Atlanta: Centers for Disease Control and Prevention, 2016).

the amount of required daily physical activity continues to decrease. As people have been lulled into a high-risk sedentary lifestyle, obesity rates have climbed.

More than a third of the population is on a diet at any given moment. People spend about $40 billion yearly attempting to lose weight, with more than $10 billion going to memberships in weight reduction centers and another $30 billion to diet food sales.

The Wellness Way to Lifetime Weight Management

This chapter will help you understand the physiological process involved in proper weight management and will help you create a positive and personalized plan to meet your body composition and body weight goals. It will also help you understand the thoughts and feelings that you are likely to experience when changing eating habits. As you clear major stressors from your life and change dietary habits, at your own pace, you should be able to use the information in this chapter to create an enjoyable healthy lifetime eating pattern.

5.2 Overweight versus Obese

Excessive body weight combined with physical inactivity is the second-leading cause of preventable death in the United States, resulting in more than 100,000 deaths each year. Furthermore, obesity is more prevalent than smoking or problem drinking. Obesity and unhealthy lifestyle habits are the most critical public health problems in the 21st century.

Overweight and obese are not the same thing. Many overweight people (who weigh about 10 to 20 pounds over the recommended weight) are not obese. Although a few pounds of excess weight may not be harmful to most people, this is not always the case. People with excessive body fat who have type 2 diabetes and other cardiovascular risk factors (elevated blood lipids, high blood pressure, physical inactivity, and poor eating habits) benefit from losing weight. People who have a few extra pounds of weight but are otherwise healthy and physically active, exercise regularly, and eat a healthy diet may not be at higher risk for early death. Such is not the case, however, with obese individuals.

Body Weight Affects Wellness

Excessive body weight and obesity are associated with poor health status and are risk factors for many physical ailments, including cardiovascular disease, type 2 diabetes, and some types of cancer. Evidence indicates that health risks associated with increased body weight start at a BMI greater than 25 and are enhanced greatly at a BMI greater than 30.

The American Heart Association has identified obesity as one of the six major risk factors for coronary heart disease. Estimates by the American Institute for Cancer Research (AICR) also indicate that 122,000 yearly cancer deaths could be prevented if Americans were not overweight or obese. Obesity in itself has been linked to nine different cancers: colorectal, esophageal, post-menopausal breast, endometrial, kidney, pancreatic, ovarian, gallbladder, and advanced prostate cancer. Excessive body weight also is implicated in psychological maladjustment and a higher accidental death rate. Extremely obese people have a lower mental health–related quality of life.

Research indicates that an individual who is 10 to 30 pounds overweight during middle age (30 to 49 years of age) loses about 3 years of life, whereas being 30 or more pounds overweight decreases the lifespan by about 7 years.[2]

Health Consequences of Excessive Body Weight

Excessive body weight increases the risk for

- High blood pressure
- Elevated blood lipids (high blood cholesterol and triglycerides)
- Type 2 (non–insulin-dependent) diabetes
- Insulin resistance
- Glucose intolerance
- Coronary heart disease
- Angina pectoris
- Congestive heart failure
- Stroke
- Gallbladder disease
- Gout
- Osteoarthritis
- Orthopedic problems
- Back pain
- Gastroesophageal reflux disease (GERD or acid reflux)
- Obstructive sleep apnea and respiratory problems
- Some types of cancer (endometrial, breast, prostate, and colon)
- Complications of pregnancy (gestational diabetes, gestational hypertension, preeclampsia, and complications during C-sections)
- Poor female reproductive health (menstrual irregularities, infertility, and irregular ovulation)
- Bladder control problems (stress incontinence)
- Skin infections
- Psychological disorders (depression, anxiety, eating disorders, distorted body image, discrimination, and low self-esteem)
- Cognitive decline
- Shortened life expectancy
- Decreased quality of life

SOURCES: Centers for Disease Control and Prevention, downloaded February 1, 2016; J. O. Hill and H. R. Wyatt, "The Myth of Healthy Obesity," *Annals of Internal Medicine*, 159 (2013): 789–790.

These decreases are similar to those seen with tobacco use. Nonetheless, severe obesity (BMI greater than 45) at a young age may cut up to 20 years off a person's life.[3]

Although the loss of years of life is significant, the decreased life expectancy doesn't begin to address the loss in quality of life, considerably compromised by obesity, and increase in illness and disability throughout the years. Even a modest reduction of 2 to 3 percent can reduce the risk for chronic diseases, including heart disease, high blood pressure, high cholesterol, and diabetes.[4]

A primary objective to achieve overall physical fitness and enhanced quality of life is to attain recommended body composition. Individuals at their recommended body weight are able to participate in a variety of moderate-to-vigorous activities without functional limitations. These people have the freedom to enjoy most of life's recreational activities to their fullest potential. Excessive body weight does not afford people the fitness level to enjoy many lifetime activities, such as basketball, soccer, racquetball, surfing, mountain cycling, or mountain climbing. Maintaining high fitness and recommended body weight gives a degree of independence throughout life that most people in developed nations no longer enjoy.

Scientific evidence also recognizes problems with being underweight. Although the social pressure to be thin has declined slightly in recent years, the pressure to attain model-like thinness is still with us and contributes to the gradual increase in the number of people who develop eating disorders (anorexia nervosa and bulimia, discussed under "Eating Disorders" on pages 176–178).

Extreme weight loss can lead to medical conditions such as heart damage, gastrointestinal problems, shrinkage of internal organs, abnormalities of the immune system, disorders of the reproductive system, loss of muscle tissue, damage to the nervous system, osteoporosis and fractures, chronic obstructive pulmonary disease, and greater risk of death following surgery. About 14 percent of people in the United States are underweight.

5.3 *Tolerable Weight*

Many people want to lose weight so that they will look better. That's a worthy goal. The problem, however, is that they have a distorted image of what they would look like if they were to reduce to what they think is their ideal weight. Hereditary factors play a big role, and only a small fraction of the population has the genes for a "perfect body."

Critical Thinking

Do you consider yourself overweight? If so, how long have you had a weight problem, what attempts have you made to lose weight, and what has worked best for you?

Body Image and Acceptance

The media have the greatest influence on people's perception of what constitutes "ideal" body weight. Most people consult fashion, fitness, and beauty magazines to determine what they should look like. The "ideal" body shapes, physiques, and proportions illustrated in these magazines are rare and are achieved mainly through airbrushing and medical reconstruction. Many individuals, primarily young women, go to extremes in attempts to achieve these unrealistic figures. Failure to attain a "perfect body" may lead to eating disorders in some individuals.

When people set their target weight, they should be realistic. Attaining the "excellent" percent of body fat shown in Table 4.11 (page 156) is extremely difficult for some people. It is even more difficult to maintain over time without a commitment to a vigorous lifetime exercise program and permanent dietary changes. Few people are willing to do that. The moderate category for percentage of body fat may be more realistic for many people.

The question you should ask yourself is, am I happy with my weight? Part of enjoying a higher quality of life is being happy with yourself. If you are not, you need to either do something about it or learn to live with it.

If your percentage of body fat is higher than the relevant percentage in the moderate category of Table 4.11 in Chapter 4, you should try to reduce it and stay in this category for health reasons. This is the category that seems to pose no detriment to health.

If you are in the moderate category but would like to reduce your percentage of body fat further, you need to ask yourself additional questions: How badly do I want it? Do I

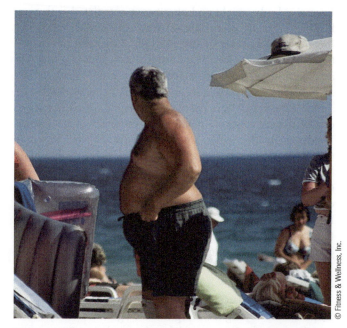

© Fitness & Wellness, Inc.

Obesity is a health hazard of epidemic proportions in industrialized nations.

Behavior Modification Planning

Preventing the Dreadful "Freshman 15!"

The infamous Freshman 15—referring to the weight gain experienced the first year in college—is for real. The transition to college life is a critical period of risk for weight gain, arbitrarily set at 15 pounds. One in four college freshmen in the United States gains at least 5 percent of their body weight, or about 10 pounds, the first semester in college.

The new-found freedom of being away from home for the first time is exciting but, at the same time, presents many challenges and temptations. As a college freshman, you are now on your own and free to eat what you want, when you want. You are free to attend as many food-filled social gatherings as you can stand, which almost always include high-calorie drinks and alcohol. You can indulge on super-sized portions in

the cafeteria, including dinners of pizza, burgers, French fries, pastries, cakes, and ice cream. You may also indulge in calorie-dense sugary/fatty/salty foods and lattes to keep you going at late-night study sessions and parties. Homesickness, friendships, dating pressures, relationships, anxiety, and school have all been documented to promote overeating. Furthermore, physical activity, exercise, and sports participation typically decline when you first attend college. To prevent the Freshman 15 syndrome you are encouraged to:

- Enroll in a fitness course every semester.
- Accumulate at least 30 minutes of physical activity every day of the week.
- Use smaller plates and fill half the plate with fruits and vegetables.
- Always "juniorsize," don't "supersize."
- Use portion control.

- Avoid skipping meals and eating late at night.
- Limit alcohol consumption.
- Avoid energy drinks and sodas; drink water instead.
- Follow the healthy eating and snack guidelines provided in Chapter 3 and in this chapter.
- Avoid fast foods, fried foods, and fatty red meat products.
- Minimize the consumption of pastries, cakes, cookies, and ice cream.
- Avoid purchasing unhealthy snacks (calorie-dense snacks such as candy bars and cookies).

Try It

Seriously consider using these recommendations to prevent weight gain not only while in college, but throughout life.

want it badly enough to implement lifetime exercise and dietary changes? If you are not willing to change, you should stop worrying about your weight and deem the moderate category "tolerable" for you.

5.4 The Weight Loss Dilemma

Unfortunately, only about 10 percent of all people who begin a traditional weight-loss program without exercise are able to lose the desired weight. Worse, only 1 in 5 people who have lost 10 percent of their body weight are able to keep the weight off for a year. The body is highly resistant to permanent weight changes through caloric restrictions alone. Short-term "on and off dieting" is not the solution to lifelong weight management. You need to adopt a sustainable strategy that involves a permanent change in eating behaviors, including healthy food choices, portion control, and regular physical activity. In addition, research indicates that most people, especially obese people, underestimate their energy intake. Those who try to lose weight but apparently fail to do so are often described as "diet resistant." A benchmark study found that while on a "diet," a group of obese individuals with a self-reported history of diet resistance underreported their average daily caloric intake by almost 50 percent (1,028 self-reported vs. 2,081 actual calories).[5] These individuals also overestimated their amount of daily physical activity by about 25 percent (1,022 self-reported vs. 771 actual calories). These differences represent an additional 1,304 calories of

energy per day unaccounted for by the subjects in the study. The findings indicate that failing to lose weight often is related to misreports of actual food intake and level of physical activity.

Consequences of Yo-Yo Dieting

Some scientists suggest that frequent fluctuations in weight, as in yo-yo dieting, send the wrong message to the brain and lead people to gain weight. They believe that repeated low-calorie diets signal frequent famines to the brain and drive the body to store more fat for future shortages.[6] This theory may explain why frequent dieters overeat when not dieting and have such a difficult time maintaining lost weight. The brain of non-dieters, on the other hand, learns that food supplies are reliable and the body has no need to store a large amount of fat.

Mathematical models developed by these scientists show that long-term weight gain by frequent dieters is greater than for people who never diet. They also suggest that avoiding frequent low-calorie diets, slightly decreasing caloric intake, and becoming much more active are most conducive to achieving and maintaining healthy body weight.

Yo-yo dieting also carries as great a health risk as being overweight and remaining overweight. Epidemiological data show that frequent fluctuations in weight (up or down) markedly increase the risk for dying from cardiovascular disease. Experts theorize that the constant shrinking and growing with yo-yo dieting causes micro tears in the blood vessels that increase their susceptibility to atherosclerosis (obstruction of the arteries; see Chapter 10).

Why Crash Diets Fail

On average, a 150-pound person stores about 1.3 pounds of **glycogen** (carbohydrate or glucose storage) in the body. This amount of glycogen is higher in aerobically trained individuals because intense training (i.e., by elite athletes) can more than double the body's capacity to store glycogen. About 80 percent of the glycogen is stored in muscles, and the remaining 20 percent is in the liver. Water, however, is required to store glycogen. About 2.6 to 3.0 pounds of water are required to store a pound of glycogen. Using the 2.6 guideline, a 150-pound person stores about 3.4 pounds of water (1.3 × 2.6), along with the 1.3 pounds of glycogen, accounting for a total of 4.7 pounds of the individual's normal body weight.

When someone is fasting or on a crash diet (typically defined as less than 800 calories per day), glycogen storage can be depleted in just a few days. This loss of weight the first few days is not in the form of body fat and is typically used to promote and guarantee rapid weight loss with many fad diets on the market today. When the person resumes a normal eating plan, the body again stores its glycogen, along with the water required to do so, and the individual subsequently gains weight.

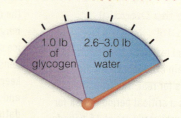

Furthermore, on a crash diet, close to half the weight loss is in lean (protein) tissue. When the body uses protein instead of a combination of fats and carbohydrates as a source of energy, weight is lost as much as 10 times faster. This is because a gram of protein produces half the amount of energy that fat does. In the case of muscle protein, one-fifth protein is mixed with four-fifths water. Therefore, each pound of muscle yields only one-tenth the amount of energy of a pound of fat. As a result, most weight lost is in the form of water, which looks good on the scale.

SOURCE: W. L. Kenney, J. H. Wilmore, and D. L. Costill, *Physiology of Sport and Exercise* (Champaign, IL: Human Kinetics, 2015).

Based on the findings that constant losses and regains can be hazardous to health, quick-fix diets should be replaced by a slow but permanent weight-loss program (as described under "Losing Weight the Sound and Sensible Way," page 184). Individuals reap the benefits of recommended body weight when they gradually achieve that weight and stay there throughout life.

Long-term or frequent crash dieting also increases the risk of heart attacks because low caloric intake eventually leads to heart muscle (protein) loss. Limiting potassium, magnesium, and copper intake as a result of very low-calorie diets may induce fatal cardiac arrhythmias. Furthermore, sodium depletion may cause a dangerous drop in blood pressure. Very low-calorie diets should always be followed under a physician's supervision. Unfortunately, most crash dieters simply consult a friend rather than seeking a physician's advice.

HOEGER KEY TO WELLNESS

We know how to take weight off, but we aren't very good at keeping it off, for good! Most diets fail because few of them incorporate permanent behavioral changes in food selection and an overall lifetime increase in physical activity.

Diet Crazes

Capitalizing on hopes that the latest diet to hit the market will work, fad diets continue to appeal to people of all shapes and sizes. These diets may work for a while, but their success is usually short-lived. Regarding the effectiveness of these diets,

Kelly Brownell, one of the foremost researchers in the field of weight management, has stated: "When I get the latest diet fad, I imagine a trick birthday cake candle that keeps lighting up and we have to keep blowing it out."

Fad diets deceive people and claim that dieters will lose weight by following all instructions. Many fad diets are very low in calories. Under these conditions, a lot of the weight lost is in the form of water and protein, not fat. Once water is rapidly lost, weight loss slows as fat begins to be metabolized. It is often at this point that the dieter gives up on the diet.

Many fad diets succeed because they restrict a large number of foods. Thus, people tend to eat less food overall. If they happen to achieve the lower weight but do not make permanent dietary changes, they regain the weight quickly once they go back to their previous eating habits.

Diet books are frequently found on best-seller lists. The market is flooded with these books. Examples include *The DASH Diet*, the *Volumetrics Eating Plan*, the *Ornish Diet*, the *Atkins Diet*, the *Zone Diet*, the *South Beach Diet*, the *Best Life Diet*, the *Abs Diet*, and *The Biggest Loser Diet*. Some of these popular diets have sound dietary principles, while others are becoming more nutritionally balanced and encourage consumption of fruits and vegetables, whole grains, some lean meat and fish, and low-fat milk and dairy products. Such plans reduce the risk for chronic diseases, including cardiovascular diseases and cancer.

While it is clear that some diets are healthier than others, strictly from a weight loss point of view, it doesn't matter what diet plan you follow: If caloric intake is lower than caloric output, weight will come off. Dropout rates for many popular diets, however, are high because of the difficulty in long-term adherence to limited dietary plans.

Low-Carb Diets

Among the most popular diets on the market in recent years were the low-carbohydrate/high-protein (LCHP) diet plans. Although they vary slightly, low-carb diets, in general, limit the intake of all sorts of carbohydrate-rich foods—bread, potatoes, rice, pasta, cereals, crackers, juices, sodas, sweets (candy, cake, cookies, etc.), and even fruits and vegetables. Dieters are allowed to eat all the protein-rich foods they desire, including steak, ham, chicken, fish, bacon, eggs, nuts, cheese, tofu, high-fat salad dressings, butter, and small amounts of a few fruits and vegetables. Typically, these diets also are high in fat content. Examples of these diets are the Atkins Diet, the Zone Diet, Protein Power, the Scarsdale Diet, the Carb Addict's Diet, the South Beach Diet, and Sugar Busters. The theory behind LCHP diets is that the body will burn more fat. With a normal mixed diet (carbohydrates, fat, and protein), the body almost exclusively uses carbohydrates (that are converted to glucose) and fat as energy substrates. When carbohydrates are depleted (as in LCHP diets), the body has to switch to fat and protein for energy. Without carbohydrates, the body must now produce glucose from muscle protein—and, to a small extent, from fat—in order to provide glucose for brain function and moderate and vigorous physical activity. Theoretically, LCHP diets result in faster weight loss by forcing the liver to produce glucose from fat stores and protein, but as you will learn in this chapter, these diets are not the best choice for weight loss.

Dieters on an LCHP diet attempt to keep blood glucose levels low. A food that has a low glycemic index, by definition, will not cause a rapid rise in blood glucose levels or the resulting release of insulin. A food that has a high **glycemic index** will cause a quick rise in blood glucose and the resulting release of insulin. A food's glycemic index is based on a 100-point rating system. At the top of the 100-point scale is glucose itself. This index is not directly related to simple and complex carbohydrates, and the glycemic values are not always what you might expect. Rather, the index is based on the actual laboratory-measured speed of absorption. Processed foods generally have a high glycemic index, whereas high-fiber foods tend to have a lower index (Table 5.1). Other factors that affect the index are the amount of carbohydrate, fat, and protein in the food; how refined the ingredients are; and whether the food was cooked.

Foods with a low glycemic index help reduce hunger later on by limiting blood-sugar spikes. The body functions best when blood sugar remains at a constant level. Although this is best accomplished by consuming low-glycemic foods (nuts, apples, oranges, low-fat yogurt, etc.), a person does not have to eliminate all high–glycemic index foods (sugar, potatoes, bread, white rice, soda drinks, etc.) from the diet. Foods with a high glycemic index along with some protein are useful to replenish depleted glycogen stores following prolonged or exhaustive aerobic exercise. Combining high– with low–glycemic index items or with some fat and protein brings down the average index.

Table 5.1 Glycemic Index of Selected Foods

Item	Index	Item	Index
All-Bran cereal	38	Milk, chocolate	43
Apples	40	Milk, chocolate, low-fat	34
Bagel, white	72	Milk, skim	32
Banana	56	Milk, whole	40
Bread, French	95	Jelly beans	80
Bread, wheat	73	Oatmeal	75
Bread, white	70	Oranges	48
Carrots, boiled (Australia)	41	Pasta, white	50
Carrots, boiled (Canada)	92	Pasta, wheat	32
Carrots, raw	47	Peanuts	20
Cherries	20	Peas	50
Colas	65	Pizza, cheese	60
Corn, sweet	60	Potato, baked	56–100
Corn Flakes	92	Potato, French fries	75
Doughnut	76	Potato, sweet	51
Frosted Flakes	55	Rice, white	56
Fruit cocktail	55	Sugar, table	65
Gatorade	78	Watermelon	72
Glucose	100	Yogurt, low-fat	32
Honey	58		

Regular consumption of high-glycemic foods by themselves may increase the risk for cardiovascular disease, especially in people at risk for diabetes. A person does not need to plan the diet around the index, as many popular diet programs indicate. The glycemic index deals with single foods eaten alone. Most people eat high–glycemic index foods with other foods as part of a meal. In combination, these foods have a lower effect on blood sugar. People who follow a healthy diet—that is, consume more fruits, non-starchy vegetables, whole grains, beans, fiber, fish, and lean meats and cut back on sugar and highly processed foods—will most likely have a diet in the low– to moderate–glycemic index category. Even people at risk for diabetes or who have the disease can eat high-glycemic foods, but in moderation.

Low-glycemic foods, nonetheless, aid with weight loss and weight maintenance. As blood sugar levels drop between snacks and meals, hunger increases. Keeping blood sugar levels constant by including low-glycemic foods in the diet helps stave off hunger, appetite, and overeating (Figure 5.4). At least

GLOSSARY

Glycogen Form in which carbohydrates (glucose molecules) are stored in the human body, predominantly in the muscles and liver.

Glycemic index A measure used to rate the plasma glucose response of carbohydrate-containing foods, comparing it with the response produced by the same amount of carbohydrates from a standard source, usually glucose or white bread.

Figure 5.4 **Effects of high- and low-glycemic carbohydrate intake on blood glucose levels.**

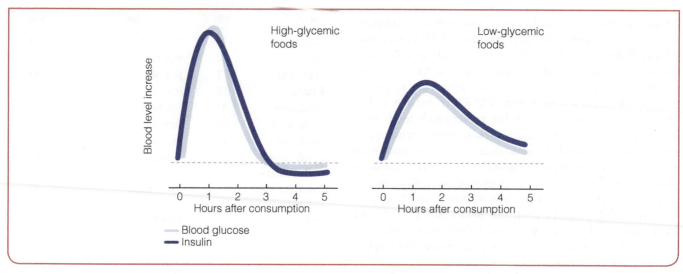

Popular Diets

The DASH Diet

The Dietary Approaches to Stop Hypertension (DASH) diet was originally designed as a heart-healthy diet to help lower high blood pressure. The diet plan is rich in fruits, vegetables, fat-free or low-fat milk and milk products, whole grains, fish, poultry, beans, seeds, and nuts. It also contains less sodium, fats, red meats, sweets, added sugars, and sugar-containing beverages than the typical American diet. Because it is such a healthy diet, the plan has been embraced by people seeking to lose weight. For weight loss purposes, the recommended daily caloric intake ranges from about 1,600 to 2,200 calories. The macronutrient composition of the diet includes 50 to 60 percent carbohydrates, less than 30 percent fat, and 15 to 20 percent protein.

The Volumetrics Eating Plan

The Volumetrics diet plan focuses on maximizing the volume of food and limiting calories by emphasizing high-water content or low-fat foods (lower energy density), low-fat cooking techniques, and extensive use of vegetables. The average daily caloric intake is reduced by 500 to 1,000 calories, with a macronutrient composition of approximately 55 percent carbohydrates, less than 30 percent fat, and more than 20 percent protein.

The Best Life Diet

The initial phase of the Best Life Diet plan encourages exercise and a recommended eating schedule. The second phase requires a reduction in caloric intake through consumption of healthful foods to satisfy hunger. The plan deals extensively with emotional eating. Caloric intake averages about 1,700 calories, with maintenance of daily moderate physical activity. The diet composition is about 50 percent carbohydrates, 30 percent fat, and 20 percent protein.

The Weight Watchers Diet

Dieters are given a daily point allowance in which calorie-dense foods with a higher fat content, simple carbohydrate content, or both are given more points. The points are determined using the patented Weight Watchers Point Calculator formula that looks to create an approximate 1,000-calorie-per-day deficit. The program encourages dieters to use points wisely by eating filling foods that keep hunger at bay, primarily foods rich in protein and fiber. The diet contains approximately 50 percent carbohydrates, 30 percent fat, and 20 percent protein.

The Ornish Diet

Ornish is a very low-fat, vegetarian-type diet. Dieters are not allowed to drink alcohol or eat meat, fish, oils, sugar, or white flour. Data indicate that strict adherence to the Ornish Diet can prevent and reverse heart disease. An average daily caloric intake is about 1,500 calories, composed of approximately 75 percent carbohydrates, less than 10 percent fat, and 15 percent protein.

The Zone Diet

The Zone Diet proposes that proper macronutrient (carbohydrate/fat/protein) distribution is critical to keep blood sugar and hormones in balance and thus prevent weight gain and disease. Daily caloric allowance is about 1,100 calories for women and 1,400 for men. All meals need to provide 40 percent carbohydrate calories, 30 percent fat calories, and 30 percent protein calories.

The Atkins Diet

In the LCHP Atkins Diet, practically all carbohydrates are eliminated during the first 2 weeks. Thereafter, very small amounts of carbohydrates are allowed, primarily in the form of limited fruits, vegetables,

(continued)

and wine. No caloric guidelines are given, but a typical daily diet plan is about 1,500 calories and is extremely high in fat (about 60 percent of calories), followed by protein (about 30 percent of calories), and limited carbohydrates (about 10 percent of calories). Dieters may not be as hungry on the Atkins Diet but may find it too restrictive for long-term adherence.

The South Beach Diet

Also an LCHP diet, the South Beach Diet is not as restrictive as the Atkins Diet. It emphasizes low-glycemic foods thought to decrease cravings for sugar and refined carbohydrates. Sugar, fruits, and grains are initially eliminated. In phase two, some high-fiber grains, fruit, and dark chocolate are permitted. No caloric guidelines are given, but a typical dietary plan provides about 1,400 calories per day, composed of 40 percent carbohydrate, 40 percent fat, and 20 percent protein calories.

The Glycemic Index Diet

The Glycemic Index Diet is based on the system of ranking carbohydrate foods according to how much each food raises the person's blood sugar level. This diet is also the basis for the Zone and South Beach diets. Dieters are encouraged to choose carbohydrate foods with a low glycemic index, such as whole fruits, vegetables, and beans. The hypothesis behind the diet is that low–glycemic index foods are absorbed more slowly, delaying hunger and making you less likely to overeat. Caloric intake ranges between 1,000 and 1,500 calories per day, and the diet composition is around 40 to 50 percent carbohydrates, 30 percent fat, and 30 percent protein.

The Biggest Loser Diet

Based on the popular TV show, The Biggest Loser Diet encourages small, frequent meals that emphasize filling calories from fruits, vegetables, lean protein sources, and whole grains; portion control; a food journal to monitor food intake; and an increase in daily physical activity and exercise. Caloric intake ranges from about 1,200 to 1,800 calories. The macronutrient composition of the diet is approximately 45 percent carbohydrate, 25 percent fat, and 30 percent protein calories.

The Mediterranean Diet

Although not specifically a dietary plan for weight reduction, the Mediterranean Diet (different cultures around the Mediterranean have slightly different patterns) emphasizes daily fruits, vegetables, whole grains, beans, nuts, legumes, olive oil, and flavorful herbs and spices; seafood at least twice a week; and poultry, eggs, cheese, yogurt, and red wine in moderation. Sweets and red meat are reserved for special occasions only, and physically activity is a part of the daily pattern. A calorie-restricted plan of the dietary pattern has been used to promote weight loss. Typically, the diet includes 40 to 50 percent carbohydrates, 25 to 40 percent fat, and 10 to 20 percent protein.

The Paleo Diet

The Paleo diet, also known as the Paleolithic or Caveman diet, is devoid of all processed foods, refined sugars, and dairy. The diet is based on animal protein; is low in carbohydrates; and includes primarily lean meats, nuts, and berries—foods that were available to ancient humans. The premise is that people today are maladapted to eating grains, legumes, gluten, dairy, and high-calorie processed foods. Although some people are gluten sensitive and processed foods should be avoided, most nutrition experts do not recommend the non-scientific Paleo diet due to major flaws to its underlying logic. Paleolithic humans most likely consumed foods that offered the highest energy for the lowest effort, including grains and legumes.

Proponents of the Paleo diet also indicate that ancient humans rarely developed cardiovascular disease or cancer. Paleolithic life expectancies, however, were much shorter than today's life expectancies, and back then, people did not live long enough to develop these chronic diseases. As compared to our 21st-century society, Paleolithic humans were much more active throughout the day and while pursuing a meal. Proponents of the Paleo diet recommend 19 to 35 percent protein, 22 to 40 percent carbohydrates, and 28 to 47 percent fat.

while attempting to lose weight, consumption of more fruit and non-starchy vegetables has been linked to better weight management. Examples of starchy vegetables include potatoes, yams, corn, zucchini, peas, squash, and pumpkin.

Proponents of LCHP diets claim that if a person eats fewer carbohydrates and more protein (and fat), the pancreas will produce less insulin; then, as insulin drops, the body will turn to its own fat deposits for energy. There is no scientific proof, however, that high levels of insulin lead to weight gain. None of the authors of these diets published studies validating their claims. Yet, these authors base their diets on the faulty premise that high insulin leads to obesity. We know the opposite to be true: Excessive body fat causes insulin levels to rise, thereby increasing the risk for developing diabetes.

Regular protein intake throughout the day helps to increase satiety and maintain lean body mass (LBM) during a weight-loss program. The main reason for rapid weight loss in very low-carbohydrate diets is that a low carbohydrate intake forces the liver to produce glucose. The source for most of this glucose is body proteins—LBM, including muscle. As indicated earlier, protein contains a lot of water; thus, weight is lost rapidly. When a person terminates the diet, the body rebuilds some protein tissue and quickly regains some weight.

Research studies indicated that individuals on an LCHP diet lose slightly more weight in the first few months than those on a low-fat diet. The effectiveness of the diet, however, seemed to dwindle over time. A year into the diet, participants in a LCHP diet regain more weight than those on a low-fat diet plan.

Low-carb diets are contrary to the nutrition advice of most leading national health organizations (which recommend a diet lower in saturated fat and trans fats and high in complex carbohydrates). Without fruits, vegetables, and whole grains, high-protein diets lack many vitamins, minerals, antioxidants, phytonutrients, and fiber—all dietary factors that protect against an array of ailments and diseases.

The major risk associated with long-term adherence to LCHP diets could be the increased risk for heart disease because many high-protein foods in the typical American diet are also high in saturated fat content (see Chapter 10). Short-term (a few weeks or months) adherence to LCHP diets does not appear to increase heart disease risk. The long-term (years) effects of these types of diets, nonetheless, have not been evaluated by scientific research (few people would be willing to adhere to such a diet for several years). A possible long-term adverse effect of adherence to an LCHP diet is a potential increase in kidney problems and cancer risk. Phytonutrients found in fruits, vegetables, and whole grains protect against certain types of cancer. A low carbohydrate intake also produces a loss of vitamin B, calcium, and potassium. Potential bone loss can accentuate the risk for osteoporosis.

Side effects commonly associated with LCHP diets include weakness, nausea, bad breath, constipation, irritability, light-headedness, and fatigue. If you choose to go on an LCHP diet for longer than a few weeks, let your physician know so that he or she may monitor your blood lipids, bone density, and kidney function.

The benefit of adding extra protein to a weight-loss program may be related to the hunger-suppressing effect of protein. Data suggest that protein curbs hunger more effectively than carbohydrates or fat.

Exercise-Related Weight Loss Myths

Cellulite and spot reducing are mythical concepts. **Cellulite** is caused by the herniation of subcutaneous fat within fibrous connective tissue, giving the tissue a padded appearance.

Spot reducing, or exercising a body part to reduce fat in that specific area, is also impossible. Doing several sets of daily sit-ups will not get rid of fat in the midsection of the body. The caloric output of a few sets of sit-ups has practically no effect on reducing total body fat. A negative caloric balance combined with exercise has to be significant enough to produce real fat loss.

Evidence shows that with initial weight gain, fat storage in the lower body is primarily accomplished by increasing the number of fat cells, whereas with abdominal weight gain, the extra fat stored is almost entirely through an increase in fat-cell size. Fat cells are thought to be capable of a fourfold increase in size. With further weight gain, nonetheless, fat-cell number also increases in the abdominal area. We all have "pre-fat cells" that fully develop when weight gain is substantial. Typically, with weight loss, abdominal weight loss comes first because of the larger cell size in this area. Lower-body fat loss comes last because most of the weight gain was the result of an increase in cell number and not size. On average, people who gain primarily leg fat tend to have a better metabolic profile.

> ### How to Recognize Fad Diets
>
> Fad diets have characteristics in common. These diets typically
> - Are nutritionally unbalanced.
> - Rely primarily on a single food (e.g., grapefruit).
> - Are based on testimonials.
> - Were developed according to "confidential research."
> - Are based on a "scientific breakthrough."
> - Promote rapid and "painless" weight loss.
> - Promise miraculous results.
> - Restrict food selection.
> - Are based on pseudoclaims that excessive weight is related to a specific condition, such as insulin resistance, combinations or timing of nutrient intake, food allergies, hormone imbalances, and certain foods (e.g., fruits).
> - Require the use of selected products.
> - Use liquid formulas instead of foods.
> - Misrepresent salespeople as individuals qualified to provide nutrition counseling.
> - Fail to provide information on risks associated with weight loss and use of the diet.
> - Do not involve physical activity.
> - Do not encourage healthy behavioral changes.
> - Are not supported by the scientific community or national health organizations.
> - Fail to provide information for weight maintenance upon completion of the diet phase.

Other touted means toward quick weight loss, such as steam baths, rubberized sweat suits, and mechanical vibrators, are misleading. When you step into a sauna, the weight lost is not fat but merely a significant amount of water. It looks nice when you step on the scale immediately afterward, but this represents a false loss of weight. As soon as you replace body fluids, you gain the weight back quickly.

Wearing rubberized sweat suits hastens the rate of body fluid that is lost—fluid that is vital during prolonged exercise—and raises core temperature at the same time. This combination puts a person in danger of dehydration, which impairs cellular function and, in extreme cases, can even cause death.

Similarly, mechanical vibrators are worthless in a weight control program. Vibrating belts and turning rollers may feel good, but they require no effort. Fat cannot be shaken off. It is lost primarily by burning it in muscle tissue.

Adopting Permanent Change

A few diets recommend exercise along with caloric restrictions—the best method for weight reduction. People who adhere to these programs succeed, so the diet has achieved its purpose. Unfortunately, if the people do not change their food selection and activity level permanently, they gain back the weight once they discontinue dieting and exercise.

If people would only accept that no magic foods provide all necessary nutrients and that they have to eat a variety of foods to be well nourished, dieters would be more successful and the diet industry would go broke. Also, people eat for pleasure and for health. Two of the most essential components of a wellness lifestyle are healthy eating and regular physical activity, and they provide the best weight management program available today.

5.5 Mental and Emotional Aspects of Weight Management

In addition to physiological needs, eating fulfills psychological, social, and cultural purposes. We eat to sustain our daily energy requirements, but we also eat at family celebrations, national holidays, social gatherings, and sporting events (as spectators) and even eat more or stop eating when we become emotional. Because food carries so many cultural and comforting associations, eating for nutritive value may seem daunting. But with the right tools, it is possible to satisfy both eating desires and nutritional needs.

Willpower versus Planning

An important concept to understand when changing eating habits is that willpower can be used only in specific, limited ways. For example, a scenario in which willpower helps is how you apply yourself to schoolwork or job responsibility. Success in either of these realms is closely associated with a person's rational self-control and long-term self-interest. Eating behavior, in contrast, is much less associated with a person's sheer rational self-control.[7] For instance, in most cases, willpower is inadequate when staring down a plate of cheese fries and not eating them (see discussion on long-term values and the prefrontal cortex in Chapter 2, page 57).

Willpower, nonetheless, can work well as a planning tool rather than a battle weapon in the moment of temptation. Use it to create deliberate lifestyle choices that fit your values. One technique is to simply change the visibility and proximity of food. Surveys indicate that a clear bowl of candy disappears faster than an opaque jar of candy and a plate of cookies at arm's reach is harder to resist than a plate of cookies across the room. Use this technique to your benefit in the environments where you make food choices. You should examine and then implement changes that you can make in your kitchen, at your work desk, or even in your breakroom.

Limiting the variety of food options is also helpful and decreases overall energy intake. Consider how you can limit food variety in positive, satisfying ways. It is likely unhelpful, for example, to wake each morning and consider whether breakfast will be a cup of yogurt or last night's leftovers of pizza and dessert cobbler. Instead, it may be helpful to create a list of healthy breakfast choices that you find satisfying and feel good about after eating them.

Implementation intention is an "if-then" planning strategy that can help you attain goals[8] (also discussed in Chapter 2 on page 58). With this technique, individuals are advised to anticipate an obstacle to their eating goals. Individuals are then directed to visualize a specific plan for overcoming that obstacle. For example, you may visualize going on a road trip and making sure any unhealthy food is out of convenient reach, perhaps allowing yourself a favorite snack toward the end of the trip. Visualizing the way you will respond greatly increases your chances of accomplishing that positive response.

When trying to lose weight, be aware that being in a bad mood (judged independently from being hungry or sleep deprived) and feeling stress decrease your chances of making healthy food choices. While you cannot control everything that happens in a day, you can be mindful of what causes stress and notice if and when it affects your eating choices. Under these circumstances, you need to plan ahead to avoid unnecessary food consumption by applying appropriate stress management techniques (see Chapter 12).

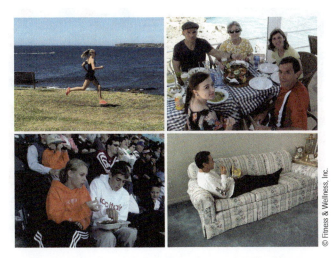

Eating is very much a part of the American way of life. We eat not only to sustain energy requirements and hunger; but often also we eat at celebrations, cultural, and sporting events; and during times of stress, boredom, and need for comfort.

© Fitness & Wellness, Inc.

---GLOSSARY---

Cellulite Term frequently used in reference to fat deposits that "bulge out," caused by the herniation of subcutaneous fat within fibrous connective tissue and giving the tissue a padded appearance.

Spot reducing Fallacious theory proposing that exercising a specific body part results in significant fat reduction in that area.

Mindful Eating versus Distracted Eating

Mindful eating is also critical to proper weight management. Keeping your nutrition goals and desired long-term outcomes in mind can improve eating behavior.[9] Before you eat, do a quick physical and emotional check. If you do not feel hungry, do you really need to eat at that moment? Note any emotions you are feeling at that point. You may discover eating cues you had never noticed before. The meals you enjoy the most take place when hunger has developed, you choose food that is appetizing to you, and the values-centered part of your brain (the prefrontal cortex) agrees that the food is wholesome, thus creating a unanimous vote that it is time to enjoy the meal.

While dieticians recommend allowing your hunger to develop before eating, they also recommend not waiting so long that you become preoccupied with thoughts of food. Long-term calorie restriction has been shown to slow the values-centered part of the brain and stimulate areas that control appetite, making food more tempting.[10] Allowing yourself to feel hunger for a few minutes, up to an hour, is reasonable for most people. You may find that if you regularly wait longer than an hour after feeling hungry, you will be more preoccupied with food and more likely to overeat.

If you find that you frequently eat for a purpose other than developed hunger, take note of these situations and brainstorm for a healthy solution. Notice any foods that you perceive have certain traits, such as foods you consider comfort foods, and take stock of whether they are necessary and contribute to a healthy lifestyle.

Be aware of the way foods you buy are presented and how they affect your mood. Studies have shown that information about food, calling it wholesome or bursting with flavor, for example, affects individuals in different ways. Perceptions about food can directly affect hormone levels. In one study, participants were given a 380-calorie milkshake on two different occasions. On one occasion it was presented as a "sensible" 140-calorie shake. On the other occasion, the same milkshake was offered as an "indulgent" 620-calorie shake. When researchers measured blood levels, they found that the hunger hormone ghrelin (which stimulates appetite) was lower after having been told the milkshake was indulgent.[11]

Allow sufficient time for your meals in a setting that lets you appreciate food flavor, texture, and appearance. Eating while distracted makes flavors less intense and the experience less satisfying.[12] Distracted eating can easily result in consuming a third or more calories than normal. Pay attention to foods that may or may not be worthwhile to you. On the few occasions when you decide to give in to a desired treat (including savory treats, alcohol, or liquid calories), take the time to mindfully enjoy your treat.

When you are trying to avoid a specific food, this is not the time to be mindful about it. Avoid thoughts about the food's texture, taste, or appearance. Rather, think as abstractly as you can about the food to help you resist eating it.[13]

Avoiding Perfectionism

In many areas of life, we do not expect perfection from ourselves. During school, we are not devastated each time we do not receive a perfect grade. To do so would be irrational. But when it comes to eating behavior, we have created a culture in which individuals set strict constraints for themselves and feel they have failed each time their compliance is less than perfect.

When teaching yourself a new eating habit, just as in teaching yourself any new skill, it is important to know you will make mistakes, even as you improve. Use failures as learning experiences to better understand yourself and your situation. Give yourself credit as you learn to rebound more quickly from each failure. Eventually, you will be able to anticipate difficult situations and have a plan for a successful outcome. In time, you will find you are able to stop a negative behavior as it begins and, someday, even before it begins.

Give yourself time to adapt to change gradually. Take on just one or two changes at a time. As you create guidelines for yourself, keep in mind that rigid eating restrictions can result in unwanted rebound eating. Find ways to limit variety without creating restrictions that you find yourself fighting all day long.

Feelings of Satisfaction versus Deprivation

To permanently change eating habits, the goal is to create new patterns that are satisfying and consistent with your own desires for well-being. Understanding how profoundly diet affects health helps to reinforce new eating habits, but it is also important to notice environments and contexts that leave you feeling resentful or deprived when turning down food. Try to make note of these feelings and brainstorm solutions. For example, if you plan to go to a party where you would rather not eat the food offered, eat a healthy meal you particularly enjoy before you go.

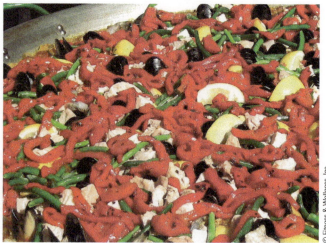

Appreciating food because of the time or skill it took to grow or prepare, its presentation on the plate, or its naturally complex and nuanced flavors can help a person feel gratified by the eating experience.

Appreciating your newfound knowledge of the benefits of wholesome foods can also help combat feelings of deprivation, especially for those who see eating healthy food as an act of self-restraint. Furthermore, appreciating food because of the time or skill it took to grow or prepare, its presentation on the plate, or its naturally complex and nuanced flavors can help a person feel gratified by the eating experience.

Eating and the Social Environment

During the weight loss process, surround yourself with people who have the same goal that you have (weight loss). Data indicate that obesity can spread through "social networks." That is, if your friends, siblings, or spouse gains weight, you are more likely to gain weight as well. People tend to accept a higher weight standard if someone they are close to or care about gains weight.

In the study, the social ties of more than 12,000 people were examined over 32 years. The findings revealed that if a close friend becomes obese, a person's risk of becoming obese during the next 2 to 4 years increases 171 percent. In addition, the risk increases 57 percent for casual friends, 40 percent for siblings, and 37 percent for the person's spouse. The reverse was also found to be true: When a person loses weight, the likelihood of friends, siblings, or a spouse losing weight is also enhanced.

Furthermore, the research found that gender plays a role in social networks. A male's weight has a greater effect on the weight of male friends and brothers than on female friends or sisters. Similarly, a woman's weight has a far greater influence on sisters and girlfriends than on brothers or male friends. Thus, if you are trying to lose weight, choose your friendships carefully: Do not surround yourself with people who either have a weight problem or are still gaining weight.

Overcoming Emotional Eating

Eating in response to emotions is a learned behavior because eating provides an instant feeling of satisfaction when you are feeling down. Food consumption as an automatic reaction to emotion is an unhealthy action on its own and does not address the problem that caused the negative emotion. The emotions return and may be compounded by a feeling of guilt from overeating.

Before eating in response to emotions, pause and notice whether you are feeling disappointed, nervous, uncertain, lonely, depressed, angry, embarrassed, guilty, stressed, bored, frustrated, tired, overwhelmed, or powerless. In some cases **emotional eating** involves the consumption of large quantities of food, especially "comfort" and junk food, almost always consumed in a distracted state. Emotional eating is more common among people who have adopted rigid dietary rules. A preference for certain foods is also present when people experience specific feelings (loneliness, anxiety, and fear).

Emotional eating can be provoked for reasons a person may not fully comprehend. Some individuals are likely to feel a compulsion to eat regardless of hunger cues when an eating occasion is limited or a particular food is seen as scarce. For example, a person who is on vacation and is in an unusual environment may feel the need to eat a great deal at a meal if uncertain as to when the next mealtime will be. Anticipating this scenario and packing healthy snacks could be enough to diffuse the eating cue.

Treatment

If you are an emotional overeater, the following list of suggestions may help:

1. Learn to differentiate between emotional and physical hunger.
2. Teach yourself the habit of noticing your emotions before picking up food.
3. Pause when you catch yourself eating in response to an emotion and ask yourself if food is really necessary.
4. Remind yourself that your choices include eating, eating and decreasing the portion size, waiting for a few minutes before you eat, eating that same food at the next meal, or using countering techniques (replacing the behavior by going for a walk, listening to music, or occupying yourself in other ways).
5. Take the time to enjoy the food mindfully if you choose to continue eating.
6. Avoid storing and snacking on unhealthy foods.
7. Keep healthy snacks handy.
8. Keep a "trigger log" and get to know what triggers your emotional food consumption.
9. Work it out with exercise instead of food.

HOEGER KEY TO WELLNESS

 There is absolutely nothing wrong with seeking professional help for an eating disorder. You may not view yourself this way, but as others recognize that you may have such a condition, you owe it to yourself to seek out the proper treatment to overcome the ailment. Your health, well-being, and quality of life are at stake if you do not exercise control over the matter.

5.6 *Physiology of Weight Loss*

Traditional concepts related to weight control have centered on three assumptions:

1. Balancing food intake against output allows a person to achieve recommended weight.
2. All fat people simply eat too much.
3. The human body doesn't care how much (or how little) fat it stores.

Although these statements contain some truth, they are open to much debate and research. We now know that the causes of excessive weight and obesity are complex, involving

---

GLOSSARY

Emotional eating The consumption of large quantities of food to suppress negative emotions.

Eating Disorders

Eating disorders are medical illnesses that involve crucial disturbances in eating behaviors thought to stem from some combination of environmental pressures. These disorders are characterized by an intense fear of becoming fat, which does not disappear even when the person is losing weight in extreme amounts. The three most common types of eating disorders are anorexia nervosa, bulimia nervosa, and binge-eating disorder. A fourth disorder, emotional eating, can also be listed under disordered eating.

Most people who have eating disorders are afflicted by significant family and social problems. They may lack fulfillment in many areas of their lives. The eating disorder then becomes the coping mechanism to avoid dealing with these problems. Taking control of their body weight helps them believe that they are restoring some sense of control over their lives.

Anorexia nervosa and bulimia nervosa are common in industrialized nations whose society encourages low-calorie diets and thinness. The female role in society has changed rapidly, which makes women more susceptible to eating disorders. Although frequently seen in young women, eating disorders are most prevalent among individuals between the ages of 25 and 50. Surveys, nonetheless, indicate that as many as 40 percent of college-age women are struggling with an eating disorder.

Eating disorders are not limited to women. One in 10 cases occur in men. But because men's role and body image are viewed differently in most societies, these cases often go unreported.

Although genetics may play a role in the development of eating disorders, most cases are environmentally related. Individuals who have clinical depression and obsessive-compulsive behavior are more susceptible. About half of all people with eating disorders have some sort of chemical dependency (alcohol and drugs), and most of them come from families with alcohol- and drug-related problems. Of reported cases of eating disorders, a large number are individuals who are, or who have been, victims of sexual molestation.

Eating disorders develop in stages. Typically, individuals who are already dealing with significant issues in life start a diet. At first, they feel in control and are happy about the weight loss, even if they are not overweight. As they are encouraged by the prospect of weight loss and the control they can exert over their weight, the dieting becomes extreme and often is combined with exhaustive exercise and overuse of laxatives and diuretics.

The syndrome typically emerges following emotional issues or a stressful life event and uncertainty about the ability to cope efficiently. Life experiences that can trigger the syndrome might be gaining weight, starting the menstrual period, beginning college, losing a boyfriend, having poor self-esteem, being socially rejected, starting a professional career, or becoming a wife or a mother.

The eating disorder then takes on a life of its own and becomes the primary focus of attention for the individual afflicted with it. Self-worth revolves around what the scale reads every day, the individual's relationship with food, and that person's perception of how she or he looks each day.

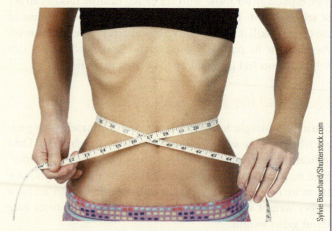

Society's unrealistic view of what constitutes recommended weight and "ideal" body image contributes to the development of eating disorders.

Anorexia Nervosa

An estimated 1 percent of the population in the United States has the eating disorder **anorexia nervosa**. Anorexic individuals seem to fear weight gain more than death from starvation. Furthermore, they have a distorted image of their bodies and think of themselves as being fat even when they are emaciated.

Anorexic patients commonly develop obsessive and compulsive behaviors and emphatically deny their condition. They are preoccupied with food, meal planning, and grocery shopping, and they have unusual eating habits. As they lose weight and their health begins to deteriorate, they feel weak and tired. They might realize they have a problem, but they will not stop the starvation and refuse to consider the behavior abnormal.

Once they have lost a lot of weight and malnutrition sets in, the physical changes become more visible. Typical changes are amenorrhea (absence of menstruation), digestive problems, extreme sensitivity to cold, hair problems, fluid and electrolyte abnormalities (which may lead to an irregular heartbeat and sudden stopping of the heart), injuries to nerves and tendons, abnormalities of immune function, anemia, growth of fine body hair, mental confusion, inability to concentrate, lethargy, depression, dry skin, lower skin and body temperature, and osteoporosis.

The following diagnostic criteria are for anorexia nervosa:

- Refusal to maintain body weight over a minimal normal weight for age and height (weight loss leading to maintenance of body weight less than 85 percent of that expected or failure to make expected weight gain during periods of growth, leading to body weight less than 85 percent of that expected).

- Intense fear of gaining weight or becoming fat, even though underweight.

- Disturbance in the way in which the individual's body weight, size, or shape is perceived; undue influences of body weight or shape on self-evaluation; or denial of the seriousness of current low body weight.

(continued)

- In postmenarcheal females, amenorrhea (absence of at least three consecutive menstrual cycles; a woman is considered to have amenorrhea if her periods occur only following estrogen therapy).

Many changes induced by anorexia nervosa can be reversed, and individuals with this condition can get better with professional therapy. However, they sometimes turn to bulimia nervosa, or they die from the disorder. Anorexia nervosa has the highest mortality rate of all psychosomatic illnesses today—20 percent of anorexic individuals die as a result of their condition. The disorder is 100 percent curable, but treatment almost always requires professional help. The sooner it is started, the better the chances for reversibility and cure. Therapy consists of a combination of medical and psychological techniques to restore proper nutrition, prevent medical complications, and modify the environment or events that triggered the syndrome.

Seldom can anorexia sufferers overcome the problem by themselves. They strongly deny their condition. They are able to hide it and deceive friends and relatives. Based on their behavior, many of them meet all characteristics of anorexia nervosa, but it goes undetected because both thinness and dieting are socially acceptable. Only a well-trained clinician is able to diagnose the ailment in its early stages.

Bulimia Nervosa

Bulimia nervosa is more prevalent than anorexia nervosa. As many as one in five women on college campuses may be bulimic. Bulimia nervosa also is more prevalent than anorexia nervosa in males, although bulimia is still more prevalent in females.

People with bulimia usually are healthy looking, well educated, and near recommended body weight. They seem to enjoy food and often socialize around it. In actuality, they are emotionally insecure, rely on others, and lack self-confidence and self-esteem. Recommended weight and food are important to them.

The binge–purge cycle usually occurs in stages. As a result of stressful life events or the simple compulsion to eat, bulimic individuals engage periodically in binge eating. With some apprehension, bulimics anticipate and plan the cycle. Next, they feel an urgency to begin large and uncontrollable food consumption, during which time they may eat for an hour or longer and may consume several thousand calories (up to 10,000 calories in extreme cases). After a short period of relief and satisfaction, feelings of deep guilt and shame and intense fear of gaining weight emerge. Purging seems to be an easy answer because the bingeing cycle can continue without fear of gaining weight.

The following diagnostic criteria are for bulimia nervosa:

- Recurrent episodes of binge eating. An episode of binge eating is characterized by both of the following: (a) eating in a discrete period (e.g., within any 2-hour period) an amount of food that is more than most people would eat during a similar period and under similar circumstances and (b) a sense of lack of control over eating during the episode (feeling unable to stop eating or control what or how much is being consumed).
- Recurring inappropriate compensatory behaviors to prevent weight gain, such as self-induced vomiting; misuse of laxatives, diuretics, other medications, or emetics; fasting; or excessive exercise.

- Occurrence of the binge eating and inappropriate compensatory behaviors occurring, on average, at least twice a week for 3 months.
- Undue influence of body shape and weight on self-evaluation.

The most typical form of purging is self-induced vomiting. Bulimics also frequently ingest strong laxatives and emetics. Near-fasting diets and strenuous bouts of exercise are common. Medical problems associated with bulimia nervosa include cardiac arrhythmias, amenorrhea, kidney and bladder damage, ulcers, colitis, tearing of the esophagus or stomach, tooth erosion, gum damage, and general muscular weakness.

Unlike anorexics, bulimia sufferers realize that their behavior is abnormal and feel shame about it. Fearing social rejection, they pursue the binge–purge cycle in secrecy and at unusual hours of the day.

Bulimia nervosa can be treated successfully when the person realizes that this destructive behavior is not the solution to life's problems. A change in attitude can prevent permanent damage or death.

Binge-Eating Disorder

Binge-eating disorder is probably the most common of the three main eating disorders. About 2 percent of American adults are afflicted with binge-eating disorder in any 6-month period. Although most people overeat occasionally, eating more than is appropriate now and then does not mean someone has binge-eating disorder. The disorder is slightly more common in women than in men; three women for every two men have the disorder.

Binge-eating disorder is characterized by uncontrollable episodes of eating excessive amounts of food within a relatively short time. The causes of binge-eating disorder are unknown, although depression, anger, sadness, boredom, and worry can trigger an episode. Unlike bulimic sufferers, binge eaters do not purge; thus, most people with this disorder are either overweight or obese.

Typical symptoms of binge-eating disorder include the following:

- Eating what most people think is an unusually large amount of food.
- Eating until uncomfortably full.
- Eating out of control.
- Eating faster than usual during binge episodes.
- Eating alone because of embarrassment about how much food is consumed.
- Feeling disgusted, depressed, or guilty after overeating.

GLOSSARY

Anorexia nervosa An eating disorder characterized by self-imposed starvation to lose weight and maintain very low body weight.

Bulimia nervosa An eating disorder characterized by a pattern of binge eating and purging in an attempt to lose weight and maintain low body weight.

Binge-eating disorder An eating disorder characterized by uncontrollable episodes of eating excessive amounts of food within a relatively short time.

(continued)

Eating Disorder Not Otherwise Specified (EDNOS)

The American Psychiatric Association introduced EDNOS, a diagnostic category for individuals who don't fall into the previously discussed categories but still have troubled relationships with food or distorted body images. EDNOS diagnoses outnumber both anorexia and bulimia nervosa cases. These conditions also lead to malnourishment.

Orthoxia This eating disorder is characterized by a fixation with healthy or righteous eating. These individuals attempt to eat organic foods only or avoid anything that isn't "pure in quality," often eliminating entire food groups. They are primarily motivated by fear of bad health and not necessarily thinness.

Pregorexia Because of the social pressure to look thin during and after child bearing, some women fear gaining the recommended 25 to 35 pounds of weight during pregnancy, resulting in excessive dieting and exercising during this time. Common health risks include anemia, hypertension, depression, and malnourished babies who may be born with birth defects or be miscarried.

Drunkorexia This disorder group includes individuals who decrease caloric intake or skip meals to save those calories for alcohol and binge drinking. One survey found that close to 30 percent of female college students engage in drunkorexic behavior. Such action increases the risk for alcohol poisoning and unplanned sexual relations; in the long term, it raises the risk for heart and liver disease.

Anorexia Athletica This group includes people who engage daily in compulsive, lengthy, and rigorous exercise routines to reach and maintain low body weight. These individuals feel extremely guilty if they miss a workout or are unable to keep up with the exercise regimen. Health risks of this behavior include depression and fatal heart disease.

Treatment Treatment for eating disorders is available on most school campuses through the school's counseling center or health center. Local hospitals also offer treatment for these conditions. Many communities have support groups, frequently led by professional personnel and often free of charge. All information and the individual's identity are kept confidential, so the person need not fear embarrassment or repercussions when seeking professional help.

SOURCE: American Psychiatric Association, *Diagnostic and Statistical Manual of Mental Disorders* (Washington, DC: APA, 2013).

a combination of genetic, metabolic, hormonal, psychological, cultural, behavioral, and socioeconomic factors.

Energy-Balancing Equation

The principle embodied in the **energy-balancing equation** is simple: As long as caloric input equals caloric output, the person does not gain or lose weight. If caloric intake exceeds output, the person gains weight; when output exceeds input, the person loses weight. If daily energy requirements could be determined accurately, caloric intake could be balanced against output. This is seldom the case because caloric balance is dynamic (it changes) and differs among individuals. The principle of **dynamic energy balance** is particularly significant during periods of weight change, as genetic and lifestyle-related differences among people determine the number of calories required to maintain, lose, or gain weight. A person's body weight, body composition (lean vs. adipose tissue), resting metabolic rate, daily exercise and physical activity patterns, composition and thermic effect of food (carbohydrates/fats/proteins), caloric content of food, fiber intake, hormonal control of fat deposition and satiety, and energy costs of fat and protein synthesis are some of the most common factors that affect the daily energy requirement.[14]

Table 5.2 (page 187) offers general guidelines to determine the **Estimated Energy Requirement (EER)** in calories per day. This is an estimated figure only and serves only as a starting point from which individual adjustments have to be made (also see "Losing Weight the Sound and Sensible Way," page 184).

The total daily energy requirement has three basic components (Figure 5.5):

1. Resting metabolic rate
2. Thermic effect of food
3. Physical activity

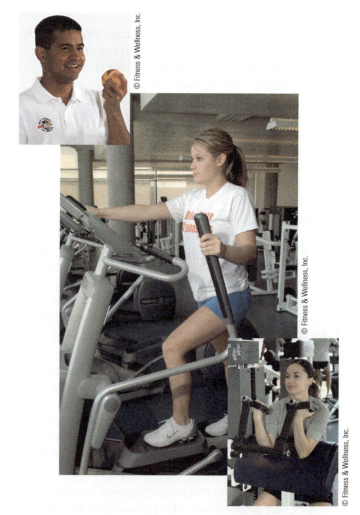

Achieving and maintaining a high physical fitness percent body fat standard requires a lifetime commitment to regular physical activity and proper nutrition.

Figure 5.5 Components of total daily energy requirement.

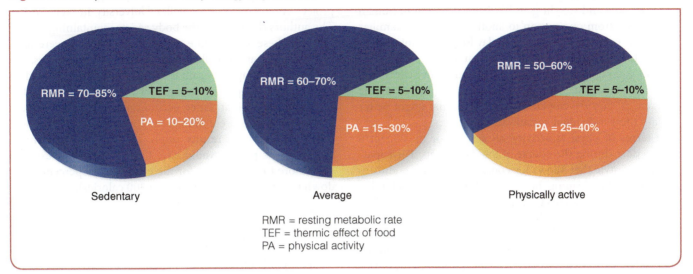

Sedentary — RMR = 70–85%, TEF = 5–10%, PA = 10–20%

Average — RMR = 60–70%, TEF = 5–10%, PA = 15–30%

Physically active — RMR = 50–60%, TEF = 5–10%, PA = 25–40%

RMR = resting metabolic rate
TEF = thermic effect of food
PA = physical activity

The **resting metabolic rate (RMR)**—the energy requirement to maintain the body's vital processes in the resting state—accounts for approximately 60 to 70 percent of the total daily energy requirement. On average, the thermic effect of food—the energy required to digest, absorb, and store food—accounts for about 5 to 10 percent of the total daily requirement. Physical activity accounts for 15 to 30 percent of the total daily requirement.

One pound of fat is said to be the equivalent of 3,500 calories. Fat is stored in adipocytes (fat cells), which contain minerals, water, and even a small amount of protein. Adipocytes are estimated to be *about* 86 percent fat (the percentage varies slightly in the literature). We know that one pound of fat equals 0.454 kg (1 ÷ 2.2046) or 454 grams. Thus, if one gram of fat provides 9 calories, one pound of fat or 454 grams contains 3,511 calories (454 × .86 × 9).

If a person decreases energy intake by 500 calories per day, theoretically, it should result in a loss of 1 pound of fat in 7 days (500 × 7 = 3,500). But research has shown—and many people have experienced—that even when dieters carefully balance caloric input against caloric output, weight loss does not always result as predicted. That is because the number of calories that must be expended to lose one pound of fat changes depending on the length of the diet, the resetting of the body's setpoint for body weight (see discussion that follows under Setpoint Theory), type of diet (food composition), amount of caloric restriction, and level and type of physical activity (activities of daily living vs. moderate-intensity aerobic exercise, vs. high-intensity interval training, vs. strength training). Also, as a person loses body weight, loss of lean tissue causes a drop in the metabolic rate and the lower overall body mass (muscle and fat) requires fewer calories to sustain the human body. Furthermore, due to genetic factors, two people with similar measured caloric intake and output seldom lose weight at the same rate.

As most people on a negative caloric intake have experienced, weight is lost at a much faster rate in the initial stages of the diet. Research looking at the energy content of weight loss found that during the first four weeks of a diet, a deficit of only 2,200 calories led to each pound of weight lost.[15] At week 6, the energy reduction to lose a pound of body weight had increased to about 2,750 calories. By week 20, the required deficit was closer to 3,500 calories per pound of weight lost. The investigators theorized that the initial weight lost included fat, water, glycogen, and protein. Subsequently, a greater proportion of the weight lost was in the form of fat, and by week 20, almost all of the weight lost was in the form of fat.

Studies have also confirmed that as people diet and lose weight, they have a natural tendency to be less active. Thus, it becomes a greater challenge to stay with the diet, most notably due to the lower caloric intake, the difference in daily physical activity, and the drop in the basal metabolic rate. Furthermore, the body burns fewer calories as weight is lost because of the lower energy cost to move a smaller body. While not a precise science, the 3,500-calorie rule is still a good guideline to work from when writing weight-loss programs.

GLOSSARY

Energy-balancing equation A principle holding that as long as caloric input equals caloric output, the person does not gain or lose weight. If caloric intake exceeds output, the person gains weight; when output exceeds input, the person loses weight.

Dynamic energy balance A principle that states that daily energy balance is a moving figure that is determined by physiological and lifestyle-related factors that regulate how many calories it takes to maintain, lose, or gain weight.

Estimated Energy Requirement (EER) Average dietary energy (caloric) intake that is predicted to maintain energy balance in a healthy adult of defined age, gender, weight, height, and level of physical activity, consistent with good health.

Resting metabolic rate (RMR) The energy requirement to maintain the body's vital processes in the resting state.

The most common explanation for individual differences in weight loss and weight gain has been variation in human metabolism from one person to another. We are all familiar with a few people who can eat "all day long" and not gain an ounce of weight, while some cannot even "dream about food" without gaining weight. Because experts did not believe that human metabolism alone could account for such extreme differences, they developed other theories that might better explain these individual variations.

In terms of physical activity, all activity or movement a person does during the course of the day counts. Participating in a lifestyle that allows for constant, small expenditures of energy, like cleaning house or filling orders behind a counter, can greatly affect weight management success (see discussion of NEAT in Chapter 1, page 17). Also playing a notable part in success at weight management is a principle is known as "spontaneous nonexercise activity," or "fidgeting." Such activity can easily account for several hundred calories a day, resulting in significant differences in weight management among people.

Setpoint Theory

Results of research studies point toward a **weight-regulating mechanism (WRM)** in the human body that has a **setpoint** for controlling both appetite and amount of fat stored. The setpoint is hypothesized to work like a thermostat for body fat, maintaining fairly constant body weight because it "knows" at all times the exact amount of adipose tissue stored in the fat cells. Some people have high settings; others have low settings.

If body weight decreases (as in dieting), the setpoint senses this change and triggers the WRM to increase appetite or make the body conserve energy to maintain the "set" weight. The opposite also may be true. Some people have a hard time gaining weight. In this case, the WRM decreases appetite or causes the body to waste energy to maintain the lower weight.

Every person has a certain body fat percentage (as established by the setpoint) that the body attempts to maintain. The genetic instinct to survive tells the body that fat storage is vital; therefore, the body sets an acceptable fat level. This level may remain somewhat constant or may climb gradually because of poor lifestyle habits.

For instance, under strict caloric reduction, the body may make extreme metabolic adjustments in an effort to maintain its setpoint for fat. The **basal metabolic rate (BMR)**, the lowest level of caloric intake necessary to sustain life, may drop dramatically when operating under a consistent negative caloric balance, and that person's weight loss may plateau for days or even weeks. A low BMR compounds a person's problems in maintaining recommended body weight. (The BMR is typically measured in a thermoneutral environment following at least 8 hours of sleep and fasting for 12 hours. The RMR does not require the aforementioned strict criteria and is commonly measured 2 to 5 hours after a meal in resting state).

These findings were substantiated by a significant research project conducted at Rockefeller University in New York.[16] The authors showed that the body resists maintaining altered weight. Obese and lifetime nonobese individuals were used in the investigation. Following a 10 percent weight loss, the body, in an attempt to regain the lost weight, compensated by burning up to 15 percent fewer calories than expected for the new reduced weight (after accounting for the 10 percent loss). The effects were similar in the obese and nonobese participants. These results imply that after a 10 percent weight loss, a person would have to eat even less or exercise even more to compensate for the estimated 15 percent slowdown (a difference of about 200 to 300 calories).

> **!**
> ### Critical Thinking
> Do you see a difference in the amount of food that you are now able to eat compared with the amount that you ate in your mid- to late-teen years? If so, to what do you attribute this difference? What actions are you taking to account for the difference?

In this same study, when the participants were allowed to increase their weight to 10 percent above their "normal" body (before weight loss) weight, the body burned 10 to 15 percent *more* calories than expected—attempting to waste energy and maintain the preset weight. This is another indication that the body is highly resistant to weight changes unless additional lifestyle changes are incorporated to ensure successful weight management. (These methods are discussed under "Losing Weight the Sound and Sensible Way," page 184.)

Dietary restriction alone does not lower the setpoint, even though the person may lose weight and fat. When the dieter goes back to the normal or even below-normal caloric intake (at which the weight may have been stable for a long time), he or she quickly regains the lost fat as the body strives to regain a comfortable fat store.

An Example

Let's use a practical illustration. A person would like to lose some body fat and assumes that his or her current stable body weight has been reached at an average daily caloric intake of 1,800 calories (no weight gain or loss occurs at this daily intake). In an attempt to lose weight rapidly, this person now goes on a **very low-calorie diet** (defined as 800 calories per day or less) or, even worse, a near-fasting diet. This immediately activates the body's survival mechanism and readjusts the metabolism to a lower caloric balance. After a few weeks of dieting at the 800-calories-per-day level, the body now can maintain its normal functions at 1,300 calories per day. This new figure (1,300 calories) represents a drop of 500 calories per day in the BMR. Having lost the desired weight, the person terminates the diet but realizes that the original intake of 1,800 calories per day has to be lower to maintain the new lower weight. To adjust to the new lower

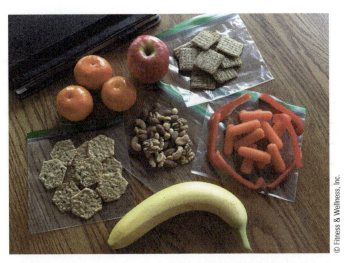

If you have a packed schedule, it is even more critical to make healthy choices to keep up with a challenging schedule. Find healthy, portable foods that work for you.

body weight, the person restricts intake to about 1,600 calories per day. The individual is surprised to find that even at this lower daily intake (200 fewer calories), the weight comes back at a rate of 1 pound every 1 to 2 weeks. After the diet is over, this new lowered BMR may take several months to kick back up to its normal level.

Based on this explanation, individuals clearly should not go on very low-calorie diets. This slows the BMR and deprives the body of basic daily nutrients required for normal function. Very low-calorie diets should be used only in conjunction with dietary supplements and under proper medical supervision. Furthermore, people who use very low-calorie diets are not as effective in keeping the weight off once the diet is terminated.

Caloric Intake Recommendation

A daily caloric intake of approximately 1,500 calories provides the necessary nutrients if a variety of nonprocessed foods are distributed properly over the basic food groups (meeting the daily recommended amounts from each group). Of course, the individual will have to learn to select healthy foods from among 100 percent whole grains, fiber-rich fruits and vegetables, beans, lean proteins, modest amounts of healthy oils (olive and canola), and nuts while on a calorie-restricted plan.

Under no circumstances should petite women go on a diet that calls for a level of 1,200 or fewer calories or should most men and women eat 1,500 or fewer calories. Weight (fat) is gained over months and years, not overnight. Likewise, weight loss should be gradual, not abrupt. At 1,200 calories per day, you may require a multivitamin supplement. Your health care professional should be consulted regarding such a supplement.

A second way in which the setpoint may work is by keeping track of the nutrients and calories consumed daily. It is thought that the body, like a cash register, records the daily food intake and that the brain does not feel satisfied until the calories and nutrients have been "registered."

This setpoint for calories and nutrients seems to operate even when people participate in moderately intense exercise. Some evidence suggests that people do not become hungrier with moderate physical activity. Therefore, people can choose to lose weight either by going hungry or by combining a sensible calorie-restricted diet with an increase in daily physical activity.

Lowering the Setpoint

The most common question regarding the setpoint is how to lower it so that the body feels comfortable at a reduced fat percentage. The following factors seem to affect the setpoint directly by lowering the fat thermostat:

- Exercise
- A diet high in complex carbohydrates
- Nicotine
- Amphetamines

The last two are more destructive than the extra fat weight, so they are not reasonable alternatives (as far as extra strain on the heart is concerned, smoking one pack of cigarettes per day is said to be the equivalent of carrying 50 to 75 pounds of excess body fat). A diet high in fats and refined carbohydrates, near-fasting diets, and perhaps even artificial sweeteners seem to raise the setpoint. Therefore, the only practical and sensible way to lower the setpoint and lose fat weight is a combination of exercise and a diet high in complex carbohydrates with only moderate amounts of healthy fats.

Because of the effects of proper food management on the body's setpoint, most of the successful dieter's effort should be spent in reforming eating habits, increasing intake of complex carbohydrates and high-fiber foods, and decreasing consumption of processed foods that are high in refined carbohydrates (sugars) and fats. This change in eating habits brings about a decrease in total daily caloric intake. Because 1 gram of carbohydrates provides only four calories, as opposed to nine calories per gram of fat, the person could eat twice the volume of food (by weight) when substituting carbohydrates for fat. Some fat, however, is recommended in the diet—primarily polyunsaturated and monounsaturated fats.

GLOSSARY

Weight-regulating mechanism (WRM) A feature of the hypothalamus of the brain that controls how much the body should weigh.

Setpoint Weight control theory that the body has an established weight and strongly attempts to maintain that weight.

Basal metabolic rate (BMR) The lowest level of oxygen consumption (and energy requirement) necessary to sustain life, typically measured in a thermoneutral environment following at least 8 hours of sleep and fasting for 12 hours.

Very-low-calorie diet A diet that allows an energy intake (consumption) of only 800 calories or less per day.

Behavior Modification Planning

Eating Right when on the Run

Current lifestyles often require people to be on the run. We don't seem to have time to eat right, but fortunately, it doesn't have to be that way. If you are on the run, it is even more critical to make healthy choices to keep up with a challenging schedule. Do you regularly consume the following foods when you are eating on the run?

I PLAN TO **I DID IT**

- ❑ ❑ Water
- ❑ ❑ Whole-grain cereal and skim milk
- ❑ ❑ Whole-grain bread and bagels
- ❑ ❑ Whole-grain bread with peanut butter
- ❑ ❑ Nonfat or low-fat yogurt
- ❑ ❑ Fresh fruits
- ❑ ❑ Frozen fresh fruit (grapes, cherries, banana slices)
- ❑ ❑ Dried fruits

- ❑ ❑ Raw vegetables (carrots, broccoli, red peppers, cucumbers, radishes, cauliflower, asparagus)
- ❑ ❑ Whole-grain crackers
- ❑ ❑ Pretzels
- ❑ ❑ Whole-grain bread sticks
- ❑ ❑ Low-fat cheese sticks
- ❑ ❑ Granola bars
- ❑ ❑ Snack-size cereal boxes
- ❑ ❑ Nuts
- ❑ ❑ Trail mix
- ❑ ❑ Light microwave popcorn
- ❑ ❑ Vegetable soups

Try It

In your online journal or class notebook, plan your fast-meal menus for the upcoming week. It may require extra shopping and some food preparation (for instance, cutting vegetables to place in snack plastic bags). At the end of the week, evaluate how many days you had a "healthy eating on the run day." What did you learn from the experience?

These so-called healthy fats do more than help protect the heart; they help delay hunger pangs.

A "diet" should not be viewed as a temporary tool to aid in weight loss but, instead, as a permanent change in eating behaviors to ensure weight management and better health. The role of increased physical activity also must be considered, because successful weight loss, weight maintenance, and recommended body composition are seldom attained without a moderate reduction in caloric intake combined with a regular exercise program.

Maintaining Metabolism and Lean Body Mass

Fat can be lost by selecting the proper foods, exercising, or restricting calories. However, when dieters try to lose weight by dietary restrictions alone, they also lose LBM (muscle protein, along with vital organ protein). The amount of LBM lost depends on caloric limitation. When people go on a near-fasting diet, up to half of the weight loss is LBM and the other half is actual fat loss (Figure 5.6).[17] When diet is combined with exercise, close to 100 percent of the weight loss is in the form of fat; lean tissue actually may increase. Loss of LBM is never good because it weakens organs and muscles and slows metabolism. Large losses in lean tissue can cause disturbances in heart function and damage to other organs. Equally important is not to overindulge (binge) following a very low-calorie diet because this may cause changes in BMR and electrolyte balance, which could trigger fatal cardiac arrhythmias.

Contrary to some beliefs, aging is not the main reason for the lower BMR. It is not so much that metabolism slows

Figure 5.6 Outcome of three forms of diet on fat loss.

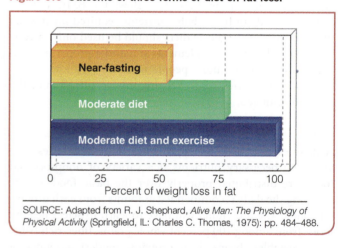

SOURCE: Adapted from R. J. Shephard, *Alive Man: The Physiology of Physical Activity* (Springfield, IL: Charles C. Thomas, 1975): pp. 484–488.

down as that people slow down. As people age, they tend to rely more on the amenities of life (remote controls, cell phones, intercoms, single-level homes, riding lawnmowers, etc.) that lull them into sedentary living.

Basal metabolism also is related to lean body weight. More lean tissue yields a higher BMR. As a consequence of sedentary living and less physical activity, the lean component decreases and fat tissue increases. The human body requires a certain amount of oxygen per pound of LBM. Given that fat is considered metabolically inert from the point of view of caloric use, the lean tissue uses most of the oxygen, even at rest. As muscle and organ mass (LBM) decrease, so do the energy requirements at rest.

Diets with caloric intakes below 1,500 calories cannot guarantee the retention of LBM. Even if you stay above the 1,500-calorie intake level, some loss is inevitable unless the diet is combined with exercise. Despite the claims of many diets that they do not alter the lean component, the simple truth is that regardless of what nutrients may be added to the diet, severe caloric restrictions always prompt the loss of lean tissue. Sadly, many people go on very low-calorie diets constantly. Every time they do, their BMR slows as more lean tissue is lost.

People in their 40s and older who weigh the same as they did when they were 20 tend to think they are at recommended body weight. During this span of 20 years or more, though, they may have dieted many times without participating in an exercise program. After they terminate each diet, they regain the weight, and much of that gain is additional body fat. Maybe at age 20 they weighed 150 pounds, of which only 15 percent was fat. Now at age 40, even though they still weigh 150 pounds, they might be 30 percent fat (Figure 5.7). At "recommended" body weight, they wonder why they are eating little and still having trouble staying at that weight.

Figure 5.7 Body composition changes as a result of frequent dieting without exercise.

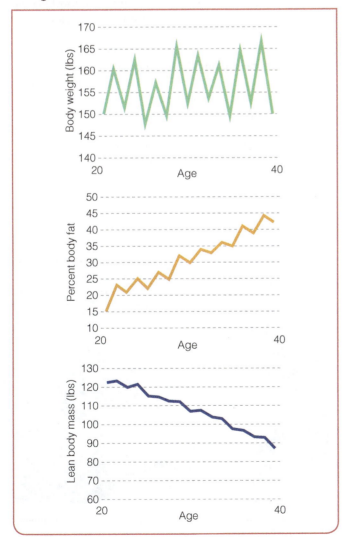

Rate of Weight Loss in Men versus Women

Traditionally, the perception has been that women lose weight at a slower rate than men. A 2014 study[18] in the prestigious *British Journal of Nutrition* put this theory to the test. Overweight and obese men and women were placed on a diet, but they did not participate in exercise (aerobic or strength-training). At 2 months, the men had lost twice as much weight as the women and also lost three times as much LBM. Thus, a difference was established not only in the amount of weight lost, but also in the composition of the lost weight. At 4 months, the rate of weight and LBM loss began to slow down for both genders, and by 6 months, both men and women were losing weight and LBM at about the same rate. The difference in fat and LBM loss during the last 4 months of the study was similar for both genders.

To an extent, the amount and rate of weight loss is related to the excess in body fat (fat mass or FM) and LBM that the person has at the start of the program. The greater the body weight, the greater the amount of weight that can be lost. Of course, physical activity and exercise should always be incorporated into a weight-loss program to prevent excessive LBM loss.

Men typically are taller and heavier and have more LBM than women (see Figure 4.1, p. 138). As a result, they have an initial edge because of their higher metabolic rate due to the greater lean tissue component and the higher total body weight. In the study, LBM losses were almost even between

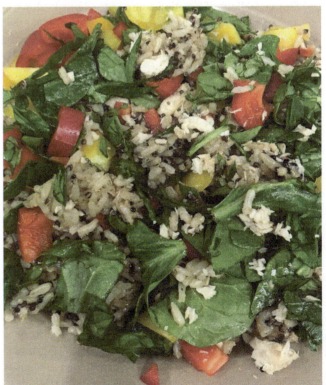

Foods that are high in volume, like spinach and rice, help your stomach feel full immediately, but adding protein to a meal along with a small amount of unsaturated fat will help you develop a complete feeling of satiety as the food is absorbed and digested.

the second and sixth months, indicating that protein-conserving adaptations were taking place, more extensively in men with increasing weight loss. By 6 months, there was practically no difference in the composition of weight loss by men or women. Consequently, women do not necessarily have the weight-loss handicap previously thought.

Protein, Fats, Fiber, and Feeling Satisfied

Feeling satisfied after you eat involves more than simply filling your stomach. The stomach, digestive organs, and fat cells are constantly sending messages to the brain that let people know when they need to eat and when they are full and satiated. Specifically, cues affecting hunger are sent to the hypothalamus.

You may have heard advice to eat slowly or to wait twenty minutes after a meal before you decide if you are still truly hungry. This advice works because different types of **satiety** signals reach the hypothalamus at different times, the first one quickly, and two additional ones more slowly as you begin to digest the food.

- The quickest feedback your brain receives is a response from stretch receptors in the stomach and intestines that react as food begins to fill these organs. Foods that have high amounts of water and fiber are **high-volume foods** that will fill the stomach on fewer calories. Though eating a plate full of lettuce will make your stomach feel full, it will not leave you feeling satiated. That is because the brain is also waiting for other signals.

- Slower feelings of satiation come as food breaks down and specialized receptors sense levels of glucose, fatty acids, and amino acids in the bloodstream. As the brain senses these nutrients, appetite slows with the cue that it is time to end the meal.

- Finally, organs in your digestive system release hormones that respond to nutrients. Different parts of your intestines respond to different combinations of protein, fat, and carbohydrates (carbohydrates are thought to contribute least to hormonal signals of satiety). When your digestive organs sense that your meal has provided enough of a certain nutrient they send messages of satiety. Scientists have also identified a neurotransmitter (oleoylethanolamide) stimulated by dietary fat in the small intestine that appears to lengthen the time a person can go between meals before feeling hungry. Nutritionists recommend meals that are between 20 and 30 percent unsaturated fat to activate this response.

Ghrelin and **leptin** are two hormones currently being extensively researched because they play a role in appetite. Ghrelin is produced by the stomach and stimulates appetite. The more ghrelin the body produces, the more you want to eat. Leptin, produced by the body's fat cells, is designed to regulate energy intake and keep you from eating too much or too little. Leptin helps the brain know when you are full; the more leptin you produce, the less you want to eat. Similar to insulin resistance (leading to type 2 diabetes), research is beginning to show that a lack of physical activity leads to leptin resistance,

setting up a vicious cycle that in turn leads to excessive eating. Other lifestyle choices that decrease sensitivity to leptin are high-fat meals, insufficient sleep, and yo-yo dieting.

5.7 Losing Weight the Sound and Sensible Way

Dieting never has been fun and never will be. People who are overweight and are serious about losing weight, however, have to include regular physical activity and exercise in their lives, along with proper food management and a sensible reduction in caloric intake.

Estimating Your Daily Energy Requirement

In addition to exercise and food management, a sensible reduction in caloric intake and careful monitoring of this intake are recommended. Research indicates that a negative caloric balance is required to lose weight for the following reasons:

1. People tend to underestimate their caloric intake and are eating more than they should be eating.
2. Developing new behaviors takes time, and most people have trouble changing and adjusting to new eating habits.
3. Many individuals are in such poor physical condition that they take a long time to increase their activity level enough to offset the setpoint and burn enough calories to aid in losing body fat.
4. Most successful dieters carefully monitor their daily caloric intake.
5. A few people simply will not alter their food selection (high-unhealthy fat foods). For those who will not, the only solution to lose weight successfully is a large increase in physical activity that will indeed yield a negative caloric balance.

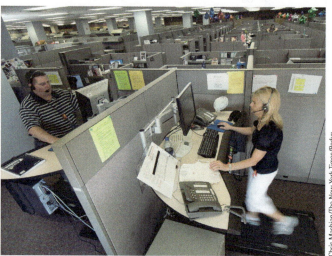

Increasing ambulatory activities throughout the day enhances fitness and is an excellent weight management strategy.

Perhaps the only exception to a decrease in caloric intake for weight loss purposes is in people who already are eating too few calories. A nutrient analysis (see Chapter 3) often reveals that long-term dieters are not consuming enough calories. These people actually need to increase their daily caloric intake and combine it with an exercise program to get their metabolism to kick back up to a normal level.

HOEGER KEY TO WELLNESS

Monitor your body weight regularly. Weigh yourself at the same time and under the same conditions each day, and do not adapt and accept a higher body weight as a new stable weight! Make immediate dietary and physical activity adjustments accordingly. It is not too difficult to lose a pound or two of increased body weight, as opposed to 10, 20, 30, or 50 pounds at a later point. Exercise restraint over calorie-dense foods; practice portion control; and maintain NEAT, physical activity, and exercise programs.

You also must learn to make wise food choices. Think in terms of long-term benefits (weight management) instead of instant gratification (unhealthy eating and subsequent weight gain). Making healthful choices allows you to eat more food, eat more nutritious food, and ingest fewer calories. For example, instead of eating a high-fat, 700-calorie scone, you could eat as much as one orange, one cup of grapes, a hardboiled egg, two slices of whole-wheat toast, two teaspoons of jam, one-half cup of honey-sweetened oatmeal, and one glass of skim milk (for other meal alternatives, see Figure 5.8).

You can estimate your daily energy requirement by consulting Table 5.2 and Table 5.3 and completing Activity 5.1. Given that this is only an estimated value, individual adjustments related to many of the factors discussed in this chapter may be necessary to establish a more precise value. And as will be discussed later in the chapter, proper food selection has a significant effect on weight management, and to a large extent, can override the estimated caloric requirement. Nevertheless, the estimated value offers beginning guidelines for weight control or reduction.

The EER without additional planned activity and exercise is based on age, total body weight, height, and gender. Individuals who hold jobs that require a lot of walking or heavy manual labor burn more calories during the day than those who have sedentary jobs (e.g., working behind a desk). To estimate your EER, refer to Table 5.2.

The daily energy requirement figure is only a target guideline for weight control. Periodic readjustments are necessary because individuals differ, and the daily requirement changes as they lose weight and modify their exercise habits.

To determine your target caloric intake to lose weight, multiply your current weight in pounds by 5 and subtract this amount from the total daily energy requirement with exercise.

For example, if a person's daily energy requirement is 2,932 calories (see "Finding the Estimated Energy Requirement," page 187), this individual would have to consume 2,132 calories per day to lose weight (160 × 5 = 800 and 2,932 − 800 = 2,132 calories).

This final caloric intake to lose weight should not be below 1,500 daily calories for most people. If distributed properly over the various food groups, 1,500 calories provide the necessary nutrients the body needs. In terms of percentages of total calories, the daily distribution should be approximately 50 to 60 percent carbohydrates (mostly complex carbohydrates), less than 30 percent fat, and about 20 to 30 percent protein.

Adjusting Your Fat Intake

Many experts believe that a person can take off weight more efficiently by reducing daily fat intake to about 20 percent of total daily caloric intake. Because 1 gram of fat supplies more than twice the number of calories that carbohydrates and protein do, the tendency when someone eats less fat is to consume fewer calories. With fat intake at 20 percent of total calories, the individual has sufficient fat in the diet to feel satisfied and avoid frequent hunger pangs.

Furthermore, it takes only 3 to 5 percent of ingested calories to store fat as fat, whereas it takes approximately 25 percent of ingested calories to convert carbohydrates to fat. Some evidence indicates that if people eat the same number of calories as carbohydrate or as fat, those on the fat diet store more fat. Long-term successful weight loss and weight management programs are lower in fat content. The carbohydrate intake, nonetheless, should be primarily in the form of complex/fiber-rich carbohydrates.

Many people have trouble adhering to a low-fat-calorie diet. During times of weight loss, however, you are strongly encouraged to do so. Refer to Table 5.4 to aid you in determining the grams of fat at 20 percent of the total calories for selected energy intakes. Also, use the form provided in Activity 3.1 (page 103) to monitor your daily fat intake. For weight maintenance, individuals who have been successful in maintaining an average weight loss of 30 pounds for more than 5 years are consuming about 24 percent of calories from fat, 56 percent from carbohydrates, and 20 percent from protein.[19]

GLOSSARY

Satiety A feeling, state, or condition of being full after eating food.

High-volume foods Foods that are low in calories but high in volume (high in water and fiber), such as fruits and vegetables, that allow a person to eat more and feel fuller on fewer calories.

Ghrelin A hormone, produced mainly in the stomach, that increases appetite ("hunger hormone").

Leptin A hormone, made by fat cells, that increases satiety ("satiety hormone").

Figure 5.8 Making wise food choices.

Breakfast	Lunch	Dinner

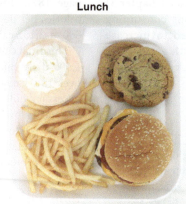

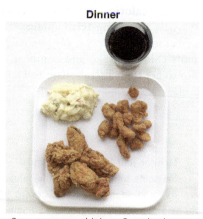

1 banana nut muffin, 1 cafe mocha
Calories: 940
Percent fat calories: 48%

1 double-decker cheeseburger, 1 serving
medium French fries, 2 chocolate chip
cookies, 1 medium strawberry milkshake
Calories: 1,790
Percent fat calories: 37%

6 oz. popcorn chicken, 3 oz. barbecue
chicken wings, 1 cup potato salad,
1 12-oz. cola drink
Calories: 1,250
Percent fat calories: 42%

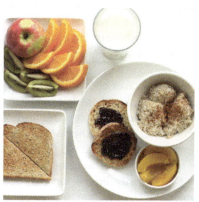

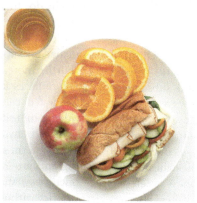

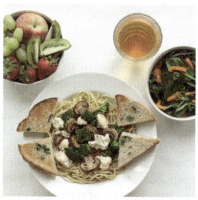

1 cup oatmeal, 1 English muffin with jelly,
1 slice whole wheat bread with honey,
½ cup peaches, 1 kiwi fruit, 1 orange,
1 apple, 1 cup skim milk
Calories: 900
Percent fat calories: 5%

6-inch turkey breast/vegetable sandwich,
1 apple, 1 orange,
1 cup sweetened green tea
Calories: 500
Percent fat calories: 10%

2 cups spaghetti with tomato sauce
and vegetables, a 2-cup salad bowl
with 2 tablespoons Italian dressing,
2 slices whole wheat bread, 1 cup
grapes, 3 large strawberries, 1 kiwi fruit,
1 peach, 1 12-oz. fruit juice drink
Calories: 1,240
Percent fat calories: 14%

These illustrations provide a comparison of how much more food you can eat when you make healthy choices. You also get more vitamins, minerals, phytonutrients, antioxidants, and fiber by making healthy choices.

Photos © Fitness & Wellness, Inc.

Reducing Evening Eating

Consuming most of the calories earlier in the day seems helpful in losing weight and in managing **atherosclerosis**. The time of day when most of the fats and cholesterol are consumed can influence blood lipids and coronary heart disease. Peak digestion time following a heavy meal is about 7 hours after that meal. If most lipids, particularly unhealthy fats, are consumed during the evening meal, digestion peaks while the person is sound asleep and the metabolism is at its lowest rate. Consequently, the body may not metabolize fats as well, leading to a higher blood lipid count and increasing the risk for atherosclerosis and coronary heart disease.

Though isolating the effects of meal timing on weight loss is difficult to do, current studies continue to focus on this lifestyle factor. While research has not been conclusive, scientists observe that obese people are more likely to eat few calories in the morning and do most of their eating in the afternoon and evening.[20]

The Importance of Breakfast

For most people, breakfast is an important meal while on a weight-loss program. People skip breakfast because it's the easiest meal to skip. Such practice may make them hungrier later in the day, and overall, they end up consuming more

Finding the Estimated Energy Requirement—an Example

For example, the EER computation for a 20-year-old man who is 71 inches tall and weighs 160 pounds would be as follows:

1. Body weight (BW) in kilograms = 72.6 kg (160 lb ÷ 2.2046)
    Height (HT) in meters = 1.8 m (71 inches × .0254)
2. EER = 662 − (9.53 × Age) + (15.91 × BW) + (539 × HT)
    EER = 662 − (9.53 × 20) + (15.91 × 72.6) + (539 × 1.8)
    EER = 662 − 190.6 + 1155 + 970
    EER = 2,596 calories/day

Thus, the EER to maintain body weight for this individual would be 2,596 calories per day.

To determine the average number of calories you burn daily as a result of exercise, figure out the total number of minutes you exercise weekly, and then figure the daily average exercise time. For instance, the man in the prior example cycling at 10 miles per hour five times a week, 60 minutes each time, exercises 300 minutes per week (5 × 60). The average daily exercise time, therefore, is 42 minutes (300 ÷ 7, rounded off to the lowest unit).

Next, from Table 5.3, find the energy expenditure for the activity (or activities) chosen for the exercise program. In the case of cycling (10 miles per hour), the expenditure is .05 calorie per pound of body weight per minute of activity (cal/lb/min). With a body weight of 160 pounds, this man would burn 8 calories each minute (body weight × .05, or 160 × .05). In 42 minutes, he would burn approximately 336 calories (42 × 8).

Now obtain the daily energy requirement, with exercise, needed to maintain body weight. To do this, add the EER obtained from Table 5.2 and the average calories burned through exercise. In our example, it is 2,932 calories (2,596 + 336).

If a negative caloric balance is recommended to lose weight, this person has to consume less than 2,932 calories daily to achieve the objective. Because of the many factors that play a role in weight control, this 2,932-calorie value is only an estimated daily requirement. Furthermore, we cannot predict that the man in the example will lose exactly one pound of fat in one week if he cuts his daily intake by 500 calories (500 × 7 = 3,500 calories, or the equivalent of 1 pound of fat).

Table 5.2 Estimated Energy Requirement (EER) Based on Age, Body Weight, and Height

Men	EER = 662 − (9.53 × Age) + (15.91 × BW) + (539 × HT)
Women	EER = 354 − (6.91 × Age) + (9.36 × BW) + (726 × HT)

NOTE: Includes activities of independent living only and no moderate physical activity or exercise.
BW = body weight in kilograms (divide BW in pounds by 2.2046).
HT = height in meters (multiply HT in inches by .0254).

SOURCE: Adapted from Dietary Reference Intakes for Energy, Carbohydrate, Fiber, Fat, Fatty Acids, Cholesterol, Protein, and Amino Acids (Institute of Medicine of the National Academies, 2002 and 2005)

total daily calories. Scientists also believe that skipping breakfast increases levels of a neurotransmitter (Neuropeptide Y) that increases a desire for simple carbohydrates. If you find that breakfast is the easiest meal to skip, at least eat a small breakfast with some protein and a slight amount of fat to avoid excessive hunger pangs later in the morning. People who follow the previous guideline tend to eat about 20 percent fewer calories for lunch and less calories throughout the entire day.

Consuming most of the calories earlier in the day seems helpful in losing weight and also in managing atherosclerosis. This concept was substantiated by researchers who found that people who eat a larger meal at breakfast are more likely to lose weight and waistline circumference than those who eat a larger meal for dinner.[21] In the 12-week study, participants were divided into two 1,400-calorie diet groups. Group one distributed the daily intake so that 700, 500, and 200 calories were consumed respectively at breakfast, lunch, and dinner; whereas group two consumed 200, 500, and 700 calories respectively over breakfast, lunch, and dinner. The participants in the larger breakfast group lost almost 18 pounds and 3 inches off their waistline as compared to only 7.3 pounds and a 1.4-inch loss for those in the larger dinner group. The larger breakfast group was also found to have lower levels of the appetite-increasing hormone ghrelin, indicating that they were more satiated

and exhibited a lower desire for snacking throughout the day. Another benefit was a significant decrease in insulin, glucose, and triglyceride levels in the larger breakfast group, and they did not experience the large spike in blood glucose level that occurs after a meal and is believed to increase cardiovascular disease risk.

Drink Water and Avoid Liquid Calories

It is well documented that replacing liquid calories with water increases chances of weight loss success.[22] Liquid calories do not take long to digest and do not require much energy to break down. As a result, they do not trigger feelings of satisfaction and fullness like calories from solid foods. Liquid calories produce a spike in blood glucose that is quickly removed from the bloodstream and leads to cravings for more food once the blood glucose level drops. This spike also encourages inflammation and visceral fat storage. Dietitians further recommend drinking water

GLOSSARY

Atherosclerosis Fatty or cholesterol deposits in the walls of the arteries leading to formation of plaque.

Table 5.3 Caloric Expenditure of Selected Physical Activities

Activity*	Cal/lb/min	Activity*	Cal/lb/min
Aerobics		Jogging/running (on a level surface)	
Moderate	0.065	11.0 min/mile	0.070
Vigorous	0.095	8.5 min/mile	0.090
Step aerobics	0.070	7.0 min/mile	0.102
Archery	0.030	6.0 min/mile	0.114
Badminton		Deep water**	0.100
Recreation	0.038	Racquetball	0.065
Competition	0.065	Rope jumping	0.060
Baseball	0.031	Rowing (vigorous)	0.090
Basketball		Skating (moderate)	0.038
Moderate	0.046	Skiing	
Competition	0.063	Downhill	0.060
Bowling	0.030	Level (5 mph)	0.078
Calisthenics	0.033	Soccer	0.059
Cross-country skiing		Stationary cycling	
Moderate	0.090	Moderate	0.055
Vigorous	0.120	Vigorous	0.070
Circuit training		Strength training	0.050
Moderate	0.070	Swimming (crawl)	
Vigorous	0.100	20 yds/min	0.031
Cycling (on a level surface)		25 yds/min	0.040
5.5 mph	0.033	45 yds/min	0.057
10.0 mph	0.050	50 yds/min	0.070
13.0 mph	0.071	Table tennis	0.030
Dance		Tennis	
Moderate	0.030	Moderate	0.045
Vigorous	0.055	Competition	0.064
Elliptical training		Volleyball	0.030
Moderate	0.070	Walking	
Vigorous	0.090	4.5 mph	0.045
Golf	0.030	Shallow pool	0.090
Gymnastics		Water aerobics	
Light	0.030	Moderate	0.050
Heavy	0.056	Vigorous	0.070
Handball	0.064	Wrestling	0.085
High-intensity interval training	0.120	Zumba	
		Moderate	0.065
Hiking	0.040	Vigorous	0.095
Judo/karate	0.086		

*Values are for actual time engaged in the activity.

**Treading water

Adapted from: P. E. Allsen, J. M. Harrison, and B. Vance, *Fitness for Life: An Individualized Approach* (Dubuque, IA: Wm. C. Brown, 1989); C. A. Bucher and W. E. Prentice, *Fitness for College and Life* (St. Louis: Times Mirror/Mosby College Publishing, 1989); C. F. Consolazio, R. E. Johnson, and L. J. Pecora, *Physiological Measurements of Metabolic Functions in Man* (New York: McGraw-Hill, 1963); R. V. Hockey, *Physical Fitness: The Pathway to Healthy Living* (St. Louis: Times Mirror/ Mosby College Publishing, 1989); W. W. K. Hoeger et al., Research conducted at Boise State University, 1986–2009.

Table 5.4 Grams of Fat at 20 and 30 Percent of Total Calories for Selected Energy Intakes

Caloric Intake	Grams of Fat		Caloric Intake	Grams of Fat	
	20%	30%		20%	30%
1,200	27	40	2,200	49	73
1,300	29	43	2,300	51	77
1,400	31	47	2,400	53	80
1,500	33	50	2,500	56	83
1,600	36	53	2,600	58	87
1,700	38	57	2,700	60	90
1,800	40	60	2,800	62	93
1,900	42	63	2,900	64	97
2,000	44	67	3,000	67	100
2,100	47	70			

Reducing Your Eating Occasions

As obesity rates have climbed in recent decades, so has the average number of eating occasions. Opportunities to consume snacks, extra meals, drinks, and treats abound. Examine your personal number of daily eating occasions. Healthy adjustments can become a permanent, lifelong key for managing weight with less effort and hunger.

Plan on eating three balanced meals and one or two healthy snacks per day. Current research shows that eating three satisfying meals is better at providing a feeling of fullness throughout the day than eating several mini meals.[23] Regular, consistent mealtimes help regulate blood lipids, regulate insulin sensitivity, and avoid weight gain. Individuals who consume two or fewer meals per day are more likely to be preoccupied with thoughts of food and more likely to overconsume food. Eating during planned times also helps you fall out of the habit of mindlessly nibbling on food. Allowing the hunger cue to develop around regular mealtimes will help you feel that hunger is not an entirely unpleasant sensation, but rather, a prelude to a satisfying meal.

Foods that Aid in Weight Loss

A well-known fact is that a low-energy dense diet plan increases satiety and is conducive to a lower daily caloric intake. Diet plans with fewer refined carbohydrates, such as sugar, white bread and rice, pasta, and potatoes; and more high-quality protein-rich foods, along with low-fat dairy, 100 percent whole grains, whole fruits, and vegetables are more conducive to weight loss. Refined carbohydrates do not promote satiety, encourage overeating, and leave you hungry sooner. You will be more successful with weight management efforts if you introduce filling and healthful foods into your meals without setting rigid eating rules. Following are recommendations for food items that make sensible eating easier, which you can fine tune to fit your personal preferences.

throughout the day and before a meal to ensure that feelings of thirst will not be confused with feelings of hunger and result in excess energy intake.

Activity 5.1   **Estimating Your Daily Caloric Requirement**

Name _____   Date _____

Course _____   Section _____   Gender _____   Age _____

A. Current body weight (BW) in kilograms (body weight in pounds ÷ 2.2046)................................... ☐

B. Current height (HT) in meters (HT in inches × .0254)... ☐

C. Estimated energy (caloric) requirement (EER) (Table 5.2, page 187)

   Men: $EER = 663 - (9.53 \times Age) + (15.91 \times BW) + (539.6 \times HT)$

   Women: $EER = 354 - (6.91 \times Age) + (9.36 \times BW) + (726 \times HT)$

   EER = ☐ − (☐ × ☐) + (☐ × ☐) + (☐ × ☐)

   EER = ☐ − ☐ + ☐ + ☐ =   ☐ calories

D. Selected physical activity (e.g., jogging)[a] .... ☐

E. Number of exercise sessions per week.. ☐

F. Duration of exercise session (in minutes).. ☐

G. Total weekly exercise time in minutes (E × F).. ☐

H. Average daily exercise time in minutes (G ÷ 7).. ☐

I. Caloric expenditure per pound per minute (cal/lb/min) of physical activity (use Table 5.3, page 188)......... ☐

J. Body weight in pounds.. ☐

K. Total calories burned per minute of physical activity (I × J)... ☐

L. Average daily calories burned as a result of the exercise program (H × K)............................ ☐

M. Total daily energy requirement with exercise to maintain body weight (C + L)...................... ☐

Stop here if no weight loss is required, otherwise proceed to items N and O.

N. Number of calories to subtract from daily requirement to achieve a negative caloric balance (J × 5).................... ☐

O. Target caloric intake to lose weight (M − N)[b]... ☐

[a] If more than one physical activity is selected, you will need to estimate the average daily calories burned as a result of each additional activity (steps D through K) and add all of these figures to L above.
[b] This figure should never be below 1,200 calories for small women or 1,500 for everyone else. See Activity 5.3 for the 1,200-, 1,500-, 1,800-, and 2,000-calorie diet plans.

© Fitness & Wellness, Inc.

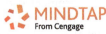 **Complete This Online**
From Cengage   Visit **www.cengagebrain.com** to access MindTap, a complete digital course that includes interactive quizzes, videos, and more.

Behavior Modification Planning

Physical Activity Guidelines for Weight Management

The following physical activity guidelines are recommended to effectively manage body weight:

- Thirty minutes of physical activity on most days of the week if you do not have difficulty maintaining body weight (more minutes and/or higher intensity if you choose to reach a high level of physical fitness).

- Between 30 and 60 minutes of light-to-moderate exercise on most days of the week if you are trying to lose weight. Incorporate as many light ambulatory activities as possible during the course of each day.

- Sixty minutes of daily activity for people with a tendency toward weight gain.

- Between 60 and 90 minutes of physical activity each day if you want to keep weight off following extensive weight loss (30 pounds of weight loss or more). Be sure to include some high-intensity/low-impact activities at least twice a week in your program.

Try It

In your Behavior Change Planner Progress Tracker, online journal, or class notebook, record how many minutes of daily physical activity you accumulate on a regular basis and record your thoughts on how effectively your activity has helped you manage your body weight. Is there one thing you could do today to increase your physical activity?

Whole Foods and High-Volume Low-Energy Dense Foods

As a general rule, choosing whole foods over processed foods will benefit you in several ways:

- By definition, whole foods have not been partially prepared or broken down, so they require more time and energy for the body to break down. This means they keep you feeling full longer and do not result in blood glucose spikes and the subsequent cravings.
- By choosing whole foods, you are likely to consume more fiber and enhance water intake, helping you feel more satiated, and likely to consume more vitamins and nutrients, including thousands of phytonutrients from plant foods.
- When cooking whole foods, you control the amount and type of fat, salt, and other ingredients in your meal.
- Whole foods naturally have complex and nuanced flavor compounds that can be interesting and satisfying to an appreciative diner. By contrast, processed foods are likely to have exaggerated flavors that dull your palate and leave you craving more.

A Calorie May Not Always Be a Calorie

While more research will be forthcoming, evidence is starting to show that not all calories are the same when it comes to weight management. A lower-calorie meal that is high in starch (white bread or rice, pasta, potatoes), sugar, and red meat leads to greater weight gain over time than a 100 to 200 higher-calorie meal that derives most of its calories from skinless poultry, fish, 100 percent whole grains, and vegetables. Chicken with skin and regular cheese have also been linked to weight gain, whereas seafood, low-fat cheese, nuts (small handful), peanut butter, and unsweetened yogurt tend to lead to weight loss. Eggs, milk, and legumes do not appear to cause either weight gain or weight loss.

Meals can be prepared with whole foods in a reasonable amount of time. If you have little experience cooking, start with whole foods that you have time to prepare and try new foods as you have time in your schedule to do so.

HOEGER KEY TO WELLNESS

 To avoid overeating, eat primarily natural, unprocessed, whole foods, and avoid all concentrated calorie-dense foods.

High-volume low-energy dense foods are foods that are high in water and/or fiber content. Vegetables, fruits, and soups are generally considered the foods with the highest volume. These foods are often high in nutrients and activate the stretch receptors in the stomach. Besides taking longer to break down in the body, they also take more time to eat, fill more of the plate, and make the meal naturally more abundant and less sparse. In general, people who eat foods that are high in volume consume fewer daily calories when allowed to eat freely. At the same time, the total volume and weight of the food consumed are greater than for people who choose energy-dense foods.

Protein Intake

To minimize the loss of LBM and hunger pangs while dieting, it is extremely important that you consume sufficient high-quality protein with each meal. It is well documented that individuals who include adequate protein in their diet (20 to 30 percent of the total daily caloric intake) spontaneously consume fewer calories throughout the day when allowed to eat freely. Unprocessed white skinless chicken and turkey, low-fat cheese and yogurt, nuts, and seafood have all been associated with relative weight loss; whereas red meats (unprocessed or processed), regardless of their fat content (lean vs. higher fat), have been associated with weight gain. The body also requires more energy to digest and store protein than either fat or carbohydrates.

You need to ensure that you are consuming between 1.5 grams and 2.0 grams of protein per kilogram of body weight per day. As explained in Chapter 3, Table 3.4 (page 94), if you weigh 141 pounds (64 kg), your total daily protein intake would be between 96 and 128 grams per day (64 × 1.5 and 64 × 2.0) or the equivalent of 384 to 512 calories from protein every day (96 × 4 and 128 × 4), distributed as 32 to 43 grams of protein for each of your three daily meals. High-protein/low-calorie foods include fat-free or low-fat dairy products, eggs, skinless white poultry, fish, soybeans and soy milk, tofu, quinoa, and beans. To help monitor your daily protein intake, you can calculate and record your daily intake at the end of this chapter in Activity 5.3 as well.

Effect of Food Choices on Long-Term Weight Gain

Although still in its infancy, research on more than 120,000 people who were evaluated every 4 years over a 20-year period showed that food choices have a significant effect on weight gain.[24] On average, study participants gained 17 pounds over the course of 20 years. Regardless of other lifestyle habits, individuals who consumed unhealthy foods gained the most weight, whereas those who made healthy food choices gained the least amount of weight. Although more research is needed, in this study, 4-year weight change was most strongly associated with consumption of potato chips, potatoes, sugar-sweetened beverages, and unprocessed and processed red meats and inversely associated with consumption of vegetables, whole grains, fruits, nuts, and yogurt. The take-home message: Consume more fruits, vegetables, whole grains, low-fat dairy products, and nuts (the latter in moderation because of their high caloric content).

Another factor that appears to affect body weight is diet drinks. People who think that consuming diet sodas will help them lose weight are actually worse off. Studies indicate that, over time, diet-soda drinkers have a much larger waist circumference, more visceral fat, and a higher BMI than non-diet-soda drinkers. Research also indicates that consumption of diet drinks does not lead to a subsequent decrease in caloric intake. That is because people feel justified in allowing themselves a larger caloric intake as a result of the low- or zero-calorie drinks they use. Diet-soda drinkers also have a higher risk of diabetes, heart disease, and stroke. Scientists believe that artificial sweeteners interfere with glucose metabolism. Furthermore, the advisory committee that developed the *2015-2020 Dietary Guidelines for Americans* does not recommend using sugar substitutes because their long-term effects are still uncertain.

Monitoring Your Diet with Daily Food Logs

To help you monitor and adhere to a weight-loss program, use the daily food logs provided in Activity 5.3. If the goal is to maintain or increase body weight, use Activity 5.4.

Evidence indicates that people who monitor daily food intake are more successful at weight loss than those who don't self-monitor. "If you eat it, record it." Most people underestimate what they eat and wonder why they aren't losing weight. One note of precaution is in order. It is important to continue to notice hunger cues even when counting calories. Use both your hunger cues and your food log to properly manage your food choices.

Before using the forms in Activity 5.3, make a master copy for your files so that you can make future copies as needed. Guidelines are provided for 1,200-, 1,500-, 1,800-, and 2,000-calorie diet plans. These plans were developed based on the MyPlate and the *Dietary Guidelines for Americans* to meet the Recommended Dietary Allowances.[25] The objective is to meet (not exceed) the number of servings allowed for each diet plan. Each time you eat a serving of a certain food, record it in the appropriate box.

To lose weight, you should use the diet plan that most closely approximates your target caloric intake. The plan is based on the following caloric allowances for these food groups:

- Grains: 80 calories per serving
- Fruits: 60 calories per serving
- Vegetables: 25 calories per serving
- Dairy (use low-fat products): 120 calories per serving
- Protein: 100 calories per serving for a 1,200 calorie-diet and 200 calories per serving for the 1,500 to 2,000-calorie diets—see Activity 3.3)

Keep in mind that most high-protein foods from animal sources also contain some fat, and possibly even a small amount of carbohydrate. Additionally, food preparation may require some oil. (Primarily vegetable oils—preferably olive or canola oil—should be used in food preparation.) As a result, in most cases, the 100 to 200 calories of protein per serving will include some fat and carbohydrate calories. You are encouraged to include as much lean/low-fat protein as possible in this serving (see Table 5.5).

As you start your diet plan, pay particular attention to food serving sizes. Take care with cup and glass sizes. A standard cup is 8 ounces, but most glasses nowadays contain between 12 and 16 ounces. If you drink 12 ounces of fruit juice, in

Table 5.5 Approximate Protein Content of Selected Foods

Food	Quantity	Calories	Protein (g)
Cheese, cheddar, shredded	¼ c	114	7
Chicken, light meat, roasted	3 oz	130	23
Cottage cheese, 2% fat	½ c	102	16
Egg	1	74	6
Greek yogurt, plain, non-fat	½ c	75	11
Fish, broiled	3 oz	155	22
Meat, red, lean, broiled	3 oz	220	22
Nuts	¼ c	200	5–8
Quinoa, dry	¼ c	160	11
Tofu, firm	3 oz	80	8

essence you are getting two servings of fruit because a standard serving is three-fourths cup of juice.

Read food labels carefully to compare the caloric value of the serving listed on the label with the caloric guidelines provided previously. Here are some examples:

- One slice of standard 100 percent whole-wheat bread has about 80 calories. A plain bagel may have 200 to 350 calories. Although it is low in fat, a 350-calorie bagel is equivalent to almost four servings in the grains group.
- The standard serving size listed on the food label for most cereals is one cup. As you read the nutrition information, however, you will find that for the same cup of cereal, one type of cereal has 120 calories and another cereal has 200 calories. Because a standard serving in the grains group is 80 calories, the first cereal would be 1.5 servings and the second would be 2.5 servings.
- A medium-size fruit is usually considered one serving. A large fruit provides more than one serving.

In the dairy group, one serving represents 120 calories. A cup of whole milk has about 160 calories, compared with a cup of skim milk, which contains 88 calories. A cup of whole milk, therefore, would provide 1.33 servings in this food group.

In your daily food logs in Activity 5.3, be sure to record the precise amount in each serving. You also can run a computerized nutrient analysis to verify your caloric intake and food distribution pattern (grams and percent of total calories from carbohydrate, fat, and protein).

5.8 *Nondietary Factors that Affect Weight Management*

The more we learn about the human body, the more we find that all lifestyle choices are interconnected. Following are nondietary guidelines that provide insight into factors beyond diet and physical activity that directly impact your body weight.

Sleep and Weight Management

As presented under the Healthy Lifestyle Habits box in Chapter 1 (see page 33), adequate sleep is one of the 12 key components that enhance health and extend life. New evidence shows that sleep is also important to adequate weight management. Sleep deprivation appears to be conducive to weight gain and may interfere with the body's capability to lose weight.

Current obesity and sleep deprivation data point toward a possible correlation between excessive body weight and sleep deprivation. About 69 percent of the U.S. population is overweight or obese, and according to the National Sleep Foundation, 63 percent of Americans report that they do not get 8 hours of sleep per night. The question must be raised: Is there a connection? Let's examine some data.

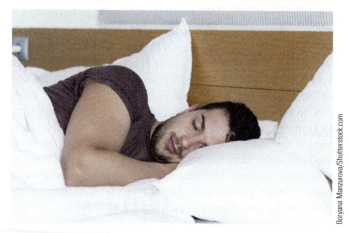

Sufficient sleep is key to healthy weight maintenance. Lack of sleep disrupts normal body hormonal balances and increases feelings of hunger.

One of the studies examining this issue showed that individuals who get less than 6 hours of sleep per night have a higher average BMI (28.3) compared with those who average 8 hours per night (24.5).[26] Another study on more than 68,000 women between the ages of 30 and 55 found that those who got 5 hours or less of sleep per night were 30 percent more likely to gain 30 or more pounds compared with women who got 8 hours per night.[27]

Researchers think that lack of sleep disrupts normal body hormonal balances. Sleep deprivation has now been shown to elevate ghrelin levels and decrease leptin levels, potentially leading to weight gain or keeping you from losing weight. Data comparing these hormone levels in 5-hour versus 8-hour sleepers found that the short sleepers had a 14.9 percent increase in ghrelin levels and a 15.5 percent decrease in leptin levels. The short sleepers also had a 3.6 percent higher BMI than the regular sleepers.[28]

Based on all these studies, the data appear to indicate that sleep deprivation has a negative impact on weight loss or maintenance. Thus, an important component in a well-designed weight management program is a good night's rest (8 hours of sleep).

Light Exposure and BMI

Although still in early stages, another piece of your weight management program may be the relationship among light exposure, timing of the exposure, and intensity of exposure. Studies are beginning to show that exposure to morning light can influence body weight and the hormones that regulate hunger. Data have shown that people who get more light exposure early in the day have lower BMIs.[29] Light exposure needs to be at least 500 lux (about the brightness of a typical office), but a higher amount could be better. Outside in full daylight exposure, a person gets approximately 10,000 lux. People who had most of their daily exposure to even moderately bright light in the morning had a significantly lower BMI than those who had most of their light exposure

Boryana Manzurova/Shutterstock.com

FTC's "7 Gut Check Claims" of Weight-Loss Gimmicks

To make it easier to spot false weight-loss representations—the "gut check" claims—the Federal Trade Commission (FTC, the nation's consumer protection agency) has compiled a list of seven statements in ads that experts say simply can't be true. If you spot one of these claims in an ad, it's likely to be a tip-off to deception.

By the way, several of the "gut check" claims refer to "substantial weight loss." This means "a lot of weight" and includes weight loss of a pound a week for more than 4 weeks or a total weight loss of more than 15 pounds in any time period. But as the examples illustrate, advertisers can convey that "substantial weight loss" message without using specific numbers. Substantial weight loss can be suggested by reference to dress size, inches, or body fat.

If one of these seven claims crosses your desk, do a "gut check:"

1. Causes weight loss of 2 pounds or more a week for a month or more without dieting or exercise
2. Causes substantial weight loss no matter what or how much the consumer eats
3. Causes permanent weight loss even after the consumer stops using the product
4. Blocks the absorption of fat or calories to enable consumers to lose substantial weight
5. Safely enables consumers to lose more than 3 pounds per week for more than 4 weeks
6. Causes substantial weight loss for all users
7. Causes substantial weight loss when a product is worn on the body or rubbed into the skin

Some gutsy con artists may repeat a gut check claim verbatim. That's a sure sign that false advertising is afoot. But gut check claims can be conveyed in more subtle ways, too. Knowing you'll be on the lookout for specific false claims, some advertisers are careful not to use the exact wording of gut check claims. Others may try to work in limiting phrases that consumers may not catch. For example, they may claim a product "*helps* consumers lose substantial weight without diet or exercise" or that people can take off "*up to* 3 pounds a week for a month or more."

You can outfox the fraudsters by understanding what makes each of those claims bogus. Fine-tuning your falsity detector will make it easier for you to spot deception when marketers try to slip a false claim past you by paraphrasing or using synonyms.

SOURCE: http://www.business.ftc.gov/documents/0492-gut-check-reference-guide-media-spotting-false-weight-loss-claims, released January 7, 2014.

later in the day, the study found. The earlier the light exposure takes place in the day, the lower the individuals' BMI. Additional research suggests that sleep-deprived individuals with ghrelin and leptin levels out of range showed improvements in their levels following 2 hours of daylight exposure shortly after waking up.[30] A third study indicated that obese women exposed to a minimum of 45 minutes of bright morning light (between 6:00 a.m. and 9:00 a.m.) for 3 weeks had a slight drop in body fat.[31] Based on these data, weight management researchers indicate that light is a powerful biological signal to the human body and that proper timing (early morning), intensity, and duration of light exposure is important in a sound weight management program.

Monitoring Body Weight

A most critical component to lifetime weight management is to regularly monitor your body weight. Get into the habit of weighing yourself, preferably at the same time of day and under the same conditions—for instance, in the morning just as you get out of bed. Data indicate that daily weigh-ins are associated with better weight maintenance and enhanced weight loss, while infrequent weighing leads to weight gain. It is much easier to make adjustments to lose small amounts of gained weight rather than having to lose a large amount.

Depending on your body size, activity patterns, rehydration level, and dietary intake on any given day, your weight will fluctuate by a pound or more from one day to the next. You do not want to be obsessed with body weight that can potentially lead to an eating disorder, but monitoring *"healthy" recommended body weight* regularly allows you to make immediate adjustments in food intake and physical activity if your weight increases and stays there for several days. Do not adapt and accept the higher weight as your new stable weight. Understand that it is easier to make sensible short-term dietary and activity changes to lose 1 or 2 pounds of weight than to make drastic long-term changes to lose 10, 20, 50, or more pounds that you allowed yourself to gain over the course of several months or years. Whenever feasible, you also want to do periodic assessments of body composition using experienced technicians and valid techniques.

5.9 Physical Activity and Weight Management

To tilt the energy-balancing equation in your favor, you need to burn more calories through physical activity (including NEAT and planned exercise). Research indicates that exercise accentuates weight loss while on a negative caloric balance (diet) as long as you do not replenish the calories expended during exercise. The debate, however, centers on what amount of exercise is best for individuals who are trying to lose weight and those who are trying to maintain weight. Nonetheless, the data are clear that exercise is the best predictor of long-term maintenance of weight loss.

Physical Activity and Energy Balance

The most important reason physical activity and exercise are vital for weight loss maintenance is that sedentary living expends no additional energy (calories) over the RMR. With limited physical activity throughout the day, sedentary people cannot afford to eat many calories; perhaps only 1,000 to 1,200 calories per day. Such a low level of energy intake is not sufficient to keep people from constantly feeling hungry. The only choice they then have is to go hungry every day, an impossible state to sustain. The only logical way to increase caloric intake and maintain weight loss is by burning more calories through exercise and by incorporating NEAT and physical activity throughout daily living.

Physical Activity Predicts Success at Weight Management

Regular exercise seems to exert control over how much a person weighs. On average, the typical adult American gradually becomes overweight by gaining 1 to 2 pounds of weight per year. A 1-pound weight gain represents a simple energy surplus of fewer than 10 calories per day (10×365 days = 3,650 calories, and 1 pound of fat represents 3,500 calories). This simple surplus of fewer than 10 calories per day is the equivalent of less than 1 teaspoon of sugar. Weight gain is clearly related to a decrease in physical activity and an increase in caloric intake. Physical inactivity, however, might well be the primary cause, leading to excessive weight and obesity. The human body was meant to be physically active, and a minimal level of activity appears to be necessary to accurately balance caloric intake to caloric expenditure. In sedentary individuals, the body seems to lose control over this fine energy balance.

Exercise enhances the rate of weight loss, enhances body composition, and is vital in maintaining the lost weight. Not only does exercise maintain lean tissue, but advocates of the setpoint theory also say that exercise resets the fat thermostat to a new, lower level.

Amount of Physical Activity Needed for Weight Loss

Most people who struggle with weight management need 60 to 90 minutes of daily physical activity to effectively manage body weight. While accumulating 30 minutes of moderate-intensity activity per day provides substantial health benefits (the minimum daily recommended amount of activity), from a weight management point of view, the Institute of Medicine of the National Academy of Sciences recommends that people accumulate 60 minutes of moderate-intensity physical activity most days of the week. Remember that this can be broken into 10-minute bouts and can include activities like walking briskly to class or washing a car. Alternatively, 30 minutes of vigorous activity can be substituted on some or all days of exercise. It is also possible to replace one to three weekly workouts with high-intensity interval training, which can provide the same benefits in an even more abbreviated time (see discussion of HIIT in Chapter 9, page 340). The evidence shows that people who maintain recommended weight typically accumulate an hour or more of daily physical activity.

According to the American College of Sports Medicine's "Position Stand on Strategies for Weight Loss and Prevention of Weight Regain for Adults" (Figure 5.9), greater weight loss is achieved by increasing the amount of weekly physical activity. Of even greater significance, physical activity is required for weight maintenance following weight loss. People who exercise regain less weight than those who do not. And those who exercise the most regain the least amount of weight. Individuals who remain physically active for 60 minutes or longer per day are able to keep the weight off.

Data from the National Weight Control Registry (www.nwcr.ws) on more than 10,000 individuals who have lost an average of 66 pounds and have kept them off for 5.5 years indicate that 90 percent of them exercise on average 1 hour per day. Furthermore, other data show that individuals who stop physical activity regain almost 100 percent of the weight within 18 months of discontinuing a weight-loss program. Most successful "weight maintainers" also show greater dietary restraint and consume less than 30 percent of their total daily calories from fat, eat breakfast, consume high-quality protein throughout the day and maintain a consistent eating pattern, engage in high levels of physical activity, and regularly monitor body weight.

The amount of exercise needed to lose weight and maintain weight loss is different from the amount of exercise needed to improve fitness. For health fitness, accumulating 30 minutes of physical activity a minimum of 5 days per week is recommended. To develop and maintain cardiorespiratory fitness, 20 to 60 minutes of vigorous exercise three to five times per week is suggested (see Chapter 6).

Figure 5.9 Approximate decrease in body weight based on total weekly minutes of physical activity without caloric restrictions.

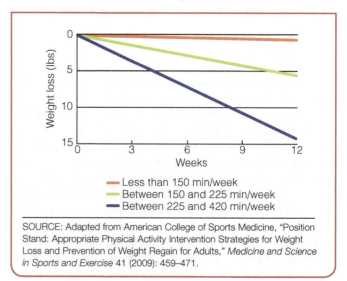

- Less than 150 min/week
- Between 150 and 225 min/week
- Between 225 and 420 min/week

SOURCE: Adapted from American College of Sports Medicine, "Position Stand: Appropriate Physical Activity Intervention Strategies for Weight Loss and Prevention of Weight Regain for Adults," *Medicine and Science in Sports and Exercise* 41 (2009): 459–471.

Behavior Modification Planning

Weight-Maintenance Benefits of Lifetime Aerobic Exercise

The two senior authors of this book have been jogging together *a minimum* of 15 miles per week (3 miles, five times per week) for the past 41 years. More recently, their exercise time has increased to 45 minutes, six times per week, and they have included a wider range of aerobic activities. Without considering the additional energy expenditure from their regular strength-training program and the myriad of other sport, recreation, and activities of daily living during all these years (walking, cycling, dance, tennis, swimming, yardwork, gardening, house cleaning), the energy cost of the regular exercise program has been approximately 3,198,000 calories (15 miles × 100 calories/mile × 52 weeks × 41 years), or the equivalent of 914 pounds of fat (3,198,000 ÷ 3,500). In essence, without this 30-minute workout five times per week, the

authors would weigh 1,054 and 1,030 pounds, respectively! Such is the long-term gratification (reward) of a lifetime exercise program—not to mention the myriad health benefits, joy, and quality of life derived through this program.

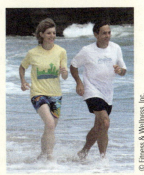

© Fitness & Wellness, Inc.

Try It

Ask yourself whether a regular aerobic exercise program is part of your long-term gratification and health enhancement program. If the answer is no, are you ready to change your behavior? Use the Behavior Change Planner to help you answer the question.

People should not try to do too much too fast. Unconditioned beginners should start with about 15 minutes of aerobic exercise three times a week and, during the next 3 to 4 weeks, gradually increase the duration by approximately 5 minutes per week and the frequency by 1 day per week.

Most experts and leading organizations now recognize that if weight management is not a consideration, 30 minutes of daily activity 5 days per week provides substantial health benefits. Nonetheless, to prevent weight gain, 60 minutes of daily activity is recommended; to maintain substantial weight loss, 90 minutes may be required. Additional light-intensity ambulation and standing throughout the day are also strongly encouraged.

Exercise and Body Composition Changes

Although size (inches) and percent body fat both decrease when sedentary individuals begin an exercise program, body weight often remains the same or may even increase during the first couple of weeks of the program. Exercise helps increase muscle tissue, connective tissue, blood volume (as much as 500 milliliters, or the equivalent of 1 pound, following the first week of aerobic exercise), enzymes and other structures within the cell, and glycogen (which binds water). All of these changes lead to a higher functional capacity of the human body. With exercise, most weight loss becomes apparent after a few weeks of training, when the lean component has stabilized.

We know that a negative caloric balance of 3,500 calories does not always result in a loss of 1 pound of fat, but the role of exercise in achieving a negative balance by burning additional calories is significant in weight reduction and maintenance programs. Sadly, some individuals claim that the number of calories burned during exercise is hardly worth the effort. They think that cutting their daily intake by 300 calories is easier than participating in some sort of exercise that would burn the same number of calories. The problem is that the willpower to cut those 300 calories lasts only a few weeks, and then people go back to the old eating patterns.

If a person gets into the habit of exercising regularly—say, three times a week, jogging 3 miles per exercise session (about 300 calories burned)—this represents 900 calories in one week, about 3,600 calories in one month, or 46,800 calories per year. This minimal amount of exercise represents as many as 13.5 extra pounds of fat in 1 year, 27 pounds in 2 years, and so on.

Does this seem hardly worth the effort? We tend to forget that our weight creeps up gradually over the years, not overnight. And we have not even taken into consideration the increase in lean tissue and metabolic rate, possible resetting of the setpoint, benefits to the cardiorespiratory system, and most important, the improved quality of life. Fundamental reasons for excessive weight and obesity, few could argue, are sedentary living and lack of a regular exercise program.

In terms of preventing disease, many health benefits that people seek by losing weight are reaped through exercise alone, even without weight loss. Exercise offers protection against premature morbidity and mortality for people who are overweight or already have risk factors for disease.

One additional benefit of exercise and physical activity is that it attenuates a person's predisposition to obesity. Genetic epidemiological studies have established that genetic factors play a role in obesity development in our 21st-century obesogenic environment abundant in energy-dense foods and labor-saving devices. The data indicate that even in the most genetically predisposed individuals, regular physical activity, exercise, and an active lifestyle significantly reduce the predisposition to obesity.[32]

HOEGER KEY TO WELLNESS

Sixty to 90 minutes of near-daily physical activity that include an aerobic exercise and a strength-training program, along with an increase in NEAT (nonexercise activity thermogenesis), are a must for a lifetime weight management program: *"Do not fear physical activity: Bring it on!"*

Diet, Exercise, and Visceral Fat

Both diet and exercise lead to reductions in visceral (intra-abdominal) fat. Visceral fat is a strong predictor of metabolic abnormalities (abnormal blood cholesterol, insulin resistance, glucose intolerance, inflammation, hypertension), chronic disease, and premature mortality.

Low-calorie diets (800 to 1,200 calories per day) often lead to a 25 to 50 percent decrease in visceral fat. Exercise further contributes to reductions in visceral fat. For any degree of excessive weight, exercisers tend to have a lower level of visceral fat as compared to sedentary people. Exercise is inversely related to intra-abdominal fat loss: the longer the exercise session, the greater the amount of visceral fat loss. Twenty minutes of daily exercise yield a 5 to 10 percent reduction, whereas 60 minutes of almost daily moderate aerobic exercise lead to a 30 to 50 percent reduction. Even in the absence of weight loss, exercise leads to a reduction in visceral fat and waist circumference, with a concomitant increase in lean body mass. The benefits are further augmented when exercisers lose weight as compared to exercisers who maintain body weight.

SOURCE: J. P. Després, "Obesity and Cardiovascular Disease: Weight Loss Is Not the Only Target," *Canadian Journal of Cardiology* 31 no.2 (2015): 216–222.

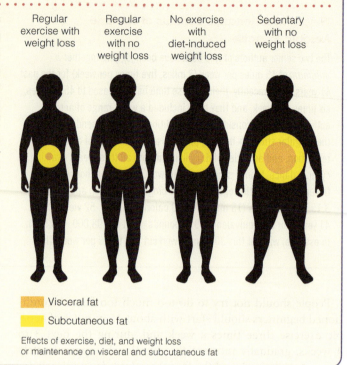

Regular exercise with weight loss   Regular exercise with no weight loss   No exercise with diet-induced weight loss   Sedentary with no weight loss

Visceral fat

Subcutaneous fat

Effects of exercise, diet, and weight loss or maintenance on visceral and subcutaneous fat

Overweight and Fit Debate

A hotly debated topic in the exercise and medical community is the topic most commonly referred to as "fit and fat." Can a person possibly be overweight/obese and still be fit?

The debate started with research indicating that the higher the aerobic fitness level, as measured by total treadmill-walking time, the lower the mortality rate, regardless of body weight. Fitness in these studies has been defined as "accumulating 30 minutes of moderate intensity activity on most days of the week." Many overweight people who reach this goal do not seem predisposed to premature death.

Data further indicate that, on average, the death rate for thin but unfit individuals (BMI $\leq$ 18.5) is twice as high as that of obese and "fit" people. Furthermore, being overweight or mildly obese may be protective, especially in people with known cardiovascular disease. Scientists refer to this finding as the "obesity paradox." And being at either extreme of the BMI continuum, very thin (BMI $\leq$ 18.5) or severely obese (class II or greater, BMI $\geq$ 35), has major negative health consequences.[33]

Looking at every category of body composition, "unfit" people have a higher rate of premature death than "fit" individuals. Thus, at least partially, lack of physical activity (fitness), and not the weight problem itself may be the cause of premature death in most overweight people. However, it's not simply a matter of fitness or fatness. Research has shown that both obesity and physical inactivity are independent risk factors for heart disease, type 2 diabetes, and other chronic ailments.

Fitness does offer substantial benefits, but regular physical activity in itself does not completely reverse chronic disease risks associated with excess body fat. Studies are encouraging because they show that overweight/obese people who focus on healthy eating and become physically active decrease the risk of premature mortality, regardless of whether they lose weight or not. Few obese people, however, eat healthy and exercise regularly for 30 minutes on most days of the week. Most obese people either choose not to exercise or are unable to do so because of functional limitations as a result of the excessive body weight.

Obese people who do not have any metabolic risk factors can be classified as "metabolically healthy." Obese individuals who are metabolically healthy at one point, however, may not stay that way in the future. Over the course of 20 years, approximately 50 percent of them will develop metabolic risk factors. And only 10 percent of metabolically healthy obese people lose weight and transition into the healthy (no metabolic risk factors) nonobese category. In most cases, long-term healthy obesity is the exception rather than the norm.

Metabolically healthy obese people are significantly more likely to have a heart attack or stroke and die at a younger age than metabolically healthy normal-weight people. The data indicate that being either overweight or obese, but otherwise metabolically healthy, increases the risk of a heart attack by 24 percent and 88 percent, respectively, as compared to metabolically healthy and normal-weight people.[34]

The answer to the question of whether a person can be fit and fat depends on the definition of fitness. If cardiorespiratory fitness is determined by "accumulating 30 minutes of moderate-intensity activity on most days of the week," then the answer is a definite "yes." If you measure fitness based on maximal oxygen uptake (VO_{2max}—see Chapter 6, page 224), the answer is a clear "no." Many fitness experts do not agree with the concept of fit and fat. And according to Dr. JoAnn Manson of Harvard Medical School, "it's a rare bird" to find someone who is truly overweight and yet truly fit from a cardiorespiratory standpoint. Most nutritionists and exercise scientists agree that healthy eating and healthy exercise contribute to healthy body weight. There are more than 50 medical conditions—from type 2 diabetes, to acid reflux, arthritis, sleep apnea, and some types of cancers—that are directly related to excessive body weight. At this point, most fitness leaders do not support the notion that people can enjoy vibrant health and good quality of life while being overweight or obese.

5.10 Types of Exercise Recommended

For people trying to lose weight, a combination of aerobic and strength-training exercises works best. Aerobic exercise is the best exercise modality to offset the setpoint, and the continuity and duration of these types of activities cause many calories to be burned in the process. The role of aerobic exercise in successful lifetime weight management cannot be overestimated.

Strength-training is critical in helping maintain and increase LBM. Fewer calories are burned during a typical hour-long strength-training session than during an hour of aerobic exercise. Because of the high intensity of strength-training, the person needs frequent rest intervals to recover from each set of exercises. In the long run, however, the person enjoys the benefits of gains in lean tissue. Guidelines for developing aerobic and strength-training programs are given in Chapter 6 and Chapter 7.

Although the increase in BMR through increased muscle mass is being debated in the literature and merits further research, data indicate that each additional pound of muscle tissue raises the BMR in the range of 6 to 35 calories per day.[35] The latter figure is based on calculations that an increase of 3 to 3.5 pounds of lean tissue through strength-training increased BMR by about 105 to 120 calories per day.[36]

Most likely, the benefit of strength-training goes beyond the new muscle tissue. Maybe a pound of muscle tissue requires only 6 calories per day to sustain itself, but as all muscles undergo strength-training, they undergo increased protein synthesis to build and repair themselves, resulting in increased energy expenditure of 1 to 1.5 calories per pound in all trained muscle tissue. Such an increase would explain the 105- to 120-calorie BMR increase in this research study.

Energy Expenditure Following a Weight-Loss Program

It is common knowledge that most people regain lost weight following a diet, most likely because they tend to conserve energy and move less while on the diet and after weight loss. To examine the effect of dieting on energy expenditure, a landmark study shed light on the role of dieting with and without exercise on post-weight loss energy expenditure.[37]

Behavior Modification Planning

Healthy Breakfast Choices

Breakfast is the most important meal of the day. Skipping breakfast makes you hungrier later in the day and leads to overconsumption and greater caloric intake throughout the rest of the day. Regular breakfast eaters have less of a weight problem, lose weight more effectively, have less difficulty maintaining lost weight, and live longer. Skipping breakfast also temporarily raises LDL (bad) cholesterol and lowers insulin sensitivity, changes that may increase the risk for heart disease and diabetes. Below are some healthy breakfast food choices. Have you tried these options for breakfast?

I PLAN TO
I DID IT

- ❑ ❑ Fresh fruit
- ❑ ❑ Low-fat or skim milk
- ❑ ❑ Low-fat yogurt with berries
- ❑ ❑ Whole-grain cereal
- ❑ ❑ Whole-grain bread or bagel with fat-free cream cheese and slices of red or green pepper
- ❑ ❑ Hummus over a whole-grain bagel
- ❑ ❑ Peanut butter with whole-grain bread or bagel
- ❑ ❑ Low-fat cottage cheese with fruit
- ❑ ❑ Oatmeal
- ❑ ❑ Reduced-fat cheese
- ❑ ❑ Egg Beaters with salsa
- ❑ ❑ A scrambled egg with veggies (limit oil or butter use)

Try It

Select a healthy breakfast choice each day for the next 7 days. Evaluate how you feel the rest of the morning. What effect did eating breakfast have on your activities of daily living and daily caloric intake? Be sure to record your food choices, how you felt, and what activities you engaged in.

How Strength-Training Affects Body Weight—an Example

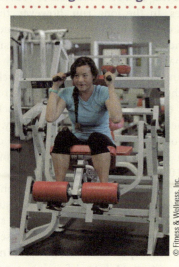

To examine the effects of a small increase in BMR on long-term body weight, let's use a conservative estimate of an additional 50 calories per day as a result of a regular strength-training program. An increase of 50 calories represents an additional 18,250 calories per year (50 × 365), or the equivalent of 5.2 pounds of fat (18,250 ÷ 3,500). This increase in BMR would more than offset the typical adult weight gain of 1 to 2 pounds per year.

This figure of 18,250 calories per year does not include the actual energy cost of the strength-training workout. If you use an energy expenditure of only 150 calories per strength-training session, done twice per week, over a year's time it would represent 15,600 calories (150 × 2 × 52), or the equivalent of another 4.5 pounds of fat (15,600 ÷ 3,500).

In addition, although the amounts seem small, the previous calculations do not account for the increase in BMR following the strength-training workout (the number of hours it takes the body to return to its preworkout resting rate, according to the intensity and duration of training). Depending on the training volume (see Chapter 7, page 267), this recovery energy expenditure ranges from 20 to 100 calories following each strength-training workout. All these "apparently small" changes make a big difference in the long run.

© Fitness & Wellness, Inc.

Study participants were on an 800-calorie diet. One group of subjects did not exercise, while a second group participated in aerobic exercise three times per week, and a third group engaged in strength training three times per week. All three groups lost about 25 pounds of body weight.

Following weight loss, however, total daily energy expenditure, RMR, and NEAT all decreased in the non-exercise group; whereas only RMR decreased in the exercise groups, attributed to the 25-pound drop in body weight. Of greater significance, however, total daily energy expenditure decreased by an average of 259 and 63 calories per day, respectively, in the non-exercise and aerobic exercise groups, while it actually increased by 63 calories per day in the strength-training group. Both exercise groups increased NEAT following the diet program. The results point to the fact that energy expenditure can be maintained or increased after weight loss if exercise is added to the program, with strength-training appearing to provide the greatest benefit, presumably due to the enhanced functional capacity provided by a greater LBM component.

The Roles of Exercise Intensity and Duration in Weight Management

A hotly debated and controversial topic is the exercise volume required for adequate weight management. Depending on the degree of the initial weight problem and the person's fitness level, there appears to be a difference in the volume of exercise that is most conducive toward adequate weight loss, weight loss maintenance, and weight management.

The Fallacy of the Fat Burning Zone

We have known for years that, compared with vigorous exercise, a greater proportion of calories burned during light-intensity exercise is derived from fat. The lower the intensity of exercise, the higher the percentage of fat utilization as an energy source. During light-intensity exercise, up to 50 percent of the calories burned may be derived from fat (the other 50 percent from glucose, which is converted from carbohydrates). With vigorous exercise, only 30 to 40 percent of the caloric expenditure comes from fat. However, you can burn twice as many calories overall—and subsequently more fat—during vigorous exercise (see Table 5.6).

Vigorous Exercise versus Exercise in the Fat Burning Zone—an Example

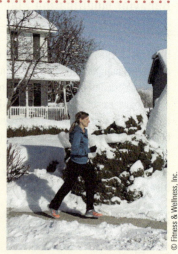

Let's look at a practical illustration of exercise intensity. If you exercised for 30 to 40 minutes at a light intensity level and burned 200 calories, about 100 of those calories (50 percent) would come from fat. If you exercised with vigorous intensity during those same 30 to 40 minutes, you could burn 400 calories, with 120 to 160 of the calories (30 to 40 percent) coming from fat. Thus, even though it is true that the percentage of fat used is greater during light-intensity exercise, the overall amount of fat used is still less during light-intensity exercise. Plus, if you were to exercise at a light intensity level, you would have to do so twice as long to burn the same number of total calories.

© Fitness & Wellness, Inc.

Table 5.6 Comparison of Approximate Energy Expenditure between 30 and 40 Minutes of Exercise at Three Intensity Levels

Exercise Intensity	Total Energy Expenditure (Calories)	Percent Calories from Fat	Total Fat Calories	Percent Calories from CHO*	Total CHO* Calories	Calories Burned per Minute	Calories per Pound per Minute
Light Intensity	200	50%	100	50%	100	6.67	0.045
Moderate Intensity	280	40%	112	60%	168	9.45	0.063
Vigorous Intensity	400	30%	120	70%	280	13.50	0.090

*CHO = Carbohydrates

Another benefit of vigorous-intensity exercise is that the metabolic rate remains at a slightly higher level longer after vigorous-intensity exercise, so you continue to burn a few extra calories following exercise. Very few calories are burned during recovery following a 45-minute moderate-intensity (50 percent or less of maximal capacity) exercise session, whereas when exercising at or above 70 percent of the maximal capacity for the same 45 minutes, nearly 40 percent of the total energy expenditure of the exercise bout is achieved during the recovery phase as the body returns to its pre-exercise baseline. A 500-calorie 45-minute vigorous exercise session will bring about another 200-calorie energy expenditure during the post-exercise recovery session.[38] Researchers believe that the extra caloric expenditure following vigorous exercise occurs because (a) the body uses more fat and less carbohydrates following a hard exercise session; (b) additional energy is required to replenish glycogen stores used during intense exercise; and (c) hormones released during vigorous exercise remain high, maintaining an elevated metabolism for several hours thereafter.

This example does not mean that light-intensity exercise is ineffective. Light-intensity exercise provides substantial health benefits, including a decrease in premature morbidity among overweight individuals. In addition, beginners are more willing to participate and stay with light-intensity programs. The risk of injury when starting out is quite low with this type of program. Light-intensity exercise does promote weight loss.

The Case for Vigorous Exercise

In terms of overall weight loss, there is additional controversy regarding the optimal duration of exercise. Early research conducted in the 1990s at Laval University in Quebec, Canada, using both men and women participants, showed that subjects who performed a high-intensity intermittent training (HIIT) program lost more body fat than participants in a light- to moderate-intensity continuous aerobic endurance group.[39] Even more surprisingly, this finding occurred despite the fact that the vigorous-intensity group burned fewer total calories per exercise session. The researchers concluded that the "results reinforce the notion that for a given level of energy expenditure, vigorous exercise favors negative energy and lipid balance to a greater extent than exercise of light to moderate intensity. Moreover, the metabolic adaptations taking place in the skeletal muscle in response to the HIIT

program appear to favor the process of lipid oxidation." If time constraints do not allow extensive exercise, to increase energy expenditure, a vigorous 20- to 30-minute exercise program is recommended.

In addition, it has been suggested that with attempts to lose weight, particularly by women, lengthy exercise sessions may not be helpful because they trigger greater food consumption following exercise, whereas shorter exercise sessions do not lead to greater caloric intake. Thus, some people think that the potential weight reduction effect of lengthy exercise sessions may be attenuated because people end up eating more food when they exercise.

A 2009 study had postmenopausal women exercise at 50 percent of their maximal aerobic capacity for about 20, 40, and 60 minutes three to four times per week.[40] On average, the groups lost 3, 4.6, and 3.3 pounds of weight, respectively. The data indicated that the 20- and 40-minute groups lost weight close to the amounts that had been predicted, whereas the 60-minute group lost significantly less than predicted. The researchers concluded that 60 minutes of exercise led this group of women to compensate with greater food intake, possibly triggered by an increase in ghrelin levels. Nonetheless, all three groups exhibited a significant decrease in waist circumference, independent of total weight lost. Researchers theorize that the biological mechanism to maintain fat stores in women is stronger than the one in men.

Choosing Physical Activity that Is Right for You

Over the years, moderate-intensity exercise is still beneficial for weight maintenance. A study of more than 34,000 women who were followed for 13 years, starting at an average age of 54, found that, on average, the women gained 6 pounds of weight. However, a small group of them who reported 60 minutes of almost daily exercise at a moderate intensity level closely maintained their body weight.[41] The routine of this group was not new, but rather exercise that they had been doing for years.

Thus, while the best exercise dose for optimal weight loss may not be a precise science, the research is quite clear that regular exercise is the best predictor of long-term weight maintenance. The data also indicate that even as little as 80 weekly minutes of aerobic or strength-training exercise prevents regain of the harmful visceral fat (also see page 141 in Chapter 4).

High-Intensity Interval Training Programs and Weight Loss

High-intensity interval training programs are becoming very popular. Do these programs really help people lose weight?

HIIT is a combined aerobic and anaerobic training program that had been used mainly by athletes but is now being embraced by fitness participants seeking better, faster, and more effective development. Following an appropriate warm-up, HIIT includes high- to very-high–intensity intervals that are interspersed with a low- to moderate-intensity recovery phase. Typically, a 1:4 or less work-to-recovery ratio is used; the more intense the interval, the longer the recovery period (for more information and for information on including HIIT in your training, see Chapter 9, pages 340–341). When looking purely at calories burned during exercise, HIIT produces the greatest improvements in aerobic capacity (VO_{2max}) and increases the capability to exercise at a higher percentage of that capacity (anaerobic threshold), thus allowing the participant to burn more calories during the exercise session. However, we now know that HIIT changes the way our bodies respond to exercise on a molecular level. Although the fuel used during high-intensity intervals is primarily glucose (carbohydrates), changes occur in the muscle that also increase the body's capability for fatty acid oxidation (fat burning).

Furthermore, following light- to moderate-intensity aerobic activity, the resting metabolism returns to normal in about 90 minutes. Depending on the volume of training (intensity and number of intervals performed), with HIIT it takes 24 to 72 hours for the body to return to its normal resting metabolic rate. Thus, a greater amount of calories (primarily from fat) are burned up to 3 days following HIIT. An added benefit, HIIT tends to suppress hunger by altering appetite-regulating hormones for up to 10 hours after exercise, thus rendering the individual less hungry following the HIIT session.

Research data indicate that HIIT programs are more effective for weight loss, as long as the individual does not compensate with greater caloric intake following exercise. While the extra calories burned during recovery do make a difference in the long run, keep in mind that the most significant factor is the number of calories actually burned during the HIIT session itself. Additionally, achieving improved levels of cardiorespiratory fitness in a shorter time will allow you to improve the level and quality of your workouts.

The take-home message from these studies is that when trying to lose weight, initial lengthy exercise sessions (longer than 60 minutes) may not be the best approach to weight loss *unless* you track daily caloric intake and avoid caloric compensation. The data show that people who carefully monitor caloric intake, instead of "guesstimating" energy intake, are by far more successful with weight loss.

Caloric compensation in response to extensive exercise in overweight individuals may be related to a low initial fitness level and an already-low caloric intake. Overall, inactive people tend to eat fewer calories, and a lengthy exercise session may well trigger a greater appetite due to the large negative caloric balance. Research confirms that energy deficit, and not exercise, is the most significant regulator of the hormonal responses seen in previously inactive individuals who begin an exercise program.[42] In active or fit individuals, lengthy exercise sessions are not counterproductive. If such were the case, health clubs and jogging trails would be full of overweight and obese people.

Because excessive body fat is a risk factor for cardiovascular disease, some precautions are in order for overweight individuals undertaking an exercise program. Depending on the extent of the weight problem, a medical examination is a good idea before undertaking the exercise program. Consult a physician in this regard.

New research is beginning to look into the role of increasing light-intensity ambulation (walking) and standing activities (doing some work on your feet instead of sitting the entire time) on weight loss. In essence, people increase light-intensity physical activity throughout the day. Light-intensity activities do not seem to trigger the

FTO: The Obesity-Associated Gene

Researchers recently discovered a variant of the fat mass and obesity-associated (FTO) gene that appears to have a strong link to BMI and increases the risk that carriers will be overweight or obese. The strength of the genetic association depends on whether the individual has inherited one or two copies of the FTO gene variant. Having one copy of the variant has a corresponding modest effect on body weight. On average, such a person weighs an extra 2.5 pounds compared to those who do not have the variant. Someone with two copies of the variant typically weighs an extra 6.5 pounds. Nonetheless, obesity is only partially driven by genes, and the genetic code does not substantially change in just a few generations. In contrast, people's lifestyles and their environment have changed significantly over the past 100 years.

People with one or two variants of the gene are not destined to be obese. The gene variant does not cause a sluggish metabolism, but rather causes them to eat more—in particular, calorie-dense foods. And lifestyle plays a crucial role in enabling or minimizing susceptibility to weight gain. Physical activity is effective in controlling weight in people with this genetic predisposition toward obesity. Shortly after the discovery of FTO in 2007, researchers found that physical activity and exercise attenuate the effect of the gene on weight gain. As little as 60 minutes of moderate- to vigorous-intensity activity per week thwarts the genetic inheritance and reduces the effects of the FTO variant. Thus, the benefits of physical activity and exercise are strong enough to keep at recommended body weight people who could otherwise become seriously overweight.

Figure 5.10 **Effects of lifestyle patterns on overall daily energy expenditure.**

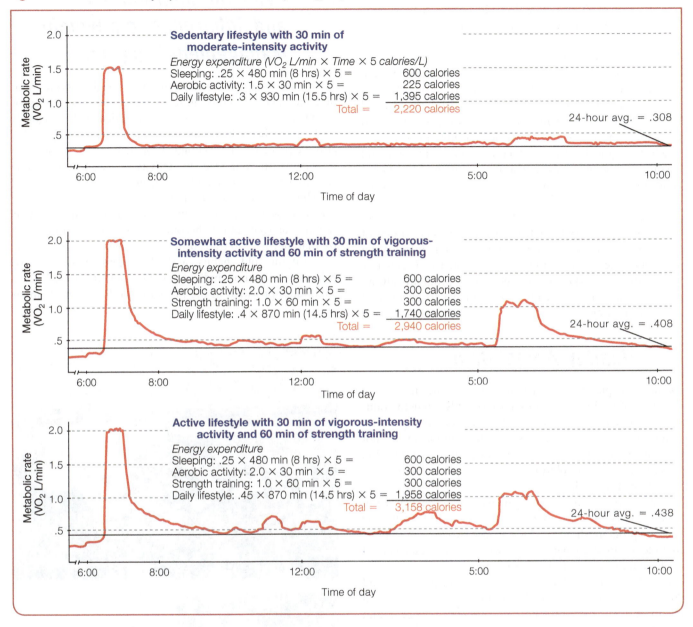

increase in ghrelin levels seen in previously inactive individuals who undertake long moderate-intensity or vigorous exercise sessions. The difference in energy expenditure by increasing light-intensity activities throughout the day can represent several hundred calories. As people achieve a higher fitness level, they can combine light-intensity activities performed throughout the day with moderate-intensity or vigorous exercise—or both. A graphic illustration of such lifestyle patterns and their effects on the metabolic rate and overall energy expenditure is provided in Figure 5.10.

Significantly overweight individuals need to choose activities in which they do not have to support their body weight but that still are effective in burning calories. Injuries to joints and muscles are common in excessively overweight

individuals who participate in weight-bearing exercises such as jogging and aerobics.

Swimming may not be a good weight loss exercise modality. Additional body fat makes a person more buoyant, and many people are not at the skill level required to swim fast enough to get a good training effect, thus limiting the number of calories burned as well as the benefits to the cardiorespiratory system. Additionally, swimmers often conduct "land training" to more effectively manage body weight. Research indicates that swimming has minimal effect on weight loss. The data further shows that swimming in cold water stimulates appetite, so people tend to eat more following their exercise session. If your preferred mode of exercise is swimming, guard against eating more after you swim. During the initial stages of exercise, better alternatives include walking, riding a bicycle (either road or stationary), elliptical training, low-impact aerobics/Zumba, or walking in a warm shallow pool. These forms of exercise aid with weight loss without fear of injuries.

If you wish to engage in vigorous-intensity exercise to either maintain lost weight or for adequate weight management, a word of caution is in order: Be sure that it is medically safe for you to participate in such activities and that you build up gradually to that level. If you are cleared to participate in vigorous exercise, do not attempt to do too much too quickly because you may incur injuries and become discouraged. You must allow your body a proper conditioning period of 8 to 12 weeks, and perhaps even longer.

In addition, keep in mind that vigorous intensity does not mean high impact. High-impact activities are the most common cause of exercise-related injuries. More information on proper exercise prescription is presented in Chapter 6. And remember, when on a weight-loss program, always carefully monitor your daily caloric intake to avoid food overconsumption.

5.11 *Healthy Weight Gain*

"Skinny" people should realize that the only healthy way to gain weight is also through exercise (mainly strength-training) and a slight increase in caloric intake. Attempting to gain weight by overeating alone raises the fat component and not the lean component—which is not the path to better health. Exercise is the best solution to weight (fat) reduction and weight (lean) gain alike.

A strength-training program, such as the one explained in Chapter 7, is the best approach to add body weight. The training program should include at least two exercises of one to three sets for each major body part. Each set should consist of about 8 to 12 repetitions maximum.

Muscle tissue contains about 75 percent water and 20 percent protein. The remainder of this tissue is composed of lipids (fat), carbohydrates, non-protein nitrogen, and inorganic compounds. Even though the metabolic cost of synthesizing a pound of muscle tissue is still unclear, consuming an estimated 500 additional calories per day is recommended to gain lean tissue.

Your diet should include a daily total intake of about 1.5 grams of protein per kilogram of body weight. If your daily protein intake already exceeds 1.5 grams per day, the extra 500 calories should be primarily in the form of complex carbohydrates. The higher caloric intake must be accompanied by a strength-training program; otherwise, the increase in body weight will be in the form of fat, not muscle tissue. (Activity 5.4 can be used to monitor your caloric intake for healthy weight gain.) Additional information on nutrition to optimize muscle growth and strength development is provided in Chapter 7 in the section "Dietary Guidelines for Strength and Muscular Development," pages 274–275.

5.12 *Behavior Modification and Adherence to a Weight Management Program*

Before you proceed to develop a thorough weight-loss program, take a moment to identify, in Activity 5.2, your current stage of change as it pertains to your recommended body weight. If applicable—that is, if you are not at recommended weight—list also the processes and techniques for change that you will use to accomplish your goal. In Activity 5.2, also outline your exercise program for weight management.

Achieving and maintaining recommended body composition is possible, but it requires desire and commitment. If weight management is to become a priority, people must realize that they have to transform their behavior to some extent.

Modifying old habits and developing new, positive behaviors takes time. Individuals who apply the management techniques provided in the Behavior Modification Planning

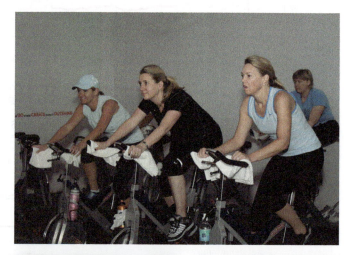

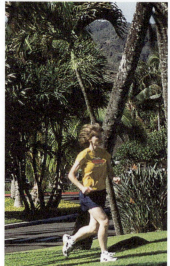

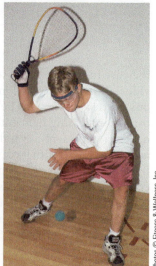

Exercising with other people and in different places helps people maintain exercise regularity.

Photos © Fitness & Wellness, Inc.

box that starts below are more successful at changing detrimental behavior and adhering to a positive lifetime weight control program. In developing a retraining program, you are not expected to incorporate all of the strategies given but should note the ones that apply to you. The form provided in Activity 5.5 will allow you to evaluate and monitor your own weight management behaviors.

> ! **Critical Thinking**
> What behavioral strategies have you used to properly manage your body weight? How do you think those strategies would work for others?

The Simple Truth

There is no quick and easy way to take off excess body fat and keep it off for good. Weight management is accomplished by making a lifetime commitment to physical activity and proper food selection. When taking part in a weight (fat)

reduction program, people also have to decrease their caloric intake moderately, use portion control, be physically active, and implement strategies to modify unhealthy eating behaviors.

During the process, relapses into past negative behaviors are almost inevitable. The three most common reasons for relapse are as follows:

1. Stress-related factors (e.g., major life changes, depression, job changes, or illness)
2. Social reasons (e.g., entertaining, eating out, or business travel)
3. Self-enticing behaviors (placing yourself in a situation to see how much you can get away with: "One small taste won't hurt" leads to "I'll eat just one slice" and finally to "I haven't done well, so I might as well eat some more")

Making mistakes is human and does not necessarily mean failure. Failure comes to those who give up and do not build on previous experiences and thereby develop skills that will prevent self-defeating behaviors in the future. *Where there's a will, there's a way*, and those who persist will reap the rewards.

Behavior Modification Planning

Weight Loss Strategies

I PLAN TO · **I DID IT**

☐ ☐ 1. **Make a commitment to change.** The first necessary ingredient is the desire to modify your behavior. You have to stop precontemplating or contemplating change and get going! You must accept that you have a problem and decide by yourself whether you really want to change. Sincere commitment increases your chances for success.

☐ ☐ 2. **Set realistic goals.** The weight problem developed over several years. Similarly, new lifetime eating and exercise habits take time to develop. A realistic long-term goal also will include short-term objectives that allow for regular evaluation and help maintain motivation and renewed commitment to attain the long-term goal.

☐ ☐ 3. **Monitor caloric intake.** Keep an accurate daily record of food consumption. "If you eat it, record it." People who keep accurate food logs are more successful at weight loss.

☐ ☐ 4. **Plan on three small meals and possibly one to two small snacks each day.** Such a plan often helps keep your blood sugar levels steady and avoid hunger pangs. Include adequate protein intake with each meal and use primarily high-volume, low-calorie foods. Space your meals and snacks so that you eat every three to four hours. Snacks need to be nutrient-rich, including fruits, vegetables, low-fat/plain yogurt, or a small amount of nuts. Avoid quick pick-me-up high-sugar and processed foods that tend to encourage overeating.

☐ ☐ 5. **Weigh yourself regularly,** preferably at the same time of day and under the same conditions. Do not adapt and accept a higher body weight as a new stable weight. Make dietary and physical activity adjustments accordingly.

☐ ☐ 6. **Incorporate exercise into the program.** Choosing enjoyable activities, places, times, equipment, and people to work out with will help you adhere to an exercise program. If time is a factor, you can easily create extra time in your day by recording your favorite TV programs and watching them later. You can then skip the commercials and end with extra time to fit in exercise.

☐ ☐ 7. **Differentiate between hunger and appetite.** Hunger is the actual physical need for food. Appetite is a desire for food, usually triggered by factors such as stress, habit, boredom, depression, availability of food, or just the thought of food. Developing and sticking to a regular meal pattern will help control hunger.

☐ ☐ 8. **Select low-energy/high-volume foods.** Soups, salads, and vegetables are more effective in promoting fullness with a meal; plus, they are lower in calories.

(continued)

❏ ❏ **9.** Increase fiber intake. Whole grains, fruits, vegetables, and legumes help you feel more satisfied and for a longer time by increasing chewing time, saliva secretion, gastric juices, and absorption time, all of which helps reduce overall caloric intake.

❏ ❏ **10.** Eat less fat. Each gram of fat provides nine calories, and protein and carbohydrates provide only four. In essence, you can eat more food by consuming primarily fruits, vegetables, and whole grains (complex carbohydrates) with each meal. Most of your fat intake should come from healthy unsaturated sources.

❏ ❏ **11.** Pay attention to calories. Just because food is labeled "low-fat" does not mean you can eat as much as you want. When reading food labels—and when eating—don't just look at the fat content. Many low-fat foods are high in calories.

❏ ❏ **12.** Cut unnecessary items from your diet. Substituting water for a daily can of soda would cut 51,100 (140 × 365) calories yearly from the diet—the equivalent of 14.6 (51,000 ÷ 3,500) pounds of fat. If you always drink water when thirsty and with your meals, instead of sugar-sweetened beverages, you can do even better and decrease caloric intake by an average of 300 daily calories. Several studies also indicate that liquid calories do not provide the same sense of satiety as a similar amount of calories from solid foods. An apple, for example, increases fullness more than a cup of apple juice. Research has shown that people who consume liquid calories do not account for those calories by eating less food during or in the subsequent meal. Liquid calories do little to suppress hunger.

❏ ❏ **13.** Maintain a daily intake of calcium-rich foods, especially low-fat or nonfat dairy products.

❏ ❏ **14.** Add foods to your diet that reduce cravings, such as oatmeal; eggs; small amounts of healthy oils and fats; salmon; poultry; tofu; avocado; almonds; Greek yogurt; and non-starchy vegetables such as lettuce, green beans, peppers, asparagus, broccoli, mushrooms, and brussels sprouts. Also, increasing the intake of low-glycemic carbohydrates with your meals helps you go longer before you feel hungry again.

❏ ❏ **15.** Avoid mindless eating. Many people make food decisions based on psychological triggers, including family and friends, packages and containers, watching television and TV ads, watching movies, computer distractions, and reading. Most foods consumed in these situations lack nutritional value or are high in sugar and fat.

❏ ❏ **16.** Stay busy. People tend to eat more when they sit around and do nothing. Occupying the mind and body with activities not associated with eating helps take away the desire to eat. Some options are walking; cycling; playing sports; gardening; sewing; or visiting a library, a museum, or a park. You also might develop other skills and interests not associated with food.

❏ ❏ **17.** Plan meals and shop sensibly. Always shop on a full stomach, because hungry shoppers tend to buy unhealthy foods impulsively—and then snack on the way home. Always use a shopping list, which should include 100 percent whole-grains (breads and cereals), fruits and vegetables, low-fat milk and dairy products, lean meats, fish, and poultry.

❏ ❏ **18.** Cook wisely:

  ❏ Use less fat and fewer refined and processed foods in food preparation.

  ❏ Trim all visible fat from meats and remove skin from poultry before cooking.

  ❏ Skim the fat off gravies and soups.

  ❏ Bake, broil, boil, or steam instead of frying.

  ❏ Sparingly use butter, cream, mayonnaise, and salad dressings.

  ❏ Avoid coconut oil, palm oil, and cocoa butter.

  ❏ Prepare plenty of foods that contain fiber.

  ❏ Include whole-grain breads and cereals, vegetables, and legumes in most meals.

  ❏ Eat fruits for dessert.

  ❏ Stay away from soda, fruit juices, fruit-flavored drinks, and sports and energy drinks.

  ❏ Use less sugar, and cut down on other refined carbohydrates, such as corn syrup, malt sugar, dextrose, and fructose (limit food items that have sugar listed as one of the top three ingredients on the food label).

  ❏ Drink plenty of water throughout the day.

❏ ❏ **19.** Do not serve more food than you should eat. Measure the food in portions and keep serving dishes away from the table. Do not force yourself or anyone else to "clean the plate" after they are satisfied (including children after they already have had a healthy, nutritious serving).

❏ ❏ **20.** Try "junior size" instead of "super size." People who are served larger portions eat more, whether they are hungry or not. Use smaller plates, bowls, cups, and glasses. Try eating half as much food as you commonly eat. Additionally, portions served on smaller plates appear bigger than they are, thus the tendency is to serve less on a small plate. People also drink less from tall/thin glasses than from large or even short/wide glasses. Watch for portion sizes at restaurants as well:

(continued)

Supersized foods create supersized people. Most restaurant meals exceed the amount of calories for a single meal. In some cases, meals provide three to four times the recommended amount of calories. Excessively large portions almost always overwhelm self-control as people do not have sufficient willpower to stop eating.

❏ ❏ 21. Use smaller and different color dishes. People tend to over-serve food on larger dinner plates. Reducing your standard dinner plate by 2 inches results in about 20 percent fewer calories served. Changing the contrast between the plate and the food—for example, pasta with red marinara sauce over a white vs. a red plate—also reduces the amount of food served by a similar 20 percent.

❏ ❏ 22. Use smaller serving spoons. People tend to serve less food when given a smaller serving spoon.

❏ ❏ 23. Eat out infrequently. The more often people eat out, the more body fat they have. People who eat out six or more times per week consume about 300 extra calories per day and 30 percent more fat than those who eat out less often.

❏ ❏ 24. Eat slowly and at the table only. Eating on the run promotes overeating because the body doesn't have enough time to "register" consumption, and people overeat before the body perceives the fullness signal.

Eating at the table encourages people to take time out to eat and deters snacking between meals. After eating, do not sit around the table but, rather, clean up and put away the food to avoid snacking.

❏ ❏ 25. Avoid social binges. Social gatherings tend to entice self-defeating behavior. Use visual imagery to plan ahead. Do not feel pressured to eat or drink and rationalize in these situations. Choose low-calorie foods and entertain yourself with other activities, such as dancing and talking.

❏ ❏ 26. Do not place unhealthy foods within easy reach. Ideally, avoid bringing high-calorie, high-sugar, or high-fat foods into the house. If they are there already, store them where they are hard to get to or see— perhaps the garage or basement.

❏ ❏ 27. Avoid evening food raids. Most people do really well during the day but then "lose it" at night. Take control. Stop and think. To avoid excessive nighttime snacking, stay busy after your evening meal. Go for a short walk, floss and brush your teeth, and get to bed earlier. Even better, close the kitchen after dinner and try not to eat anything 3 hours prior to going to sleep.

❏ ❏ 28. Practice stress management techniques (discussed in Chapter 12). Many people snack and increase their food consumption in stressful situations.

❏ ❏ 29. Get support. People who receive support from friends, relatives, and formal support groups are much more likely to lose and maintain weight loss than those without such support. The more support you receive, the better off you will be.

❏ ❏ 30. Monitor changes and reward accomplishments. Being able to exercise without interruption for 15, 20, 30, or 60 minutes; swimming a certain distance; running a mile— all these accomplishments deserve recognition. Create rewards that are not related to eating: new clothing, a tennis racquet, a bicycle, exercise shoes, or something else that is special and you would not have acquired otherwise.

❏ ❏ 31. Prepare for slipups. Most people will slip and occasionally splurge. Do not despair and give up. Reevaluate and continue with your efforts. An occasional slip won't make much difference in the long run.

❏ ❏ 32. Think positive. Avoid negative thoughts about how difficult changing past behaviors might be. Instead, think of the benefits you will reap, such as feeling, looking, and functioning better, plus enjoying better health and improving the quality of life. Avoid negative environments and unsupportive people.

Try It

In your online journal or class notebook, answer the following questions: How many of these strategies do you use to help you maintain recommended body weight? Do you feel that any of these strategies specifically help you manage body weight more effectively? If so, explain why.

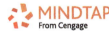 **MINDTAP** **Complete This Online**
From Cengage Visit **www.cengagebrain.com** to access MindTap, a complete digital course that includes interactive quizzes, videos, and more.

Assess Your Behavior

1. Are you satisfied with your current body composition (including body weight) and quality of life? If not, are you willing to do something about it to properly resolve the problem?

2. Are physical activity, aerobic exercise, and strength-training a regular part of your lifetime weight management program?

3. Do you weigh yourself regularly and make adjustments in energy intake and physical activity habits if your weight starts to shift upward?

4. Do you exercise portion control, watch your overall fat intake, and plan ahead before you eat out or attend social functions that entice overeating?

Assess Your Knowledge

1. During the past three decades, the rate of obesity in the United States has
   a. been on the decline.
   b. increased at an alarming rate.
   c. increased slightly.
   d. remained steady.
   e. increased in men and decreased in women.

2. Obesity is defined as a BMI equal to or above
   a. 10.
   b. 25.
   c. 30.
   d. 45.
   e. 50.

3. Obesity increases the risk for
   a. hypertension.
   b. congestive heart failure.
   c. atherosclerosis.
   d. type 2 diabetes.
   e. All of the choices are correct.

4. Tolerable weight is a body weight
   a. that is not ideal but one that you can live with.
   b. that tolerates the increased risk for chronic diseases.
   c. with a BMI range between 25 and 30.
   d. that meets both ideal values for percent body weight and BMI.
   e. All of the choices are correct.

5. When the body uses protein instead of a combination of fats and carbohydrates as a source of energy,
   a. weight loss is very slow.
   b. a large amount of weight loss is in the form of water.
   c. muscle turns into fat.
   d. fat is lost rapidly.
   e. fat cannot be lost.

6. Eating disorders
   a. are characterized by an intense fear of becoming fat.
   b. are physical and emotional conditions.
   c. almost always require professional help for successful treatment of the disease.
   d. are common in societies that encourage thinness.
   e. All of the choices are correct.

7. The most effective physical activity program to use during a weight-loss program is
   a. HIIT.
   b. low-intensity aerobic exercise.
   c. moderate-intensity aerobic exercise.
   d. yoga.
   e. low-resistance strength-training.

8. The key to maintaining weight loss successfully is
   a. frequent dieting.
   b. very low-calorie diets when "normal" dieting doesn't work.
   c. a lifetime physical activity program.
   d. regular LCHP meals.
   e. All of the choices are correct.

9. The recommended amount of daily physical activity for people who struggle with weight management is
   a. 15 to 20 minutes.
   b. 20 to 30 minutes.
   c. 30 to 60 minutes.
   d. 60 to 90 minutes.
   e. Any duration is sufficient as long as physical activity is done daily.

10. A daily energy expenditure of 300 calories through physical activity represents approximately ___ pounds of fat per year.
    a. 12
    b. 15
    c. 22
    d. 27
    e. 31

Correct answers can be found at the back of the book.

MINDTAP **Complete This Online**
From Cengage   Visit **www.cengagebrain.com** to access MindTap, a complete digital course that includes interactive quizzes, videos, and more.

Activity 5.2	Weight-Loss Behavior Modification Plan

Name _____ **Date** _____

Course _____ **Section** _____ **Gender** _____ **Age** _____

1. Using Figure 2.7 (page 73) and Table 2.3 (page 73), identify your current stage of change regarding **recommended body weight:** [_____]

2. How much weight do you want to lose? [_____]   Is it a realistic goal? [_____]

3. Target caloric intake to lose weight (diet plan—see Activity 5.1, item O) [_____].

4. Based on the processes and techniques of change discussed in Chapter 2, indicate what you can do to help yourself implement a weight management program.

_____

_____

5. How much effort are you willing to put into reaching your weight loss goal? _____

   Indicate your feelings about participating in an exercise program.

_____

6. Will you commit to participate in a combined aerobic and strength-training program?[a]   Yes [____]   No [____]

   If your answer is "Yes," proceed to the next question; if you answered "No," please read Chapters 3–9.

7. Select one or two aerobic activities in which you will participate regularly: [_____]

   List facilities available to you where you can carry out the aerobic and strength-training programs.

_____

8. Indicate days and times you will set aside for your aerobic and strength-training program (5 or 6 days per week should be devoted to aerobic exercise and 1 to 3 nonconsecutive days per week to strength training).

Monday:	
Tuesday:	
Wednesday:	
Thursday:	
Friday:	
Saturday:	

Sunday: A complete day of rest once a week is recommended to allow your body to fully recover from exercise.

Behavior Modification

Briefly describe whether you think you can meet the goals of your aerobic and strength-training program. What obstacles will you have to overcome, and how will you overcome them?

_____

[a]*Flexibility programs are necessary for adequate fitness, possible injury prevention, and good health but do not help with weight loss. Stretching exercises can be conducted regularly during the cool-down phase of your aerobic and strength-training programs (see Chapter 8).*

© Fitness & Wellness, Inc.

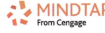

MINDTAP From Cengage   **Complete This Online**
Visit **www.cengagebrain.com** to access MindTap, a complete digital course that includes interactive quizzes, videos, and more.

<table>
<tr><td>**Activity 5.3**</td><td>**Calorie-Restricted Diet Plans**</td></tr>
</table>

Name _____ **Date** _____

Course _____ **Section** _____ **Gender** _____ **Age** _____

1,200 CALORIE DIET PLAN
Instructions:
The objective of the diet plan is to meet (not exceed) the number of servings allowed for the food groups listed. Each time that you eat a particular food, record it in the space provided for each group along with the amount you ate. Refer to the number of calories below to find out what counts as one serving for each group listed. Make additional copies of this form as needed.

Dairy: 2 servings
Grains: 6 servings
Fruits: 2 servings
Veggies: 3 servings
Protein: 3 servings

ChooseMyPlate.gov

Grains (80 calories/serving): 6 servings

1	
2	
3	
4	
5	
6	

Vegetables (25 calories/serving): 3 servings

1	
2	
3	

Fruits (60 calories/serving): 2 servings

1	
2	

Dairy (120 calories/serving, use low-fat milk and milk products): 2 servings

1	
2	

Protein (100 calories/serving): 3 servings

1	
2	
3	

Today's physical activity: [____]   Intensity: [__]   Duration: [__] min   Number of steps: [____]

Grams of protein consumed with each meal: Breakfast : _____ g, Lunch:_____ g, Dinner: _____ g

© Fitness & Wellness, Inc.

Activity 5.3 **Calorie-Restricted Diet Plans** (continued)

1,500 CALORIE DIET PLAN

Instructions:

The objective of the diet plan is to meet (not exceed) the number of servings allowed for the food groups listed. Each time that you eat a particular food, record it in the space provided for each group along with the amount you ate. Refer to the number of calories below to find out what counts as one serving for each group listed. Make additional copies of this form as needed.

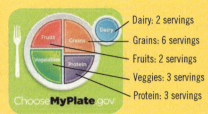

Dairy: 2 servings
Grains: 6 servings
Fruits: 2 servings
Veggies: 3 servings
Protein: 3 servings

Grains (80 calories/serving): 6 servings

1	
2	
3	
4	
5	
6	

Vegetables (25 calories/serving): 3 servings

1	
2	
3	

Fruits (60 calories/serving): 2 servings

| 1 | |
| 2 | |

Dairy (120 calories/serving, use low-fat milk and milk products): 2 servings

| 1 | |
| 2 | |

Protein (200 calories/serving): 3 servings

1	
2	
3	

Today's physical activity: ☐   Intensity: ☐   Duration: ☐ min   Number of steps: ☐

Grams of protein consumed with each meal: Breakfast : _____ g, Lunch: _____ g, Dinner: _____ g

Activity 5.3 Calorie-Restricted Diet Plans *(continued)*

1,800 CALORIE DIET PLAN

Instructions:

The objective of the diet plan is to meet (not exceed) the number of servings allowed for the food groups listed. Each time that you eat a particular food, record it in the space provided for each group along with the amount you ate. Refer to the number of calories below to find out what counts as one serving for each group listed. Make additional copies of this form as needed.

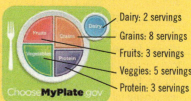

Dairy: 2 servings
Grains: 8 servings
Fruits: 3 servings
Veggies: 5 servings
Protein: 3 servings

ChooseMyPlate.gov

Grains (80 calories/serving): 8 servings

1	
2	
3	
4	
5	
6	
7	
8	

Vegetables (25 calories/serving): 5 servings

1	
2	
3	
4	
5	

Fruits (60 calories/serving): 3 servings

1	
2	
3	

Dairy (120 calories/serving, use low-fat milk and milk products): 2 servings

1	
2	

Protein (200 calories/serving): 3 servings

1	
2	
3	

Today's physical activity: _____ Intensity: ___ Duration: ___ min Number of steps: _____

Grams of protein consumed with each meal: Breakfast : _____ g, Lunch: _____ g, Dinner: _____ g

Activity 5.3 **Calorie-Restricted Diet Plans** *(continued)*

2,000 CALORIE DIET PLAN
Instructions:
The objective of the diet plan is to meet (not exceed) the number of servings allowed for the food groups listed. Each time that you eat a particular food, record it in the space provided for each group along with the amount you ate. Refer to the number of calories below to find out what counts as one serving for each group listed. Make additional copies of this form as needed.

Dairy: 2 servings
Grains: 10 servings
Fruits: 4 servings
Veggies: 5 servings
Protein: 3 servings

ChooseMyPlate.gov

Grains (80 calories/serving): 10 servings

1	
2	
3	
4	
5	
6	
7	
8	
9	
10	

Vegetables (25 calories/serving): 5 servings

1	
2	
3	
4	
5	

Fruits (60 calories/serving): 4 servings

1	
2	
3	
4	

Dairy (120 calories/serving, use low-fat milk and milk products): 2 servings

| 1 | |
| 2 | |

Protein (200 calories/serving): 3 servings

1	
2	
3	

Today's physical activity: [   ]   Intensity: [ ]   Duration: [ ] min   Number of steps: [   ]

Grams of protein consumed with each meal: Breakfast : _____ g, Lunch: _____ g, Dinner: _____ g

MINDTAP **Complete This Online**
From Cengage   Visit **www.cengagebrain.com** to access MindTap, a complete digital course that includes interactive quizzes, videos, and more.

Activity 5.4   Healthy Plan for Weight Maintenance or Gain

Name _____ **Date** _____

Course _____ **Section** _____ **Gender** _____ **Age** _____

I. Daily Caloric Requirement

A. Current body weight in pounds... ☐

B. Current percent body fat... ☐

C. Current body composition classification (Table 4.11, page 156)... ☐

D. Total daily energy requirement with exercise to maintain body weight (use item M from Activity 5.1). Use this figure and stop further computations if the goal is to maintain body weight... ☐

E. Target body weight (if your goal is to increase body weight)... ☐

F. Number of additional daily calories to increase body weight (combine this increased caloric intake with a strength-training program, see Chapter 7)... **500**

G. Total daily energy (caloric) requirement with exercise to increase body weight (D + 500) ☐

II. Strength-Training Program

For weight gain purposes, indicate three days during the week and the time when you will engage in a strength-training program.

_____

_____

III. Healthy Diet Plan

Design a sample healthy daily diet plan according to the total daily energy requirement computed in D (maintenance) or G (weight gain) in Part I. Using Appendix A, list all individual food items that you can consume on that day, along with their caloric, carbohydrate, fat, and protein content. Be sure that the diet meets the recommended number of servings from the five food groups.

Breakfast

	Food item	Amount	Calories	Carbohydrates (gr)	Fat (gr)	Protein (gr)
1.						
2.						
3.						
4.						
5.						
6.						
7.						
8.						

© Fitness & Wellness, Inc.

Activity 5.4 **Healthy Plan for Weight Maintenance or Gain** *(continued)*

Lunch	Food item	Amount	Calories	Carbohydrates (gr)	Fat (gr)	Protein (gr)
1.						
2.						
3.						
4.						
5.						
6.						
7.						
8.						
Snack						
1.						
Dinner						
1.						
2.						
3.						
4.						
5.						
6.						
7.						
8.						
		Totals:				

IV. Percent of Macronutrients

Determine the percent of total calories that are derived from carbohydrates, fat, and protein.

A. Total calories = [ ]

B. Grams of carbohydrates [ ] × 4 ÷ [ ] (total calories) = [ ] %

C. Grams of fat [ ] × 9 ÷ [ ] (total calories) = [ ] %

D. Grams of protein [ ] × 4 ÷ [ ] (total calories) = [ ] %

E. Body weight (BW) in kilograms (BW in pounds divided by 2.2046) = [ ] kg

F. Grams of protein per kilogram of body weight [ ] (grams of protein) ÷ [ ] (BW in kg) = [ ] gr/kg

G. Please summarize your diet and protein intake to either maintain or gain weight.

_____

_____

Activity 5.5   Weight Management: Measuring Progress

Name _____ Date _____

Course _____ Section _____ Gender _____ Age _____

I. Please answer all of the following:

1. State your own feelings regarding your current body weight, your target body composition, and a completion date for this goal.

_____

_____

_____

_____

2. Do you have an eating disorder? If so, express your feelings about it. Can your instructor help you find professional advice so that you can work toward resolving this problem?

_____

_____

_____

_____

_____

3. Is your present diet adequate according to the nutrient analysis? Yes _____ No _____

4. State dietary changes necessary to achieve a balanced diet and/or to lose weight (increase or decrease caloric intake, decrease fat intake, increase intake of complex carbohydrates, etc.). List specific foods that will help you improve in areas where you may have deficiencies and food items to avoid or consume in moderation to help you achieve better nutrition.

Changes to make: _____

_____

Foods that will help: _____

_____

Foods to avoid: _____

_____

© Fitness & Wellness, Inc.

Activity 5.5 **Weight Management: Measuring Progress** *(continued)*

II. Behavior Modification Progress Form

Instructions: Read the section on tips for behavior modification and adherence to a weight management program (pages 203–205). On a weekly or biweekly basis, go through the list of strategies and provide a "Yes" or "No" answer to each statement. If you are able to answer "Yes" to most questions, you have been successful in implementing positive weight management behaviors. (Make additional copies of this page as needed.)

Strategy	Date						
1. I have made a commitment to change.							
2. I set realistic goals.							
3. I monitor body weight on a regular basis.							
4. I exercise regularly.							
5. I exercise control over my appetite.							
6. I am consuming less fat in my diet.							
7. I pay attention to the number of calories in food.							
8. I have eliminated unnecessary food items from my diet.							
9. I include calcium-rich foods in my diet.							
10. I use craving-reducing foods in my diet.							
11. I avoid automatic eating.							
12. I stay busy.							
13. I plan meals ahead of time and shop sensibly.							
14. I cook wisely.							
15. I do not serve more food than I should eat.							
16. I use portion control in my diet and when dining out.							
17. I do not eat out more than once per week. When I do, I eat low-fat meals.							
18. I eat slowly and at the table only.							
19. I avoid social binges.							
20. I avoid temptation by relocating or removing unhealthy foods.							
21. I avoid evening food raids.							
22. I practice stress management.							
23. I have a strong support group.							
24. I monitor changes and reward my accomplishments.							
25. I prepare for lapses/relapses.							
26. I think positive.							
27. I make sensible adjustments in caloric intake and physical activity if my weight increases and stabilizes there for several days.							

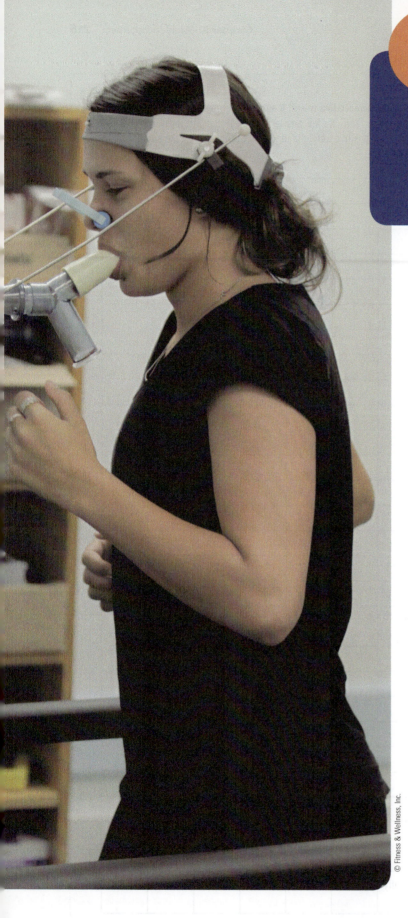

© Fitness & Wellness, Inc.

Cardiorespiratory Endurance

Physical activity is the miracle medication that people are looking for. It should be a nonnegotiable priority in daily life. It makes you look and feel younger, boosts energy, provides lifetime weight management, improves self-confidence and self-esteem, and enhances independent living, health, and quality of life. It further allows you to enjoy a longer life by decreasing the risk of many chronic conditions, including heart disease, high blood pressure, stroke, diabetes, some cancers, and osteoporosis. Your attitude should be: **I do not fear nor will I avoid physical activity: Bring it on!**

Objectives

6.1 **Define** cardiorespiratory (CR) endurance and describe the benefits of CR endurance training in maintaining health and well-being.

6.2 **Define** and give examples of aerobic and anaerobic exercise.

6.3 **Understand** the concept of oxygen uptake (VO_2) and its role in determining cardiorespiratory fitness and energy (caloric) expenditure.

6.4 **Assess** CR fitness through five test protocols: 1.5-Mile Run Test, 1.0-Mile Walk Test, Step Test, Astrand-Ryhming Test, and 12-Minute Swim Test.

6.5 **Interpret** the results of CR endurance assessments according to health fitness and physical fitness standards.

6.6 **Determine** your readiness to start an exercise program.

6.7 **Explain** the principles that govern CR exercise prescription: intensity, mode, duration, frequency, volume, and rate of progression.

6.8 **Learn** to write a comprehensive cardiorespiratory exercise prescription.

6.9 **Understand** the benefits of and differences between moderate-intensity and vigorous-intensity cardiorespiratory exercise.

6.10 **Learn** ways to foster adherence to exercise.

FAQ

Does aerobic exercise make people immune to heart and blood vessel disease?

Although aerobically fit individuals as a whole have a lower incidence of cardiovascular disease, a regular aerobic exercise program by itself does not guarantee immunity. The best way to minimize the risk for cardiovascular disease is to manage the risk factors. Many factors, including a genetic predisposition, can increase the risk. Research data, however, indicate that a regular aerobic exercise program delays the onset of cardiovascular problems and improves the chances of surviving a heart attack. Even moderate increases in aerobic fitness significantly lower the incidence of premature cardiovascular deaths. Data from a research study on death rates by physical fitness groups (illustrated in Figure 1.7, page 10) indicate that the decrease in cardiovascular mortality is greatest between the unfit and the moderately fit groups. A further decrease in cardiovascular mortality is observed between the moderately fit and the highly fit groups.

Is light-, moderate-, or high-intensity aerobic exercise most effective in burning fat?

During light- and moderate-intensity exercise, a greater percentage of energy is derived from fat than during high-intensity exercise. It is also true, however, that an even greater percentage of the energy comes from fat when doing nothing (resting or sleeping). And when someone does nothing, as in a sedentary lifestyle, that person doesn't burn many calories.

Let's examine this issue. During resting conditions, the human body is an efficient "fat-burning machine." That is, most energy, approximately 70 percent, is derived from fat, and only 30 percent comes from carbohydrates. But we burn few calories per minute at rest, about 1.5 calories compared with 3 to 4 calories during light-intensity exercise, 5 to 7 calories during moderate-intensity exercise, and 8 to 10 (or more) calories during vigorous exercise. As we begin to exercise and subsequently increase exercise intensity, we progressively rely more on carbohydrates and less on fat for energy until we reach maximal intensity, when 100 percent of the energy is derived from carbohydrates. Even though a lower percentage of the energy is derived from fat during vigorous exercise, the total caloric expenditure is so much greater (twice as high or more) that the total fat burned overall is still higher than it is during activities of moderate intensity.

A word of caution, nonetheless: Do not start vigorous, intense exercise without several weeks of proper and gradual conditioning. Effects can be even worse if such exercise is a weight-bearing activity. If you do high-intensity exercise from the outset, you increase the risk of injury and may have to stop exercising. Also, people with an initial low level of fitness often compensate with greater caloric intake following vigorous exercise, thus defeating the added energy expenditure obtained through exercise (additional information on this subject is provided on pages 198–202).

Do energy drinks enhance performance?

People associate energy with work. If an energy drink can enhance work capacity, the benefits of such drinks would surpass plain thirst-quenching drinks. Energy drinks typically contain sugar (discussed in Chapter 3), herbal extracts, large amounts of caffeine, and water-soluble vitamins. Consumers are led to believe that these ingredients increase energy metabolism, provide an energy boost, improve endurance, and aid in weight loss. These purported benefits are yet to be proven through scientific research.

The energy content of many of these drinks is around 60 grams of sugar and 240 calories in a 16-ounce drink, with little additional nutritive value. If you are going to participate in an intense and lengthy workout, the carbohydrate content can boost performance and help you get through the workout. If, however, you are concerned with weight management, 240 calories is an extraordinarily large amount of calories in a two-cup drink. Weight gain may be the end result if you drink a few of these throughout the day to give you a boost while studying or while at work. Sugar-free energy drinks provide little or no energy (calories), although they are packed with nervous system stimulants. The high caffeine content in energy drinks can also cause adverse health effects, including excessive use and abuse, which can lead to life-threatening complications (See Chapter 13, pages 488–489 for more information on the danger of energy drinks).

REAL LIFE STORY | Yumiko's Experience

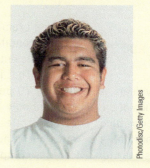

I never really noticed how much walking I did (or did not do) each day until our whole class got pedometers and started tracking our steps as part of an assignment for class. At first I was shocked that my number of steps was so low. I would have guessed that I was a lot more active than that. But after a while, wearing the pedometer made me want to walk more so that I could break my previous record. I set a goal each day for the number of steps I was aiming for. I started taking the stairs instead of elevators, parking farther away from wherever I was going, and walking to friends' dorm rooms to talk to them rather than calling or texting them, just to try to get more steps in. If at the end of the day my total number of steps was under the goal, I would go outside and walk around the block until I got to the goal number. I was surprised to find how much seeing that number on the pedometer would motivate me. Eventually, after continuing to increase my number of steps over the semester, I started hitting the recommended amount of 10,000 steps per day, and even increased to 12,000. Though the semester has ended and I am no longer in the fitness class, I have still kept up my walking habit, hitting my goal number most days, and sometimes jogging a portion of my steps. I have really noticed a difference in my cardiorespiratory fitness, and am hoping to keep my new habit up for life. I would recommend that anyone else who has trouble getting motivated purchase a pedometer and start walking!

Photodisc/Getty Images

PERSONAL PROFILE: My Personal Cardiorespiratory Fitness Profile

I. Have you ever experienced the feeling of being aerobically fit? ____ Yes ____ No

II. Do you understand the concept of oxygen uptake and the difference between absolute and relative oxygen uptake? ____ Yes ____ No

III. At 70 percent training intensity, your exercise prescription requires a heart rate of 156 beats per minute. Is there a difference between jogging, cycling, or doing Zumba when exercising at this same heart rate? ____ Yes ____ No

IV. Can you identify and relate to the factors that motivated Yumiko to become aerobically fit and what helped him stay with the exercise program? ____ Yes ____ No
What factors do you think can help you start or stay with aerobic exercise?

V. Your cardiorespiratory fitness test indicates that your maximal oxygen uptake (VO_{2max}) is 48 mL/kg/min. If you chose to exercise at 50 percent of your VO_{2max} (moderate intensity, as most people like to do during aerobic exercise), can you compute how many calories you burn per minute at this intensity level and the total minutes that you'd have to exercise to burn the equivalent of one pound of fat? ____ Yes ____ No

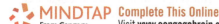

MINDTAP **Complete This Online**
From Cengage   Visit **www.cengagebrain.com** to access MindTap, a complete digital course that includes interactive quizzes, videos, and more.

Cardiorespiratory (CR) endurance is the most important component of health-related physical fitness. For the majority of life, people can get by without high levels of strength and flexibility, but they cannot do without a good CR system, facilitated by aerobic exercise. The exception occurs among older adults, for whom muscular fitness is particularly important.

Aerobic exercise is especially important in preventing cardiovascular disease. A poorly conditioned heart, which has to pump more often just to keep a person alive, is subject to more wear and tear than a well-conditioned heart. In situations that place strenuous demands on the heart, such as doing yard work, lifting heavy objects or weights, or running to catch a bus, the unconditioned heart may not be able to sustain the strain. Regular participation in CR endurance activities also helps a person achieve and maintain

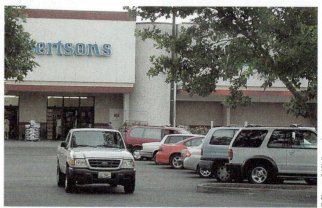

The epitome of physical inactivity: driving around a parking lot for several minutes in search of a parking spot 20 yards closer to the store's entrance.

© Fitness & Wellness, Inc.

recommended body weight—the fourth component of health-related physical fitness.

Physical activity, unfortunately, is no longer a natural part of human existence. Technological developments have driven most people in developed countries into sedentary lifestyles. For instance, when many people go to a store only a couple of blocks away, they drive their automobiles and then spend a couple of minutes driving around the parking lot to find a spot 20 yards closer to the store's entrance. At times, they don't even have to carry the groceries to the car because an employee working at the store offers to do this for them.

Similarly, during a visit to a multilevel shopping mall, almost everyone chooses to take the escalator instead of the stairs (which are sometimes inaccessible). Automobiles, elevators, escalators, telephones, intercoms, remote controls, electric garage door openers—all are modern-day conveniences that minimize the amount of movement and effort required of the human body.

One of the most harmful effects of modern-day technology is an increase in chronic conditions related to a lack of physical activity. These **hypokinetic diseases** include hypertension, heart disease, chronic low back pain, and obesity. ("Hypo" means low or little, and "kinetic" implies motion.) Lack of adequate physical activity is a fact of modern life that most people can no longer avoid. To enjoy modern-day conveniences and still expect to live life to its fullest, people have to make a personalized lifetime exercise program a part of daily living.

6.1 *Basic Cardiorespiratory Physiology: A Quick Survey*

Before people begin to overhaul their bodies with an exercise program, they should understand the mechanisms they propose to alter and survey the ways in which they can measure how well they perform these mechanisms. CR endurance is a measure of how the pulmonary (lungs), cardiovascular (heart and blood vessels), and muscular systems work together during aerobic activities. As people breathe, part of the oxygen in the air is taken up by the **alveoli** in the lungs. As blood passes through the alveoli, oxygen is picked up by **hemoglobin** and transported in the blood to the heart. The heart then is responsible for pumping the oxygenated blood through the circulatory system to all organs and tissues of the body.

At the cellular level, oxygen is used to convert food substrates (primarily carbohydrates and fats) through aerobic metabolism into **adenosine triphosphate (ATP)**. This compound provides the energy for physical activity, body functions, and maintenance of a constant internal equilibrium. During physical exertion, more ATP is needed to perform the activity. As a result, the lungs, heart, and blood vessels have to deliver more oxygen to the muscle cells to supply the required energy.

During prolonged exercise, an individual with a high level of CR endurance is able to deliver the required amount of

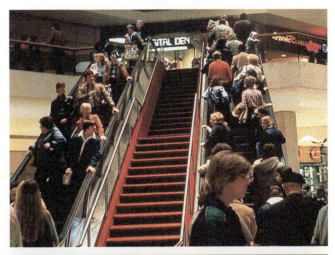

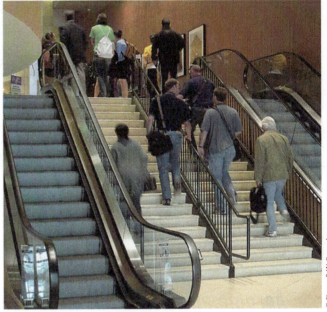

Advances in modern technology have almost completely eliminated the need for physical activity, but you can choose to be physically active and greatly decrease the risk for premature mortality.

oxygen to the tissues with relative ease. In contrast, the CR system of a person with a low level of endurance has to work harder, the heart has to work at a higher rate, less oxygen is

---

GLOSSARY

Cardiorespiratory (CR) endurance Ability of the lungs, heart, and blood vessels to deliver adequate amounts of oxygen to the cells to meet the demands of prolonged physical activity.

Hypokinetic diseases Hypo denotes "lack of"; therefore, chronic ailments that result from a lack of physical activity.

Alveoli Air sacs in the lungs where oxygen is taken up and carbon dioxide (produced by the body) is released from the blood.

Hemoglobin Protein-iron compound in red blood cells that transports oxygen in the blood.

Adenosine triphosphate (ATP) High-energy chemical compound that the body uses for immediate energy.

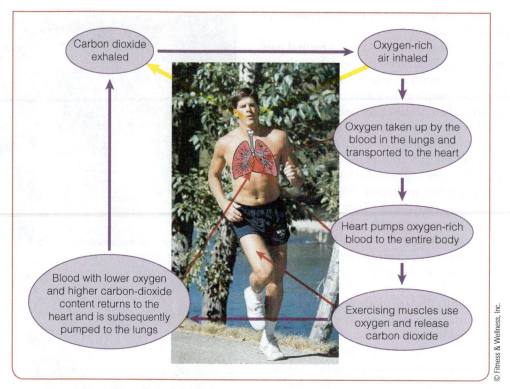

Carbon dioxide exhaled

Oxygen-rich air inhaled

Oxygen taken up by the blood in the lungs and transported to the heart

Heart pumps oxygen-rich blood to the entire body

Blood with lower oxygen and higher carbon-dioxide content returns to the heart and is subsequently pumped to the lungs

Exercising muscles use oxygen and release carbon dioxide

© Fitness & Wellness, Inc.

CR endurance refers to the ability of the lungs, heart, and blood vessels to deliver adequate amounts of oxygen to the cells to meet the demands of prolonged physical activity.

delivered to the tissues, and, consequently, the individual fatigues faster. Hence, a higher capacity to deliver and utilize oxygen—called **oxygen uptake,** or **VO₂**—indicates a more efficient CR system. Therefore, measuring VO_2—volume (V) of oxygen (O_2)—is an important way to evaluate CR health.

6.2 *Aerobic and Anaerobic Exercise*

CR endurance activities often are called **aerobic** exercises. Examples are walking, jogging, swimming, cycling, cross-country skiing, aerobics (including water aerobics), and rope skipping. By contrast, the intensity of **anaerobic** exercise is so high that oxygen cannot be delivered and utilized to produce energy. Because energy production is limited in the absence of oxygen, anaerobic activities can be carried out for only short periods—2 to 3 minutes. The higher the intensity of the activity, the shorter the duration.

Critical Thinking

Your friend Joe is not physically active and doesn't exercise. He manages to keep his weight down by dieting and tells you that because he feels and looks good, he doesn't need to exercise. How do you respond to your friend?

Good examples of anaerobic activities are races of 100, 200, and 400 meters in track and field, a 100-meter race in

swimming, gymnastics routines, and strength-training. Anaerobic activities do not contribute much to developing the CR system. Only aerobic activities increase CR endurance. The basic guidelines for CR exercise prescription are set forth later in this chapter.

6.3 *Benefits of Aerobic Exercise*

Everyone who participates in a CR or aerobic exercise program can expect a number of beneficial physiological adaptations from training (Figure 6.1). Among them are the following:

1. A higher **maximal oxygen uptake (VO₂max)**. The amount of oxygen that the body is able to use during exercise increases significantly. This allows the individual to exercise longer and more intensely before becoming fatigued. Depending on the initial fitness level, the increases in VO_{2max} average 15 to 20 percent, although increases greater than 50 percent have been reported in people who have very low initial levels of fitness or who were significantly overweight prior to starting the aerobic exercise program.

2. An increase in the oxygen-carrying capacity of the blood. As a result of training, the red blood cell count goes up. Red blood cells contain hemoglobin, which transports oxygen in the blood.

3. A decrease in **resting heart rate (RHR)** and an increase in cardiac muscle strength. During resting conditions, the heart ejects between 5 and 6 liters of

Figure 6.1 Selected benefits of cardiorespiratory (aerobic) fitness.

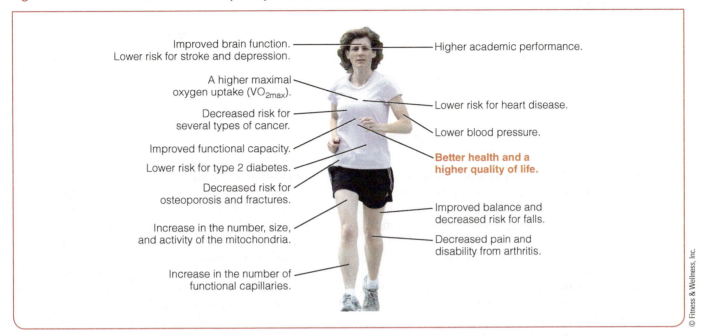

Improved brain function. Lower risk for stroke and depression.

A higher maximal oxygen uptake (VO_{2max}).

Decreased risk for several types of cancer.

Improved functional capacity.

Lower risk for type 2 diabetes.

Decreased risk for osteoporosis and fractures.

Increase in the number, size, and activity of the mitochondria.

Increase in the number of functional capillaries.

Higher academic performance.

Lower risk for heart disease.

Lower blood pressure.

Better health and a higher quality of life.

Improved balance and decreased risk for falls.

Decreased pain and disability from arthritis.

© Fitness & Wellness, Inc.

blood per minute (a liter is slightly larger than a quart). This amount of blood, also referred to as **cardiac output**, meets the body's energy demands in the resting state. Like any other muscle, the heart responds to training by increasing in strength and size. As the heart gets stronger, the muscle can produce a more forceful contraction, which helps the heart to eject more blood with each beat. This **stroke volume** yields a lower heart rate. The lower heart rate also allows the heart to rest longer between beats. Average resting and maximal cardiac outputs, stroke volumes, and heart rates for sedentary, trained, and highly trained (elite) males are shown in Table 6.1. RHRs frequently decrease by 10 to 20 beats per minute (bpm) after only 6 to 8 weeks of training. A reduction of 20 bpm saves the heart about 10,483,200 beats per year. The average heart beats between 70 and 80 bpm. As seen in Table 6.1, RHRs in highly trained athletes are often around 45 bpm.

4. A lower heart rate at given workloads. When compared with untrained individuals, trained people have a lower heart rate response to a given task because of greater efficiency of the CR system. Individuals are surprised to find that following several weeks of training, a given **workload** (let's say a 10-minute mile) elicits a lower heart rate response than their response when they first started training.

5. An increase in the number, size, and capacity of mitochondria. All energy necessary for cell function is produced in the **mitochondria**. As their size and numbers increase, so does their potential to produce energy for muscular work.

6. An increase in the number of functional capillaries. **Capillaries** allow exchange of oxygen and carbon

dioxide between the blood and the cells. As more vessels open up, more gas exchange can take place, delaying the onset of fatigue during prolonged exercise. This increase in capillaries speeds the rate at which waste products of cell metabolism can be removed as well. This increased capillarization occurs in the heart as well, which enhances the oxygen delivery capacity to the heart muscle.

7. An increase in fat-burning enzymes. These enzymes are significant because fat is lost primarily by burning

GLOSSARY

Oxygen uptake (VO_2) The amount of oxygen the human body uses.

Aerobic Exercise that requires oxygen to produce the necessary energy (ATP) to carry out the activity.

Anaerobic Exercise that does not require oxygen to produce the necessary energy (ATP) to carry out the activity.

Maximal oxygen uptake (VO_{2max}) Maximum volume of oxygen the body is able to utilize per minute of physical activity, commonly expressed in milliliters per kilogram per minute (mL/kg/min); the best indicator of CR or aerobic fitness.

Resting heart rate (RHR) Heart rate after a person has been sitting quietly for 15 to 20 minutes.

Cardiac output Amount of blood pumped by the heart in 1 minute.

Stroke volume Amount of blood pumped by the heart in one beat.

Workload Load (or intensity) placed on the body during physical activity.

Mitochondria Structures within the cells where energy transformations take place.

Capillaries Smallest blood vessels carrying oxygenated blood and nutrients to the tissues in the body.

Table 6.1 Average Resting and Maximal Cardiac Output, Stroke Volume, and Heart Rate for Sedentary, Trained, and Highly Trained Young Males

	Resting			Maximal		
	Cardiac Output (L/min)	Stroke Volume (mL)	Heart Rate (bpm)	Cardiac Output (L/min)	Stroke Volume (mL)	Heart Rate (bpm)
Sedentary	5–6	68	74	20	100	200
Trained	5–6	90	56	30	150	200
Highly trained	5–6	110	45	35	175	200

NOTE: Cardiac output and stroke volume in women are about 25 percent lower than in men.

it in muscle. As the concentration of the enzymes increases (along with the number and size of mitochondria), so does the ability to burn fat (triglycerides) as opposed to carbohydrates (glucose/glycogen) during submaximal workloads (below a pace that you can comfortably sustain for at least 20 minutes).

8. Ability to recover rapidly. Trained individuals have a faster **recovery time** after exercising. A fit body system is able to more quickly restore any internal equilibrium disrupted during exercise.

9. Lower blood pressure and blood lipid levels. A regular aerobic exercise program leads to lower blood pressure (thereby reducing a major risk factor for stroke) and lower levels of fats (e.g., cholesterol and triglycerides), which have been linked to the formation of atherosclerotic plaque that obstructs the arteries (see Chapter 10). Regular aerobic exercise leads to a decrease in "bad" low-density lipoprotein (LDL) cholesterol and an increase in "good" high-density lipoprotein (HDL) cholesterol. These beneficial changes lower the risk for coronary heart disease (see Chapter 10).

10. Better health and wellness. Aerobic exercise is viewed by scientists and sportsmedicine specialists as *medicine of motion*. We know that aerobic exercise is one of the most effective, affordable, and readily accessible "medications" available to all. Most chronic diseases improve and can be prevented though a daily routine of aerobic exercise. The myriad of immediate and long-term health benefits start as soon as the individual begins the first exercise session (see Chapter 1 page 13).

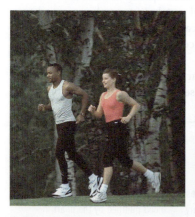
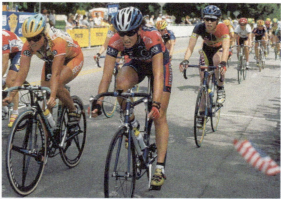
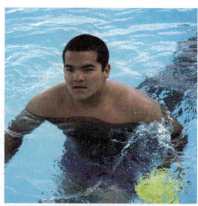

Aerobic activities.

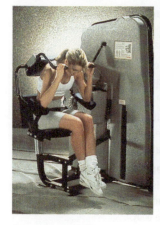
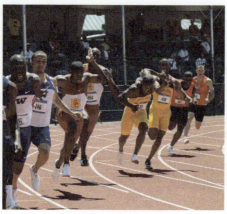
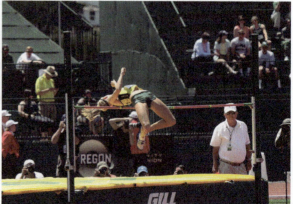

Anaerobic activities.

© Fitness & Wellness, Inc.

Behavior Modification Planning

Tips to Increase Daily Physical Activity

Adults need recess, too! There are 1,440 minutes in every day. Schedule a minimum of 30 of these minutes for physical activity. With a little creativity and planning, even the person with the busiest schedule can make room for physical activity. For many folks, before or after work or meals is often an available time to cycle, walk, or play. Think about your weekly or daily schedule and look for or make opportunities to be more active. Every little bit helps. Consider the following suggestions:

I PLAN TO / **I DID IT**

❑ ❑ Walk, cycle, jog, skate, etc., to school, work, the store, or a place of worship.

❑ ❑ Use a fitness tracker to count daily steps, mileage, total activity time, and estimated calories used through physical activity.

❑ ❑ Walk while doing errands.

❑ ❑ Get on or off the bus several blocks away.

❑ ❑ Park the car farther away from your destination.

❑ ❑ At work, walk to nearby offices instead of sending e-mails or using the phone.

❑ ❑ Walk or stretch a few minutes every hour that you are at your desk.

❑ ❑ Take fitness breaks—walking or doing desk exercises—instead of taking cigarette breaks or coffee breaks.

❑ ❑ Incorporate activity into your lunch break (walk to the restaurant).

❑ ❑ Take the stairs instead of the elevator or escalator.

❑ ❑ Play with children, grandchildren, or pets. Everybody wins. If you find it too difficult to be active after work, try it before work.

❑ ❑ Do household tasks.

❑ ❑ Work in the yard or garden.

❑ ❑ Avoid labor-saving devices. Turn off the self-propelled option on your lawnmower or vacuum cleaner.

❑ ❑ Use leg power. Take small trips on foot to get your body moving.

❑ ❑ Walk extra laps around the supermarket or mall before you start shopping.

❑ ❑ Exercise while watching TV (e.g., use hand weights or stationary bicycle/treadmill, elliptical training, or stretch).

❑ ❑ Spend more time playing sports than sitting in front of the TV or the computer.

❑ ❑ Dance or exercise to music. Pick some songs that inspire you to dance, then do it.

❑ ❑ Pace while talking on the phone.

❑ ❑ Keep a pair of comfortable walking or running shoes in your car and office. You'll be ready for activity wherever you go!

❑ ❑ Make a Saturday morning walk a group habit.

❑ ❑ Learn a new sport or join a sports team.

❑ ❑ Avoid carts when golfing.

❑ ❑ When out of town, stay in hotels with fitness centers.

❑ ❑ Use positive self-talk: I can do this, I am getting fitter, I am strong, I can finish, I am getting healthier, I am managing my weight.

Try It

Keep a 3-day log of all your activities. List the activities performed, time of day, and how long you were engaged in these activities. You may be surprised by your findings.

SOURCE: Adapted from Centers for Disease Control and Prevention, Atlanta, 2014.

MINDTAP From Cengage **Complete This Online**
Visit **www.cengagebrain.com** to access MindTap, a complete digital course that includes interactive quizzes, videos, and more.

6.4 Assessing Physical Fitness

The assessment of physical fitness serves several purposes:

- To educate participants regarding their present fitness levels and compare them with health fitness and physical fitness standards
- To motivate individuals to participate in exercise programs
- To provide a starting point for an individualized exercise prescription and establish realistic goals
- To evaluate improvements in fitness achieved through exercise programs and adjust exercise prescription and fitness goals accordingly
- To monitor changes in fitness throughout the years

Responders versus Nonresponders

Individuals who follow similar training programs show wide variation in physiological responses. Heredity plays a crucial role in how each person responds to and improves after beginning an exercise program. Several studies have documented that following exercise training, most individuals, called **responders**, readily show improvements but a few, the

---

GLOSSARY

Recovery time Amount of time that the body takes to return to resting levels after exercise.

Responders Individuals who exhibit improvements in fitness as a result of exercise training.

nonresponders, exhibit small or no improvements. This concept is referred to as the **principle of individuality**.

After several months of aerobic training, increases in VO_{2max} are between 15 and 20 percent on the average, although individual responses can range from 0 percent (in a few cases) to more than 50 percent improvement, even when all participants follow the same training program. Nonfitness and low-fitness participants, however, should not label themselves as nonresponders based on the previous discussion. Nonresponders constitute less than 5 percent of exercise participants. Although additional research is necessary, lack of improvement in CR endurance among nonresponders might be related to low levels of leg strength. A lower-body strength-training program has been shown to help these individuals improve VO_{2max} through aerobic exercise.[1]

If, through your self-assessment of CR fitness, you find your fitness level is less than adequate, do not let that discourage you; rather, set a priority to be physically active every day. In addition to regular exercise, lifestyle behaviors—walking, taking stairs, cycling to work, parking farther from the office, doing household tasks, gardening and doing yard work, for example—provide substantial benefits. In this regard, daily **physical activity** and **exercise** habits should be monitored, in conjunction with fitness testing, to evaluate adherence among nonresponders. After all, it is through increased daily activity that you will reap the health benefits that improve your quality of life.

HOEGER KEY TO WELLNESS

In today's primarily sedentary society, a person cannot afford not to be physically active. The research is clear: The benefits of increasing daily physical activity (NEAT—see Chapter 1, page 17) and engaging in a regular aerobic exercise program are far too impressive to be ignored.

6.5 Assessing Cardiorespiratory Endurance

CR endurance, CR fitness, or aerobic capacity is determined by the maximal volume of oxygen the human body is able to utilize (oxygen uptake) per minute of physical activity (VO_{2max}).

This value can be expressed in liters per minute (L/min) or milliliters per kilogram per minute (mL/kg/min). The relative value in mL/kg/min is used most often for VO_{2max}, because it considers total body mass (weight) in kilograms. When comparing two individuals with the same absolute value, the one with the lesser body mass will have a higher relative value, indicating that more oxygen is available to each kilogram (2.2 pounds) of body weight. Because all tissues and organs of the body need oxygen to function, higher oxygen consumption indicates a more efficient CR system.

Components of VO₂

The amount of oxygen the body uses at rest or during submaximal (VO_2) or maximal (VO_{2max}) exercise is determined by heart rate, stroke volume, and the amount of oxygen removed from the vascular system (for use by all organs and tissues of the body, including the muscular system).

Heart Rate

Normal heart rate ranges from about 45 bpm or lower during resting conditions in trained athletes to 200 bpm or higher during maximal exercise. The **maximal heart rate (MHR)** that a person can achieve starts to drop by about one beat per year beginning around 12 years of age. The MHR in trained endurance athletes is sometimes slightly lower than in an untrained individual. This adaptation to training is thought to allow the heart more time to effectively fill with blood so as to produce a greater stroke volume.

Stroke Volume

Stroke volume can range from 50 milliliters (mL) per beat (stroke) during resting conditions in highly sedentary people to as high as 200 mL per beat at maximum in elite endurance-trained athletes (Table 6.1). Following endurance training, stroke volume increases significantly. Some of the increase is the result of a stronger heart muscle, but it also is related to an increase in total blood volume and a greater filling capacity of the ventricles during the resting phase (diastole) of the cardiac cycle. As more blood enters the heart, more blood can be ejected with each heartbeat (systole). The increase in stroke volume is primarily responsible for the increase in VO_{2max} with endurance training.

Estimating Energy Expenditure from Oxygen Uptake in L/min

VO_2 expressed in liters per minute is valuable in determining the caloric expenditure of physical activity. The human body burns about five calories for each liter of oxygen consumed. If you know your VO_{2max} in mL/kg/min, you can easily determine your VO_{2max} in L/min by multiplying the value in mL/kg/min by your body weight in kg and dividing it by 1,000. For example, if you weigh 150 lbs (68 kg or 150 ÷ 2.2046) and after your assessment of CR fitness you find out that your VO_{2max} is 47.0 mL/kg/min, your absolute VO_{2max} would be 3.2 L/min (47 × 68 ÷ 1,000).

During aerobic exercise the average person trains around 50 percent of VO_{2max}. A person with an absolute VO_{2max} of 3.5 L/min who trains at 50 percent of maximum uses 1.75 (3.5 × .50) liters of oxygen per minute of physical activity. This indicates that 8.75 calories are burned during each minute of exercise (1.75 × 5). If the activity is carried out for 30 minutes, 263 calories (8.75 × 30) have been burned. Because a pound of body fat represents about 3,500 calories, the previous example indicates that this individual would have to exercise for a total of 400 minutes (3,500 ÷ 8.75) to burn the equivalent of a pound of body fat. At 30 minutes per exercise session, slightly over 13 sessions (400 ÷ 30) would be required to expend the 3,500 calories.

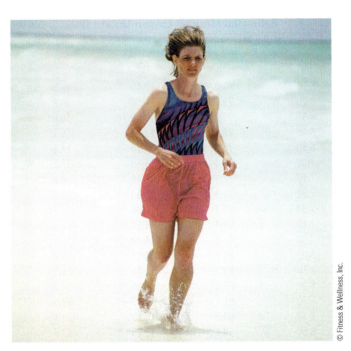

Aerobic fitness leads to better health and a higher quality of life.

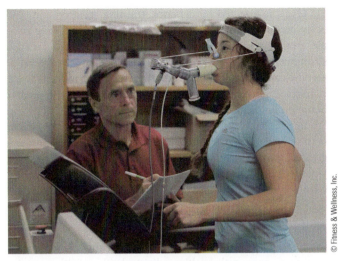

Oxygen uptake (VO_2), as determined through direct gas analysis.

Amount of Oxygen Removed from Blood

The amount of oxygen removed from the vascular system is known as the **arterial-venous oxygen difference ($a-\overline{v}O_{2diff}$)**. The oxygen content in the arteries at sea level is typically 20 mL of oxygen per 100 mL of blood. (This value decreases at higher altitudes because of the drop in barometric pressure, which affects the amount of oxygen picked up by hemoglobin.) The oxygen content in the veins during a resting state is about 15 mL per 100 mL. Thus, the $a-\overline{v}O_{2diff}$ —the amount of oxygen in the arteries minus the amount in the veins—at rest is 5 mL per 100 mL. The arterial value remains constant during both resting and exercise conditions. Because of the additional oxygen removed during maximal exercise, the venous oxygen content drops to about 5 mL per 100 mL, yielding an $a-\overline{v}O_{2diff}$ of 15 mL per 100 mL. The latter value may be slightly higher in endurance athletes.

These three factors are used to compute VO_2 using the following equation:

$$VO_2 \text{ in L/min} = (HR \times SV \times a-\overline{v}O_{2diff}) \div 100,000$$

where HR is the heart rate and SV is the stroke volume. For example, the resting VO_2 (also known as the resting metabolic rate) of an individual with an RHR of 76 bpm and a stroke volume of 79 mL would be

$$VO_2 \text{ in L/min } 5 (76 \times 79 \times 5) \div 100,000 = .3 \text{ L/min.}$$

Likewise, the VO_{2max} of a person exercising maximally who achieves a heart rate of 190 bpm and a maximal stroke volume of 120 mL would be

$$VO_{2max} \text{ in L/min } 5 (190 \times 120 \times 15) \div 100,000 = 3.42 \text{ L/min.}$$

To convert L/min to mL/kg/min, multiply the L/min value by 1,000 and divide by body weight in kilograms. In the preceding example, if the person weighs 70 kilograms, the VO_{2max} would be 48.9 mL/kg/min ($3.42 \times 1000 \div 70$).

Because the actual measurement of the stroke volume and the $a-\overline{v}O_{2diff}$ is impractical in the fitness setting, VO_2 also is determined through gas (air) analysis. To do so, the air exhaled by a person being tested is analyzed by a metabolic cart that measures the difference in oxygen content between the person's exhaled air and the atmosphere. The air we breathe contains 21 percent oxygen; thus, VO_2 can be assessed by establishing the difference between 21 percent and the percentage of oxygen left in the air the person exhales, according to the total volume of air taken into the lungs. This type of equipment, however, is expensive. Consequently, several alternative methods of estimating VO_{2max} using limited equipment have been developed. These methods are discussed next.

GLOSSARY

Nonresponders Individuals who exhibit small or no improvements in fitness compared to others who undergo the same training program.

Principle of individuality Training concept holding that genetics plays a role in individual responses to exercise training and these differences must be considered when designing exercise programs for different people.

Physical activity Bodily movement produced by skeletal muscles, which requires expenditure of energy and produces progressive health benefits. Examples include walking, taking the stairs, dancing, gardening, working in the yard, cleaning the house, shoveling snow, washing the car, and all forms of structured exercise.

Exercise Type of physical activity that requires planned, structured, and repetitive bodily movement with the intent of improving or maintaining one or more components of physical fitness.

Maximal heart rate (MHR) Highest heart rate for a person, related primarily to age.

Arterial-venous oxygen difference ($a-\overline{v}O_{2diff}$) Amount of oxygen removed from the blood as determined by the difference in oxygen content between arterial and venous blood.

VO_{2max} is affected by genetics, training, gender, age, and body composition. Although aerobic training can help people attain good or excellent CR fitness, only those with a strong genetic component are able to reach an "elite" level of aerobic capacity (60 to 80 mL/kg/min). Furthermore, VO_{2max} is 15 to 30 percent higher in men. This is related to a greater hemoglobin content, lower body fat (see "Essential and Storage Fat" in Chapter 4, page 137), and larger heart size in men (a larger heart pumps more blood and thus produces a greater stroke volume). VO_{2max} also decreases by about 1 percent per year starting at age 25. This decrease, however, is only .5 percent per year in physically active individuals.

Tests to Estimate VO₂max

Even though most CR endurance tests probably are safe to administer to apparently healthy individuals (those with no major coronary risk factors or symptoms), a health history questionnaire (including the PAR-Q), such as found in Activity 1.3 in Chapter 1, should be used as a minimum screening tool prior to exercise testing or participation. The American College of Sports Medicine (ACSM) also recommends that individuals at risk, with signs or symptoms suggestive of or diagnosed with cardiovascular, kidney, or **metabolic disease**, undergo a medical examination prior to exercise testing or exercise participation.[2]

Five exercise tests used to assess CR fitness are introduced in this chapter: the 1.5-Mile Run Test, the 1.0-Mile Walk Test, the Step Test, the Astrand-Ryhming Test, and the 12-Minute Swim Test. The procedures for each test are explained in detail in Figure 6.2, Figure 6.3, Figure 6.4, Figure 6.5, and Figure 6.6, respectively. The 1.5-Mile Run Test and the Swim Test are considered maximal tests because they require an all-out or nearly all-out effort on the part of the participant. Submaximal exercise tests do not require all-out efforts.

You may choose one or more of these tests depending on time, equipment, and individual physical limitations. For

Figure 6.2 Procedure for the 1.5-Mile Run Test.

1. Make sure you qualify for this test. This test is contraindicated for unconditioned beginners, individuals with symptoms of heart disease, and those with known heart disease or risk factors.
2. Select the testing site. Find a school track (each lap is one-fourth of a mile) or a premeasured 1.5-mile course.
3. Have a stopwatch available to determine your time.
4. Conduct a few warm-up exercises prior to the test. Do some stretching exercises, some walking, and slow jogging.
5. Initiate the test and try to cover the distance in the fastest time possible (walking or jogging). Time yourself during the run to see how fast you have covered the distance. If any unusual symptoms arise during the test, do not continue. Stop immediately and retake the test after another 6 weeks of aerobic training.
6. At the end of the test, cool down by walking or jogging slowly for another 3 to 5 minutes. Do not sit or lie down after the test.
7. According to your performance time, look up your estimated maximal oxygen uptake (VO_{2max}) in Table 6.2.

Example: A 20-year-old male runs the 1.5-mile course in 10 minutes and 20 seconds. Table 6.2 shows a VO_{2max} of 49.5 mL/kg/min for a time of 10:20. According to Table 6.8, this VO_{2max} would place him in the "good" cardiorespiratory fitness category.

Table 6.2 Estimated Maximal Oxygen Uptake (VO₂max) for the 1.5-Mile Run Test

Time	VO₂max (mL/kg/min)	Time	VO₂max (mL/kg/min)
6:10	80.0	12:40	39.8
6:20	79.0	12:50	39.2
6:30	77.9	13:00	38.6
6:40	76.7	13:10	38.1
6:50	75.5	13:20	37.8
7:00	74.0	13:30	37.2
7:10	72.6	13:40	36.8
7:20	71.3	13:50	36.3
7:30	69.9	14:00	35.9
7:40	68.3	14:10	35.5
7:50	66.8	14:20	35.1
8:00	65.2	14:30	34.7
8:10	63.9	14:40	34.3
8:20	62.5	14:50	34.0
8:30	61.2	15:00	33.6
8:40	60.2	15:10	33.1
8:50	59.1	15:20	32.7
9:00	58.1	15:30	32.2
9:10	56.9	15:40	31.8
9:20	55.9	15:50	31.4
9:30	54.7	16:00	30.9
9:40	53.5	16:10	30.5
9:50	52.3	16:20	30.2
10:00	51.1	16:30	29.8
10:10	50.4	16:40	29.5
10:20	49.5	16:50	29.1
10:30	48.6	17:00	28.9
10:40	48.0	17:10	28.5
10:50	47.4	17:20	28.3
11:00	46.6	17:30	28.0
11:10	45.8	17:40	27.7
11:20	45.1	17:50	27.4
11:30	44.4	18:00	27.1
11:40	43.7	18:10	26.8
11:50	43.2	18:20	26.6
12:00	42.3	18:30	26.3
12:10	41.7	18:40	26.0
12:20	41.0	18:50	25.7
12:30	40.4	19:00	25.4

Adapted from K. H. Cooper, "A Means of Assessing Maximal Oxygen Intake," *Journal of the American Medical Association*, 203 (1968): 201–204; M. L. Pollock, J. H. Wilmore, and S. M. Fox III, *Health and Fitness Through Physical Activity* (New York: John Wiley & Sons, 1978); and J. H. Wilmore and D. L. Costill, *Training for Sport and Activity* (Dubuque, IA: Wm. C. Brown Publishers, 1988).

example, people who can't jog or walk can take the Astrand-Ryhming (bicycle) Test or 12-Minute Swim Test. However, because these tests are different and only estimate VO_{2max}, they may not yield the same results. Therefore, to make valid comparisons, you should take the same test when doing pre- and postassessments. You can record the results of your test or tests in Activity 6.1.

1.5-Mile Run Test

The 1.5-Mile Run Test is used most frequently to predict VO_{2max}, according to the time the person takes to run or walk

Figure 6.3 Procedure for the 1.0-Mile Walk Test.

1. Select the testing site. Use a 440-yard track (4 laps to a mile) or a premeasured 1.0-mile course.
2. Determine your body weight in pounds prior to the test.
3. Have a stopwatch available to determine total walking time and exercise heart rate.
4. Walk the 1.0-mile course at a brisk pace (the exercise heart rate at the end of the test should be above 120 beats per minute).
5. At the end of the 1.0-mile walk, check your walking time and immediately count your pulse for 10 seconds. Multiply the 10-second pulse count by 6 to obtain the exercise heart rate in beats per minute.
6. Convert the walking time from minutes and seconds to minute units. Because each minute has 60 seconds, divide the seconds by 60 to obtain the fraction of a minute. For instance, a walking time of 12 minutes and 15 seconds would equal 12 + (15 ÷ 60), or 12.25 minutes.
7. To obtain the estimated maximal oxygen uptake (VO_{2max}) in mL/kg/min, plug your values in the following equation:
   $$VO_{2max} = 88.768 - (0.0957 \times W) + (8.892 \times G) - (1.4537 \times T) - (0.1194 \times HR)$$

Where:

W = Weight in pounds
G = Gender (use 0 for women and 1 for men)
T = Total time for the one-mile walk in minutes (see item 6)
HR = Exercise heart rate in beats per minute at the end of the 1.0-mile walk

Example: A 19-year-old female who weighs 140 pounds completed the 1.0-mile walk in 14 minutes 39 seconds with an exercise heart rate of 148 beats per minute. Her estimated VO_{2max} would be:

W = 140 lbs
G = 0 (female gender = 0)
T = 14:39 = 14 + (39 ÷ 60) = 14.65 min
HR = 148 bpm
VO_{2max} = 88.768 − (0.0957 × 140) + (8.892 × 0) − (1.4537 × 14.65) − (0.1194 × 148)
VO_{2max} = 36.4 mL/kg/min

SOURCE: F. A. Dolgener, L. D. Hensley, J. J. Marsh, and J. K. Fjelstul, "Validation of the Rockport Fitness Walking Test in College Males and Females," *Research Quarterly for Exercise and Sport* 65 (1994): 152–158.

a 1.5-mile course (Figure 6.2). VO_{2max} is estimated based on the time the person takes to cover the distance (Table 6.2).

The only equipment necessary to conduct this test is a stopwatch and a track or premeasured 1.5-mile course. This perhaps is the easiest test to administer, but a note of caution is in order when conducting the test: Given that the objective is to cover the distance in the shortest time, it is considered a maximal exercise test. The 1.5-Mile Run Test should be limited to conditioned individuals who have been cleared for exercise. The test is not recommended for unconditioned beginners, men over age 45 and women over age 55 without proper medical clearance, symptomatic individuals, or those with known disease or risk factors for heart disease. A program of at least 6 weeks of aerobic training is recommended before unconditioned individuals take this test.

1.0-Mile Walk Test

The 1.0-Mile Walk Test can be used by individuals who are unable to run because of low fitness levels or injuries. All that is required is a brisk 1.0-mile walk that elicits an exercise heart rate of at least 120 bpm at the end of the test.

You need to know how to take your heart rate by counting your pulse. You can do this by gently placing the middle and index fingers over the radial artery on the inside of the wrist on the side of the thumb or over the carotid artery in the neck just below the jaw next to the voice box. You should not use the thumb to check the pulse because it has a strong pulse of its own, which can make you miscount. When checking the carotid pulse, do not press too hard because it may cause a reflex action that slows the heart. For checking the pulse over the carotid artery, some exercise experts recommend that the hand on the same side of the neck (right hand over right carotid artery) be used to avoid excessive pressure on the artery. With minimum experience, however, you can be accurate using either hand as long as you apply only gentle pressure. If available, heart rate monitors can be used to increase the accuracy of heart rate assessment.

VO_{2max} is estimated according to a prediction equation that requires the following data: 1.0-mile walk time, exercise heart rate at the end of the walk, gender, and body weight in pounds. The procedure for this test and the equation are given in Figure 6.3.

Step Test

The Step Test requires little time and equipment and can be administered to almost anyone, because a submaximal workload is used to estimate VO_{2max}. Symptomatic and diseased individuals should not take this test. Significantly overweight individuals and those with joint problems in the lower extremities may have difficulty performing the test.

The actual test takes only 3 minutes. A 15-second recovery heart rate is taken between 5 and 20 seconds following the test (Figure 6.4 and Table 6.3). The required equipment

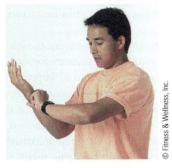

Pulse taken at the radial artery.

© Fitness & Wellness, Inc.

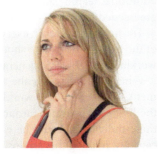

Pulse taken at the carotid (right) artery.

© Fitness & Wellness, Inc.

GLOSSARY

Metabolic disease Any condition that disrupts normal metabolism.

Figure 6.4 **Procedure for the step test.**

1. Conduct the test with a bench or gymnasium bleacher 16¼ inches high.
2. Perform the stepping cycle to a four-step cadence (up-up-down-down). Men should perform 24 complete step-ups per minute, regulated with a metronome set at 96 beats per minute. Women perform 22 step-ups per minute, or 88 beats per minute on the metronome.
3. Allow a brief practice period of 5 to 10 seconds to familiarize yourself with the stepping cadence.
4. Begin the test and perform the step-ups for exactly 3 minutes.
5. Upon completing the 3 minutes, remain standing and take your heart rate for a 15-second interval from 5 to 20 seconds into recovery. Convert recovery heart rate to beats per minute (multiply 15-second heart rate by 4).
6. Maximal oxygen uptake (VO_{2max}) in mL/kg/min is estimated

according to the following equations:
Men:
$VO_{2max} = 111.33 - (0.42 \times \text{recovery heart rate in bpm})$
Women:
$VO_{2max} = 65.81 - (0.1847 \times \text{recovery heart rate in bpm})$

Example: The recovery 15-second heart rate for a male following the 3-minute step test is found to be 39 beats. His VO_{2max} is estimated as follows:
15-second heart rate = 39 beats
Minute heart rate = 39 × 4 = 156 bpm
$VO_{2max} = 111.33 - (0.42 \times 156) = 45.81$ mL/kg/min
VO_{2max} also can be obtained according to recovery heart rates in Table 6.3.

SOURCE: McArdle, W.D., et al. *Exercise Physiology: Energy, Nutrition, and Human Performance* (Philadelphia: Lea & Febiger, 1986).

Table 6.3 **Predicted Maximal Oxygen Uptake for the Step Test**

15-Sec HR	HR (bpm)	Men (mL/kg/min)	Women (mL/kg/min)
30	120	60.9	43.6
31	124	59.3	42.9
32	128	57.6	42.2
33	132	55.9	41.4
34	136	54.2	40.7
35	140	52.5	40.0
36	144	50.9	39.2
37	148	49.2	38.5
38	152	47.5	37.7
39	156	45.8	37.0
40	160	44.1	36.3
41	164	42.5	35.5
42	168	40.8	34.8
43	172	39.1	34.0
44	176	37.4	33.3
45	180	35.7	32.6
46	184	34.1	31.8
47	188	32.4	31.1
48	192	30.7	30.3
49	196	29.0	29.6
50	200	27.3	28.9

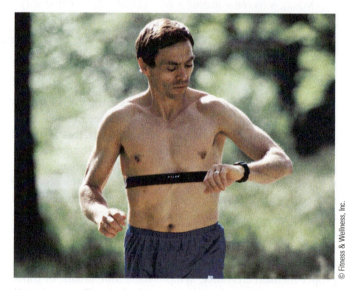

Heart rate monitors increase the accuracy of heart rate assessment.

© Fitness & Wellness, Inc.

consists of a bench or gymnasium bleacher 16¼ inches high, a stopwatch, and a metronome.

People taking this test also need to know how to take their heart rate by counting their pulse, as just discussed for the 1.0-Mile Walk Test. Once people learn to take their own heart rate, a large group of people can be tested at once, using gymnasium bleachers for the steps.

Astrand-Ryhming Test

Because of its simplicity and practicality, the Astrand-Ryhming Test is one of the most popular tests used to estimate VO_{2max} in a laboratory setting. The test is conducted on a bicycle ergometer and, similar to the Step Test, requires only submaximal workloads and little time to administer.

The cautions given for the Step Test also apply to the Astrand-Ryhming Test. Nevertheless, because the participant does not have to support his or her own body weight while riding the bicycle, overweight individuals and those with limited joint problems in the lower extremities can take this test.

The bicycle ergometer to be used for this test should allow the regulation of workloads (see the test procedure in Figure 6.5). Besides the bicycle ergometer, a stopwatch and an additional technician to monitor the participant's heart rate are needed to conduct the test.

The heart rate is taken every minute for 6 minutes. At the end of the test, the heart rate should be in the range given for each workload in Table 6.5 (generally between 120 and 170 bpm).

When administering the test to older people, good judgment is essential. Low workloads should be used, because if the higher heart rates (around 150 to 170 bpm) are reached, these individuals could be working near or at their maximal capacity, making this an unsafe test without adequate medical supervision. When testing older people, choose workloads so that the final exercise heart rates do not exceed 130 to 140 bpm.

Figure 6.5 Procedure for the Astrand-Ryhming Test.

1. Adjust the bike seat so the knees are almost completely extended as the foot goes through the bottom of the pedaling cycle.
2. During the test, keep the speed constant at 50 revolutions per minute. Test duration is 6 minutes.
3. Select the appropriate workload for the bike based on gender, age, weight, health, and estimated fitness level. For unconditioned individuals: women, use 300 kpm (kilopounds per meter) or 450 kpm; men, 300 kpm or 600 kpm. Conditioned adults: women, 450 kpm or 600 kpm; men, 600 kpm or 900 kpm.*
4. Ride the bike for 6 minutes and check the heart rate every minute during the last 15 seconds of each minute. Determine heart rate by recording the time it takes to count 30 pulse beats and then converting to beats per minute using Table 6.4.
5. Average the final two heart rates (5th and 6th minutes). If these two heart rates are not within 5 beats per minute of each other, continue the test for another few minutes until this is accomplished. If the heart rate continues to climb significantly after the 6th minute, stop the test and rest for 15 to 20 minutes. You may then retest, preferably at a lower workload. The final average

heart rate should also fall between the ranges given for each workload in Table 6.5 (men: 300 kpm = 120 to 140 beats per minute; 600 kpm = 120 to 170 beats per minute).
6. Based on the average heart rate of the final 2 minutes and your workload, look up the maximal oxygen uptake (VO_{2max}) in Table 6.5 (for example: men: 600 kpm and average heart rate = 145, VO_{2max} = 2.4 L/min).
7. Correct VO_{2max} using the correction factors found in Table 6.6 (if VO_{2max} = 2.4 and age 35, correction factor = .870. Multiply 2.4 × .870 and final corrected VO_{2max} = 2.09 L/min).
8. To obtain VO_{2max} in mL/kg/min, multiply the VO_{2max} by 1,000 (to convert liters to milliliters) and divide by body weight in kilograms (to obtain kilograms, divide your body weight in pounds by 2.2046).

Example: Corrected VO_{2max} = 2.09 L/min
Body weight = 132 pounds ÷ 2.2046 = 60 kilograms

$$VO_{2max} \text{ in mL/kg/min} = \frac{2.09 \times 1,000}{60} = 34.8 \text{ mL/kg/min}$$

*On the Monark bicycle ergometer, at a speed of 50 revolutions per minute, a load of 1 kp = 300 kpm, 1.5 kp = 450 kpm, 2 kp = 600 kpm, and so forth, with increases of 150 kpm to each half kp.

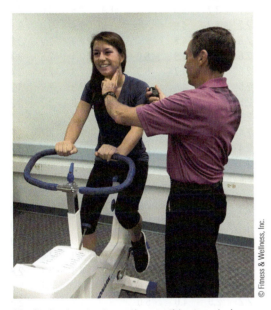

Monitoring heart rate on the carotid artery during the Astrand-Ryhming Test.

than an unskilled swimmer. Unskilled and unconditioned swimmers can expect lower CR fitness ratings than can be obtained with a land-based test. In addition, improper breathing patterns cause premature fatigue. Overweight individuals are more buoyant in the water, and the larger surface area (body size) produces more friction against movement in the water medium.

Lack of conditioning affects swimming test results as well. An unconditioned yet skilled swimmer who is in good CR shape because of a regular jogging program will not perform as effectively in a swimming test.

Because of these limitations, VO_{2max} cannot be estimated for a swimming test, and the fitness categories given in Table 6.7 are only estimated ratings.

> **!**
> ## Critical Thinking
> Should fitness testing be a part of a fitness program? Why or why not? Does preparticipation fitness testing have benefits, or should fitness testing be done at a later date?

12-Minute Swim Test

Similar to the 1.5-Mile Run Test, the 12-Minute Swim Test is considered a maximal exercise test, and the same precautions apply. The objective is to swim as far as possible during the 12-Minute Swim Test (Figure 6.6).

Unlike with land-based tests, predicting VO_{2max} through a swimming test is difficult. A swimming test is practical only for those who are planning to take part in a swimming program or who cannot perform any of the other tests. Differences in skill level, swimming conditioning, and body composition greatly affect the energy requirements (VO_2) of swimming. A skilled swimmer is able to swim more efficiently and expend less energy

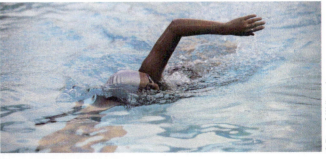

Only those with swimming skill and proper conditioning should take the 12-Minute Swim Test.

Table 6.4 Conversion of the Time for 30 Pulse Beats to Pulse Rate per Minute

Sec	Bpm	Sec	bpm	Sec	Bpm
22.0	82	17.3	104	12.6	143
21.9	82	17.2	105	12.5	144
21.8	83	17.1	105	12.4	145
21.7	83	17.0	106	12.3	146
21.6	83	16.9	107	12.2	148
21.5	84	16.8	107	12.1	149
21.4	84	16.7	108	12.0	150
21.3	85	16.6	108	11.9	151
21.2	85	16.5	109	11.8	153
21.1	85	16.4	110	11.7	154
21.0	86	16.3	110	11.6	155
20.9	86	16.2	111	11.5	157
20.8	87	16.1	112	11.4	158
20.7	87	16.0	113	11.3	159
20.6	87	15.9	113	11.2	161
20.5	88	15.8	114	11.1	162
20.4	88	15.7	115	11.0	164
20.3	89	15.6	115	10.9	165
20.2	89	15.5	116	10.8	167
20.1	90	15.4	117	10.7	168
20.0	90	15.3	118	10.6	170
19.9	90	15.2	118	10.5	171
19.8	91	15.1	119	10.4	173
19.7	91	15.0	120	10.3	175
19.6	92	14.9	121	10.2	176
19.5	92	14.8	122	10.1	178
19.4	93	14.7	122	10.0	180
19.3	93	14.6	123	9.9	182
19.2	94	14.5	124	9.8	184
19.1	94	14.4	125	9.7	186
19.0	95	14.3	126	9.6	188
18.9	95	14.2	127	9.5	189
18.8	96	14.1	128	9.4	191
18.7	96	14.0	129	9.3	194
18.6	97	13.9	129	9.2	196
18.5	97	13.8	130	9.1	198
18.4	98	13.7	131	9.0	200
18.3	98	13.6	132	8.9	202
18.2	99	13.5	133	8.8	205
18.1	99	13.4	134	8.7	207
18.0	100	13.3	135	8.6	209
17.9	101	13.2	136	8.5	212
17.8	101	13.1	137	8.4	214
17.7	102	13.0	138	8.3	217
17.6	102	12.9	140	8.2	220
17.5	103	12.8	141	8.1	222
17.4	103	12.7	142	8.0	225

Table 6.5 Maximal Oxygen Uptake (VO_{2max}) Estimates for the Astrand-Ryhming Test

Heart Rate	Men Workload					Women Workload				
	300	600	900	1200	1,500	300	450	600	750	900
120	2.2	3.4	4.8			2.6	3.4	4.1	4.8	
121	2.2	3.4	4.7			2.5	3.3	4.0	4.8	
122	2.2	3.4	4.6			2.5	3.2	3.9	4.7	
123	2.1	3.4	4.6			2.4	3.1	3.9	4.6	
124	2.1	3.3	4.5	6.0		2.4	3.1	3.8	4.5	
125	2.0	3.2	4.4	5.9		2.3	3.0	3.7	4.4	
126	2.0	3.2	4.4	5.8		2.3	3.0	3.6	4.3	
127	2.0	3.1	4.3	5.7		2.2	2.9	3.5	4.2	
128	2.0	3.1	4.2	5.6		2.2	2.8	3.5	4.2	4.8
129	1.9	3.0	4.2	5.6		2.2	2.8	3.4	4.1	4.8
130	1.9	3.0	4.1	5.5		2.1	2.7	3.4	4.0	4.7
131	1.9	2.9	4.0	5.4		2.1	2.7	3.4	4.0	4.6
132	1.8	2.9	4.0	5.3		2.0	2.7	3.3	3.9	4.5
133	1.8	2.8	3.9	5.3		2.0	2.6	3.2	3.8	4.4
134	1.8	2.8	3.9	5.2		2.0	2.6	3.2	3.8	4.4
135	1.7	2.8	3.8	5.1		2.0	2.6	3.1	3.7	4.3
136	1.7	2.7	3.8	5.0		1.9	2.5	3.1	3.6	4.2
137	1.7	2.7	3.7	5.0		1.9	2.5	3.0	3.6	4.2
138	1.6	2.7	3.7	4.9		1.8	2.4	3.0	3.5	4.1
139	1.6	2.6	3.6	4.8		1.8	2.4	2.9	3.5	4.0
140	1.6	2.6	3.6	4.8	6.0	1.8	2.4	2.8	3.4	4.0
141		2.6	3.5	4.7	5.9	1.8	2.3	2.8	3.4	3.9
142		2.5	3.5	4.6	5.8	1.7	2.3	2.8	3.3	3.9
143		2.5	3.4	4.6	5.7	1.7	2.2	2.7	3.3	3.8
144		2.5	3.4	4.5	5.7	1.7	2.2	2.7	3.2	3.8
145		2.4	3.4	4.5	5.6	1.6	2.2	2.7	3.2	3.7
146		2.4	3.3	4.4	5.6	1.6	2.2	2.6	3.2	3.7
147		2.4	3.3	4.4	5.5	1.6	2.1	2.6	3.1	3.6
148		2.4	3.2	4.3	5.4	1.6	2.1	2.6	3.1	3.6
149		2.3	3.2	4.3	5.4		2.1	2.6	3.0	3.5
150		2.3	3.2	4.2	5.3		2.0	2.5	3.0	3.5
151		2.3	3.1	4.2	5.2		2.0	2.5	3.0	3.4
152		2.3	3.1	4.1	5.2		2.0	2.5	2.9	3.4
153		2.2	3.0	4.1	5.1		2.0	2.4	2.9	3.3
154		2.2	3.0	4.0	5.1		2.0	2.4	2.8	3.3
155		2.2	3.0	4.0	5.0		1.9	2.4	2.8	3.2
156		2.2	2.9	4.0	5.0		1.9	2.3	2.8	3.2
157		2.1	2.9	3.9	4.9		1.9	2.3	2.7	3.2
158		2.1	2.9	3.9	4.9		1.8	2.3	2.7	3.1
159		2.1	2.8	3.8	4.8		1.8	2.2	2.7	3.1
160		2.1	2.8	3.8	4.8		1.8	2.2	2.6	3.0
161		2.0	2.8	3.7	4.7		1.8	2.2	2.6	3.0
162		2.0	2.8	3.7	4.6		1.8	2.2	2.6	3.0
163		2.0	2.8	3.7	4.6		1.7	2.2	2.6	2.9
164		2.0	2.7	3.6	4.5		1.7	2.1	2.5	2.9
165		2.0	2.7	3.6	4.5		1.7	2.1	2.5	2.9
166		1.9	2.7	3.6	4.5		1.7	2.1	2.5	2.8
167		1.9	2.6	3.5	4.4		1.6	2.1	2.4	2.8
168		1.9	2.6	3.5	4.4		1.6	2.0	2.4	2.8
169		1.9	2.6	3.5	4.3		1.6	2.0	2.4	2.8
170		1.8	2.6	3.4	4.3		1.6	2.0	2.4	2.7

SOURCE: I. Astrand, *Acta Physiologica Scandinavica* 49 (1960). Supplementum 169: 45–60.

Table 6.6 Age-Based Correction Factors for Maximal Oxygen Uptake

Age	Correction Factor	Age	Correction Factor	Age	Correction Factor	Age	Correction Factor	Age	Correction Factor	Age	Correction Factor
14	1.11	23	1.02	32	.909	41	.820	50	.750	59	.686
15	1.10	24	1.01	33	.896	42	.810	51	.742	60	.680
16	1.09	25	1.00	34	.883	43	.800	52	.734	61	.674
17	1.08	26	.987	35	.870	44	.790	53	.726	62	.668
18	1.07	27	.974	36	.862	45	.780	54	.718	63	.662
19	1.06	28	.961	37	.854	46	.774	55	.710	64	.656
20	1.05	29	.948	38	.846	47	.768	56	.704	65	.650
21	1.04	30	.935	39	.838	48	.762	57	.698		
22	1.03	31	.922	40	.830	49	.756	58	.692		

Adapted from I. Astrand, *Acta Physiologica Scandinavica Supplementum* 169: 45–60.

Table 6.7 12-Minute Swim Test Fitness Categories

Distance (yards)	Fitness Category
≥700	Excellent
500–700	Good
400–500	Average
200–400	Fair
≤200	Poor

Adapted from K. H. Cooper, *The Aerobics Program for Total Well-Being* (New York: Bantam Books, 1982).

Table 6.8 Cardiorespiratory Fitness Classification According to Maximal Oxygen Uptake (VO_{2max})

		Fitness Category (based on VO_{2max} in mL/kg/min)				
Gender	Age	Poor	Fair	Average	Good	Excellent
Men	<29	< 24.9	25–33.9	34–43.9	44–52.9	>53
	30–39	<22.9	23–30.9	31–41.9	42–49.9	>50
	<40–49	<19.9	20–26.9	27–38.9	39–44.9	>45
	50–59	<17.9	18–24.9	25–37.9	38–42.9	>43
	60–69	< 15.9	16–22.9	23–35.9	36–40.9	>41
	≥70	≤12.9	13–20.9	21–32.9	33–37.9	≥38
Women	<29	<23.9	24–30.9	31–38.9	39–48.9	>49
	30–39	<19.9	20–27.9	28–36.9	37–44.9	>45
	40–49	<16.9	17–24.9	25–34.9	35–41.9	>42
	50–59	<14.9	15–21.9	22–33.9	34–39.9	>40
	60–69	<12.9	13–20.9	21–32.9	33–36.9	>37
	≥70	≤11.9	12–19.9	20–30.9	31–34.9	≥35

▢ High physical fitness standard   ▢ Health fitness standard

NOTE: See the Chapter 1 discussion on health fitness versus physical fitness.

Interpreting the Results of Your VO_{2max}

After obtaining your VO_{2max}, you can determine your current level of CR fitness by consulting Table 6.8. Locate the VO_{2max} in your age category; then, on the top row, find your present level of CR fitness. For example, a

Figure 6.6 Procedure for the 12-Minute Swim Test.

1. Enlist a friend to time the test. The only other requisites are a stopwatch and a swimming pool. Do not attempt to do this test in an unsupervised pool.
2. Warm up by swimming slowly and doing a few stretching exercises before taking the test.
3. Start the test and swim as many laps as possible in 12 minutes. Pace yourself throughout the test and do not swim to the point of complete exhaustion.
4. After completing the test, cool down by swimming another 2 or 3 minutes at a slower pace.
5. Determine the total distance you swam during the test and look up your fitness category in Table 6.7.

19-year-old male with a VO_{2max} of 35 mL/kg/min would be classified in the average CR fitness category. After you initiate your personal CR exercise program (Activity 6.3), you may wish to retest yourself periodically to evaluate your progress.

HOEGER KEY TO WELLNESS

If, following your cardiorespiratory endurance test, your fitness level is less than adequate, do not let that discourage you, but do set a priority to be physically active on most days of the week and participate in aerobic exercise at least 20 minutes three times per week.

6.6 Ready to Start an Exercise Program?

Before proceeding with the principles of exercise prescription, you should ask yourself if you are willing to give exercise a try. A low percentage of the U.S. population is

Activity 6.1　Cardiorespiratory Endurance Assessment

Name _____ **Date** _____

Course _____ **Section** _____ **Gender** _____ **Age** _____

OBJECTIVE
To estimate maximal oxygen uptake (VO_{2max}) and cardiorespiratory endurance classification.

NECESSARY EQUIPMENT
1.5-Mile Run and 1.0-Mile Walk Test: School track or premeasured course and a stopwatch.

Step Test: A bench or gymnasium bleachers 16¼ inches high, a metronome, and a stopwatch.

Astrand-Ryhming Test: A bicycle ergometer that allows for regulation of workloads and a stopwatch.
12-Minute Swim Test: Swimming pool and a stopwatch.

PREPARATION
Wear appropriate exercise clothing including jogging shoes and/or a swimsuit if required. Avoid vigorous physical activity 24 hours prior to this activity.

I.　1.5-Mile Run Test

1.5-Mile Run Time: _____ min and _____ sec　　VO_{2max} (see Table 6.2, page 226): _____ mL/kg/min

Cardiorespiratory Fitness Category (Table 6.8, page 231): _____

II.　1.0-Mile Walk Test

Weight (W) = _____ lbs　　Gender (G) = _____ (female = 0, male = 1)　　Time = _____ min and _____ sec

Heart Rate (HR) = _____ bpm　　Time in minutes (T) = min + (sec ÷ 60) = _____ + (_____ ÷ 60) = _____ min

$VO_{2max} = 88.768 - (0.0957 \times W) + (8.892 \times G) - (1.4537 \times T) - (0.1194 \times HR)$

$VO_{2max} = 88.768 - (0.0957 \times$ _____ $) + (8.892 \times$ _____ $) - (1.4537 \times$ _____ $) - (0.1194 \times$ _____ $)$

$VO_{2max} = 88.768 - ($ _____ $) + ($ _____ $) - ($ _____ $) - ($ _____ $) =$ _____ mL/kg/min

Cardiorespiratory Fitness Category (Table 6.8, page 231): _____

III.　Step Test

15-second recovery heart rate: _____ beats　　　VO_{2max} (Table 6.3, page 228): _____ mL/kg/min

Cardiorespiratory Fitness Category (Table 6.8, page 231): _____

Activity 6.1 Cardiorespiratory Endurance Assessment *(continued)*

IV. Astrand–Ryhming Test

Weight (W) = _____ lbs   Weight (BW) in kilograms = (W ÷ 2.2046) = _____ kg   Workload = _____ kpm

Exercise Heart Rates	Time to count 30 beats	Heart Rate (bpm) (from Table 6.4, page 230)		Time to count 30 beats	Heart Rate (bpm) (from Table 6.4, page 230)
First minute:	[ ]	[ ]	Fourth minute:	[ ]	[ ]
Second minute:	[ ]	[ ]	Fifth minute:	[ ]	[ ]
Third minute:	[ ]	[ ]	Sixth minute:	[ ]	[ ]

Average heart rate for the fifth and sixth minutes = _____ bpm

VO_{2max} in L/min (Table 6.5, page 230) = _____ L min   Correction factor (from Table 6.6, page 231) = _____

Corrected VO_{2max} = VO_{2max} in L/min × correction factor = _____ × _____ = _____ L/min

VO_{2max} in mL/kg/min = corrected VO_{2max} in L/min × 1000 ÷ BW in kg = _____ × 1000 ÷ _____ = _____ mL/kg/min

Cardiorespiratory Fitness Category (Table 6.8, page 231): _____

V. 12-Minute Swim Test

Distance swum in 12 minutes: _____ yards   Cardiorespiratory Fitness Category (Table 6.7, page 231): _____

© Fitness & Wellness, Inc.

MINDTAP From Cengage   **Complete This Online**
Visit **www.cengagebrain.com** to access MindTap, a complete digital course that includes interactive quizzes, videos, and more.

---

truly committed to exercise. The first 6 weeks of the program are most critical. Adherence to exercise is greatly enhanced if you are able to make it through 4 to 6 weeks of training. The benefits of exercise cannot help unless you commit and participate in a lifetime program of physical activity.

The first step is to ask yourself: Am I ready to start an exercise program? The information provided in Activity 6.2 can help you answer this question. You are evaluated in four categories: mastery (self-control), attitude, health, and commitment. The higher you score in any category—mastery, for example—the more important that reason for exercising is to you.

Scores can vary from 4 to 16. A score of 12 or above is a strong indicator that the factor is important to you, whereas 8 or below is low. If you score 12 or more points in each category, your chances of initiating and sticking to an exercise program are good. If you do not score at least 12 points in each of any three categories, your chances of succeeding at exercise may be slim. You need to be better informed about

the benefits of exercise, and a retraining process might be helpful to change core values regarding exercise. More tips on how you can become committed to exercise are provided in the section "Getting Started and Adhering to a Lifetime Exercise Program" (page 246).

Next you have to decide positively that you will try. As per the instructions in item II of Activity 6.2, you can list the advantages and disadvantages of incorporating exercise into your lifestyle. Your list might include the following advantages:

- It will make me feel better.
- I will lose weight.
- I will have more energy.
- It will lower my risk for chronic diseases.

Your list of disadvantages might include the following:

- I don't want to take the time.
- I'm too out of shape.
- There's no good place to exercise.
- I don't have the willpower to do it.

Activity 6.2   Exercise Readiness Questionnaire

Name _____   Date _____

Course _____   Section _____   Gender _____   Age _____

> Carefully read each statement and circle the number that best describes your feelings in each statement. Please be completely honest with your answers.

I. Questionnaire

	Strongly Agree	Mildly Agree	Mildly Disagree	Strongly Disagree
1. I can walk, ride a bike (or use a wheelchair), swim, or walk in a shallow pool.	4	3	2	1
2. I enjoy exercise.	4	3	2	1
3. I believe exercise can help decrease the risk for disease and premature mortality.	4	3	2	1
4. I believe exercise contributes to better health.	4	3	2	1
5. I have previously participated in an exercise program.	4	3	2	1
6. I have experienced the feeling of being physically fit.	4	3	2	1
7. I can envision myself exercising.	4	3	2	1
8. I am contemplating an exercise program.	4	3	2	1
9. I am willing to stop contemplating and give exercise a try for a few weeks.	4	3	2	1
10. I am willing to set aside time at least three times a week for exercise.	4	3	2	1
11. I can find a place to exercise (the streets, a park, a YMCA, a health club).	4	3	2	1
12. I can find other people who would like to exercise with me.	4	3	2	1
13. I will exercise when I am moody, fatigued, and even when the weather is bad.	4	3	2	1
14. I am willing to spend a small amount of money for adequate exercise clothing (shoes, shorts, leotards, swimsuit).	4	3	2	1
15. If I have any doubts about my present state of health, I will see a physician before beginning an exercise program.	4	3	2	1
16. Exercise will make me feel better and improve my quality of life.	4	3	2	1

Scoring Your Test:

This questionnaire allows you to examine your readiness for exercise. You have been evaluated in four categories: mastery (self-control), attitude, health, and commitment. Mastery indicates that you can be in control of your exercise program. Attitude examines your mental disposition toward exercise. Health measures the strength of your convictions about the wellness benefits of exercise. Commitment shows dedication and resolution to carry out the exercise program. Write the number you circled after each statement in the corresponding spaces below. Add the scores on each line to get your totals. Scores can vary from 4 to 16. A score of 12 and above is a strong indicator that that factor is important to you, and 8 and below is low. If you score 12 or more points in each category, your chances of initiating and adhering to an exercise program are good. If you fail to score at least 12 points, you need to be better informed about the benefits of exercise, and a retraining process may be required.

Mastery: 1. [   ] + 5. [   ] + 6. [   ] + 9. [   ] = [   ]

Attitude: 2. [   ] + 7. [   ] + 8. [   ] + 13. [   ] = [   ]

Health: 3. [   ] + 4. [   ] + 15. [   ] + 16. [   ] = [   ]

Commitment: 10. [   ] + 11. [   ] + 12. [   ] + 14. [   ] = [   ]

II. On a separate sheet of paper list the advantages and disadvantages of starting an exercise program, your stage of change for aerobic exercise, and specific processes and techniques for change to help you implement your exercise program.

© Fitness & Wellness, Inc.

When your reasons for exercising outweigh your reasons for not exercising, you will find it easier to try. You should also determine your stage of change for aerobic exercise. Using the information learned in Chapter 2, you can outline specific processes and techniques for change (also see the example in Chapter 9, page 370–371).

6.7 *Guidelines for Developing Cardiorespiratory Endurance*

As far back as 380 BCE, Plato, the renowned Greek philosopher, stated: *"Lack of activity destroys the good condition of every human being, while movement and methodical physical exercise save it and preserve it."* In the 20th century, Dr. Calvin Wells, a scholar in the study of ancient disease indicates in his book *Bones, Bodies, and Disease*: "The pattern of disease or injury that affects any group of people is never a matter of chance. It is invariably the expression of stresses and strains to which they were exposed, a response to everything in their environment and behaviour…It is influenced by their daily occupations, their habits of diet…Man is a whole with his environment." These statements are more applicable than ever in our modern-day technologically driven culture.

In spite of the release of the U.S. Surgeon General's statement on physical activity and health in 1996 indicating that regular moderate physical activity provides substantial health benefits,[3] and the overwhelming evidence validating the benefits of exercise on health, longevity, and quality of life, the majority of adults in the United States still do not meet the minimum recommendations for the improvement and maintenance of CR fitness.

To develop the CR system, the heart muscle has to be overloaded like any other muscle in the human body. Just as the biceps muscle in the upper arm is developed through strength-training exercises, the heart muscle has to be exercised to increase in size, strength, and efficiency. To better understand how the CR system can be developed, you have to be familiar with the different variables that govern exercise prescription.[4]

Be aware that the ACSM recommends that exercise participants complete a cardiovascular disease risk factor assessment for the development of a comprehensive lifestyle modification program.[5] Particular attention should be paid to the following risk factors: men 45 or older and women 55 or older, family history of cardiovascular disease, cigarette smoking, sedentary lifestyle, obesity, high blood pressure, high LDL cholesterol, low HDL cholesterol, and diabetes (see Chapter 10). They may, however, initiate a light- to moderate-intensity exercise program without medical clearance if they have no signs or symptoms or known cardiovascular, metabolic, or renal disease. The ACSM has defined light-to-moderate intensity as exercise intensity below 60 percent of heart rate reserve. Anyone at high risk, symptomatic, or diagnosed with disease should undergo a medical examination prior to initiating even a **moderate-intensity exercise** program (one that noticeably increases heart rate and breathing or between 40 percent and 60 percent of heart rate reserve).

For exercise prescription purposes, the ACSM uses the **FITT-VP** principle. This acronym stands for Frequency, Intensity, Time (duration), Type (mode), Volume, and Progression Rate. A discussion of each of these principles follows. For practicability and ease of understanding, these principles are discussed in a different order.

Intensity

When trying to develop the CR system, many people ignore **intensity** of exercise. For muscles to develop, they have to be overloaded to a given point. The training stimulus to develop the biceps muscle, for example, can be accomplished with arm curl exercises with increasing weights. Likewise, the CR system is stimulated by making the heart pump faster for a specified period.

Health and CR fitness benefits result when the person is working between 30 and 90 percent of **heart rate reserve (HRR)** in combination with an appropriate duration and frequency of training (discussed next).[6] Health benefits are achieved when training at a lower exercise intensity, that is, between 30 and 60 percent of the person's HRR. Even greater health and cardioprotective benefits, as well as higher and faster improvements in CR fitness (VO_{2max}), are achieved primarily through vigorous programs.[7]

Most people who initiate exercise programs have a difficult time adhering to **vigorous exercise**. Thus, unconditioned individuals (those in the poor CR fitness category of Table 6.8) and older adults should start at a 30 to 40 percent training intensity (TI). For people in the fair fitness category, training is recommended between 40 and 50 percent TI. For those in the average category, a 50 to 60 percent TI is recommended. Active and fit people in the good category should exercise between 60 and 70 percent TI, while active people in the excellent fitness category can exercise at the higher TIs between 70 and 90 percent.

GLOSSARY

Moderate-intensity exercise CR exercise that noticeably increases heart rate and breathing, one that requires an intensity level of approximately 50 percent of capacity.

FITT-VP Acronym used to describe the CR exercise prescription variables: frequency, intensity, type (mode), time (duration), volume, and progression.

Intensity In CR exercise, how hard a person has to exercise to improve or maintain fitness.

Heart rate reserve (HRR) The difference between the MHR and the RHR.

Vigorous exercise CR exercise that requires an intensity level of approximately 70 percent of capacity.

Following 4 to 8 weeks of progressive training (depending on your starting TI) at light to moderate (30 to 60 percent) intensities, exercise can be performed between 60 and 90 percent TI. Increases in VO_{2max} are accelerated when the heart is working closer to 90 percent of HRR. Exercise training above 90 percent is recommended only for healthy, performance-oriented individuals and competitive athletes. For most people, training above 90 percent is discouraged to avoid potential cardiovascular problems associated with very high-intensity exercise. As intensity increases, exercise adherence decreases and the risk of orthopedic injuries increases.

Intensity of exercise can be calculated easily, and training can be monitored by checking your pulse. To determine the intensity of exercise or **cardiorespiratory (CR) training zone** according to HRR, follow these steps (also refer to Activity 6.3):

1. Estimate your MHR according to the following formula[8]:

$$MHR = 207 - (.7 \times age)$$

2. Check your RHR for a full minute in the evening, after you have been sitting quietly for about 30 minutes reading or watching a relaxing TV show. As previously explained, you can check your pulse on the wrist by placing two fingers over the radial artery or in the neck, using the carotid artery.

3. Determine the HRR by subtracting the RHR from the MHR:

$$HRR = MHR - RHR$$

4. Calculate the TIs at 30, 40, 50, 60, 70, and 90 percent. Multiply the HRR by the respective .30, .40, .50, .60, .70, and .90, and then add the RHR to all six of these figures (e.g., 60% TI = HRR × .60 + RHR).

Example. The 30, 40, 50, 60, 70, and 90 percent TIs for a 20-year-old with an RHR of 68 bpm would be as follows:

MHR = 207 − (.70 × 20) = 193 bpm
RHR = 68 bpm
HRR = 193 − 68 = 125 beats
30% TI = (125 × .30) + 68 = 106 bpm
40% TI = (125 × .40) + 68 = 118 bpm
50% TI = (125 × .50) + 68 = 131 bpm
60% TI = (125 × .60) + 68 = 143 bpm
70% TI = (125 × .70) + 68 = 155 bpm
90% TI = (125 × .90) + 68 = 181 bpm

Light-intensity CR training zone: 106 to 118 bpm
Moderate-intensity CR training zone: 118 to 143 bpm
Vigorous CR training zone: 143 to 181 bpm

Once you reach the vigorous-intensity CR training zone, continue to exercise between the 60 and 90 percent TIs to further improve or maintain your CR fitness (Figure 6.7).

Following a few weeks of training, you may have a considerably lower RHR (10 to 20 beats fewer in 8 to 12 weeks). Therefore, you should recompute your target zone periodically. You

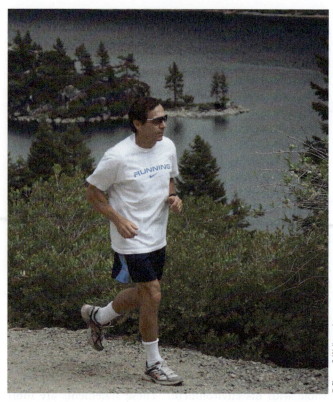

High-intensity exercise is required to achieve the high physical fitness standard (good or excellent category) for CR endurance.

© Fitness & Wellness, Inc.

can compute your CR training zone using Activity 6.3. Once you have reached an ideal level of CR endurance, frequent training in the 60 to 90 percent range allows you to maintain your fitness level.

Moderate- versus Vigorous-Intensity Exercise

As fitness programs became popular in the 1970s, vigorous exercise (about 70 percent TI) was routinely prescribed for all fitness participants. Following extensive research in the late 1980s and 1990s, we learned that moderate-intensity physical activity (about 50 percent TI) provided many health benefits, including decreased risk for cardiovascular mortality—a statement endorsed by the U.S. Surgeon General in 1996.[9] Thus, the emphasis switched from vigorous to moderate-intensity training in the late 1990s. In the 1996 report, the Surgeon General also stated that vigorous exercise would provide even greater benefits. Limited attention, however, was paid to this recommendation.

Vigorous-intensity programs yield higher improvements in VO_{2max} than do moderate-intensity programs, especially in people with higher fitness levels.[10] Furthermore, a comprehensive review of research articles looking at the protective benefits of physical fitness versus the weekly amount of physical activity found that higher levels of aerobic fitness are associated with a lower incidence of cardiovascular disease (Figure 6.8), even when the duration of

Figure 6.7 **Recommended cardiorespiratory or aerobic training pattern.**

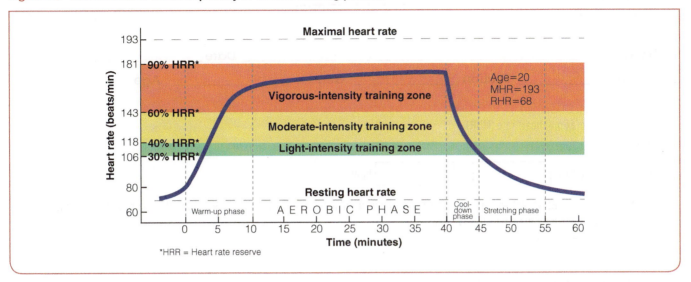

Figure 6.8 **Decrease in relative risk of cardiovascular disease (CVD) based on weekly volume of physical activity and aerobic fitness (VO_{2max}).**

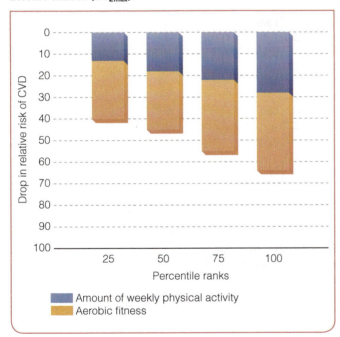

moderate-intensity activity is prolonged to match the energy expenditure performed during a shorter vigorous effort.[11] The results showed that people who accumulate the greatest amount of weekly physical activity (the 100th percentile rank in Figure 6.8) have a 28 percent reduction in the risk of cardiovascular disease; whereas the individuals with the highest level of aerobic fitness (also the 100th percentile rank in Figure 6.8) reduce their risk by 64 percent, more than twice the level of risk reduction in the most active group (timewise).

Another review of several clinical studies substantiated that vigorous, compared with moderate-intensity, exercise leads to better improvements in coronary heart disease risk factors, including aerobic endurance, blood pressure, and blood glucose control.[12] As a result, the pendulum is again swinging toward vigorous intensity because of the added aerobic benefits, greater protection against disease, and larger energy expenditure that helps with weight management.

Monitoring Exercise Heart Rate

During the first few weeks of an exercise program, you should monitor your exercise heart rate regularly to make sure you are training in the proper zone. Wait until you are about 5 minutes into the aerobic phase of your exercise session before taking your first reading. When you check your heart rate, count your pulse for 10 seconds, and then multiply by 6 to get the per minute pulse rate. The exercise heart rate will remain at the same level for about 15 seconds following aerobic exercise but then drop rapidly. Do not hesitate to stop during your exercise bout to check your pulse. If the rate is too low, increase the intensity of exercise. If the rate is too high, slow down.

When determining the TI for your program, you need to consider your personal fitness goals and possible cardiovascular risk factors. Individuals who exercise around 50 percent TI will reap significant health benefits—in particular, improvements in the metabolic profile (see "Health Fitness Standards" in Chapter 1, page 20). Training at this

GLOSSARY

Cardiorespiratory (CR) training zone Recommended TI range, in terms of exercise heart rate, to obtain adequate CR endurance development.

Activity 6.3   Cardiorespiratory Exercise Prescription

Name _____   Date _____

Course _____   Section _____   Gender _____   Age _____

I. Intensity of Exercise

1. Estimate your maximal heart rate (MHR)

    MHR = 207 − (.70 × age)

    MHR = 207 − (.70 × [_____]) = [_____] bpm

2. Resting Heart Rate (RHR). Determine your RHR by counting your pulse for a full minute in the evening after you have been sitting quietly, reading, or watching a relaxing TV show.

    RHR = [_____] bpm

3. Heart Rate Reserve (HRR) = MHR − RHR

    HRR = [_____] − [_____] = [_____] beats

4. Training Intensities (TI) = HRR × TI + RHR

    30 Percent TI = [_____] × .30 + [_____] = [_____] bpm

    40 Percent TI = [_____] × .40 + [_____] = [_____] bpm

    50 Percent TI = [_____] × .50 + [_____] = [_____] bpm

    60 percent TI = [_____] × .60 + [_____] = [_____] bpm

    70 percent TI = [_____] × .70 + [_____] = [_____] bpm

    90 Percent TI = [_____] × .90 + [_____] = [_____] bpm

5. Current cardiorespiratory fitness category (see Activity 6.1, pp. 232–233): [_____]

    Cardiorespiratory Training Zone: unconditioned individuals, persons in the poor cardiorespiratory fitness category, and older adults starting an exercise program should use a 30% to 40% TI. Individuals in fair and average fitness are encouraged to exercise between 40% and 60% TI. Active individuals in the good or excellent categories should exercise between 60% and 90% TI.

    Light-intensity cardiorespiratory training zone (30% to 40% TI): [_____] to [_____] bpm

    Moderate-intensity cardiorespiratory training zone (40% to 60% TI): [_____] to [_____] bpm

    Vigorous-intensity cardiorespiratory training zone (60% to 90% TI): [_____] to [_____] bpm

II. Mode of Exercise

Select any activity or combination of activities that you enjoy doing. The activity has to be continuous in nature and must get your heart rate up to the cardiorespiratory training zone and keep it there for as long as you exercise. Indicate your preferred mode(s) of exercise:

1. [_____]   2. [_____]   3. [_____]

4. [_____]   5. [_____]   6. [_____]

Activity 6.3 **Cardiorespiratory Exercise Prescription** *(continued)*

III. Cardiorespiratory Exercise Program

The following is your weekly program for development of cardiorespiratory endurance. If you are in the poor or fair cardiorespiratory fitness category, start with week 1. If you are in the average category, you may start at week 5. If you are already active and in the good or excellent category, you may start at week 9 (otherwise start at week 5). After completing the goal for week 12, you can maintain fitness by training between a 70% and 85% TI for about 20 to 30 minutes, a minimum of three times per week, on nonconsecutive days. You should also recompute your TIs periodically because you will experience a significant reduction in resting heart rate with aerobic training (approximately 10 to 20 beats in 8 to 12 weeks).

Week	Duration (min)	Frequency	Training Intensity	Heart Rate (bpm)	Physical Activity Perceived Exertion*
1	15	3	Between 30% and 40%	[ ] to [ ]	[ ] to [ ] beats
2	15	4	Between 30% and 40%		
3	20	4	Between 30% and 40%		
4	20	5	Between 30% and 40%		
5	20	4	Between 40% and 60%	[ ] to [ ]	[ ] to [ ] beats
6	20	5	Between 40% and 60%		
7	30	4	Between 40% and 60%		
8	30	5	Between 40% and 60%		
9	30	4	Between 60% and 90%	[ ] to [ ]	[ ] to [ ] beats
10	30	5	Between 60% and 90%		
11	30–40	5	Between 60% and 90%		
12	30–40	5	Between 60% and 90%		

*See Figure 6.9, page 240.

Maintenance cardiorespiratory training zone (60% to 90% TI): [ ] to [ ] bpm

IV. Briefly State Your Experiences and Feelings Regarding Aerobic Exercise:

_____

_____

_____

_____

_____

_____

_____

_____

_____

V. Monitoring Daily Physical Activity

How many minutes of physical activity do you accumulate (in at least 10-min segments) on a daily basis: _____

What is your average total number of daily steps (use a 7-day average): [ ]

Do you accumulate 10,000 steps on most days of the week (at least five days)? [ ] Yes [ ] No

© Fitness & Wellness, Inc.

Health and Fitness Apps

Apps are now a part of our ever-changing world. As you search for a personal health/fitness app, take into consideration your desired activities and outcome, current fitness level, personal budget, and whether you wish to use a device other than your smartphone (wrist band, chest strap, clip on, arm band). Apps provide motivation, training guidance, activity tracking, nutrition recommendations, and health advice.

Be careful when selecting apps. Many people with limited or no knowledge in the related field are designing apps. When it comes to fitness, one size doesn't fit all because fitness levels and needs vary widely among participants. An instructor or personal trainer may be a better option when getting started. If you are looking for apps, search for those designed by health and fitness experts who hold degrees and certifications in the related field. A good place to start is the government's app store (apps.usa.gov) that lists apps designed by experts.

Some apps involve a cost, while others are free. An Internet search can help identify apps in your area of need and interest. As a consumer, you are strongly encouraged to research available apps and search for the best that fit your interests but still follow recommended exercise guidelines by leading national health, fitness, and sports medicine organizations.

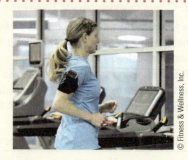

© Fitness & Wellness, Inc.

---

lower percentage, however, may place you in only the "average" (moderate fitness) category (Table 6.8). Exercising at this lower intensity will not allow you to achieve a good or excellent CR endurance fitness rating (the physical fitness standard). The latter ratings, and even greater health benefits, are obtained by exercising closer to the 90 percent threshold.

Rate of Perceived Exertion

Because many people do not check their heart rate during exercise, an alternative method of prescribing intensity of exercise has been devised using the **physical activity perceived exertion (or H-PAPE) scale** (Figure 6.9). This

Figure 6.9 Physical activity perceived exertion scale.

The H-PAPE (Hoeger-Physical Activity Perceived Exertion) Scale provides a subjective rating of the perceived exertion or difficulty of physical activity and exercise when training at a given intensity level. The intensity level is associated with the corresponding perceived exertion phrase provided. These phrases are based on common terminology used in physical activity and exercise prescription guidelines.

Perceived exertion	Training intensity
Light	40%
Moderate	50%
Somewhat hard	60%
Vigorous	70%
Hard	80%
Very hard	90%
All-out effort	100%

SOURCE: Adapted from Werner W. K. Hoeger, "Training for a Walkathon," *Diabetes Self-Management* 24, no. 4 (2007): 56–68.

scale uses phrases based on terminology common in physical activity and exercise prescription guidelines. Using the scale, a person subjectively rates the perceived exertion or difficulty of exercise when training at different intensity levels. The exercise heart rate then is associated with the corresponding perceived exertion phrase provided.

For example, if someone is training between 143 bpm (60 percent TI) and 155 bpm (70 percent TI), the person may associate this with training between "somewhat hard" and "vigorous." Some individuals perceive less exertion than others when training at a certain intensity level. Therefore, people have to associate their inner perception of the task with the phrases given on the scale. They then may proceed to exercise at that rate of perceived exertion.

Be sure to cross-check your target zone with your perceived exertion during the first weeks of your exercise program. To help you develop this association, you should regularly keep a record of your activities, using the form provided in Activity 6.4. After several weeks of training, you should be able to predict your exercise heart rate just by your perceived exertion during exercise.

Whether you monitor the intensity of exercise by checking your pulse or using the H-PAPE scale, you should be aware that changes in normal exercise conditions affect the TI. For example, exercising on a hot, humid day or at a high altitude increases the heart rate response to a given task, requiring adjustments in the intensity of your exercise.

Type (Mode)

The type, or **mode**, of exercise that develops the CR system has to be aerobic in nature. Once you have established your CR training zone, any activity or combination of activities that get your heart rate up to that zone and keep it there for as long as you exercise gives you adequate development.

Examples of these activities are walking, jogging, aerobics, water aerobics, road cycling, spinning, elliptical training, and stationary jogging or cycling. The latter activities require little skill to perform and can be enjoyed by most adults to improve health and fitness. Other aerobic activities—such as swimming, cross-country skiing, mountain cycling, rope skipping, racquetball, basketball, and soccer—can also be used and are recommended for individuals who already possess the skills to perform these activities or have adequate fitness to learn the necessary skills to safely perform them.

To be aerobic, exercise has to involve the major muscle groups of the body, and it has to be rhythmic and continuous. As the amount of muscle mass involved during exercise increases, so do the demands on the CR system. The activity you choose should be pleasant—based on your personal preferences, what you most enjoy doing, and your physical limitations. Low-impact activities greatly reduce the risk for injuries. Most injuries to beginners result from high-impact activities. Also, general strength conditioning (see Chapter 7) is recommended prior to initiating an aerobic exercise program for individuals who have been inactive. Strength conditioning can significantly reduce the incidence of injuries.

The amount of strength or flexibility you develop through various activities differs. In terms of CR development, though, the heart doesn't know whether you are walking, swimming, or cycling. All the heart knows is that it has to pump at a certain rate, and as long as that rate is in the desired range, your CR fitness will improve. From a health fitness point of view, training in the lower end of the CR zone yields substantial health benefits. The closer the heart rate is to the higher end of the CR training zone, however, the greater the health benefits and improvements in VO_{2max} (high physical fitness).

Because of the specificity of training, to ascertain changes in fitness, it is recommended that you use the same mode of exercise for training and testing. If your primary mode of training is cycling, it is best to assess your VO_{2max} using a bicycle test. For joggers, a field or treadmill running test is ideal. Swimmers should use a swim test.

Time (Duration)

The general recommendation is that a person exercise between 20 and 60 minutes per session. For vigorous-intensity exercise, a minimum of 75 total minutes per week are recommended, while those in a moderate-intensity program should accumulate at least 150 minutes per week (see Figure 6.11).

The duration of exercise is based on how intensely a person trains. The variables are inversely related. If the training intensity is around 90 percent, a session of 20 to 30 minutes is sufficient. With intensity around 50 percent, the person should train close to 60 minutes. As mentioned in the section "Intensity of Exercise," an unconditioned person or older adult should train at a lower percentage;

therefore, the activity should be carried out over a longer period.

Although the recommended guideline is 20 to 60 minutes of aerobic exercise per session, in the early stages of conditioning and for individuals who are pressed for time, accumulating 30 minutes or more of moderate-intensity physical activity throughout the day still provides health benefits. Three 10-minute exercise sessions per day, separated by at least 4 hours, and at approximately 70 percent of MHR, have been shown to produce training benefits.[13] Although the increases in VO_{2max} with the latter program were not as large (57 percent) as those found in a group performing a continuous 30-minute bout of exercise per day, the researchers concluded that the accumulation of 30 minutes of moderate-intensity physical activity, conducted for at least 10 minutes three times per day, benefits

Getting Fit Fast

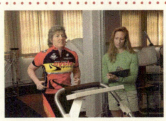

© Fitness & Wellness, Inc.

A popular myth that is often pitched through mass media (TV infomercials, radio advertisements, the Internet, magazines, and newspapers) is the "get fit fast" gimmick. This myth has been built into mass marketing to deceive consumers into buying products that purportedly provide fast and miraculous results. Statements such as "the 10-minute fitness program," "lose 16 pounds in a month," "tone up in just 5 minutes a day," and "fit into your bikini in just 30 days" are often used to catch consumers' attention.

It is time to get over this quick-fix mentality. There are no shortcuts to fitness. If it sounds too good to be true, it is! Getting fit is a process that takes commitment and perseverance, to be done according to exercise guidelines. The American College of Sports Medicine guidelines for exercise prescription are quoted extensively throughout this book. They are quite clear as to the mode, intensity, duration, and frequency of exercise required to achieve optimal results. Thus, if you are looking to get in shape overnight or in just a few days, you are only setting yourself up for failure. Furthermore, 5 to 10 minutes of daily physical activity will not make a dent in the current obesity epidemic afflicting most developed countries throughout the world.

GLOSSARY

Physical activity perceived exertion (or H-PAPE) scale A perception scale to monitor or interpret the intensity of aerobic exercise.

Mode Form or type of exercise.

the CR system significantly. Activity bouts of less than 10 minutes in duration do not count toward the 30-minute daily guideline.

Results of this and other similar studies are meaningful because people often mention lack of time as the reason they do not take part in an exercise program. Many think they have to exercise at least 20 continuous minutes to get any benefits at all. Even though a duration of 20 to 30 minutes of continuous vigorous-intensity activity is ideal, short, intermittent physical activity bouts of at least 10 minutes each are beneficial to the CR system.

Exercising for Weight Management

From a weight management point of view, the recommendation to prevent weight gain is for people to accumulate 60 minutes of moderate-intensity physical activity most days of the week,[14] whereas 60 to 90 minutes of daily moderate-intensity activity is necessary to prevent weight regain.[15] These recommendations are based on evidence that people who maintain healthy weight typically accumulate this amount of physical activity at least five times per week. The duration of exercise should be increased gradually to avoid undue fatigue and exercise-related injuries.

Exercising for Maximum Time Efficiency

If lack of time is a concern, you should exercise at a vigorous intensity for about 30 minutes, which can burn as many calories as 60 minutes of moderate-intensity exercise (also see "The Role of Exercise Intensity and Duration in Weight Management," Chapter 5, page 198). Unfortunately, only 19 percent of adults in the United States typically exercise at a vigorous intensity level. Novice and overweight exercisers also need proper conditioning prior to vigorous exercise to avoid injuries or cardiovascular-related problems.

Warm-Up and Cool-Down

Exercise sessions always should be preceded by a 5- to 10-minute **warm-up** and be followed by a 5- to 10-minute **cool-down** period (Figure 6.7). The purpose of the warm-up is to aid in the transition from rest to exercise. A good warm-up increases extensibility of the muscles and connective tissue, extends joint range of motion, and enhances muscular activity. A warm-up consists of general calisthenics, mild stretching exercises, and walking, jogging, or cycling for a few minutes at a lower intensity than the actual target zone. The concluding phase of the warm-up is a gradual increase in exercise intensity to the lower end of the target training zone.

In the cool-down, the intensity of exercise is decreased gradually to help the body return to near resting levels, followed by stretching and relaxation activities. Stopping abruptly causes blood to pool in the exercised body parts, diminishing the return of blood to the heart. The pressure in the veins of the limbs is too low to effectively pump the blood back to the heart against gravity. Immediately

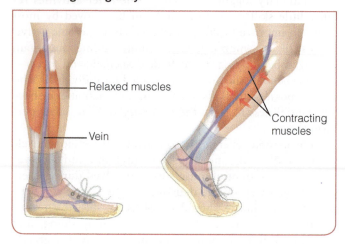

Figure 6.10 Skeletal muscle pump. Contraction of surrounding muscles aids with venous blood return toward the heart against gravity.

Relaxed muscles

Vein

Contracting muscles

following exercise, the veins in the limbs depend on the contraction of the surrounding muscles to squeeze the large amount of blood used during physical activity back to the heart, also known as the skeletal muscle pump (see Figure 6.10). Less blood return can cause a sudden drop in blood pressure, dizziness, and faintness, or it can bring on cardiac abnormalities. The cool-down phase also helps dissipate body heat and aids in removing the lactic acid produced during high-intensity exercise.

In its latest guidelines, the ACSM recommends at least 10 minutes of stretching exercises performed immediately following the warm-up phase (prior to exercising in the appropriate target zone) or after the cool-down phase. The reason for stretching following either the warm-up or the cool-down phase is because warm muscles achieve a greater range of motion, thus helping enhance the flexibility program (discussed in Chapter 8). While two to three stretching sessions per week are recommended, near daily stretching is most effective.

Frequency

The recommended exercise **frequency** for aerobic exercise is 3 to 5 days per week. When performing vigorous-intensity exercise, three 20- to 30-minute exercise sessions per week, on nonconsecutive days, are sufficient to improve or maintain VO_{2max}. When exercising at a moderate intensity, 30 to 60 minutes 5 days per week are required. A combination of moderate- and vigorous-intensity may also be used 3 to 5 days per week. Research indicates that when vigorous training is conducted more than 5 days a week, further improvements in VO_{2max} are minimal. Although endurance athletes often train 6 or 7 days per week (often twice per day), their training programs are designed to increase training mileage to endure long-distance races (6 to 100 miles) at a high percentage of VO_{2max}, frequently at or above the **anaerobic threshold**.

Behavior Modification Planning

Tips for People Who Have Been Physically Inactive

I PLAN TO

I DID IT

☐ ☐ Make exercise a priority in your daily life. Schedule exercise time as you do for any other important event of the day.

☐ ☐ Take the sensible approach by starting slowly.

☐ ☐ Begin by choosing moderate-intensity activities you enjoy the most. By choosing activities you enjoy, you'll be more likely to stick with them.

☐ ☐ Gradually build up the time spent exercising by adding a few minutes every few days or so until you can comfortably perform a minimum recommended amount of exercise (30 minutes per day).

☐ ☐ As the minimum amount becomes easier, gradually increase either the length of time exercising or increase the intensity of the activity, or both.

☐ ☐ Vary your activities, both for interest and to broaden the range of benefits.

☐ ☐ Explore new physical activities.

☐ ☐ If you have children, exercise with the kids at home. It is a win-win situation. For them it is play time. For you, exercise time. You get to spend quality time with the kids, and they will view you as a caring parent.

☐ ☐ Reward and acknowledge your efforts.

Try It

Fill out the cardiorespiratory exercise prescription in Activity 6.3 either in your text or online. In your Online Journal or class notebook, describe how well you implement the above suggestions.

Although three vigorous exercise sessions per week maintain CR fitness, when exercising at a moderate intensity, 30 to 60 minutes 5 days per week are recommended. The importance of almost daily physical activity in preventing disease and enhancing quality of life has been stated clearly by the ACSM, the U.S. Centers for Disease Control and Prevention, and the President's Council on Fitness, Sports & Nutrition. These organizations, along with the U.S. Surgeon General, advocate at least 30 minutes of moderate-intensity physical activity on most (defined as 5 days) or preferably all days of the week. This routine has been promoted as an effective way to improve health and quality of life. Furthermore, the Surgeon General states that no one, including older adults, is too old to enjoy the benefits of regular physical activity. Also, be aware that most benefits of exercise and activity diminish within 2 weeks of substantially decreased physical activity and the benefits are lost within a few months of inactivity.

"Physical Stillness": A Deadly Proposition

As introduced in Chapter 1 and Chapter 2 under "Sitting Disease" (page 14–15) and "Environmental Influence on Physical Activity" (pages 48–50), if you meet the guidelines and you are physically active five times per week, but spend most of your day sitting, your sedentary lifestyle may be voiding the health benefits of exercise. The nature of our society nowadays is such that physical activity is not required in our environment. Even people with excellent exercise habits tend to spend most of the remainder of their day in a sedentary environment: commuting to and from work, riding escalators and elevators, sitting behind a desk, sitting at a computer, reading, watching TV, and lying down. In essence, people spend most of their nonexercise time not moving.

HOEGER KEY TO WELLNESS

 Determining your exercise prescription is the easy task. The difficult part is starting and adhering to a lifetime aerobic exercise program. It will take a lifelong commitment, dedication, and perseverance to reap and maintain good cardiorespiratory fitness. The rewards, nonetheless, will be worth it: Improved health and quality of life.

If you are physically active or exercise seven times per week for 30 minutes a day, you will accumulate 210 weekly minutes of intentional activity. Even though you perceive yourself as being physically active because of the daily 30 minutes of activity, the issue at hand is the physical stillness the rest of the day. Two hundred and ten minutes translates into just 2 percent of the total 10,080 minutes available to you on a weekly basis. Thus, the difference between a regular exerciser and a sedentary individual is 30 minutes of activity per day. The other 98 percent of the time, most exercisers and sedentary people spend their time in very similar nonmoving activities.

GLOSSARY

Warm-up Starting a workout slowly.

Cool-down Tapering off an exercise session slowly.

Frequency Number of times per week a person engages in exercise.

Anaerobic threshold The highest percentage of VO_{2max} at which an individual can exercise (maximal steady state) for an extended time without accumulating significant amounts of lactic acid, which forces an individual to reduce exercise intensity or stop exercising.

Research indicates that people who spend most of their day sitting have a greater risk of dying prematurely from all causes and an even greater risk of dying from cardiovascular disease.[16] The data further indicate that death rates are still high for people who spend most of their day sitting, even though they meet the current minimum moderate-physical activity recommendations (30 minutes, at least five times per week).[17]

Thirty daily minutes of activity per day are certainly a good step toward decreasing absolute sedentarism, but it's only a small step. Your challenge is not only to exercise for a minimum of 30 minutes on most days of the week, but to consciously incorporate as much physical activity throughout the day as possible—at least 10 minutes every waking hour of the day. To meet this challenge, a change in attitude is required on your part. Your frame of mind should be: *"I do not fear nor will I avoid physical activity: Bring it on!"* Thus, increase your frequency of physical activity by learning to move as much as possible all through the day for health, quality of life, wellness, and a long life.

Volume

A relatively new concept, volume of exercise is the product of frequency, intensity, and duration. The recommended absolute minimum volume is an energy expenditure of 1,000 calories per week or the equivalent of 150 minutes of moderate-intensity exercise each week. Volume can also be measured using a pedometer and achieving 10,000 or more steps each day. This minimal amount of volume is essential to achieve health benefits and help regulate body weight. A minimum of 75 minutes of vigorous-intensity activity along with at least 2 days of 30 minutes of moderate-intensity activity are required for substantial fitness benefits.

Training volume is also used as an indicator of excessive exercise. Too much exercise and physical activity lead to overtraining, muscle soreness, undue fatigue, shortness of breath, and increased risk for injury. Should you experience any adverse effects as a result of your physical activity/exercise program, downward adjustments to the exercise prescription, including the rate of exercise progression (discussed next), are recommended.

Progression Rate

How quickly an individual progresses through an exercise program depends on the person's health status, fitness status, exercise tolerance, training responses, and exercise program goals.[18] Initially, only three weekly training sessions of 15 to

Figure 6.11 **The physical activity pyramid.**

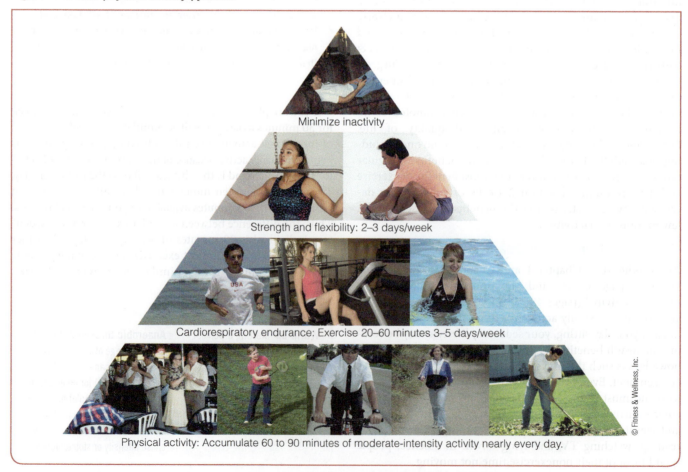

Minimize inactivity

Strength and flexibility: 2–3 days/week

Cardiorespiratory endurance: Exercise 20–60 minutes 3–5 days/week

Physical activity: Accumulate 60 to 90 minutes of moderate-intensity activity nearly every day.

© Fitness & Wellness, Inc.

20 minutes are recommended to avoid excessive muscle soreness and musculo-skeletal injuries. You may then increase the duration by 5 to 10 minutes per week and the frequency so that by the fourth or fifth week you are exercising five times per week (see Activity 6.3). Thereafter, you can adjust frequency, duration, and intensity of exercise until you reach your fitness and maintenance goals. All increases in FITT-VP variables should be gradual to minimize the risk of overtraining and injuries.

A slow and gradual rate of progression is most important for people who have been significantly inactive for several years and those who suffer from major chronic diseases such as fibromyalgia and systemic exertion intolerance disease (SEID—more commonly known as chronic fatigue syndrome). A graded exercise program, starting with 2- to 5-minute walks, may be all that is initially possible for these people. Such a minimum level of conditioning needs to be followed up with adequate rest, up to two days, before proceeding to the next activity session. The increase in duration may be limited to 1 to 2 minutes per session, and the intensity can be progressively increased as functional capacity improves over the course of several weeks or months. To sum up: Ideally, a person should engage in physical activity six or seven times per week. Based on the previous discussion (with few exceptions), to reap both the high physical fitness and the health fitness benefits of exercise, a person should do vigorous exercise three times per week for high physical fitness maintenance and moderate-intensity activities two to four additional times per week (Figure 6.11) for overall health benefits. Depending on the intensity of the activity and the health and fitness goals, all exercise sessions should last between 20 and 60 minutes. For adequate weight-management purposes, additional daily physical activity, up to 90 minutes, may be necessary. A summary of the CR exercise prescription guidelines according to the ACSM is provided in Figure 6.12.

Figure 6.12 **FITT-VP cardiorespiratory exercise prescription guidelines.**

Frequency:	3 to 5 days per week for vigorous-intensity aerobic activity or 5 days per week of moderate-intensity aerobic activity
Intensity:	30% to 90% of heart rate reserve (the training intensity is based on age, health status, initial fitness level, exercise tolerance, and exercise program goals)
Time (duration):	Be active 20 to 90 minutes. At least 20 minutes of continuous vigorous-intensity or 30 minutes of moderate-intensity aerobic activity (the latter may be accumulated in segments of at least 10 minutes in duration each over the course of the day)
Type (mode):	Moderate- or vigorous-intensity aerobic activity (examples: walking, jogging, stair climbing, elliptical activity, aerobics, water aerobics, cycling, stair climbing, swimming, cross-country skiing, racquetball, basketball, and soccer)
Volume:	Accumulate at least 150 minutes of moderate-intensity or 75 minutes of vigorous-intensity aerobic activity per week. You may also accumulate a minimum of 10,000 steps per day each day of the week (at least 70,000 steps per week)
Progression rate:	• Start with three training sessions per week of 15 to 20 minutes • Increase the duration by 5 to 10 minutes per week and the frequency so that by the fourth or fifth week you are exercising five times per week • Progressively increase frequency, duration, and intensity of exercise until you reach your fitness goal prior to exercise maintenance

SOURCE: Adapted from American College of Sports Medicine, *ACSM's Guidelines for Exercise Testing and Prescription* (Philadelphia, PA: Wolters Kluwer/Lippincott Williams & Wilkins, 2018).

6.8 *Rating the Fitness Benefits of Aerobic Activities*

The contributions of different aerobic activities to the health-related components of fitness vary. Although an accurate assessment of the contributions to each fitness component is difficult to establish, a summary of likely benefits of several activities is provided in Table 6.9. Instead of a single rating or number, ranges are given for some categories. The benefits derived are based on the person's effort while participating in the activity.

The nature of the activity often dictates the potential aerobic development. For example, jogging is more strenuous than walking. The effort during exercise also affects the amount of physiological development. For example, during a

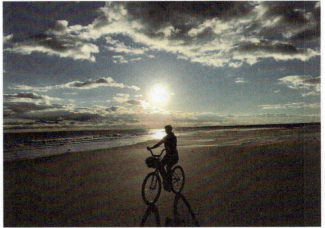

Being aerobically fit provides the freedom to enjoy most of life's leisure and recreational activities without functional limitations—a feeling difficult to explain to someone who has never reached good aerobic fitness.

low-impact aerobics routine, accentuating all movements (instead of just going through the motions) increases training benefits by orders of magnitude.

Table 6.9 indicates a starting fitness level for each aerobic activity. Attempting to participate in vigorous activities without proper conditioning often leads to injuries, not to mention discouragement. Beginners should start with light-intensity activities that carry a minimum risk for injuries.

In some cases, such as high-impact aerobics and rope skipping, the risk for orthopedic injuries remains high even if the participants are adequately conditioned. These activities should be supplemental only and are not recommended as the sole mode of exercise. Most exercise-related injuries occur as a result of high-impact activities, not high intensity of exercise.

An alternative method of prescribing exercise intensity is through **metabolic equivalents (METs)**. One MET represents the rate of energy expenditure at rest, that is, 3.5 mL/kg/min. METs are used to measure the intensity of physical activity and exercise in multiples of the resting metabolic rate. At an intensity level of 10 METs, the activity requires a 10-fold increase in the resting energy requirement (or approximately 35 mL/kg/min). MET levels for a given activity vary according to the effort expended. The MET range for various activities is included in Table 6.9. The harder a person exercises, the higher the MET level.

The effectiveness of various aerobic activities in weight management is also charted in Table 6.9. As a rule, the greater the muscle mass involved in exercise, the better the results. Rhythmic and continuous activities that involve large amounts of muscle mass are most effective in burning calories.

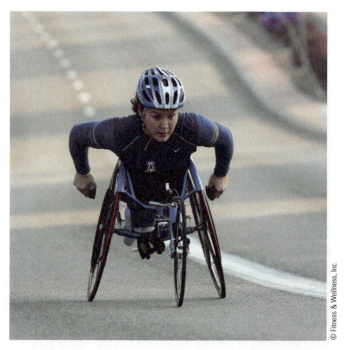

Physically challenged people can participate in and derive health and fitness benefits through a vigorous-intensity exercise program.

© Fitness & Wellness, Inc.

! Critical Thinking

Mary started an exercise program last year as a means to lose weight and enhance her body image. She now runs about 6 miles every day, strength-trains daily, participates in dance aerobics twice per week, and plays tennis or racquetball twice a week. Evaluate her program and make suggestions for improvements.

Vigorous activities increase caloric expenditure as well. Exercising longer, however, compensates for lower intensities. If carried out long enough (45 to 60 minutes five or six times per week), even walking can help with weight management. Additional information on a comprehensive weight management program was given in Chapter 5.

6.9 Getting Started and Adhering to a Lifetime Exercise Program

Following the guidelines provided in Activity 6.3, you may proceed to initiate your own CR endurance program. If you have not been exercising regularly, you might begin by attempting to train five or six times a week for 30 minutes at a time. You might find this discouraging and be tempted to drop out before getting too far because you will probably develop some muscle soreness and stiffness and possibly incur minor injuries. However, muscle soreness and stiffness and the risk for injuries can be lessened or eliminated by increasing the intensity, duration, and frequency of exercise progressively, as outlined in Activity 6.3.

Once you have determined your exercise prescription, the difficult part begins: starting and sticking to a lifetime exercise program. Exercise is not like putting money in the bank. It doesn't help much to exercise 4 or 5 hours on Saturday and not do anything else the rest of the week. If anything, exercising only once a week is not safe for unconditioned adults.

The time involved in losing the benefits of exercise varies among the components of physical fitness and depends on the person's condition before the interruption. In regard to CR endurance, it has been estimated that 4 weeks of aerobic training are reversed in 2 consecutive weeks of physical inactivity. But if someone has been exercising regularly for months or years, 2 weeks of inactivity won't hurt that person as much as it will someone who has exercised only a few weeks. As a rule, after 48 to 72 hours of aerobic inactivity, the CR system starts to lose some of its capacity.

To maintain fitness, you should keep up a regular exercise program, even during vacations. If you have to interrupt your program for reasons beyond your control, you should not attempt to resume training at the same level you left off; rather, build up gradually again.

Table 6.9 Ratings of Selected Aerobic Activities

Activity	Recommended Starting Fitness Level[1]	Injury Risk[2]	Potential Cardiorespiratory Endurance Development (VO_{2max})[3,4]	Upper Body Strength Development[3]	Lower Body Strength Development[3]	Upper Body Flexibility Development[3]	Lower Body Flexibility Development[3]	Weight Management[3]	MET Level[4,5,6]	Caloric Expenditure (cal/hour)[4,6]
Aerobics										
High-Impact Aerobics	A	H	3–4	2	4	3	2	4	6–12	450–900
Moderate-Impact Aerobics	I	M	2–4	2	3	3	2	3	6–12	450–900
Low-Impact Aerobics	B	L	2–4	2	3	3	2	3	5–10	375–750
Step Aerobics	I	M	2–4	2	3–4	3	2	3–4	5–12	375–900
Circuit Training	B	M	2–3	3–4	3–4	2	2–3	3–4	5–12	375–900
Cross-Country Skiing	B	M	4–5	4	4	2	2	4–5	8–16	600–1,200
Cross-Training	I	M	3–5	2–3	3–4	2–3	1–2	3–5	6–15	450–1,125
Cycling										
Road	I	M	2–5	1	4	1	1	3	6–12	450–900
Stationary	B	L	2–4	1	4	1	1	3	6–10	450–750
Functional Fitness	B	L	2–3	2–3	2–3	2–3	2–3	2–3	5–10	375–750
High-Intensity Interval Training	I	M	4–5	2	3-4	1	1	4-5	8–16	600–1,200
Jogging	I	M	3–5	1	3	1	1	5	6–15	450–1,125
Jogging, Deep Water	I	L	3–5	2	2	1	1	5	5–12	375–900
Racquet Sports	I	M	2–4	3	3	3	2	3	6–10	450–750
Rowing	B	L	3–5	4	2	3	1	4	8–14	600–1,050
Elliptical training/Stair Climbing	B	L	3–5	1	4	1	1	4–5	8–15	600–1,125
Strength Training	B	L	1	4–5	4–5	2–3	2–3	3–4	4–8	300–600
Swimming (front crawl)	B	L	3–5	4	2	3	1	3	6–12	450–900
Walking	B	L	1–2	1	2	1	1	3	4–6	300–450
Walking, Water, Chest-Deep	I	L	2–4	2	3	1	1	3	5–10	375–750
Water Aerobics	B	L	2–4	3	3	3	2	3	6–10	450–750
Yoga	B	L	1	1–2	1–2	3–5	3–5	1–3	4–8	300–600
Zumba	B	M	3–4	2	3	3	2	3-4	6–12	450–900

[1] B = Beginner, I = Intermediate, A = Advanced

[2] L = Low, M = Moderate, H = High

[3] 1 = Low, 2 = Fair, 3 = Average, 4 = Good, 5 = Excellent

[4] Varies according to the person's effort (intensity) during exercise.

[5] 1 MET represents the rate of energy expenditure at rest (3.5 mL/kg/min). Each additional MET is a multiple of the resting value. For example, 5 METs represents an energy expenditure equivalent to five times the resting value, or about 17.5 mL/kg/min.

[6] Varies according to body weight.

Even the greatest athletes, if they were to stop exercising, would be around the same risk for disease after just a few years as someone who has never done any physical activity. Staying with a physical fitness program long enough brings about positive physiological and psychological changes. Once you are there, you will not want to have it any other way.

A Lifetime Commitment to Fitness

The benefits of fitness can be maintained only through a regular lifetime program. Although you may be motivated after reading about the benefits to be gained from physical activity, lifelong dedication and perseverance are necessary to reap and maintain good fitness. Just reading and thinking about fitness will not provide benefits; you need active participation to derive benefits.

GLOSSARY

Metabolic equivalent (MET) Rate of energy expenditure at rest; 1 MET is the equivalent of a VO_2 of 3.5 mL/kg/min.

Activity 6.4 **Cardiorespiratory Exercise Record Form**

Name: _____ Date: _____ Course: _____ Section: _____ Gender: _____ Age: _____

Month: _____

Date	Body Weight	Exercise HR	Type of Activity	Dist. in Miles	Time in Min.	H-PAPE*	Daily Steps
1							
2							
3							
4							
5							
6							
7							
8							
9							
10							
11							
12							
13							
14							
15							
16							
17							
18							
19							
20							
21							
22							
23							
24							
25							
26							
27							
28							
29							
30							
31							
Total							

*Physical activity perceived exertion.

Month: _____

Date	Body Weight	Exercise HR	Type of Activity	Dist. in Miles	Time in Min.	H-PAPE*	Daily Steps
1							
2							
3							
4							
5							
6							
7							
8							
9							
10							
11							
12							
13							
14							
15							
16							
17							
18							
19							
20							
21							
22							
23							
24							
25							
26							
27							
28							
29							
30							
31							
Total							

*Physical activity perceived exertion.

© Fitness & Wellness, Inc.

MINDTAP From Cengage **Complete This Online**
Visit **www.cengagebrain.com** to access MindTap, a complete digital course that includes interactive quizzes, videos, and more.

Behavior Modification Planning

Tips to Enhance Exercise Compliance

I PLAN TO **I DID IT**

1. Set aside a regular time for exercise. If you don't plan ahead, it is a lot easier to skip. On a weekly basis, using red ink, schedule your exercise time into your day planner. Next, hold your exercise hour "sacred." Give exercise priority equal to the most important school or business activity of the day.

   If you are too busy, attempt to accumulate 30 to 60 minutes of daily activity by doing separate 10-minute sessions throughout the day. Try reading the mail while you walk, taking stairs instead of elevators, walking the dog, or riding the stationary bike as you watch the evening news.

2. Exercise early in the day, when you will be less tired and the chances of something interfering with your workout are minimal; thus, you will be less likely to skip your exercise session.

3. Do some activity every day. Early on, you may have a difficult time getting your workout under way. When such happens, tell yourself, "I will only exercise for 10 minutes. If I don't feel right, I will stop." Almost every single time that you apply this strategy, you will keep going and complete your entire workout. At times, the most difficult part is to get started, but once you do so, it's easy to complete the workout.

4. Select aerobic activities you enjoy. Exercise should be as much fun as your favorite hobby. If you pick an activity you don't enjoy, you will be unmotivated and less likely to keep exercising. Don't be afraid to try out a new activity, even if that means learning new skills.

5. Combine different activities. You can train by doing two or three different activities the same week. This cross-training may reduce the monotony of repeating the same activity every day. Try lifetime sports. Many endurance sports, such as racquetball, basketball, soccer, badminton, roller skating, cross-country skiing, and body surfing (paddling the board), provide a nice break from regular workouts.

6. Use the proper clothing and equipment for exercise. A poor pair of shoes, for example, can make you more prone to injury, discouraging you from the beginning.

7. Find a friend or group of friends to exercise with. Social interaction will make exercise more fulfilling. Besides, exercise is harder to skip if someone is waiting to go with you.

8. Set goals and share them with others. Quitting is tougher when someone else knows what you are trying to accomplish. When you reach a targeted goal, reward yourself with a new pair of shoes or a jogging suit.

9. Purchase a fitness or activity tracker. Build up to 10,000 steps per day or monitor your heart rate, miles logged, calories expended, or total movement time. Fitness trackers motivate people toward activity because they track daily activity, provide feedback on activity level, and remind you to enhance daily activity.

10. Don't become a chronic exerciser. Overexercising can lead to chronic fatigue and injuries. Exercise should be enjoyable, and in the process you should stop and smell the roses.

11. Exercise in different places and facilities. This will add variety to your workouts.

12. Exercise to music. People who listen to fast-tempo music tend to exercise more vigorously and longer. Using headphones when exercising outdoors, however, can be dangerous. Even indoors, it is preferable not to use headphones so that you are still aware of your surroundings.

13. Use positive self-talk. When you are tired or depressed and choose to lie down and watch TV instead of exercising, it's like telling yourself: "I am thirsty, so I can't drink anything." Instead tell yourself, "Since I am not feeling good, exercise is just what I need. I know how much better I feel afterward."

14. Keep a regular record of your activities. Keeping a record allows you to monitor your progress and compare it against previous months and years.

15. Conduct periodic assessments. Improving to a higher fitness category is often a reward in itself, and creating your own rewards is even more motivating.

16. Listen to your body. If you experience pain or unusual discomfort, stop exercising. Pain and aches are an indication of potential injury. If you do suffer an injury, don't return to your regular workouts until you are fully recovered. You may cross-train using activities that don't aggravate your injury (e.g., swimming instead of jogging).

17. If a health problem arises, see a physician. When in doubt, it's better to be safe than sorry.

Try It

The most difficult challenge about exercise is to keep going once you start. The preceding behavioral change tips will enhance your chances for exercise adherence. In your Online Journal or class notebook, describe which suggestions were most useful.

The first few weeks probably will be the most difficult for you, but where there's a will, there's a way. Once you begin to see positive changes, it won't be as hard. Soon you will develop a habit of exercising that will be deeply satisfying and will bring about a sense of self-accomplishment. The suggestions provided in the Behavior Modification Planning box (see page 249) have been used successfully to help people change behavior and adhere to a lifetime exercise program.

HOEGER KEY TO WELLNESS

Substantial health benefits are derived by being more active throughout the day (increasing NEAT). Bouts of moderate physical activity lasting 10 continuous minutes or longer provide additional benefits. Thirty minutes of nonstop moderate-intensity activity five days per week are even better. And 20 to 60 minutes of vigorous-intensity activity three to five days per week combined with everyday NEAT are best for cardiorespiratory fitness, greater health benefits, and chronic disease prevention.

Assess Your Behavior

1. Do you consciously attempt to incorporate as much physical activity as possible in your daily living (walk, take stairs, cycle, participate in sports and recreational activities)?

2. Are you accumulating at least 30 minutes of moderate-intensity physical activity over a minimum of five days per week?

3. Is aerobic exercise in the appropriate target zone a priority in your life a minimum of three times per week for at least 20 minutes per exercise session?

4. Do you own a pedometer or activity tracker and do you accumulate 10,000 or more steps on most days of the week?

5. Have you evaluated your aerobic fitness, and do you meet at least the health fitness category?

Assess Your Knowledge

1. CR endurance is determined by
   a. the amount of oxygen the body is able to utilize per minute of physical activity.
   b. the length of time it takes the heart rate to return to 120 bpm following the 1.5-Mile Run Test.
   c. the difference between the MHR and the RHR.
   d. the product of heart rate and blood pressure at rest versus exercise.
   e. the time it takes a person to reach a heart rate between 120 bpm and 170 bpm during the Astrand-Ryhming Test.

2. Which of the following is not a benefit of aerobic training?
   a. higher VO_{2max}
   b. increase in red blood cell count
   c. decrease in RHR
   d. increase in heart rate at a given workload
   e. increase in functional capillaries

3. The VO_2 for a person with an exercise heart rate of 130 bpm, a stroke volume of 100 mL, and an a-$\bar{v}O_{2diff}$ of 10 mL per 100 mL is
   a. 130,000 mL/kg/min.
   b. 1,300 L/min.
   c. 1.3 L/min.
   d. 130 mL/kg/min.
   e. 13 mL/kg/min.

4. The VO_2 in mL/kg/min for a person with a VO_2 of 2.0 L/min who weighs 60 kilograms is
   a. 120 mL/kg/min.
   b. 26.5 mL/kg/min.
   c. 33.3 mL/kg/min.
   d. 30 mL/kg/min.
   e. 120,000 mL/kg/min.

5. The Step Test estimates VO_{2max} according to
   a. how long a person is able to sustain the proper Step Test cadence.
   b. the lowest heart rate achieved during the test.
   c. the recovery heart rate following the test.
   d. the difference between the MHR achieved and the RHR.
   e. the exercise heart rate and the total stepping time.

6. An "excellent" CR fitness rating for young male adults is about
   a. 10 mL/kg/min.
   b. 20 mL/kg/min.
   c. 30 mL/kg/min.
   d. 40 mL/kg/min.
   e. 50 mL/kg/min.

7. How many minutes would a person training at 2.0 L/min have to exercise to burn the equivalent of 1 pound of fat?
   a. 700 minutes
   b. 350 minutes
   c. 120 minutes
   d. 60 minutes
   e. 20 minutes

8. The vigorous CR training zone for a 22-year-old individual with an RHR of 68 bpm is
   a. 120 to 148 bpm.
   b. 132 to 156 bpm.
   c. 138 to 164 bpm.
   d. 142 to 180 bpm.
   e. 154 to 188 bpm.

9. Which of the following activities does not contribute to the development of CR endurance?
   a. light-impact aerobics
   b. jogging
   c. 400-yard dash
   d. racquetball
   e. All of these activities contribute to its development.

10. The recommended duration for each CR training session is
   a. 10 to 20 minutes.
   b. 15 to 30 minutes.
   c. 20 to 60 minutes.
   d. 45 to 70 minutes.
   e. 60 to 120 minutes.

Correct answers can be found at the back of the book.

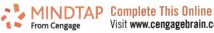 **MINDTAP** From Cengage **Complete This Online**
Visit **www.cengagebrain.com** to access MindTap, a complete digital course that includes interactive quizzes, videos, and more.

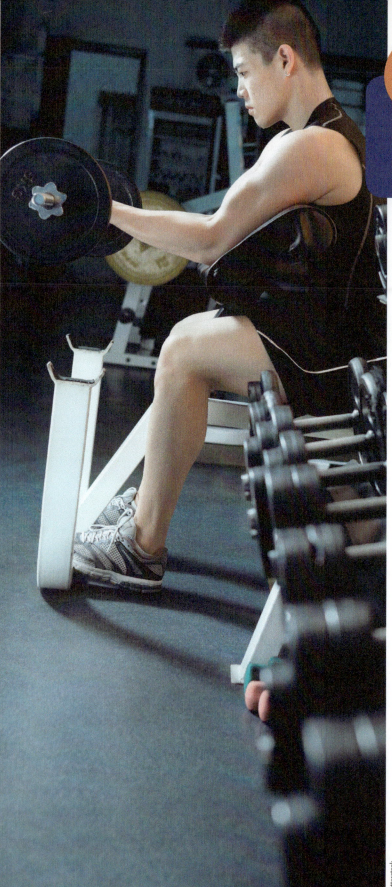

ifong/Shutterstock

7

Muscular Fitness

Progressive resistance strength-training enhances fitness, health, self-esteem and self-confidence, functional capacity, and overall well-being.

Objectives

7.1 **Explain** the importance of adequate muscular fitness levels in maintaining good health and well-being.

7.2 **Clarify** misconceptions about strength fitness.

7.3 **Define** muscular fitness, muscular strength, and muscular endurance.

7.4 **Assess** muscular strength and endurance, and learn to interpret test results according to health fitness and physical fitness standards.

7.5 **Identify** the factors that affect strength.

7.6 **Understand** the principles of overload and specificity of training for strength development.

7.7 **Learn** dietary guidelines for optimum strength development.

7.8 **Become familiar** with core strength-training and realize its importance for overall quality of life.

7.9 **Become acquainted** with two distinct strength training programs—with weights and without weights.

FAQ

Which is more important for good health: aerobic fitness or muscular fitness?

They are both important. During the initial fitness boom in the 1970s and 1980s, the emphasis was almost exclusively on aerobic fitness. We now know that a comprehensive training routine that combines aerobic fitness and muscular strength (along with regular flexibility training) contribute to health, fitness, work capacity, independent living, and overall quality of life. Among many health benefits, aerobic fitness is important in the prevention of cardiovascular diseases and some types of cancer, whereas muscular fitness builds strong muscles and bones, prevents sarcopenia (age-related muscle loss), increases functional capacity, helps prevent osteoporosis and type 2 diabetes, and decreases the risk for low back pain and other musculoskeletal injuries.

Should I do aerobic exercise or strength-training first?

If you can't afford the time, the training order should be based on your fitness goals and preferences. Aerobic training first can help improve cardiorespiratory performance and VO_{2max} to a larger extent than following the strength-training segment of exercise. Aerobic exercise followed by strength-training also has been shown to enhance post-exercise energy expenditure (calories burned during recovery from exercise). If you are trying to develop the cardiorespiratory system or enhance caloric expenditure for weight-loss purposes, heavy lower body lifting will make it very difficult to sustain a good cardio workout thereafter.

Resistance training first is more effective for developing strength, power, and muscular hypertrophy. Vigorous-intensity aerobic training has been shown to diminish strength and

power gains. Aerobic training is believed to decrease the amount of tension that can be developed during a subsequent resistance training session and may also lessen the hormonal response for muscular growth. In adults over the age of 65, strength-training first seems more effective in enhancing aerobic power because in older adults VO_{2max} is somewhat limited due to age-related loss of muscle and strength.

If strength-development is the primary objective, unless exhausting, aerobic exercise provides a sound warm-up prior to resistance training. Excessive fatigue from vigorous aerobic exercise, however, can lead to bad form while lifting and may result in injury. Thus, you need to evaluate your goals and select the training order accordingly.

The lone exception is when performing heavy-resistance strength-training. Some research indicates that heavy-resistance strength-training contributes to arterial stiffness, a contributing factor to cardiovascular problems (see box on page 280). When the ultimate goal is to maximize strength and power, for health reasons and until more definite data are available, one should always end the strength-training program with a light- to moderate-intensity aerobic workout.

Do big muscles turn into fat when you stop training?

Muscle and fat tissue are two different types of tissue. Just as an apple will not turn into an orange, muscle tissue cannot turn into fat, or vice versa. Muscle cells increase and decrease in size according to your training program. If you train quite hard, muscle cells increase in size. This increase is limited in women compared with men due to hormonal differences. When you stop training, muscle cells again decrease in size. If you maintain a

high caloric intake without physical training, however, fat cells will increase in size as weight (fat) is gained.

What strength-training exercises are best to get an abdominal "six-pack"?

Most men tend to store body fat around the waist, while women do so around the hips. There are, however, no "miracle" exercises to spot reduce. Multiple sets of abdominal curl-ups, crunches, reverse crunches, or sit-ups performed three to five times per week strengthen the abdominal musculature but are not sufficient to allow the muscles to appear through the layer of fat between the skin and the muscles. The total energy (caloric) expenditure of a few sets of abdominal exercises is not sufficient to lose a significant amount of weight (fat). If you want to get a "washboard stomach" (or, for women, achieve shapely hips), you need to engage in a moderate to vigorous aerobic and strength-training program combined with a moderate reduction in daily caloric intake (diet).

Can I use CrossFit (or a similar program) to replace a traditional strength-training program?

CrossFit is a conditioning and competitive fitness program that aims to develop overall fitness. The program focuses on constantly varied, high-intensity, and functional movements to improve fitness. Some exercise specialists have expressed concerns about the safety of CrossFit for novice participants (see box on the CrossFit exercise program provided in Chapter 9, page 353). Invariably, proper and progressive performance of CrossFit under competent supervision will lead to both strength and

(continued)

cardiorespiratory development. Because of the constant exercise variations, the fitness level achieved, however, may never equal that reached through a complete and well-executed traditional strength-training program. CrossFit and similar programs excel at addressing a wide spectrum of fitness training needs in a single high-intensity workout. Meanwhile, traditional training programs allow an individual to progressively increase weight resistance and to repeat workouts according to a schedule that maximizes improvement. Strength-fitness development achieved through CrossFit, nonetheless, will be substantial and more than adequate to achieve the excellent strength-fitness classification given in this chapter. If you like CrossFit, can safely perform the activity, can include periods of recovery as needed, and can progressively move up through the conditioning phase, by all means enjoy this exercise modality.

REAL LIFE STORY | Nathan's Experience

I started strength-training 2 years ago because I wanted to get stronger and have a more muscular build. I got a membership to a gym near my house and started using the free weights and machines there. The problem was, after a year of going off and on, I still didn't see the improvements I was hoping for. I then decided to take a strength training course at my college, and there I learned all the things that I had been doing wrong that had prevented me from getting results. My biggest mistake was that when I would go to the gym, I would try to do too much, working out for almost 2 hours, pushing myself to use heavy weights, and doing 20 different exercises. Afterwards, I would get very sore, and sometimes I wouldn't feel like going back to the gym for the rest of the week or even a couple weeks. So my workouts were off and on, and I was never consistent enough to really progress in the amount of weight I could lift. Another big mistake I made was that I didn't watch what I ate. In fact, since I had started to lift weights, I figured I could eat whatever I wanted, so I would go ahead and take an extra slice of pizza or two. The only thing I did, nutrition-wise, to try to help my efforts to get a stronger body was to buy a box of chocolate and peanut butter supplement bars that my gym sells and eat a couple a day. But my weight lifting teacher says that the ones I was buying were not much better than candy bars, and eating them in that amount was just causing me to take in way more sugar and calories than I needed. Once I changed my habits to work out moderately and consistently, to slowly increase the amount of weight I lift, and to support my routine with healthy meals and snacks, I really started to get the toned and muscular body I want!

Flashon Studio/Shutterstock.com

PERSONAL PROFILE: Personal Understanding of Muscular Fitness Concepts

I. In terms of health and wellness, is muscular fitness or aerobic fitness more important?

II. Body weight may not drop or even increase as a result of a progressive resistance strength-training program; nonetheless, circumference measurements and percent body fat may decrease. Can you describe the reason for these changes? ____ Yes ____ No

III. Performing at least one set of each strength-training exercise within the repetition maximum zone produces substantial strength development. Is this a program you could follow? ____ Yes ____ No   How does it differ from traditional programs?

IV. A periodized strength-training program is frequently used to maximize muscular strength and endurance gains. Have you ever used such an approach? ____ Yes ____ No How did it contribute to your muscular fitness?

V. In your training, have single-joint exercises been more effective than multiple-joint exercises in developing strength? ____ Yes ____ No Share your experience.

The benefits of **muscular fitness**, achieved through **strength-training** or **resistance training**, on health and well-being are well documented. Muscular fitness, achieved through **progressive resistance training**, involves both muscular strength and muscular endurance, with the corresponding improvements in **muscular power** and tone.

The need for muscular fitness is not confined to highly trained athletes, fitness enthusiasts, or individuals who have jobs that require heavy muscular work. All people need adequate muscular fitness for good health, improved functional capacity, and a better quality of life. Unfortunately, according to the 2013 survey released by the Centers for Disease Control and Prevention (CDC), only 27 percent of men and 19 percent of women meet the Federal Physical Activity Guidelines for muscular fitness. Worse yet, almost 74 percent or nearly three out of every four American adults did not participate in any type of muscular fitness activity; that is, they did not strength train or take a class that required some sort of muscular strength activity such as cardio/strength-training, Pilates, boot camp, PX90, TRX, CrossFit, or even a single push-up during their available leisure time.

7.1 Benefits of Strength-Training

A well-rounded fitness program includes aerobic exercise, strength-training, and flexibility exercises. Because of the many health benefits provided by a regular muscular-fitness training program, the American Medical Association (AMA), the American Heart Association (AHA), the American College of Sports Medicine, the American Diabetes Association (ADA), and the CDC have offered strong support of strength-training as an exercise modality to promote overall health, prevent disease, and decrease the risk for premature mortality.

Improves Functional Capacity

A well-planned strength-training program leads to increased muscle strength and endurance, power, muscle tone, and tendon and ligament strength—all of which help improve and maintain everyday functional physical capacity. Muscular fitness is a basic health-related fitness component and is an important wellness component for optimal performance in **activities of daily living** such as sitting, walking, running, lifting and carrying objects, doing housework, and enjoying recreational activities. With time, the heart rate and blood pressure response to lifting a resistance (a weight) also decreases. This adaptation reduces the demands on the cardiovascular system when you perform activities such as carrying a child, the groceries, or a suitcase.

Strength also is of great value in improving posture, personal appearance, and self-image; in developing sports skills; in promoting stability of joints; and in meeting certain emergencies in life.

Improves Overall Health

From a health standpoint, experts believe that poor muscle strength and mass make premature mortality more likely in people who develop chronic diseases. Good muscular fitness, on the other hand, improves the cardiovascular risk factor profile (better cholesterol, triglycerides, and blood pressure), decreases cardiovascular mortality, improves blood glucose and insulin sensitivity, and is as effective as aerobic exercise in the prevention and management of type 2 diabetes. Good strength fitness also helps increase or maintain muscle and a higher resting metabolic rate; encourages weight loss and maintenance, which prevents obesity; lessens the risk for injury; reduces chronic low back pain; reduces pressure on the joints, alleviating arthritic pain; aids in childbearing; improves bone density, which prevents osteoporosis; and may help prevent some types of cancer. Furthermore, it decreases the risk of developing physical function limitations and the overall risk of nonfatal disease, helps with anxiety and depression, improves energy, and reduces fatigue, thus promoting psychological well-being.[1]

Increases Muscle Mass and Resting Metabolism

Another benefit of maintaining a good strength level is its relationship to human **metabolism**. A primary outcome of a strength-training program is an increase in muscle mass or size (lean body mass), known as muscle **hypertrophy**.

Muscle tissue uses more energy than does fatty tissue. That is, your body expends more calories to maintain muscle than to maintain fat. All other factors being equal, if two individuals both weigh 150 pounds but have different amounts of muscle mass, the one with more muscle mass will have a higher **resting metabolism**. Even small increases in muscle mass have a long-term positive effect on metabolism.

GLOSSARY

Muscular fitness A term used in reference to the general health, strength, endurance, and power of a person's muscular system.

Strength-training A program designed to improve muscular strength and/or endurance through a series of progressive resistance (weight) training exercises that overload the muscular system and cause physiological development.

Resistance training See strength-training.

Progressive resistance training A gradual increase of resistance used during strength-training over a period of time.

Muscular power The ability of muscles to generate maximal force as quickly as possible.

Activities of daily living Everyday behaviors that people normally do to function in life (cross the street, carry groceries, lift objects, do laundry, sweep floors, etc.).

Metabolism All energy and material transformations that occur within living cells and are necessary to sustain life.

Hypertrophy An increase in the size of the cell, as in muscle hypertrophy.

Resting metabolism Amount of energy (expressed in milliliters of oxygen per minute or total calories per day) an individual requires during resting conditions to sustain proper body function.

Figure 7.1 Changes in body composition as a result of a combined aerobic and strength-training program.

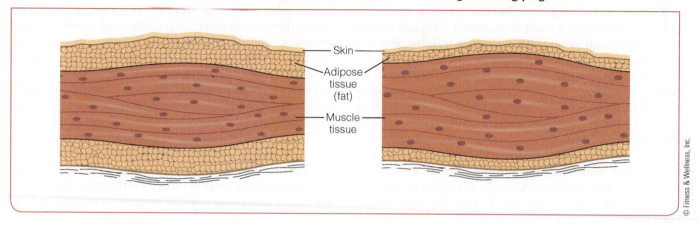

Skin

Adipose tissue (fat)

Muscle tissue

© Fitness & Wellness, Inc.

Loss of lean tissue is thought to be a primary reason for the decrease in metabolism as people grow older. Contrary to some beliefs, metabolism does not have to slow down significantly as you age. It is not so much that metabolism slows down, it's that we slow down. Lean body mass decreases with sedentary living, which in turn slows down the resting metabolic rate. Thus, if people continue eating at the same rate as they age, body fat increases. A good strength-training program can help curb that trend by increasing both muscle mass and resting metabolism.

Improves Body Composition

One of the most desirable benefits of strength-training, accentuated even more when combined with aerobic exercise, is a decrease in adipose or fatty tissue around muscle fibers. This decrease is often greater than the amount of muscle hypertrophy (Figure 7.1). Therefore, losing inches but not body weight is common. Research data have also confirmed significant drops in unhealthy visceral fat (intra-abdominal fat) through strength-training, despite little or no change in total body weight (the loss of fat is compensated for by an increase in muscle mass).

Because muscle tissue is denser than fatty tissue (and even though inches are lost during a combined strength-training and aerobic program), people, especially women, often become discouraged because they cannot see the results readily on the scale. They can offset this discouragement by determining body composition regularly to monitor their changes in percent body fat rather than simply measuring changes in total body weight (see Chapter 4).

Although it does not result in a greater amount of weight loss (because of the concomitant increase in lean body mass), research has shown that regular strength-training contributes to a greater decrease in the dangerous type of intra-abdominal visceral fat (see Chapter 4, page 141) than a similar time spent doing regular aerobic exercise. Visceral fat is thought to secrete harmful inflammatory substances that pose a greater risk for disease and premature mortality.

Helps Control Blood Sugar

Regular strength-training also helps control blood sugar. Glucose is the preferred energy fuel used by the muscles during strength-training. Much of the blood glucose from food consumption goes to the muscles, where it is used or stored as glycogen. If the glycogen stores are full, the remaining glucose will not enter the muscles but will be stored as fat in adipose tissue.

When muscles are not used, muscle cells may become insulin resistant, and glucose cannot enter the cells, thereby increasing the risk for type 2 diabetes. Research indicates that even a single strength-training exercise session enhances insulin sensitivity for the next 24 hours. Additionally, with regular strength-training, diabetic men and women improve their blood sugar control, gain strength, increase lean body mass, lose body fat, and lower blood pressure. Furthermore, across all ages, the greater the amount of muscle mass, relative to body size, the better the insulin sensitivity and the lower the risk for diabetes. Individuals with the most muscle mass cut their risk for diabetes by more than half as compared to those with the least amount.

HOEGER KEY TO WELLNESS

 Regular strength-training helps control blood sugar, decreasing the risk for type 2 diabetes. Even a single strength-training exercise session enhances insulin sensitivity for the next 24 hours.

Enhances Quality of Life as You Age

In the older adult population (65 and older), muscular fitness may be the most important health-related component of physical fitness. Although proper cardiorespiratory endurance is necessary to help maintain a healthy heart, good strength contributes more to independent living than any other fitness component. The two fundamental reasons older adults end up in assisted living are because either the brain or the muscles fail.

Studies indicate that, on average, a 30-year-old loses 25 percent of muscle strength by age 70 and about half by age 90. Once in their 50s, older adults who strength train and have adequate protein throughout the day can successfully perform most activities of daily living. Those who don't become weaker and less functional.

A common occurrence as people age is **sarcopenia**—loss of muscle mass, strength, and function. How much of this loss of muscle mass is related to the aging process itself or to actual physical inactivity and faulty nutrition is unknown. Sarcopenia leads to mobility disability and loss of independence. Muscle mass loss is also related to a lower metabolic rate, high prevalence of obesity, insulin resistance, type 2 diabetes, abnormal blood lipids, and high blood pressure. Muscular strength has also been shown to be inversely associated with all-cause mortality; the lower the strength level, the higher the risk for early mortality.[2] Estimates indicate that half of all adults 65 and older in the United States currently suffer from age-related muscle loss. Early muscle loss doesn't appear to bother them or hold them back. They think they are fine until they lose functional independence; at that point they recognize the serious mistake made and subsequent loss of quality of life.

Studies[3] further indicate that adults who do not strength train lose between 4 and 6 pounds of muscle tissue per decade of life. After age 30, inactive adults lose muscle mass at a rate of 3 percent to 8 percent per decade of life. At age 50, this loss accelerates to 5 percent to 10 percent per decade.[4] As a result, a person who has maintained body weight but did not strength train between the ages of 40 and 60 can remain at the same body mass index (BMI), but their percent body fat can easily go up 7 to 10 percentage points (i.e., 20 percent to 27 to 30 percent). A summary of 49 research studies also indicates that older adults gain an average of 2.42 pounds of lean body mass following 20 weeks of strength-training.[5] The findings are significant because so many older adults are affected by sarcopenia and strength-training can prevent much of this loss and allow these older adults to preserve independent living throughout the aging process.

More than anything else, older adults want to enjoy good health and to function independently. Many of them, however, are confined to nursing homes because they lack sufficient muscular fitness to move about. They cannot walk very far, and many have to be helped in and out of beds, chairs, and bathtubs.

A strength-training program can enhance quality of life tremendously, and nearly everyone can benefit from it. As muscular fitness improves, so does the ability to move about, the capacity for independent living, and enjoyment of life during the "golden years." In their muscular fitness training program, older adults are encouraged to regularly include repetitions at a faster speed so as to help increase muscular power. The latter component is known to decrease at a much faster rate than other fitness components during the aging process.

Specifically, good muscular fitness in older adults enhances quality of life in that it

- Improves balance and restores mobility
- Makes lifting and reaching easier
- Decreases the risk for injuries and falls
- Stresses the bones and preserves bone mineral density, thereby decreasing the risk for osteoporosis

7.2 *Gender Differences*

A common misconception about physical fitness concerns women in strength-training. Because of the increase in muscle mass typically seen in men, some women still think that a strength-training program will result in the development of large musculature.

Even though the quality of muscle in men and women is the same, endocrinological differences do not allow women to achieve the same amount of muscle hypertrophy (size) as men. Men also have more muscle fibers, and because of the sex-specific male hormones, each individual fiber has more potential for hypertrophy. On the average, following 6 months of training, women can achieve up to a 50 percent increase in strength but only a 10 percent increase in muscle size.

The idea that strength-training allows women to develop muscle hypertrophy to the same extent as men is as false as the notion that playing basketball turns women into giants. Masculinity and femininity are established by genetic inheritance, not by amount of physical activity. Variations in the extent of masculinity and femininity are determined by individual differences in hormonal secretions of androgen, testosterone, estrogen, and progesterone. Women with a bigger-than-average build often are inclined to participate in sports because of their natural physical advantage. As a result, many people have associated women's participation in sports and strength-training with large muscle size.

As the number of females who participate in sports has increased steadily, the myth of strength-training in women leading to large increases in muscle size has abated somewhat. For example, per pound of body weight, female gymnasts are among the strongest athletes in the world. These athletes engage regularly in vigorous strength-training programs. Yet, female gymnasts have some of the most well-toned and graceful figures of all women.

Improved body appearance has become the rule rather than the exception for women who participate in strength-training programs. Some of the most attractive female movie stars also train with weights to further improve their personal image.

Nonetheless, you may ask: If weight training does not masculinize women, why do so many women body builders

---

GLOSSARY

Sarcopenia Age-related loss of lean body mass, strength, and function.

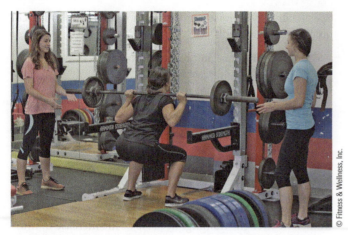

Improved body appearance has become the rule rather than the exception for women who participate in strength-training exercises.

develop such heavy musculature? In the sport of body building, the athletes follow intense training routines consisting of 2 or more hours of constant weight lifting with short rest intervals between sets. Many body-building training routines call for back-to-back exercises using the same muscle groups. The objective of this type of training is to cause sarcoplasmic hypertrophy (see page 265) and to pump extra blood into the muscles. This additional fluid makes the muscles appear much bigger than they do in a resting condition. Based on the intensity and the length of the training session, the muscles can remain filled with blood, appearing measurably larger for an hour or longer after completing the training session. Performing such routines is a common practice before competitions. Therefore, in real life, these women are not as muscular as they seem to be when they are participating in a contest.

> **! Critical Thinking**
>
> What role should strength-training have in a fitness program? Should people be motivated for the health fitness benefits, or should they participate to enhance their body image? What are your feelings about individuals (male or female) with large body musculature?

In the sport of body building (among others), a big point of controversy is the use of **anabolic steroids** and human growth hormones. These hormones produce detrimental and undesirable side effects, even more so in women (e.g., hypertension, fluid retention, decreased breast size, deepening of the voice, and whiskers and other atypical body hair growth). Anabolic steroid use in general—except for medical reasons and when carefully monitored by a physician—can lead to serious health consequences.

Use of anabolic steroids by female body builders and female track-and-field athletes is not uncommon. Athletes use anabolic steroids to remain competitive at the highest level. Even at the 2012 Olympic Games in London, the woman shot

Selected Detrimental Effects from Using Anabolic Steroids

- Liver tumors
- Hepatitis
- Hypertension
- Reduction of high-density lipoprotein (HDL) cholesterol
- Elevation of low-density lipoprotein (LDL) cholesterol
- Hyperinsulinism
- Impaired pituitary function
- Impaired thyroid function
- Mood swings
- Aggressive behavior
- Increased irritability
- Acne
- Fluid retention
- Decreased libido
- HIV infection (via injectable steroids)

- Prostate problems (men)
- Testicular atrophy (men)
- Reduced sperm count (men)
- Clitoral enlargement (women)
- Decreased breast size (women)
- Increased body and facial hair (nonreversible in women)
- Deepening of the voice (nonreversible in women)

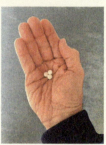

put gold medal winner was expelled from the games and stripped of her medal for using steroids. Women who take steroids undoubtedly will build heavy musculature, and if they take them long enough, the steroids will produce masculinizing effects.

To prevent steroid use, the International Federation of Body Building and Fitness instituted a mandatory steroid-testing program for women participating in the Ms. Olympia contest. When drugs are not used to promote development, improved body image is the rule rather than the exception among women who participate in body building, strength-training, and sports in general.

7.3 Assessing Muscular Strength and Endurance

Although muscular strength and endurance are interrelated, they do differ. **Muscular strength** is the ability to exert maximum force against resistance. **Muscular endurance** is the ability of a muscle to exert submaximal force repeatedly over time.

Muscular endurance (also referred to as localized muscular endurance) largely depends on muscular strength. Weak muscles cannot repeat an action several times or sustain it. Based on these principles, strength tests and training programs have been designed to measure and develop absolute muscular strength, muscular endurance, or a combination of the two.

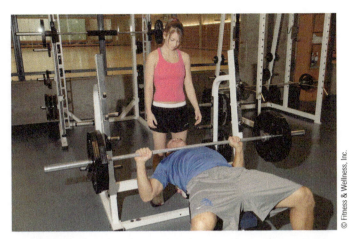

The maximal amount of resistance that an individual is able to lift in one single effort (1 RM) is a measure of absolute strength.

Muscular strength is usually determined by the maximal amount of resistance (weight)—**one repetition maximum, or 1 RM**—that an individual is able to lift in a single effort. Although this assessment yields a good measure of absolute strength, it requires considerable time, because the 1 RM is determined through trial and error. For example, strength of the chest muscles is frequently measured through the bench press exercise. If a man has not trained with weights, he may try 100 pounds and lift this resistance easily. After adding 50 pounds, he may fail to lift the resistance. Then he decreases resistance by 20 or 30 pounds. Finally, after several trials, the 1 RM is established.

Using this method, a true 1 RM might be difficult to obtain the first time an individual is tested because fatigue becomes a factor. By the time the 1 RM is established, the person already has made several maximal or near-maximal attempts.

In contrast, muscular endurance typically is established by the number of repetitions an individual can perform against a submaximal resistance or by the length of time a given contraction can be sustained. For example: How many push-ups can an individual do? Or how many times can a 30-pound resistance be lifted? Or how long can a person hold a chin-up?

If time is a factor and only one test item can be done, the Hand Grip Strength Test, described in Figure 7.2, is commonly used to assess strength. This test, though, provides only a weak correlation with overall body strength. Two additional strength tests are provided in Figure 7.3 and Figure 7.4. Activity 7.1 also offers you the opportunity to assess your level of muscular strength or endurance with all three tests. You may take one or more of these tests, according to your time and the facilities available.

In strength testing, several body sites should be assessed because muscular strength and muscular endurance are both highly specific. A high degree of strength or endurance in one body part does not necessarily indicate similarity in other parts, so no single strength test provides a good assessment of overall body strength. Accordingly, exercises for the strength tests were selected to include the upper body, lower body, and abdominal regions.

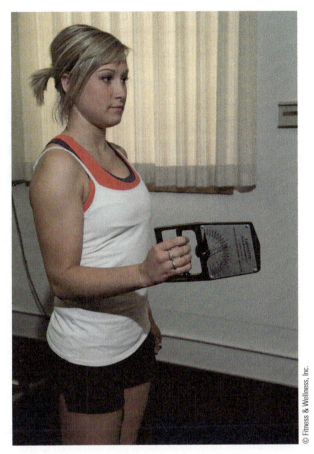

The hand grip tests strength.

Before strength testing, you should become familiar with the procedures for the respective tests. For safety reasons, always take at least one friend with you whenever you train with weights or undertake any type of strength assessment. Also, these are different tests, so to make valid comparisons, you should use the same test for pre- and post-assessments. The following are your options.

Muscular Strength: Hand Grip Strength Test

As indicated previously, when time is a factor, the Hand Grip Strength Test can be used to provide a rough estimate of strength. Unlike the next two tests, this one is isometric

---

GLOSSARY

Anabolic steroids Synthetic versions of the male sex hormone testosterone, which promotes muscle development and hypertrophy.

Muscular strength The ability of a muscle to exert maximum force against resistance (e.g., 1 repetition maximum [or 1 RM] on the bench press exercise).

Muscular endurance The ability of a muscle to exert submaximal force repeatedly over time.

One repetition maximum (1 RM) The maximum amount of resistance an individual is able to lift in a single effort.

Figure 7.2 Procedure for the Hand Grip Strength Test.

1. Adjust the width of the dynamometer* so the middle bones of your fingers rest on the distant end of the dynamometer grip.
2. Use your dominant hand for this test. Place your elbow at a 90° angle and about 2 inches away from the body.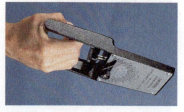
3. Now grip as hard as you can for a few seconds. Do not move any other body part as you perform the test (do not flex or extend the elbow, do not move the elbow away or toward the body, and do not lean forward or backward during the test).
4. Record the dynamometer reading in pounds (if reading is in kilograms, multiply by 2.2046).
5. Three trials are allowed for this test. Use the highest reading for your final test score. Look up your percentile rank for this test in Table 7.1.
6. Based on your percentile rank, obtain the hand grip strength fitness category according to the following guidelines:

Percentile Rank	Fitness Category
≥90	Excellent
70–80	Good
50–60	Average
30–40	Fair
≤20	Poor

*A Lafayette model 78010 dynamometer is recommended for this test (Lafayette Instruments Co., Sagamore and North 9th Street, Lafayette, IN 47903).

© Fitness & Wellness, Inc.

provided in Table 7.1. You can record your results of this test in Activity 7.1.

Changes in strength are more difficult to evaluate with the Hand Grip Strength Test than with other muscular strength tests. Most strength-training programs are dynamic (body segments are moved through a range of motion), whereas this test provides an isometric assessment.

Although more research will be required, a study of significant interest that included more than 140,000 adult participants in 17 countries over a span of 4 years showed that each 11-pound decrease in grip strength led to a 16 percent increase in risk of dying from any cause, and a 17 percent and 9 percent higher risk of dying from heart disease and stroke, respectively.[6] The association between grip strength, cardiovascular disease, and premature death prevailed even after adjusting for other cardiovascular disease risk factors.

Muscular Endurance Test

Three exercises were selected to assess the endurance of the upper body, lower body, and midbody muscle groups (Figure 7.3). The advantage of the Muscular Endurance Test is that it does not require strength-training equipment—only a stopwatch, a metronome, a bench or gymnasium bleacher $16\frac{1}{4}$ inches high, a cardboard strip $3\frac{1}{2}$ inches wide by 30 inches long, and a partner. A percentile rank is given for each exercise according to the number of repetitions performed (Table 7.2). An overall endurance rating can be obtained by totaling the number of points obtained on each exercise. Record your results of this test in Activity 7.1 and Appendix A.

Muscular Strength and Endurance Test

In the Muscular Strength and Endurance Test, you lift a submaximal resistance as many times as possible using the six

(involving static contraction, discussed later in the chapter). If the proper grip is used, no finger motion or body movement is visible during the test. The test procedure is given in Figure 7.2, and percentile ranks based on results are

Table 7.1 Scoring Table for Hand Grip Strength Test (Pounds)

Percentile Rank	Men	Women
99	153	101
95	145	94
90	141	91
80	139	86
70	132	80
60	124	78
50	122	74
40	114	71
30	110	66
20	100	64
10	91	60
5	76	58

High physical fitness standard

Health fitness standard

© Fitness & Wellness, Inc.

Figure 7.3 Muscular Endurance Test.

Three exercises are conducted on this test: bench jumps, modified dips (men) or modified push-ups (women), and bent-leg curl-ups or abdominal crunches. All exercises should be conducted with the aid of a partner. The correct procedure for performing each exercise is as follows:

Bench jump. Using a bench or gymnasium bleacher 16¼" high, attempt to jump up onto and down off of the bench as many times as possible in 1 minute. If you cannot jump the full minute, you may step up and down. A repetition is counted each time both feet return to the floor.

Modified dip. **Men only:** Using a bench or gymnasium bleacher, place the hands on the bench with the fingers pointing forward. Have a partner hold your feet in front of you. Bend the hips at approximately 90° (you also may use three sturdy chairs: Put your hands on two chairs placed by the sides of your body and place your feet on the third chair in front of you). Lower your body by flexing the elbows until they reach a 90° angle, then return to the starting position (also see Exercise 6 at the end of this chapter). Perform the repetitions to a two-step cadence (down-up) regulated with a metronome set at 56 beats per minute. Perform as many continuous repetitions as possible. Do not count any more repetitions if you fail to follow the metronome cadence.

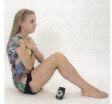

Figure 7.3a Bench jump

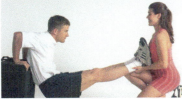

Figure 7.3b Modified dip

Modified push-up. **Women only:** Lie down on the floor (face down), bend the knees (feet up in the air), and place the hands on the floor by the shoulders with the fingers pointing forward. The lower body will be supported at the knees (as opposed to the feet) throughout the test (see Figure 7.3c). The chest must touch the floor on each repetition. As with the modified dip exercise (above), perform the repetitions to a two-step cadence (up-down) regulated with a metronome set at 56 beats per minute. Perform as many continuous repetitions as possible. Do not count any more repetitions if you fail to follow the metronome cadence.

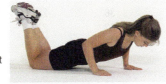

Figure 7.3c Modified push-up

Bent-leg curl-up. Lie down on the floor (face up) and bend both legs at the knees at approximately 100°. The feet should be on the floor, and you must hold them in place yourself throughout the test. Cross the arms in front of the chest, each hand on the opposite shoulder. Now raise the head off the floor, placing the chin against the chest. This is the starting and finishing position for each curl-up (see Figure 7.3d). **The back of the head may not come in contact with the floor, the hands cannot be removed from the shoulders, nor may the feet or hips be raised off the floor at any time during the test. The test is terminated if any of these four conditions occur.** When you curl up, the upper body must come to an upright position before going back down (see Figure 7.3e). The repetitions are performed to a two-step cadence (up-down)

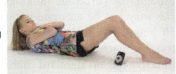

Figure 7.3d Bent-leg curl-up

regulated with the metronome set at 40 beats per minute. For this exercise, you should allow a brief practice period of 5 to 10 seconds to familiarize yourself with the cadence (the *up* movement is initiated with the first beat, then you must wait for the next beat to initiate the *down* movement; one repetition is accomplished every two beats of the metronome). Count as many repetitions as you are able to perform following the proper cadence. The test is

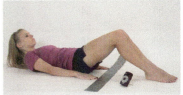

Figure 7.3e Bent-leg curl-up

also terminated if you fail to maintain the appropriate cadence or if you accomplish 100 repetitions. Have your partner check the angle at the knees throughout the test to make sure to maintain the 100° angle as close as possible.

Abdominal crunch. **This test is recommended only for individuals who are unable to perform the bent-leg curl-up test because of susceptibility to low back injury. Exercise form must be carefully monitored during the test.** Several authors and researchers have indicated that proper form during this test is extremely difficult to control. Subjects often slide their bodies, bend their elbows, or shrug their shoulders during the test. Such actions facilitate the performance of the test and misrepresent the actual test results. Biomechanical factors also limit the ability to perform this test. Further, lack of spinal flexibility keeps some individuals from being able to move the full 3½" range of motion. Others are unable to keep their heels on the floor during the test. The validity of this test as an effective measure of abdominal strength or abdominal endurance has also been questioned through research.

Tape a 3½" × 30" strip of cardboard onto the floor. Lie down on the floor in a supine position (face up) with the knees bent at approximately 100°. The feet should be on the floor, and you must hold them in place yourself throughout the test. Straighten out your arms and place them on the floor alongside the trunk with the palms down and the fingers fully extended. The fingertips of both hands should barely touch the closest edge of the cardboard (see Figure 7.3f). Bring the head off the floor until the chin is 1" to 2" away from your chest. Keep the head in this position during the entire test (do not move the head by flexing or extending the neck). You are now ready to begin the test.

Perform the repetitions to a two-step cadence (up-down) regulated with a metronome set at 60 beats per minute. As you curl up, slide the fingers over the cardboard until the fingertips reach the far edge (3½") of the board (see Figure 7.3g), then return to the starting position.

Allow a brief practice period of 5 to 10 seconds

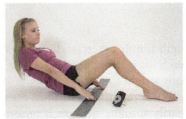

Figure 7.3f Abdominal crunch test

Figure 7.3g Abdominal crunch test

to familiarize yourself with the cadence. Initiate the *up* movement with the first beat and the *down* movement with the next beat. Accomplish one repetition every two beats of the metronome. Count as many repetitions as you are able to perform following the proper cadence. You may not count a repetition if the fingertips fail to reach the distant edge of the cardboard.

Terminate the test if you (a) fail to maintain the appropriate cadence, (b) bend the elbows, (c) shrug the shoulders, (d) slide

(continued)

Photos © Fitness & Wellness, Inc.

Figure 7.3 Muscular Endurance Test. *(continued)*

the body, (e) lift heels off the floor, (f) raise the chin off the chest, (g) accomplish 100 repetitions, or (h) no longer can perform the test. Have your partner check the angle at the knees throughout the test to make sure that the 100° angle is maintained as closely as possible.

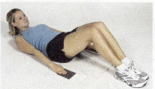 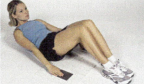

Figure 7.3h   Figure 7.3i

Abdominal crunch test performed with a Crunch-Ster Curl-Up Tester.

For this test you may also use a Crunch-Ster Curl-Up Tester, available from Novel Products.* An illustration of the test performed with this equipment is provided in Figures 7.3h and 7.3i.

According to the results, look up your percentile rank for each exercise in the far left column of Table 7.2 and determine your

muscular endurance fitness category according to the following classification:

Average Score	Fitness Category	Points
≥90	Excellent	5
70–80	Good	4
50–60	Average	3
30–40	Fair	2
≤20	Poor	1

Look up the number of points assigned for each fitness category above. Total the number of points and determine your overall strength endurance fitness category according to the following ratings:

Total Points	Strength Endurance Category
≥13	Excellent
10–12	Good
7–9	Average
4–6	Fair
≤3	Poor

*Novel Products, Inc. Figure Finder Collection, P.O. Box 408, Rockton, IL 61072-0408. 1-800-323-5143, Fax 815-624-4866.

Table 7.2 Muscular Endurance Scoring Table

	Men				Women			
Percentile Rank	Bench Jumps	Modified Dips	Bent-Leg Curl-Ups	Abdominal Crunches	Bench Jumps	Modified Push-Ups	Bent-Leg Curl-Ups	Abdominal Crunches
99	66	54	100	100	58	95	100	100
95	63	50	81	100	54	70	100	100
90	62	38	65	100	52	50	97	69
80	58	32	51	66	48	41	77	49
70	57	30	44	45	44	38	57	37
60	56	27	31	38	42	33	45	34
50	54	26	28	33	39	30	37	31
40	51	23	25	29	38	28	28	27
30	48	20	22	26	36	25	22	24
20	47	17	17	22	32	21	17	21
10	40	11	10	18	28	18	9	15
5	34	7	3	16	26	15	4	0

▨ High physical fitness standard   ▨ Health fitness standard

© Fitness & Wellness, Inc.

strength-training exercises listed in Figure 7.4. The resistance for each lift is determined according to selected percentages of body weight shown in Figure 7.4 and Activity 7.1.

With this test, if an individual does only a few repetitions, primarily absolute strength is measured. For those who are able to do a lot of repetitions, the test is an indicator of muscular endurance. If you are not familiar with the different lifts, see the illustrations provided at the end of this chapter.

A strength/endurance rating is determined according to the maximum number of repetitions you are able to perform on each exercise. Fixed-resistance strength units are necessary to administer all but the abdominal exercises in this test (see "Dynamic Training" on pages 268–270 for an explanation of fixed-resistance equipment).

A percentile rank for each exercise is given based on the number of repetitions performed (Table 7.3). As with the Muscular Endurance Test, an overall muscular strength/endurance rating is obtained by totaling the number of points obtained on each exercise.

If no fixed-resistance equipment is available, you can still perform the test using different equipment. In that case, though, the percentile rankings and strength fitness categories may not be accurate because a certain resistance (e.g., 50 pounds) is seldom the same on two different strength-training machines (e.g., Universal Gym versus Nautilus). The industry has no standard calibration procedure for strength equipment. Consequently, if you lift a certain resistance for a specific exercise (e.g., bench press) on one machine, you may

Figure 7.4 Muscular Strength and Endurance Test.

1. Familiarize yourself with the six lifts used for this test: lat pull-down, knee extension, bench press, bent-leg curl-up or abdominal crunch,* leg curl, and arm curl. Graphic illustrations for each lift are given at the end of this chapter. For the leg curl exercise, the knees should be flexed to 90°. A description and illustration of the bent-leg curl-up and the abdominal crunch exercises are provided in Figure 7.3. On the knee extension lift, maintain the trunk in an upright position.
2. Determine your body weight in pounds.
3. Determine the amount of resistance to be used on each lift. To obtain this number, multiply your body weight by the percent given below for each lift.

Lift	Percent of Body Weight	
	Men	**Women**
Lat Pull-Down	.70	.45
Knee Extension	.65	.50
Bench Press	.75	.45
Bent-Leg Curl-Up or Abdominal Crunch*	NA**	NA**
Leg Curl	.32	.25
Arm Curl	.35	.18

*The abdominal crunch exercise should be used only by individuals who suffer or are susceptible to low back pain.
**NA = not applicable—see Figure 7.3.

4. Perform the maximum continuous number of repetitions possible.
5. Based on the number of repetitions performed, look up the percentile rank for each lift in the left column of Table 7.3.
6. The individual strength fitness category is determined according to the following classification:

Percentile Rank	Fitness Category	Points
≥90	Excellent	5
70–80	Good	4
50–60	Average	3
30–40	Fair	2
≤20	Poor	1

7. Look up the number of points assigned for each fitness category under item 6 above. Total the number of points and determine your overall strength fitness category according to the following ratings:

Total Points	Strength Category
≥25	Excellent
19–24	Good
13–18	Average
7–12	Fair
≤6	Poor

8. Record your results in Activity 7.1.

© Fitness & Wellness, Inc.

Table 7.3 Muscular Strength and Endurance Scoring Table

Percentile Rank	Men							Women						
	Lat Pull-Down	Knee Extension	Bench Press	Bent-Leg Curl-Up	Abdominal Crunch	Leg Crunch	Arm Curl	Lat Pull-Down	Knee Extension	Bench Press	Bent-Leg Curl-Up	Abdominal Crunch	Leg Curl	Arm Curl
99	30	25	26	100	100	24	25	30	25	27	100	100	20	25
95	25	20	21	81	100	20	21	25	20	21	100	100	17	21
90	19	19	19	65	100	19	19	21	18	20	97	69	12	20
80	16	15	16	51	66	15	15	16	13	16	77	49	10	16
70	13	14	13	44	45	13	12	13	11	13	57	37	9	14
60	11	13	11	31	38	11	10	11	10	11	45	34	7	12
50	10	12	10	28	33	10	9	10	9	10	37	31	6	10
40	9	10	7	25	29	8	8	9	8	5	28	27	5	8
30	7	9	5	22	26	6	7	7	7	3	22	24	4	7
20	6	7	3	17	22	4	5	6	5	1	17	21	3	6
10	4	5	1	10	18	3	3	3	3	0	9	15	1	3
5	3	3	0	3	16	1	2	2	1	0	4	0	0	2

▢ High physical fitness standard   ▢ Health fitness standard

© Fitness & Wellness, Inc.

or may not be able to lift the same amount for this exercise on a different machine.

Even though the percentile ranks may not be valid across different equipment, test results can be used to evaluate changes in fitness. For example, you may be able to do 7 repetitions during the initial test, but if you can perform 14 repetitions after 12 weeks of training, that's a measure of improvement. Results of the Muscular Strength and Endurance Test can be recorded in Activity 7.1.

7.4 Basic Muscle Physiology

The capacity of muscle cells to exert force increases and decreases according to the demands placed upon the muscular system. If muscle cells are overloaded beyond their normal use, such as in strength-training programs, the cells increase in size (hypertrophy) and strength. If the demands placed on the muscle cells decrease, such as in sedentary living or required rest because of illness or injury, the cells

Activity 7.1 Muscular Fitness Assessment

Name _____ Date _____

Course _____ Section _____ Gender _____ Age _____

I. Hand Grip Strength Test

The instructions for the Hand Grip Strength Test are provided in Figure 7.2, page 260. Perform the test according to the instructions and look up your results in Table 7.1, page 260.

Hand used: _____ Right _____ Left Reading: _____ lbs. Fitness category (see Figure 7.2, page 260): _____

II. Muscular Endurance Test

Conduct this test using the guidelines provided in Figure 7.3, pages 261–262, and Table 7.2, page 262. Record your repetitions, fitness category, and points in the spaces provided below.

Exercise	Metronome Cadence	Repetitions	Fitness Category	Points
Bench jumps	none			
Modified dips—men only	56 bpm			
Modified push-ups—women only	56 bpm			
Bent-leg curl-ups	40 bpm			
Abdominal crunches	60 bpm			
			Total Points:	

Overall muscular endurance fitness category (see Figure 7.3, pages 261–262): _____

III. Muscular Strength and Endurance Test

Perform the Muscular Strength and Endurance Test according to the procedure outlined in Figure 7.4 and the percentile ranks in Table 7.3, page 263. Record the results, fitness category, and points in the appropriate blanks provided below.

Body weight: _____ lbs. Lift	Percent of Body Weight (pounds) Men	Women	Resistance	Repetitions	Fitness Category	Points
Lat pull-down	.70	.45				
Knee extension	.65	.50				
Bench press	.75	.45				
Bent-leg curl-up or abdominal crunch	NA*	NA*				
Leg curl	.32	.25				
Arm curl	.35	.18				

*Not applicable—no resistance required. Use test described in Figure 7.3, pages 261–262.   Total Points: [ ]

Overall muscular strength fitness category (see Figure 7.4, page 263) [   ]

IV. Muscular Strength and Endurance Goals

Indicate the muscular strength/endurance category that you would like to achieve by the end of the term (see Figure 7.4): [   ]

© Fitness & Wellness, Inc.

Figure 7.5 Skeletal muscle structure.

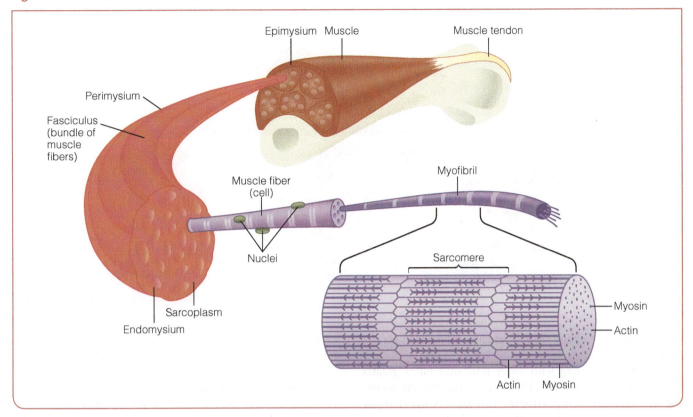

atrophy and lose strength. A good level of muscular fitness is important to develop and maintain fitness, health, and total well-being.

Types of Muscle Hypertrophy

There are two known types of muscular hypertrophy. People who train for strength and power will be training for **myofibrillar hypertrophy**. People who train to increase muscle size will be training for **sarcoplasmic hypertrophy**. The differences between these two types of hypertrophy can be explained on a molecular level. Looking at the smallest element that makes up a muscle will help explain why muscles respond differently depending on the way a person trains.

Myosin and actin are protein filaments that slide past each other and temporarily lock together when a muscle needs to contract. These filaments make up sarcomeres (see Figure 7.5). Sarcomeres are the basic contractile element of the muscle. Sarcomeres are put together end to end to make myofibrils, which are a long rod that goes the entire length of the muscle fiber. Myofibrils are important because they are the basic sub-unit of muscle cells. It takes several hundred of these myofibrils together to make up a single muscle fiber (which is a muscle cell). A bundle of muscle fibers (about 10 to 100) make up a fasciculus. In turn, many of these bundles together (called fasciculi in plural) make up an entire muscle.

Inside the muscle fiber is a substance called **sarcoplasm**. The sarcoplasm in muscle is comparable to the cytoplasm in other cells. Sarcoplasm is a semifluid substance in muscle (noncontractile muscle cell fluid) that contains primarily myosin and actin myofibrils, but also large amounts of glycosomes (organelles that store glycogen and enzymes) and myoglobin (the oxygen-binding protein in muscle).

Now think back to the smallest element of a muscle, the actin and myosin that make up a myofibril. When there is greater synthesis of these protein filaments of myosin and actin that temporarily lock together to produce a muscle contraction, the result is myofibrillar hypertrophy, the type of hypertrophy that produces power and strength. With this type of hypertrophy, the number and the area density (size) of the myofibrils increases and results in a greater ability of the muscle to generate tension (exert muscle strength). This type of hypertrophy is achieved by training with heavy resistance and low repetitions (1 to 6). Strength and power

---

GLOSSARY

Atrophy Decrease in the size of a cell.

Myofibrillar hypertrophy Muscle hypertrophy as a result of increased protein synthesis in the myosin and actin myofibrils.

Sarcoplasmic hypertrophy Muscle hypertrophy as a

result of an increase in sarcoplasm.

Sarcoplasm The equivalent of the cytoplasm in other cells—a semifluid substance that contains myosin and actin filaments, as well as other muscle cell organelles.

Figure 7.6 Myofibrillar hypertrophy vs. sarcoplasmic hypertrophy.

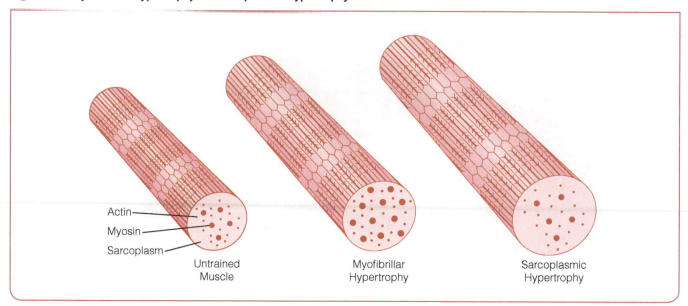

Actin
Myosin
Sarcoplasm

Untrained Muscle

Myofibrillar Hypertrophy

Sarcoplasmic Hypertrophy

athletes use this training method because it results in greater strength increases.

In contrast, training with lower resistance but a greater number of repetitions (8 to 15) increases sarcoplasm, resulting in sarcoplasmic hypertrophy. This type of hypertrophy results in greater muscle size than myofibrillar hypertrophy but yields lower increases in strength. Although muscle size increases (the added fluid accounts for 25 to 30 percent), the density of the muscle fibers actually decreases (see Figure 7.6). Because muscular strength is primarily dependent on the amount and the density of the muscle fibers, adding more muscle fluid does not increase strength to the same extent as myofibrillar hypertrophy. Body builders typically rely on training that leads to sarcoplasmic hypertrophy as they are judged by appearance and not by the amount of resistance lifted.

7.5 *Factors that Affect Muscular Fitness*

Several physiological factors combine to create muscle contraction and subsequent strength gains: neural stimulation, type of muscle fiber, overload, specificity of training, training volume, and periodization. Basic knowledge of these concepts is important for understanding the principles involved in strength development.

Neural Function

Within the neuromuscular system, single **motor neurons** branch and attach to multiple muscle fibers. The motor neuron and the fibers it innervates (supplies with nerves) form a **motor unit**. The number of fibers that a motor neuron can innervate varies from just a few in muscles that require precise control (e.g., eye muscles) to as many as 1,000 or more in large muscles that do not perform refined or precise movements.

Stimulation of a motor neuron causes the muscle fibers to contract maximally or not at all. Variations in the number of fibers innervated and the frequency of their stimulation determine the strength of the muscle contraction. As the number of fibers innervated and frequency of stimulation increase, so does the strength of the muscular contraction.

Neural adaptations are prominent in the early stages of strength-training. In novice participants, significant strength increases seen during the first 2 to 3 weeks of training are largely related to enhanced neural function by increasing motor neuron stimulation and muscle fiber recruitment (skill acquisition). Long-term strength development is primarily related to increased physiological adaptation within the muscle(s) and to a lesser extent to continued neural adaptations.

Types of Muscle Fiber

The human body has two basic types of muscle fibers: (1) slow-twitch or red fibers and (2) fast-twitch or white fibers. **Slow-twitch fibers** have a greater capacity for aerobic work. **Fast-twitch fibers** have a greater capacity for anaerobic work and produce more overall force. The latter are important for quick and powerful movements commonly used in strength-training activities.

The proportion of slow- and fast-twitch fibers is determined genetically and consequently varies from one person to another. Nevertheless, training increases the functional capacity of both types of fiber, and more specifically, strength-training increases their ability to exert force.

During muscular contraction, slow-twitch fibers always are recruited first. As the force and speed of muscle contraction increase, the relative importance of the fast-twitch fibers increases. To activate the fast-twitch fibers, an activity must be intense and powerful.

Overload

Strength gains are achieved in two ways:

1. Through increased ability of individual muscle fibers to generate a stronger contraction
2. By recruiting a greater proportion of the total available fibers for each contraction

These two factors combine in the **overload principle**. The demands placed on the muscle must be increased systematically and progressively over time, and the resistance must be of a magnitude significant enough to cause physiological adaptation. In simpler terms, just like all other organs and systems of the human body, to increase in physical capacity, muscles have to be taxed repeatedly beyond their accustomed loads. Because of this principle, strength-training also is called progressive resistance training.

Several procedures can be used to overload in strength-training[7]:

1. Increasing the intensity (the resistance or the amount of weight used)
2. Increasing the number of repetitions at the current intensity
3. Increasing the number of sets
4. Increasing or decreasing the speed at which the repetitions are performed
5. Decreasing the rest interval for endurance improvements (with lighter resistances) or lengthening the rest interval for strength and power development (with higher resistances)
6. Increasing the volume (the sum of the repetitions performed multiplied by the resistance used)
7. Increasing training sessions per week
8. Using any combination of the above

Specificity of Training

Training adaptations are specific to the impetus applied. In strength-training, the principle of **specificity of training** holds that for a muscle to increase in strength, endurance, or power, the training program must be specific to obtain the desired effects (see also the discussion on resistance on page 270).

The principle of specificity also applies to activity- or sport-specific development and is commonly referred to as **specific adaptation to imposed demand (SAID) training**. The SAID principle implies that if an individual is attempting to improve specific activity or sport skills, the strength-training exercises performed should resemble as closely as possible the movement patterns encountered in that particular activity or sport.

For example, a soccer player who wishes to become stronger and faster emphasizes exercises that develop leg strength and power. In contrast, an individual recovering from a lower-limb fracture initially exercises to increase strength and stability and subsequently to improve muscle endurance.

Training Volume

Volume is the sum of all repetitions performed multiplied by the resistances used during a strength-training session. Volume frequently is used to quantify the amount of work performed in a given training session. For example, an individual who does three sets of six repetitions with 150 pounds has performed a training volume of 2,700 ($3 \times 6 \times 150$) for this exercise. The total training volume can be obtained by totaling the volume of all exercises performed.

The volume of training done in a strength-training session can be modified by changing the total number of exercises performed, the number of sets done per exercise, or the number of repetitions performed per set. Athletes typically use high training volumes and low intensities to achieve muscle hypertrophy and low volumes and high intensities to increase strength and power.

Periodization

The concept of **periodization** (variation) entails systematically altering training variables over time to keep the program challenging and lead to greater strength development. Periodization means cycling training objectives (hypertrophy, strength, and endurance), with each phase of the program, which lasts anywhere from 2 to 12 weeks. Training variables that can be altered include resistance (weight lifted), number of repetitions, number of sets, and number of exercises performed.

GLOSSARY

Motor neurons Nerves connecting the central nervous system to the muscle.

Motor unit The combination of a motor neuron and the muscle fibers that neuron innervates.

Slow-twitch fibers Muscle fibers with greater aerobic potential and slow speed of contraction.

Fast-twitch fibers Muscle fibers with greater anaerobic potential and fast speed of contraction.

Overload principle Training concept that the demands placed on a system (cardiorespiratory or muscular) must be increased systematically and progressively over time to cause physiological adaptation (development or improvement).

Specificity of training Principle that training must be done with the specific muscle(s) the person is attempting to improve.

Specific adaptation to imposed demand (SAID) training Training principle stating that, for improvements to occur in a specific activity, the exercises performed during a strength-training program should resemble as closely as possible the movement patterns encountered in that particular activity.

Volume (in strength-training) The sum of all repetitions performed multiplied by resistances used during a strength-training session.

Periodization A training approach that divides the season into three cycles (macrocycles, mesocycles, and microcycles) using systematic variation in intensity and volume of training to enhance fitness and performance.

The periodized training approach is popular among athletes and is frequently used to prevent **overtraining**. Training volume should not increase by more than 5 percent from one phase to the next. Periodization is now popular among fitness participants who wish to achieve maximal strength gains. Over the long run, for intermediate and advanced participants, the periodized approach has been shown to be superior to nonperiodized training (using the same exercises, sets, and repetitions repeatedly).

Three types of periodized training, based on program design and objectives, are commonly used:

1. *Classical periodization,* used by individuals seeking maximal strength development. It starts with an initial high volume of training using low resistances. In subsequent cycles, the program gradually switches to a lower volume and higher resistances.
2. *Reverse periodization,* used primarily by individuals seeking greater muscular endurance. Also a linear model, it is opposite of the classical model: The resistances are highest at the beginning of training, with a low volume, and subsequently followed by progressive decreases in resistances and increases in training volume.
3. *Undulating periodization,* using a combination of volumes and resistances within a cycle by alternating now (randomly or systematically) among the muscular fitness components: strength, hypertrophy, power, and endurance. The undulating model compares favorably, and in some cases is superior to, the classical and reverse models.

Understanding all five training concepts that affect strength (neural stimulation, muscle fiber types, overload, specificity, and periodization) discussed thus far is required to design an effective strength-training program.

7.6 Guidelines for Strength-Training

Because muscular strength and endurance are important in developing and maintaining overall fitness and well-being, the principles necessary to develop a strength-training program have to be understood, just as in the prescription for cardiorespiratory endurance (see Chapter 6). In addition to volume of training (as described previously), the FITT-VP principles of frequency, intensity (resistance), time (sets), type (mode) of exercise, volume, and progression can also be applied to strength-training. The key factor in successful muscular fitness development, however, is the individualization of the program according to these principles and the person's goals, as well as the magnitude of the individual's effort during training.

Type (Mode) of Training

Two types of training methods are used to improve strength: isometric (static) and dynamic (previously called "isotonic").

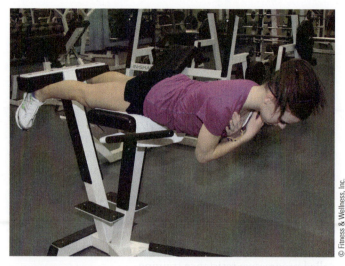

In isometric (static) training, muscle contraction produces little or no movement.

In **isometric training**, muscle contractions produce little or no movement, such as when pushing or pulling against an immovable object or holding a given position against resistance for a given period. In **dynamic training**, the muscle contractions produce movement, such as when extending the knees with resistance on the ankles (knee extension). The specificity of training principle applies here too. To increase isometric versus dynamic strength, an individual must use static instead of dynamic training to achieve the desired results.

Isometric Training

Isometric training does not require much equipment. Because strength gains with isometric training are specific to the angle of muscle contraction, this type of training is beneficial in a sport such as gymnastics, which requires regular static contractions during routines. Selected isometric exercises, in particular core exercises, are recommended as a part of a comprehensive strength-training program.

As presented in Chapter 8, isometric training is a critical component of health conditioning programs for the low back (see "Preventing and Rehabilitating Low Back Pain," page 314–321) and for spinal-stabilization musculature and healthy posture. Furthermore, several studies indicate that light- to moderate-intensity isometric training appears to be more effective in decreasing both systolic and diastolic blood pressure in normotensive and hypertensive individuals than aerobic exercise or dynamic resistance strength-training.[8] Systolic and diastolic blood pressure reductions were approximately 6 mm Hg and 4 mm Hg, respectively.

Dynamic Training

Dynamic training is the most common mode for strength-training. The primary advantage is that strength is gained through the full **range of motion (ROM)**. Most daily activities are dynamic. We are constantly lifting, pushing, and pulling objects, and strength is needed through a complete ROM. Another advantage is that improvements are measured easily by the amount lifted.

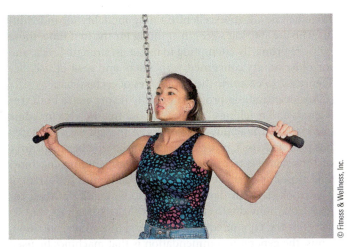

In dynamic training, muscle contraction produces movement in the respective joint(s).

Dynamic training consists of two action phases when an exercise is performed: (1) **concentric** or **positive resistance** and (2) **eccentric** or **negative resistance**. In the concentric phase, the muscle shortens as it contracts to overcome the resistance. In the eccentric phase, the muscle lengthens to overcome the resistance. For example, during a bench press exercise, when the person lifts the resistance from the chest to full-arm extension, the triceps muscle on the back of the upper arm shortens to extend (straighten) the elbow. During the eccentric phase, the same triceps muscle is used to lower the weight during elbow flexion, but the muscle lengthens slowly to avoid dropping the resistance. Both motions work the same muscle against the same amount of resistance.

Eccentric muscle contractions allow you to lower weights in a smooth, gradual, and controlled manner. Without eccentric contractions, weights would be suddenly dropped on the way down. Because the same muscles work when you lift and lower a resistance, always be sure to execute both actions in a controlled manner. Failure to do so diminishes the benefits of the training program and increases the risk for injuries. Eccentric contractions seem to be more effective in producing muscle hypertrophy but result in greater muscle soreness. High-intensity eccentric training, greater than 100 percent of the 1 RM, is not recommended because such can lead to injury and severe muscle damage.

Dynamic training programs can be conducted with **free weights**, **fixed-resistance** machines, **variable-resistance** machines, or isokinetic equipment; or without weights with programs such as elastic-band resistive exercise, stability exercise balls, body weight resistance training, CrossFit, TRX (Total Resistance eXercise), Pilates, boot camp, PX90, functional fitness, and circuit training, among others. A description of some of the latter exercise programs without weights is given on pages 285–289 in Chapter 9. When you perform dynamic exercises without weights (e.g., pull-ups and push-ups), with free weights, or with fixed-resistance machines, you move a constant resistance through a joint's full ROM. The greatest resistance that can be lifted equals the maximum weight that can be moved at the weakest angle of the joint. This is because of changes in length of muscle and angle of pull as the joint moves through its ROM. This type of training is also referred to as **dynamic constant external resistance,** or **DCER**.

As strength-training became more popular, new strength-training machines were developed. This technology brought

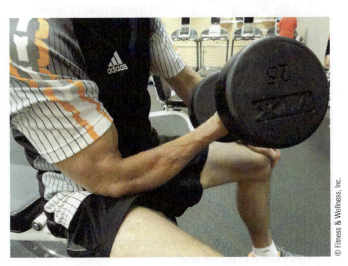

Strength-training can be done using free weights.

GLOSSARY

Overtraining An emotional, behavioral, and physical condition marked by increased fatigue, decreased performance, persistent muscle soreness, mood disturbances, and feelings of "staleness" or "burnout" as a result of excessive physical training.

Isometric training Strength-training method referring to a muscle contraction that produces little or no movement, such as pushing or pulling against an immovable object.

Dynamic training Strength-training method referring to a muscle contraction with movement.

Range of motion (ROM) Entire arc of movement of a given joint.

Concentric Refers to shortening of a muscle during muscle contraction.

Positive resistance The lifting, pushing, or concentric phase of a repetition during a strength-training exercise.

Eccentric Refers to lengthening of a muscle during muscle contraction.

Negative resistance The lowering or eccentric phase of a repetition during a strength-training exercise.

Free weights Barbells and dumbbells.

Fixed resistance Type of exercise in which a constant resistance is moved through a joint's full range of motion (dumbbells, barbells, and machines using a constant resistance).

Variable resistance Training using special machines equipped with mechanical devices that provide differing amounts of resistance through the range of motion.

Dynamic constant external resistance (DCER) See **fixed resistance.**

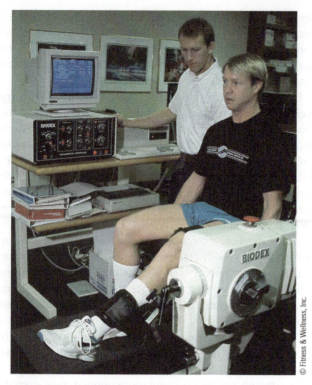

In isokinetic training, the speed of muscle contraction is constant.

about **isokinetic training** and variable-resistance training programs, which require special machines equipped with mechanical devices that provide differing amounts of resistance, with the intent of overloading the muscle group maximally through the entire ROM. A distinction of isokinetic training is that the speed of the muscle contraction is kept constant because the machine provides resistance to match the user's force through the ROM. The mode of training that an individual selects depends mainly on the type of equipment available and the specific objective the training program is attempting to accomplish.

The benefits of isokinetic and variable-resistance training are similar to those of the other dynamic training methods. Theoretically, strength gains should be better because maximum resistance is applied at all angles. Research, however, has not shown this type of training to be more effective than other modes of dynamic training.

Free Weights versus Machines in Dynamic Training The most popular weight-training devices available during the first half of the 20th century were plate-loaded barbells (free weights). Strength-training machines were developed in the middle of the century but did not become popular until the 1970s. With subsequent technological improvements to these machines, a debate arose over which of the two training modalities was better.

Free weights require that the individual balance the resistance through the entire lifting motion. Free weights are thought to provide greater strength development because additional muscles are needed to balance the resistance as it is moved through the ROM. Strength-training machines,

nonetheless, are an excellent training modality for individuals who are starting strength-training for the first time, those who are primarily attempting to maintain strength levels, and for older adults concerned with safety and ease of use. See Figure 7.7 to examine the advantages of each system.

An ideal training program actually incorporates both free weights and machines. You can choose free weights for some exercises and machines for others. Although each modality has pros and cons, muscles do not know whether the source of a resistance is free weights or a strength-training machine. The most important components that determine the extent of a person's strength development are the quality of the program, the individual's effort during the training program itself (not the type of equipment used), and proper nutrition. Thus, the general recommendation is that machines be used early on. Subsequently, both machines and free weights can be used by intermediate and advanced participants.

Intensity (Resistance)

Resistance in strength-training is the equivalent of intensity in cardiorespiratory exercise prescription. To stimulate strength development, the general recommendation has been to use a resistance of approximately 80 percent of the maximum capacity (the 1 RM). For example, a person with a 1 RM of 150 pounds should work with about 120 pounds (150 × .80).

I Have Been Told That Certain Types of Equipment Are Better for Strength Development. Which One Is Best?

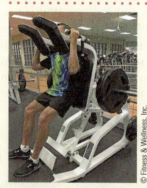

Free weights, as opposed to strength-training machines, require that the individual balance the resistance through the entire lifting motion. We could logically assume that free weights are a better training modality because additional stabilizing muscles are needed to balance the resistance as it is moved through the range of motion. Research, however, has not shown any differences in strength development among different exercise modalities. Proper technique and degree of effort are more important than the specific type of equipment used. Muscles do not know whether the source of a resistance is a barbell, a dumbbell, a weight machine, or a simple cinder block. What determines the extent of a person's strength development is the quality of the program (number of exercises, sets, reps, frequency, and progression), the individual's effort during the training program (not the type of equipment used), and proper nutrition. Selection comes down to personal preference, equipment availability, and a program that fits personal lifestyle.

Figure 7.7 Strength-training guidelines. Advantages of free weights vs. machines in strength-training.

Advantages of Free Weights

Following are the advantages of using free weights instead of machines in a strength-training program:

- **Cost:** Free weights are less expensive than most exercise machines. On a limited budget, free weights are a better option.
- **Variety:** A bar and a few plates can be used to perform many exercises to strengthen most muscles in the body.
- **Portability:** Free weights can be easily moved from one area or station to another.
- **Coordination:** Free weights require greater muscular coordination to mimic movement requirements of specific tasks.
- **Balance:** Free weights require that a person balance the weight through the entire range of motion. This feature involves additional support and stabilizing muscles to keep the weight moving properly.
- **One size fits all:** People of almost all ages can use free weights. A drawback of machines is that individuals who are at the extremes in terms of height or limb length often do not fit into the machines. In particular, small women and adolescents are at a disadvantage.

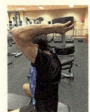

Advantages of Machines

Strength-training machines have the following advantages over free weights:

- **Safety:** Machines are safer because spotters are rarely needed to monitor lifting.
- **Ease of use:** Only a minimal amount of skill is required because the machines guide and control the movement through the entire range of motion.
- **Selection:** A few exercises—such as hip flexion, hip abduction, leg curls, lat pull-downs, and neck exercises—can be performed only with machines.
- **Variable resistance:** Most machines provide variable resistance. Free weights provide only fixed resistance.
- **Isolation:** Individual muscles are better isolated with machines, because stabilizing muscles are not used to balance the weight during the exercise.
- **Time:** Exercising with machines requires less time, because you can set the resistance quickly by using a selector pin instead of having to manually change dumbbells or weight plates on both sides of a barbell.
- **Flexibility:** Most machines can provide resistance over a greater range of movement during the exercise, thereby contributing to more flexibility in the joints. For example, a barbell pullover exercise provides resistance over a range of 100 degrees, whereas a weight machine may allow for as much as 260 degrees.
- **Rehabilitation:** Machines are more useful during injury rehabilitation. A knee injury, for instance, is practically impossible to rehab using free weights, whereas with a weight machine, small loads can be easily selected through a limited range of motion.
- **Skill acquisition:** Learning a new exercise movement—and performing it correctly—is faster, because the machine controls the direction of the movement.

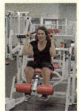

Photos © Fitness & Wellness, Inc.

The number of repetitions that someone can perform at 80 percent of the 1 RM, however, varies among exercises (i.e., bench press, lat pull-down, and leg curl; Table 7.4). Data indicate that the total number of repetitions performed at a certain percentage of the 1 RM depends on the amount of muscle mass involved (bench press versus triceps extension) and whether it is a single or multi-joint exercise (leg press versus leg curl). In trained and untrained subjects alike, the number of repetitions is greater with larger muscle mass involvement and multi-joint exercises.[9]

Because of the time factor involved in constantly determining the 1 RM on each lift to ensure that the person is indeed working around 80 percent, the accepted rule for many years has been that individuals perform between 8 and 12 repetitions maximum (or in the 8 to 12 RM zone) for adequate muscle hypertrophy and strength gains. For example, if a person is training with a resistance of 120 pounds and cannot

Table 7.4 Number of Repetitions Performed at 80 Percent of the One Repetition Maximum (1 RM)

Exercise	Trained		Untrained	
	Men	Women	Men	Women
Leg press	19	22	15	12
Lat pull-down	12	10	10	10
Bench press	12	14	10	10
Knee extension	12	10	9	8
Sit-up*	12	12	8	7
Arm curl	11	7	8	6
Leg curl	7	5	6	6

*Sit-up exercise performed with weighted plates on the chest and feet held in place with an ankle strap.

SOURCE: W. W. K. Hoeger, D. R. Hopkins, S. L. Barette, and D. F. Hale, "Relationship between Repetitions and Selected Percentages of One Repetition Maximum: A Comparison between Untrained and Trained Males and Females," *Journal of Applied Sport Science Research* 4, no. 2 (1990): 47–51.

GLOSSARY

Isokinetic training Strength-training method in which the speed of the muscle contraction is kept constant because the equipment (machine) provides an accommodating resistance to match the user's force (maximal) through the range of motion.

Resistance Amount of weight lifted.

lift it more than 12 times—that is, the person reaches volitional fatigue at or before 12 repetitions—the training stimulus (weight used) is adequate for strength and hypertrophy development. It is important to note that volitional fatigue means to the point of muscle fatigue but not muscle failure. Exerting muscles to failure substantially increases the risk of excessive soreness and injury among beginner lifters and older adults. Once the person can lift the resistance more than 12 times, the resistance is increased by 5 to 10 pounds and the person again should build up to 12 repetitions. This is referred to as *progressive resistance training*.

Strength development, however, also occurs when working with less than 80 percent of the 1 RM (60 to 80 percent). Although the 8 to 12 RM zone is the most commonly prescribed resistance training zone, benefits still accrue when working with less than 8 RM or above 12 RM (i.e., the greater the resistance, the fewer the number of repetitions that will be performed). Some research has found small differences in muscular fitness between individuals who train with lighter resistances (≤+ 60 percent of 1 RM) as compared to heavier resistances (≥ 65 percent of 1 RM), but all sets must be done to the point where the last few repetitions are difficult to perform (volitional exhaustion is reached with each set). In all cases, nonetheless, heavy resistances provide greater strength gains, while differences in muscular hypertrophy are not as significant.

Older adults and individuals susceptible to musculoskeletal injuries are encouraged to work with 10 to 25 repetitions using moderate resistances (about 50 to 60 percent of the 1 RM). To increase muscular power, perform a similar number of repetitions but at a faster cadence (speed). If the main objective of the training program is muscular endurance, 15 to 25 repetitions per set are recommended.

In both young and older individuals, all repetitions should be performed at a moderate velocity (about 1 second concentric and 1 second eccentric), which yields the greatest strength gains. For advanced training, varying training velocity among sets, from very slow to fast, is recommended.

Elite strength and power athletes typically work between 1 and 6 RM, but they often shuffle training (periodized training) with a different number of repetitions and sets for selected periods (weeks). Body builders tend to work with moderate resistance levels (60 to 85 percent of the 1 RM) and perform 8 to 15 repetitions to near fatigue. A foremost objective of body building is to increase muscle size. Moderate resistance promotes blood flow to the muscles, "pumping up the muscles" (also known as "the pump"), which makes them look larger than they do in a resting state.

From a general fitness point of view, a moderate resistance of only about 50 percent should be used initially while learning proper form and lifting technique. Following the first 2 weeks of training, working near a 10-repetition threshold seems to improve overall performance most effectively. We live in a dynamic world in which muscular strength and endurance are both required to lead an enjoyable life. Working around 10 RM produces good balanced results between strength, endurance, and hypertrophy. To maximize training development, advanced participants are encouraged to cycle between 1 and 12 RM.

HOEGER KEY TO WELLNESS

Two to four sets of 8 to 12 repetitions maximum (RM) performed two to three times per week, using 8 to 10 dynamic strength-training exercises, are sufficient to elicit significant muscular fitness and health benefits.

Time (Sets)

In strength-training, a **set** is the number of repetitions performed for a given exercise. For example, a person lifting 120 pounds eight times has performed one set of eight repetitions ($1 \times 8 \times 120$). For general fitness, muscular strength, and muscular hypertrophy, the recommendation is two to four sets per exercise with 2 to 3 minutes' rest interval between sets (advanced participants often train with up to six sets per exercise). For a person looking to improve muscular endurance, no more than two sets (of 15 to 25 repetitions each) per exercise are recommended.

When performing multiple sets using the RM zone with the same resistance, if the person truly performs 12 RM to muscle fatigue (or close to it), in subsequent sets fewer RM will be performed (perhaps 10, 8, and 6 RM). Because of the characteristics of muscle fiber, the number of sets the exerciser can do is limited. As the number of sets increases, so does the amount of muscle fatigue and subsequent recovery time. While significant strength gains are reaped performing just one RM set per muscle group, strength gains tend to peak at four sets per muscle group.

When time is a factor, and although multiple-set training is most beneficial, single-set programs are still effective, as long as the single set is performed within the RM zone to muscular fatigue. You may also choose to do two sets for multi-joint exercises (bench press, leg press, lat pull-down, etc.) and a single RM-zone set for single-joint exercises (arm curl, triceps extension, knee extension, etc.).

A recommended program for beginners in their first few weeks of training is one or two light warm-up sets per exercise, using about 50 percent of the 1 RM (no warm-up sets are necessary for subsequent exercises that use the same muscle group), followed by one to four sets to near fatigue per exercise. Maintaining resistance and effort that temporarily fatigue the muscle (volitional exhaustion) from the number of repetitions selected in at least one of the sets is crucial to achieve optimal progress. Because of the lower resistances used in body building, three to eight sets can be done for each exercise.

To avoid muscle soreness and stiffness, new participants should build up gradually to the three to four sets of maximal repetitions. They can do this by performing only one set of each exercise with a lighter resistance on the first day of training and two sets of each exercise on the second day—the first light and the second with the required resistance to volitional exhaustion. They then could choose to increase to three sets on the third day—one light and two with the prescribed resistance. After that, they should be able to perform anywhere from two to four sets as planned.

The time necessary to recover between sets depends mainly on the resistance used during each set. In strength-training, the energy to lift heavy weights is derived primarily from the system involving adenosine triphosphate (ATP) and creatine phosphate (CP) or phosphagen [see "Energy (ATP) Production," Chapter 3, page 126]. Ten seconds of maximal exercise nearly depletes the CP stores in the exercised muscle(s). These stores are replenished in about 3 to 5 minutes of recovery.

Based on this principle, rest intervals between sets vary in length depending on the program goals and are dictated by the amount of resistance used in training. Short rest intervals of less than 2 minutes are commonly used when people are trying to develop local muscular endurance. Moderate rest intervals of 2 to 4 minutes are used for strength development. Long intervals of more than 4 minutes are used when people are training for power development.[10] Using these guidelines, individuals training for health fitness purposes might allow 2 minutes of rest between sets. Body builders, who use lower resistances, should rest no more than 1 minute to maximize the "pumping" effect.

You can also work smarter to save time. The exercise program is more time effective if two or three exercises are alternated that require different muscle groups, called **circuit training**. In this way you can go directly from one exercise to another and will not have to wait 2 to 3 minutes before proceeding to a new set on a different exercise. For example, the bench press, knee extension, and abdominal curl-up exercises may be combined so that the person can go almost directly from one exercise set to the next.

Men and women alike should observe the guidelines given previously. However, many women do not follow them. They erroneously believe that training with low resistances and many repetitions is best to enhance body composition and maximize energy expenditure. Unless people are seeking to

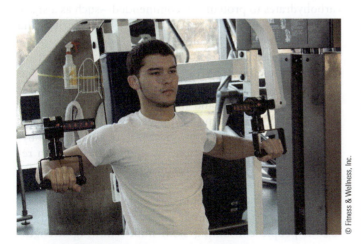

From a health-fitness standpoint, one to two strength-training sessions per week are sufficient to maintain strength.

Figure 7.8 FITT-VP strength-training guidelines.

Frequency: 2 to 3 days per week on nonconsecutive days. More frequent training can be done if different muscle groups are exercised on different days. (Allow at least 48 hours between strength-training sessions of the same muscle group.)

Intensity (Resistance): Sufficient resistance to perform 8 to 12 repetitions maximum for muscular strength and 15 to 25 repetitions to near fatigue for muscular endurance. Older adults and injury prone individuals should use 10 to 15 repetitions with moderate resistance (50% to 60% of their 1 RM).

Time (Sets): 2 to 4 sets per exercise with 2 to 3 minutes recovery between sets for optimal strength development. Less than 2 minutes per set if exercises are alternated that require different muscle groups (chest and upper back) or between muscular endurance sets.

Type (Mode): Select 8 to 10 dynamic strength-training exercises that involve the body's major muscle groups and include opposing muscle groups (chest and upper back, abdomen and lower back, front and back of the legs).

Volume: The sum of all repetitions performed multiplied by the resistance used in training.

Progression: Gradually increase the resistance, and/or: the number of repetitions per set, training frequency, speed at which the repetitions are performed, and/or volume per training session.

SOURCE: Adapted from American College of Sports Medicine, *ACSM's Guidelines for Exercise Testing and Prescription* (Philadelphia, PA: Wolters Kluwer/Lippincott Williams & Wilkins, 2018).

increase muscular endurance for a specific sport-related activity, the use of low resistances and high repetitions is not recommended to achieve optimal strength fitness goals and maximize long-term energy expenditure.

Frequency

Strength-training should be done through a total body workout two to three times a week. Strength-training two times per week produces about 80 percent of the strength gains seen in a traditional three-times-per-week program. Training can be performed more frequently if using a split-body routine, that is, upper body one day and lower body the next. After a maximum strength workout, a rest interval of 48 to 72 hours between sessions is recommended to promote the adaptations required for optimal muscle hypertrophy and the respective strength gains. If not recovered in 2 to 3 days, the person most likely is overtraining and therefore not reaping the full benefits of the program. In that case, the person should do fewer sets of exercises than in the previous workout. A summary of strength-training guidelines for health fitness purposes is provided in Figure 7.8.

GLOSSARY

Set A fixed number of repetitions; one set of bench presses might be 10 repetitions.

Circuit training Alternating exercises by performing them in a sequence of three to six or more.

Table 7.5 Guidelines for Various Strength-Training Programs

Strength-Training Program	Resistance	Sets	Rest Between Sets*	Frequency (workouts per week)**
General fitness	8–12 reps max	2–4	2–3 min	2–3
Muscular endurance	15–25 reps	1–2	1–2 min	2–3
Maximal strength	1–6 reps max	2–5	3 min	2–3
Body building	8–15 reps near max	3–8	up to 1 min	4–12

*Recovery between sets can be decreased by alternating exercises that use different muscle groups.

**Weekly training sessions can be increased by using a split-body routine.

To achieve significant strength gains, a minimum of 8 weeks of consecutive training is recommended. After an individual has achieved an adequate strength level, from a health fitness standpoint, one to two training sessions per week are sufficient to maintain it. Highly trained athletes have to train twice a week to maintain their strength levels.

Frequency of strength-training for body builders varies from person to person. Because body builders use moderate resistance, daily or even two-a-day workouts are common. The frequency depends on the amount of resistance, number of sets performed per session, and the person's ability to recover from the previous exercise bout (Table 7.5). The latter often is dictated by level of conditioning.

Results in Strength Gain

A common question among many strength-training participants is: How quickly can strength gains be observed? Strength-training studies have revealed that most strength gains are seen in the first 8 weeks of training. The amount of improvement, however, is related to previous training status. Increases of 40 percent are seen in individuals with no previous strength-training experience, 16 percent in previously strength-trained people, and 10 percent in advanced individuals.[11] Using a periodized strength-training program can yield further improvements (see "Periodization," Chapter 9, page 344).

7.7 Dietary Guidelines for Strength and Muscular Development

Individuals who wish to enhance muscle growth and strength during periods of intense strength-training should increase protein to 1.2 to 2.0 grams per kilogram of body weight per day. The selected amount should be based on the volume of the undertaken strength-training program. Adequate dietary protein (at least 1.2 g per kilogram of body weight per day) distributed throughout the day is particularly important for older adults. Unless protein intake is adequate, even strength-training is associated with lower muscle mass. For a 140-pound older adult, 1.2 g per kilogram of body weight translates into 76 total g of protein per day or 25 g per meal.

The timing, dose, and type of protein are all important in promoting muscle growth. Studies suggest that consuming a pre-exercise snack consisting of a combination of carbohydrates and protein leads to greater amino acid (the building blocks of protein) uptake by the muscle cells. The carbohydrates supply energy for training, and the availability of amino acids in the blood during training enhances muscle building. A peanut butter, turkey, or tuna sandwich; milk or yogurt and fruit; or nuts and fruit consumed 20 to 60 minutes before training are excellent choices for a pre-workout snack. As an added benefit, research showed that a whey protein (18 grams) supplement ingested 20 minutes prior to strength-training resulted in a greater increase in resting energy expenditure during the 24 hours following the exercise session as compared to a carbohydrate-only (19 grams) supplement.[12]

Consuming a carbohydrate/protein snack immediately following strength-training and a meal or second snack an hour thereafter further promotes muscle growth and strength development. Post-exercise carbohydrates help restore muscle glycogen depleted during training and, in combination with protein, induce an increase in blood insulin and growth hormone levels. These hormones are essential to the muscle-building process. The higher level of circulating amino acids in the bloodstream immediately following training is believed to increase protein synthesis to a greater extent than amino acids made available later in the day. People who consume a carbohydrate/protein supplement immediately before and right after strength training gain significantly more muscle mass than those who consume a similar supplement morning and evening (6.2 pounds vs. 3.3 pounds).[13] A ratio of 4 to 1 grams of carbohydrates to protein is recommended—such as a snack containing 40 grams of carbohydrates (160 calories) and 10 grams of protein (40 calories).

The type of protein you consume is also important for optimal development. Whey protein, found in milk, has been shown to be the most effective type of protein for strength development and myofibrillar hypertrophy. Milk contains two major types of proteins: whey and casein. Whey can be separated from the casein or formed as a by-product of cheese production. Whey protein has been reported to be superior to casein, soy, or egg proteins for muscular development. An effective and cheaper alternative to a protein supplement is a simple glass of skim milk. The data show greater muscle mass gain and more body fat loss in people consuming skim milk following strength-training as opposed to those consuming a carbohydrate-only supplement.

HOEGER KEY TO WELLNESS

 The timing, dose, and type of protein are all important in promoting muscle growth through a strength-training program. A pre-exercise carbohydrate/protein snack, and one immediately following strength-training, followed by regular protein intake during the next 48 hours are all critical for adequate muscular development.

The relatively immediate pre-exercise/post-exercise carbohydrate/protein consumption is critical, but muscle fibers do continue to absorb a greater amount of amino acids up to 48 hours following strength-training. Thus, while attempting to increase muscular strength and size, proper distribution of protein intake at regular intervals throughout the day is important. Research indicates that further myofibrillar protein synthesis and muscle development are best accomplished with a 20-gram dose of whey protein taken every 3 hours throughout the day.[14] The latter has proven to be more effective than taking a similar total amount of protein with morning and evening meals.

Once you have reached your strength and hypertrophy goals, do not neglect your daily protein intake. Spreading the intake over three meals (about 20 to 40 grams of high-quality protein per meal based on your body size and level of activity) is most effective in keeping you satisfied, maintaining your muscle tissue, and helping reduce your caloric intake the rest of the day.

Critical Thinking

A friend started a strength-training program last year and has seen good results. He is now strength-training nearly daily and taking performance-enhancing supplements, hoping to accelerate results. What are your feelings about his program? What would you say (and not say) to him?

7.8 Strength-Training Exercises

The strength-training programs introduced on pages 285–301 provide a complete body workout. The major muscles of the human body referred to in the exercises are pointed out in Figure 7.9 and within the exercises themselves at the end of the chapter.

Only a minimum of equipment is required for the first program, Strength-Training Exercises without Weights (Bodyweight Training—see Exercises 1 through 14). You can conduct this program at home. Your body weight is used as the primary resistance for most exercises. A few exercises call for a friend's help or some basic implements from around your house to provide greater resistance.

Strength-Training Exercises with Weights (Exercises 15 through 37) require machines, as shown in the accompanying photographs. These exercises can be conducted on either fixed- or variable-resistance equipment. Many of these exercises also can be performed with free weights. The first 13 of these exercises (Exercises 15 through 27) are recommended to get a complete workout. You can do these exercises as circuit training. If time is a factor, as a minimum perform the first nine exercises (Exercises 15 through 23). Exercises 28 through 37 are supplemental or can replace some of the basic 13 (e.g., substitute Exercise 29 or 30 for 15; 31 for 16; 33 for 19; 34 for 24; 35 for 26; 32 for 27). Exercises 38 through 46 are stability ball exercises that can be used to complement your workout. Some of these exercises can also take the place of others that you use to strengthen similar muscle groups.

Selecting different exercises for a given muscle group is recommended between training sessions (e.g., chest press for bench press). No evidence indicates that a given exercise is best for a given muscle group. Changing exercises works the specific muscle group through a different ROM and may change the difficulty of the exercise. Alternating exercises is also beneficial to avoid the monotony of repeating the same training program each training session.

Exercise Variations

Multiple- and single-joint exercises are used in strength-training. Multiple-joint exercises, such as the squat, bench press, and lat pull-down, require more skill and complex neural responses than single-joint exercises. Multiple-joint exercises also allow you to lift more weight and develop more strength. Single-joint exercises, such as the arm curl or knee extension, are used to target specific muscles for further development. Both are recommended for a comprehensive training program.

Many strength-training exercises can be performed bilaterally and unilaterally. Muscle activation differs between the two modes. Unilateral training can enhance selected sport skills, such as single-leg jumping, high jumping, and single-arm throwing. Unilateral training is also used extensively in rehab programs. For example, bilateral concentric knee extension followed by unilateral eccentric knee flexion is strongly recommended for individuals with weak knees and to prevent potential knee problems (see Exercise 28B). Both modes of training are recommended to maximize strength gains.

Plyometric Exercise

Strength, speed, and explosiveness are all crucial for success in athletics. All three of these factors are enhanced with a progressive resistance training program, but greater increases in speed and explosiveness are thought to be possible with **plyometric exercise**. The objective is to generate the greatest

---

GLOSSARY

Plyometric exercise Explosive jump training, incorporating speed and strength training to enhance explosiveness.

Figure 7.9 Major muscles of the human body.

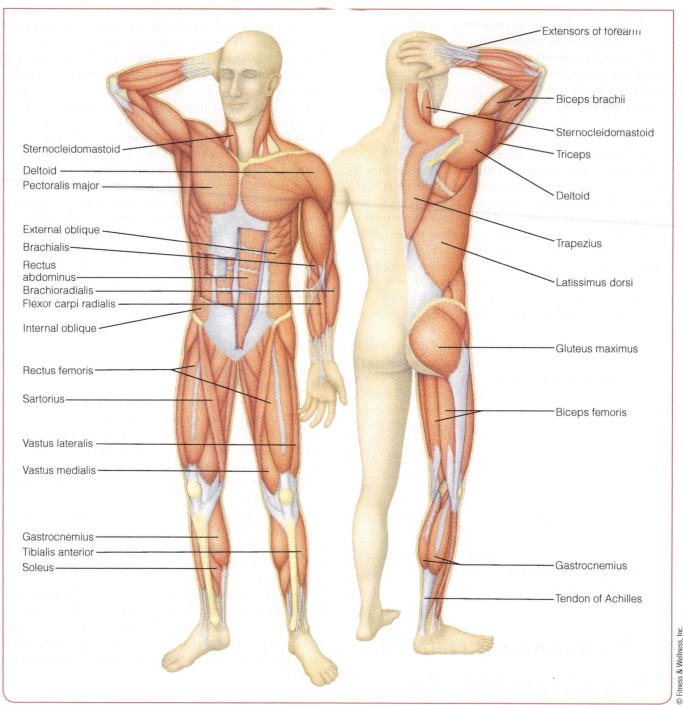

Extensors of forearm

Biceps brachii

Sternocleidomastoid

Triceps

Deltoid

Trapezius

Latissimus dorsi

Gluteus maximus

Biceps femoris

Gastrocnemius

Tendon of Achilles

Sternocleidomastoid

Deltoid

Pectoralis major

External oblique

Brachialis

Rectus abdominus

Brachioradialis

Flexor carpi radialis

Internal oblique

Rectus femoris

Sartorius

Vastus lateralis

Vastus medialis

Gastrocnemius

Tibialis anterior

Soleus

© Fitness & Wellness, Inc.

amount of force in the shortest time. A solid strength base is necessary before attempting plyometric exercises.

Plyometric training is popular in sports that require powerful movements, such as basketball, volleyball, sprinting, jumping, and gymnastics. A typical plyometric exercise involves jumping off and back onto a box, attempting to rebound as quickly as possible on each jump. Box heights are increased progressively from about 12 to 22 inches.

The bounding action attempts to take advantage of the stretch–recoil and stretch reflex characteristics of muscle. The rapid stretch applied to the muscle during contact with the ground is thought to augment muscle contraction, leading to more explosiveness. Plyometrics also can be used for strengthening upper body muscles. An example is doing push-ups so that the extension of the arms is forceful enough to drive the hands (and body) off the floor during each repetition.

A drawback of plyometric training is its higher risk for injuries compared with conventional modes of progressive resistance training. For instance, the potential for injury in rebound exercise escalates with the increase in box height or the number of repetitions.

Behavior Modification Planning

Healthy Strength-Training

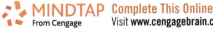

❏	❏	Make a progressive resistance strength-training program a priority in your weekly schedule.
❏	❏	Strength-train at least once a week; even better, two to three times per week.
❏	❏	Find a facility where you feel comfortable training and where you can get good professional guidance.
❏	❏	Learn the proper technique for each exercise.
❏	❏	Train with a friend or group of friends.
❏	❏	Consume a pre-exercise snack consisting of a combination of carbohydrates and some protein about 20 to 60 minutes before each strength-training session.

❏	❏	Use a minimum of 8 to 10 exercises that involve all major muscle groups of your body.
❏	❏	Perform at least one set of each exercise to near muscular fatigue.
❏	❏	To enhance protein synthesis, consume one post-exercise snack with a 4-to-1 gram ratio of carbohydrates to protein (preferably whey protein) immediately following strength-training; eat a second snack or meal with some whey protein 1 hour thereafter; and then continue to consume 20 grams of whey protein every 3 hours throughout the day.
❏	❏	Allow at least 48 hours between strength-training sessions that involve the same muscle groups.

Try It

Attend the school's fitness or recreation center and have an instructor or fitness trainer help you design a progressive resistance strength-training program. Train twice a week for the next 4 weeks. Thereafter, evaluate the results and write down your feelings about the program.

MINDTAP From Cengage **Complete This Online**
Visit www.cengagebrain.com to access MindTap, a complete digital course that includes interactive quizzes, videos, and more.

Core Strength-Training

The trunk (spine) and pelvis are referred to as the "core" of the body. Core muscles include the abdominal muscles (rectus, transversus, and internal and external obliques), hip muscles (front and back), and spinal muscles (lower and upper back muscles). These muscle groups are responsible for maintaining the stability of the spine and pelvis.

Many major muscle groups of the legs, shoulders, and arms attach to the core. A strong core allows a person to perform activities of daily living with greater ease, improve sports performance through a more effective energy transfer from large to small body parts, and decrease the incidence of low back pain. **Core strength-training** also contributes to better posture and balance.

A major objective of core training is to exercise the abdominal and lower back muscles in unison. Furthermore, individuals should spend as much time training the back muscles as they do the abdominal muscles. Besides enhancing stability, core training improves dynamic balance, which is often required during physical activity and participation in sports.

Key core training exercises include the abdominal crunch and bent-leg curl-up, reverse crunch, pelvic tilt, side plank, plank, leg press, seated back, lat pull-down, back extension, lateral trunk flexion, supine bridge, and pelvic clock (Exercises 4, 11, 12, 13, 14, 16, 20, 24, 36, and 37 in this chapter and Exercises 26 and 27 in Chapter 8, respectively). Stability ball Exercises 38 through 46 are also used to strengthen the core.

When core training is used in athletic conditioning programs, athletes attempt to mimic the dynamic skills they use in their sport. To do so, they use special equipment such as balance boards, stability balls, and foam pads. Using this equipment allows the athletes to train the core while seeking balance and stability in a sport-specific manner.

Stability Exercise Balls

A stability exercise ball is a large, flexible, inflatable ball used for exercises that combine the principles of Pilates with core strength-training. Stability exercises are specifically designed to develop abdominal, hip, chest, and spinal muscles by addressing core stabilization while the exerciser maintains a balanced position over the ball. Emphasis is placed on correct movement and maintenance of proper body alignment to involve as much of the core as possible. Although the primary objective is core strength and stability, many stability exercises can be performed to strengthen other body areas as well.

Stability exercises are thought to be more effective than similar exercises on the ground. For example, just sitting on the ball requires the use of stabilizing core muscles (including the rectus abdominis and the external and internal obliques) to keep the body from falling off the ball. Traditional strength-training exercises are primarily for strength and power development and do not contribute as much to body balance.

When performing stability exercises, choose a ball size based on your height. Your thighs should be parallel to the floor when you sit on the ball. A slightly larger ball may be

---GLOSSARY---

Core strength-training A program designed to strengthen the abdominal, hip, and spinal muscles (the core of the body).

used if you suffer from back problems. Several stability ball exercises are provided on pages 209–301. For best results, have a trained specialist teach you the proper technique and watch your form while you learn the exercises. Individuals who have a weak muscular system or poor balance or who are over the age of 65 should perform stability exercises under the supervision of a qualified trainer.

Elastic-Band Resistive Exercise

Elastic bands and tubing can also be used for strength-training. This type of constant-resistance training has increased in popularity and can be used to supplement traditional strength-training because it has been shown to help increase strength, mobility, and functional ability (particularly in older adults) and to aid in the rehab of many types of injuries. Some advantages to using this type of training include low cost, versatility (you can create resistance in almost all angles and directions of the ROM), use of a large number of exercises to work all joints of the body, and accessibility to a

workout while traveling (exercise bands and tubes can be easily packed in a suitcase). This type of resistance training can also add variety to your routine workout.

Elastic-band resistive exercise workouts can be just as challenging as those with free weights or machines. Due to the constant resistance provided by the bands or tubing, the training may appear more difficult to some individuals because the resistance is used during both the eccentric and the concentric phases of the repetition. In addition, the bands can be used by beginners and strength-trained individuals. This is because several tension cords (up to eight bands) are available and all participants can progress through various resistance levels.

At the beginning, it may be a little confusing to determine how to use the bands and create the proper loops to grip the bands. The assistance of a training video, an instructor, or a personal trainer is helpful. The bands can be wrapped around a post or a doorknob, or you can stand on them for some exercises. A few sample elastic-band resistive exercises are provided in Figure 7.10. Instructional booklets are available for purchase with elastic bands or tubing.

Figure 7.10 Sample elastic-band resistive exercises.

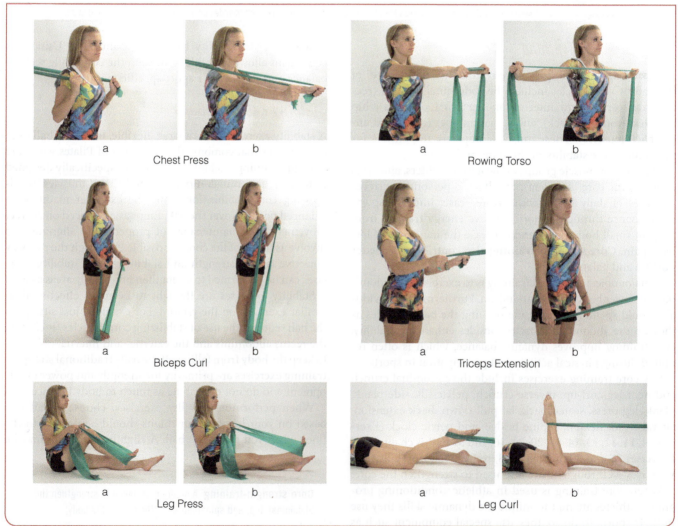

a b	a b
Chest Press	Rowing Torso
a b	a b
Biceps Curl	Triceps Extension
a b	a b
Leg Press	Leg Curl

© Fitness & Wellness, Inc.

HOEGER KEY TO WELLNESS

To maximize health and fitness benefits, always end a heavy-resistance strength-training session with a 30-minute light- to moderate-intensity aerobic workout.

7.9 Exercise Safety Guidelines

As you prepare to design your strength-training program, keep the following guidelines in mind:

- *Safety is the most important component in strength-training.* If you are new to strength-training or if you are lifting alone, strength-training machines are the best option for you. Experienced lifters like to use a combination of both free weights and strength-training machines.
- *Select exercises that will involve all major muscle groups:* chest, shoulders, back, legs, arms, hip, and trunk.
- *Select exercises that will strengthen the core.* Use controlled movements and start with light to moderate resistances. (Later, athletes may use explosive movements with heavier resistances.)
- *Never lift weights alone.* Always have someone work out with you in case you need a spotter or help with an injury. When you use free weights, one to two spotters are recommended for certain exercises (e.g., bench press, squats, and overhead press).
- *Prior to lifting weights, warm up properly* by performing a light- to moderate-intensity aerobic activity (5 to 7 minutes) and some gentle stretches for a few minutes.
- *Use proper lifting technique for each exercise.* The correct lifting technique will involve only those muscles and joints intended for a specific exercise. Involving other muscles and joints to "cheat" during the exercise to complete a repetition or to be able to lift a greater resistance decreases the long-term effectiveness of the exercise and can lead to injury (such as arching the back during the push-up, squat, or bench press exercises). Proper lifting technique also implies performing the exercises in a controlled manner and throughout the entire ROM. Perform each repetition in a rhythmic manner and at a moderate speed. Avoid fast and jerky movements, and do not throw the entire body into the lifting motion. Do not arch the back when lifting a weight.
- *Don't lock your elbows and knee joints while lifting.* See that you always leave a slight bend in the elbows and knees when straightening out the legs and arms.
- *Maintain proper body balance while lifting.* Proper balance involves good posture, a stable body position, and correct seat and arm/leg settings on exercise machines. Loss of balance places undue strain on smaller muscles and leads to injuries because of the high resistances suddenly placed on them. In the early stages of a program, first-time lifters often struggle with bar control and balance when using free weights. This problem is overcome quickly with practice following a few training sessions.
- *Exercise larger muscle groups (multi-joint groups such as those in the chest, back, and legs) before exercising smaller muscle groups (single-joint groups such as the arms, abdominals, ankles, and neck).* For example, the bench press exercise works the chest, shoulders, and back of the upper arms (triceps), whereas the triceps extension works the back of the upper arms only.
- *Exercise opposing muscle groups for a balanced workout.* When you work the chest (bench press), also work the back (rowing torso). If you work the biceps (arm curl), also work the triceps (triceps extension).
- *Breathe naturally.* Inhale during the eccentric phase (bringing the weight down), and exhale during the concentric phase (lifting or pushing the weight up). Practice proper breathing with lighter weights when you are learning a new exercise.
- *Avoid holding your breath while straining to lift a weight.* Holding your breath increases the pressure inside the chest and abdominal cavity greatly, making it nearly impossible for the blood in the veins to return to the heart, and can cause arterial stiffness (see insert box on page 280). Although rare, a sudden high intrathoracic pressure may lead to dizziness, blackout, stroke, heart attack, deadly aneurism, or hernia.
- *Based on the program selected, allow adequate recovery time between sets of exercises* (see Table 7.5).
- *If you experience unusual discomfort or pain, discontinue training.* Strength-training exercises should not cause pain while lifting. Stay within a ROM that is comfortable and as you progress along, you can gradually extend the range. The high-tension loads used in strength-training can exacerbate potential injuries. Discomfort and pain are signals to stop and determine what's wrong. Be sure to evaluate your condition properly before you continue training.
- *Use common sense on days when you feel fatigued or when you are performing sets to complete fatigue.* Excessive fatigue affects lifting technique, body balance, muscles involved, and ROM—all of which increase the risk for injury. Learn to listen to your body and decrease exercise intensity and volume if you are not feeling right. A spotter is recommended when sets are performed to complete fatigue. The spotter's help through the most difficult part of the repetition will relieve undue stress on muscles, ligaments, and tendons—and help ensure that you perform the exercise correctly.
- *At the end of each strength-training workout, stretch for a few minutes* to help your muscles return to their normal resting length and to minimize muscle soreness and risk for injury.

7.10 Setting Up Your Own Strength-Training Program

The same pre-exercise guidelines outlined for cardiorespiratory endurance training apply to strength-training (see Activity 1.3 "PAR-Q," pages 39–42). If you have concerns about your present health status or ability to participate safely in strength-training, consult a physician before you start. Strength-training is not advised for people with advanced heart disease.

Before you proceed to write your strength-training program, you should determine your stage of change for this fitness component in Activity 7.2 at the end of the chapter. Next, if you are prepared to do so, and depending on the facilities available, you can choose one of the training programs outlined in this chapter (use Activity 7.2). Once you begin your strength-training program, you may use the form provided in Activity 7.3 to keep a record of your training sessions.

You should base the resistance, number of repetitions, and sets you use with your program on your current muscular fitness level and the amount of time that you have for your strength workout. If you are training for reasons other than general health fitness, review Table 7.5 for a summary of the guidelines.

Recommendations to Minimize the Risk of Arterial Stiffness with Heavy-Resistance Strength-Training

Regular strength-training provides substantial health benefits. Among other benefits it includes a decrease in risk for diabetes, hypertension, cardiovascular disease, osteoporosis, and premature mortality. It further helps with weight management, overall fat and visceral fat loss, and an increase in lean body mass and resting metabolic rate.

Because of several research reports, concerns have risen in recent years regarding *heavy-resistance* strength-training and increased arterial stiffness (hardening of the arteries). Heavy-resistance strength-training can be defined as the regular execution of multiple sets of exercises with fewer than 10 reps all out (1 RM to <10 RM performed to muscular failure). Blood vessels are made of elastic/muscular walls that aid the heart as it contracts and relaxes. Decreased arterial compliance (increased stiffness) is frequently seen with advancing age and in people suffering from atherosclerosis, abnormal blood lipids, coronary heart disease, high blood pressure, diabetes, chronic kidney disease, obesity, and high cholesterol. It is also a risk factor for strokes.

Aerobic exercise has been shown to enhance arterial compliance, whereas some data indicate that heavy-resistance strength-training is associated with increased arterial stiffness. Furthermore, aerobically trained people have better blood vessel compliance than either sedentary or strength-trained (only) individuals.

Heavy-resistance strength-training can be performed using different breathing-control techniques. The two most common techniques involve exhalation during exertion and the Valsalva maneuver during exertion. The former does not require holding your breath during the exertion phase. On an exercise like the bench press, for example, the person inhales during the down phase and exhales during the up (exertion) phase of lifting. The Valsalva maneuver implies inhaling fully and then exhaling against a closed airway (holding your breath) that is aided by the contraction of the diaphragm, the abdominal muscles, and other expiratory muscles during the exertion phase. Such great intra-abdominal pressure causes an extraordinary rise in blood pressure.

Arterial stiffness is one of the markers that reflect blood-vessel-wall health. A healthy blood vessel expands and recoils in response to changes in blood pressure and is able to withstand high-pressure blood flow through distention during each heart contraction. When arteries stiffen, the blood vessel wall is unable to distend sufficiently. Such a condition increases the load on the heart as the myocardium (heart muscle) now has to generate a stronger contraction to provide the amount of blood needed for the activity. Although rare, high blood pressure increases the risk of deadly aneurysms. An aneurysm is a

bulge in the blood vessel that may rupture, form blood clots, or cause the layers of the blood vessel to come apart. Ruptured aneurysms are one of the top 10 causes of death in men over 50. Some physicians state that older men have weakened arterial walls and thus are more likely to have an aneurysm.

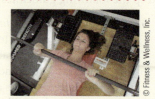
© Fitness & Wellness, Inc.

Normal blood pressure is any pressure at or below 120/80 mm Hg. Blood pressure may rise to an average of 320/250 mm Hg among individuals performing at or close to 1 RM lifts. Healthy arteries can withstand high blood pressure for a few seconds, the time required to complete an intense set of lifting. An unhealthy blood vessel, however, may not withstand such extremely high blood pressure.

Increases in blood vessel stiffness have been found following acute (a single bout) and chronic (long-term) heavy-resistance strength-training. Of particular concern is the cardiovascular health of middle-aged and older adults who perform heavy-resistance strength-training for years. Although the data are still debatable, some research indicates that even young, strength-trained athletes who do not participate in aerobic exercise have stiffer arteries. Furthermore, athletes who have trained with heavy resistances for longer than a year, without engaging in aerobic exercise, have greater arterial stiffness than sedentary people who do not strength train or perform aerobic exercise.

The good news is that arterial stiffness does not increase to the same extent in strength-trained individuals who use the exhalation technique during exertion. And even better news, research shows that performing aerobic exercise immediately following heavy-resistance training prevents blood vessel stiffness. Thirty to 60 minutes of aerobic exercise is recommended after intense strength-training. A practical example, Jack LaLanne, known as "the godfather of fitness," and a successful body builder, died in 2011 at the age of 96. He opened one of the nation's first fitness gyms in Oakland, California in 1936 and is also credited with inventing several strength-training machines. Jack was known to lift weights for 90 minutes and always followed his strength-training session with 30 to 60 minutes of swimming. Until more data and definite guidelines become available, if you choose not to do aerobic exercise following heavy strength-training, you are encouraged to use the exhalation on exertion technique and perform sets of 10 to 15 repetitions, with sufficient resistance to build muscle tone and derive strength-training benefits without stressing the arteries. A combination of both strength-training and aerobic exercise, however, is best to derive the full benefits of both activities.

Activity 7.2   Strength-Training Program

Name _____ Date _____

Course _____ Section _____ Gender _____ Age _____

I. Stage of Change for Muscular Strength or Endurance

Using Figure 2.7 (page 73) and Table 2.3 (page 73), identify your current stage of change for participation in a muscular strength or muscular endurance program:

II. Instructions

Select one of the two strength-training exercise programs. Perform all of the recommended exercises and, with the exception of the abdominal curl-up exercises, determine the resistance required to do approximately 10 repetitions maximum. For "Strength-Training Exercises without Weights," simply indicate the total number of repetitions performed. For the abdominal crunches or curl-up exercises, perform or build up to about 20 repetitions.

1. Strength-Training Exercises without Weights

Exercise	Repetitions
Step-up	
Rowing torso	
Push-up	
Abdominal crunch or bent-leg curl-up	
Leg curl	
Modified dip	
Pull-up or arm curl	
Heel raise	
Leg abduction and adduction	
Reverse crunch	
Pelvic tilt	
Side plank	
Plank	

2. Strength-Training Exercises with Weights

Exercise	Repetitions	Resistance
Bench press, shoulder press, or chest press (select and circle one)		
Leg press or squat (select one)		
Abdominal crunch or bent-leg curl-up		N/A
Rowing torso		
Arm curl or upright rowing (select one)		
Leg curl or seated leg curl (select one)		
Seated back		
Heel raise		
Lat pull-down or bent-arm pullover (select one)		
Rotary torso		
Triceps extension or dip (select one)		
Knee extension		
Back extension		

Activity 7.2 Strength-Training Program *(continued)*

3. Stability Ball Exercises

Exercise	Length of hold (if applicable)	Repetitions
The plank	☐	☐
Abdominal crunches	☐	☐
Supine bridge or reverse supine bridge	☐	N/A
Push-ups	☐	☐
Back extension	☐	☐
Wall squats	☐	☐
Jackknives	☐	☐
Hamstring roll	☐	☐
Lateral trunk flexion	☐	☐

III. Your Personalized Strength-Training Program

Once you have performed the strength-training exercises in this lab, and depending on your personal preference (strength vs. endurance), design your strength-training program selecting a minimum of 8 to 10 exercises. Indicate the number of sets, repetitions, and approximate resistance that you will use. Also state the days of the week, time, and facility that will be used for this program.

Strength-training days: M ☐ T ☐ W ☐ Th ☐ F ☐ Sa ☐ Su ☐ Time of day: ☐ Facility: ☐

	Exercise	Sets / Reps / Resistance		Exercise	Sets / Reps / Resistance
1.			9.		
2.			10.		
3.			11.		
4.			12.		
5.			13.		
6.			14.		
7.			15.		
8.			16.		

© Fitness & Wellness, Inc.

Activity 7.3 **Strength-Training Record Form**

Name: _____ Date: _____ Course: _____ Section: _____ Gender: _____ Age: _____

Date											
Exercise	St/Reps/Res*	St/Reps/Res*	St/Reps/Res*	St/Reps/Res*	St/Reps/Res*	St/Reps/Res*	St/Reps/Res*	St/Reps/Res*	St/Reps/Res*	St/Reps/Res*	St/Reps/Res*

*St/Reps/Res = Sets, Repetitions, and Resistance (e.g., 1/6/125 = 1 set of 6 repetitions with 125 pounds)

MINDTAP From Cengage **Complete This Online**
Visit **www.cengagebrain.com** to access MindTap, a complete digital course that includes interactive quizzes, videos, and more.

© Fitness & Wellness, Inc.

Assess Your Behavior

1. Are your strength levels sufficient to perform tasks of daily living (climbing stairs, carrying a backpack, opening jars, doing housework, mowing the yard, etc.) without requiring additional assistance or feeling unusually fatigued?

2. Do you regularly participate in a strength-training program that includes all major muscle groups of the body, and do you perform at least one set of each exercise to near fatigue?

Assess Your Knowledge

1. The ability of a muscle to exert submaximal force repeatedly over time is known as
   a. muscular strength.
   b. plyometric training.
   c. muscular endurance.
   d. isokinetic training.
   e. isometric training.

2. Muscle hypertrophy as a result of a similar strength-training program is greater in men than in women
   a. due to endocrinological differences.
   b. because the former have more muscle fibers.
   c. due to differences in muscle quality between both genders.
   d. Choices a and b are correct.
   e. Choices a through c are correct.

3. The Hand Grip Strength Test is an example of
   a. an isometric test.
   b. an isotonic test.
   c. a dynamic test.
   d. an isokinetic test.
   e. a plyometric test.

4. A 70th percentile rank places an individual in the ___ fitness category.
   a. excellent
   b. good
   c. average
   d. fair
   e. poor

5. During an eccentric muscle contraction,
   a. the muscle shortens as it overcomes the resistance.
   b. there is little or no movement during the contraction.
   c. a joint has to move through the entire range of motion.
   d. the muscle lengthens as it contracts.
   e. the speed is kept constant throughout the range of motion.

6. The training concept stating that the demands placed on a system must be increased systematically and progressively over time to cause physiological adaptation is referred to as
   a. the overload principle.
   b. positive-resistance training.
   c. specificity of training.
   d. variable-resistance training.
   e. progressive resistance.

7. A set in strength-training refers to
   a. the starting position for an exercise.
   b. the recovery time required between exercises.
   c. a given number of repetitions.
   d. the starting resistance used in an exercise.
   e. the sequence in which exercises are performed.

8. For health fitness, the recommendation of the American College of Sports Medicine is that a person should perform a maximum of between
   a. 1 and 6 reps.
   b. 4 and 10 reps.
   c. 8 and 12 reps.
   d. 10 and 25 reps.
   e. 20 and 30 reps.

9. Nutrition guidelines for optimum myofibrillar hypertrophy indicate that
   a. the timing, dose, and type of protein following strength-training are all important.
   b. you should consume a carbohydrate/protein snack immediately following strength-training.
   c. you should consume between 1.2 and 2.0 grams of protein per kilogram of body weight per day.
   d. whey protein is superior to other types of protein.
   e. All of the choices are correct.

10. The posterior deltoid, rhomboids, and trapezius muscles can be developed with the
    a. bench press.
    b. lat pull-down.
    c. rotary torso.
    d. squat.
    e. rowing torso.

Correct answers can be found at the back of the book.

MINDTAP **Complete This Online**
From Cengage   Visit **www.cengagebrain.com** to access MindTap, a complete digital course that includes interactive quizzes, videos, and more.

Strength-Training Exercises without Weights

EXERCISE 1 Step-Up

ACTION Step up and down using a box or chair approximately 12 to 15 inches high (a). Conduct one set using the same leg each time you step up, and then conduct a second set using the other leg. You also could alternate legs on each step-up cycle. You may increase the resistance by holding an object in your arms (b). Hold the object close to the body to avoid increased strain in the lower back.

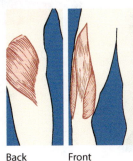
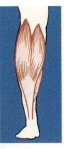

Back · Front · Back

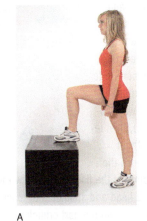
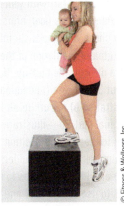

A · B

MUSCLES DEVELOPED Gluteal muscles, quadriceps, gastrocnemius, and soleus

EXERCISE 2 Rowing Torso

ACTION Raise your arms laterally (abduction) to a horizontal position and bend your elbows to 90 degrees. Have a partner apply enough pressure on your elbows to gradually force your arms forward (horizontal flexion) while you try to resist the pressure. Next, reverse the ACTION, horizontally forcing the arms backward as your partner applies sufficient forward pressure to create resistance.

MUSCLES DEVELOPED Posterior deltoid, rhomboids, and trapezius

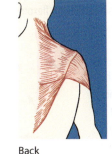
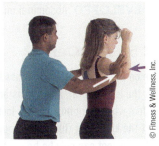

Back

EXERCISE 3 Push-Up

ACTION Maintaining your body as straight as possible (a), flex the elbows, lowering the body until you almost touch the floor (b), then raise yourself back up to the starting position. If you are unable to perform the push-up as indicated, decrease the resistance by supporting the lower body with the knees rather than the feet (c).

MUSCLES DEVELOPED Triceps, deltoid, pectoralis major, abdominals, and erector spinae

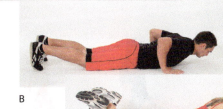

A

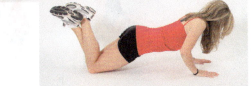

B

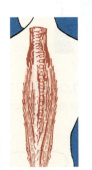

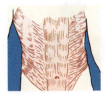

Back · Back · Front · Front · C

Strength-Training Exercises without Weights *(continued)*

EXERCISE 4
Abdominal Crunch and Bent-Leg Curl-Up

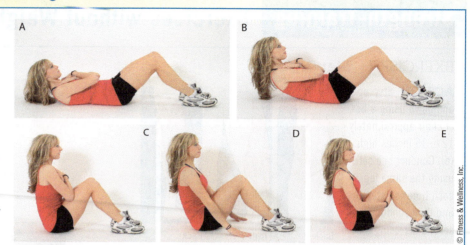

ACTION Start with your head and shoulders off the floor, arms crossed on your chest, and knees slightly bent (a). The greater the flexion of the knee, the more difficult the curl-up. Now curl up to about 30 degrees (abdominal crunch—illustration b) or curl up all the way (abdominal curl-up—illustration c), then return to the starting position without letting the head or shoulders touch the floor or allowing the hips to come off the floor. If you allow the hips to rise off the floor and the head and shoulders to touch the floor, you most likely will "swing up" on the next crunch or curl-up, which minimizes the work of the abdominal muscles. If you cannot curl up with the arms on the chest, place the hands by the side of the hips or even help yourself up by holding on to your thighs (d and e). Do not perform the sit-up exercise with your legs completely extended, because this will strain the lower back.

MUSCLES DEVELOPED Abdominal muscles and hip flexors

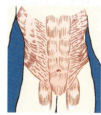

Front

NOTE The abdominal curl-up exercise should be used only by individuals of at least average fitness without a history of lower back problems. New participants and those with a history of lower back problems should use the abdominal crunch exercise in its place.

EXERCISE 5   Leg Curl

ACTION Lie on the floor face down. Cross the right ankle over the left heel (a). Apply resistance with your right foot while you bring the left foot up to 90 degrees at the knee joint (b). Apply enough resistance so the left foot can only be brought up slowly. Repeat the exercise, crossing the left ankle over the right heel.

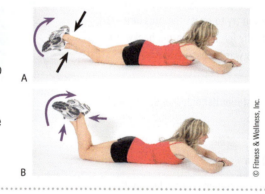

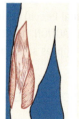

Front   Back

MUSCLES DEVELOPED
Hamstrings (and quadriceps)

EXERCISE 6   Modified Dip

ACTION Using a gymnasium bleacher or box and with the help of a partner, dip down at least to a 90-degree angle at the elbow joint and then return to the initial position.

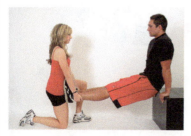

A

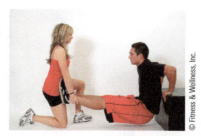

B

Back   Front

MUSCLES DEVELOPED
Triceps, deltoid, and pectoralis major

© Fitness & Wellness, Inc.

Strength-Training Exercises without Weights *(continued)*

EXERCISE 7 Pull-Up

ACTION Suspend yourself from a bar with a pronated (thumbs-in) grip (a). Pull your body up until your chin is above the bar (b), then lower the body slowly to the starting position. If you are unable to perform the pull-up as described, have a partner hold your feet to push off and facilitate the movement upward (c and d).

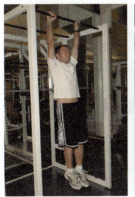

A

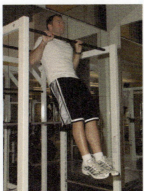

B

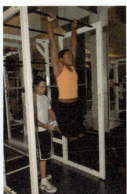

C

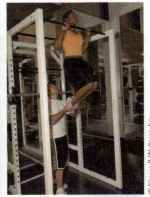

D

MUSCLES DEVELOPED
Biceps, brachioradialis, brachialis, trapezius, and latissimus dorsi

Front   Front

EXERCISE 8 Arm Curl

ACTION Using a palms-up grip, start with the arm completely extended and, with the aid of a sandbag or bucket filled (as needed) with sand or rocks (a), curl up as far as possible (b), then return to the initial position. Repeat the exercise with the other arm.

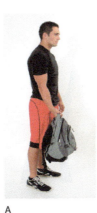

A

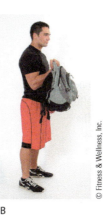

B

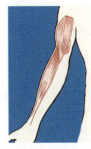

Front

MUSCLES DEVELOPED
Biceps, brachioradialis, and brachialis

EXERCISE 9 Heel Raise

ACTION From a standing position with feet flat on the floor or at the edge of a step (a), raise and lower your body weight by moving at the ankle joint only (b). For added resistance, have someone else hold your shoulders down as you perform the exercise.

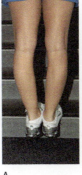

A

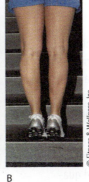

B

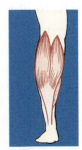

MUSCLES DEVELOPED
Gastrocnemius and soleus

Back

Strength-Training Exercises without Weights (continued)

EXERCISE 10   Leg Abduction and Adduction

ACTION Both participants sit on the floor. The person on the left places the feet on the inside of the other person's feet. Simultaneously, the person on the left presses the legs laterally (to the outside—abduction), while the person on the right presses the legs medially (adduction). Hold the contraction for 5 to 10 seconds. Repeat the exercise at all three angles, and then reverse the pressing sequence: The person on the left places the feet on the outside and presses inward while the person on the right presses outward.

MUSCLES DEVELOPED Hip abductors (rectus femoris, sartori, gluteus medius and minimus) and adductors (pectineus, gracilis, adductor magnus, adductor longus, and adductor brevis)

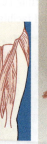

Back

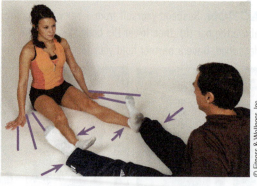

© Fitness & Wellness, Inc.

EXERCISE 11
Reverse Crunch

ACTION Lie on your back with arms to the sides and knees and hips flexed at 90 degrees (a). Now attempt to raise the pelvis off the floor by lifting vertically from the knees and lower legs (b). This is a challenging exercise that may be difficult for beginners to perform.

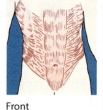

Front

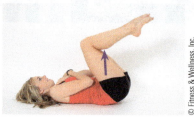

A   B

MUSCLES DEVELOPED
Abdominals

© Fitness & Wellness, Inc.

EXERCISE 12   Pelvic Tilt

ACTION Lie flat on the floor with the knees bent at about a 90-degree angle (a). Tilt the pelvis by tightening the abdominal muscles, flattening your back against the floor, and raising the lower gluteal area ever so slightly off the floor (b). Hold the final position for several seconds.

AREAS STRETCHED Low back muscles and ligaments

AREAS STRENGTHENED Abdominal and gluteal muscles

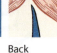

Front   Back

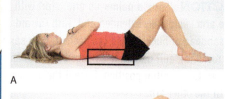

A

B

© Fitness & Wellness, Inc.

EXERCISE 13   Side Plank

ACTION Lie on your side with legs bent (a: easier version) or straight (b: harder version) and support the upper body with your arm. Straighten your body by raising the hip off the floor and hold the position for several seconds. Repeat the exercise with the other side of the body.

MUSCLES DEVELOPED Abdominals (obliques and transversus abdominus) and quadratus lumborum (lower back)

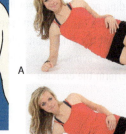

Front   Back

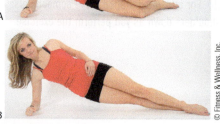

A

B

© Fitness & Wellness, Inc.

Strength-Training Exercises without Weights *(continued)*

EXERCISE 14 Plank

ACTION Starting in a prone position on a floor mat, balance yourself on the tips of your toes and elbows while attempting to maintain a straight body from heels to shoulders (do not arch the lower back) (a). You can increase the difficulty of this exercise by placing your hands in front of you and straightening the arms (elbows off the floor) (b).

MUSCLES DEVELOPED Anterior and posterior muscle groups of the trunk and pelvis

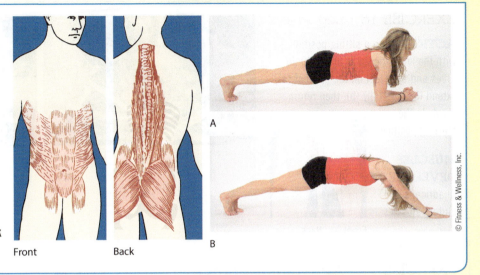

Front   Back

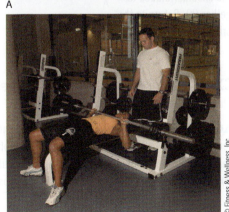

A

B

© Fitness & Wellness, Inc.

Strength-Training Exercises with Weights

EXERCISE 15 Chest/Bench Press

MUSCLES DEVELOPED Pectoralis major, triceps, and deltoid

MACHINE From a seated position, grasp the bar handles (a) and press forward until the arms are completely extended (b), then return to the original position. Do not arch.

FREE WEIGHTS Lie on the bench with arms extended and have one or two spotters help you place the barbell directly over your shoulders (a). Lower the weight to your chest (b) and then push it back up until you achieve full extension of the arms. Do not arch the back during this exercise.

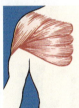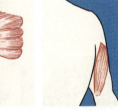

Front   Back

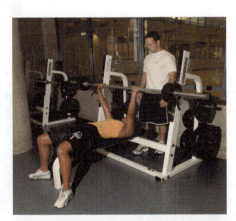

A

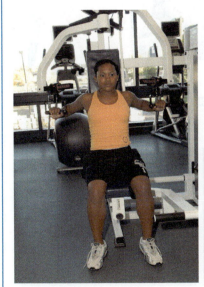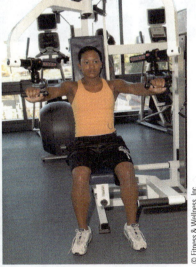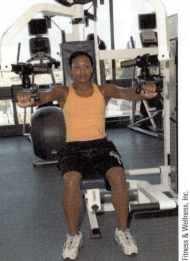

A   B

B

© Fitness & Wellness, Inc.

© Fitness & Wellness, Inc.

Strength-Training Exercises with Weights *(continued)*

EXERCISE 16   Leg Press

ACTION From a sitting position with the knees flexed at about 90 degrees and both feet on the footrest (a), extend the legs fully (b); then return slowly to the starting position.

MUSCLES DEVELOPED Quadriceps and gluteal muscles

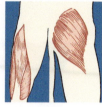

Front   Back

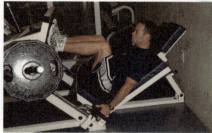

A

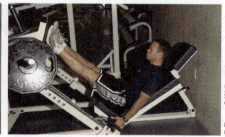

B

EXERCISE 17   Abdominal Crunch

ACTION Sit in an upright position. Grasp the handles in front of you and crunch forward. Return slowly to the original position.

MUSCLES DEVELOPED Abdominals

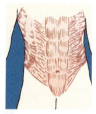

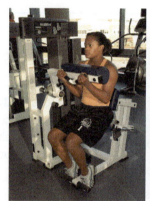

A

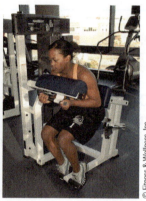

B

EXERCISE 18A Rowing Torso

ACTION Sit in the machine and grasp the handles in front of you (a). Press back as far as possible, drawing the shoulder blades together (b). Return to the original position.

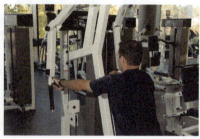

A

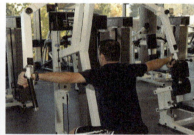

B

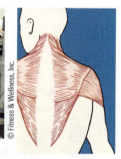

Back

MUSCLES DEVELOPED Posterior deltoid, rhomboids, and trapezius

EXERCISE 18B Bent-over Lateral Raise

ACTION Bend over with your back straight and knees bent at about 5 to 10 degrees (a). Hold one dumbbell in each hand. Raise the dumbbells laterally to about shoulder level (b) and then slowly return them to the starting position.

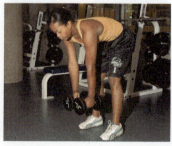

A

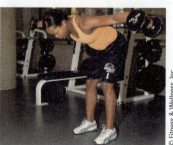

B

Strength-Training Exercises with Weights *(continued)*

EXERCISE 19   Leg Curl

ACTION Lie face down on the bench, legs straight, and place the back of the feet under the padded bar (a). Curl up to at least 90 degrees (b), then return to the original position.

MUSCLES DEVELOPED
Hamstrings

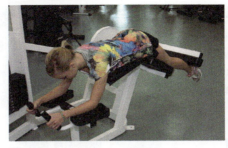

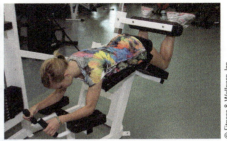

A   B

© Fitness & Wellness, Inc.

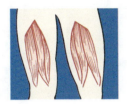

Back

EXERCISE 20   Seated Back

ACTION Sit in the machine with your trunk flexed and the upper back against the shoulder pad. Place the feet under the padded bar and hold on with your hands to the bars on the sides (a). Start the exercise by pressing backward, simultaneously extending the trunk and hip joints (b). Slowly return to the original position.

MUSCLES DEVELOPED Erector spinae and gluteus maximus

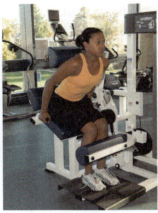

Back

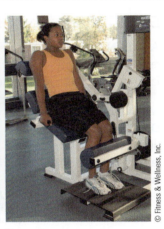

A   B

© Fitness & Wellness, Inc.

EXERCISE 21   Calf Press

MACHINE Start with your feet flat on the plate (a). Now extend the ankles by pressing on the plate with the balls of your feet (b). Return to the starting position.

FREE WEIGHTS In a standing position, place a barbell across the shoulders and upper back. Grip the bar by the shoulders (a). Raise your heels off the floor or step box as far as possible (b) and then slowly return them to the starting position.

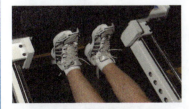

A

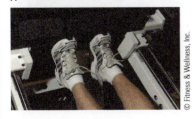

B

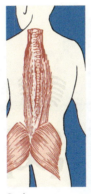

Back

MUSCLES DEVELOPED
Gastrocnemius, soleus

© Fitness & Wellness, Inc.

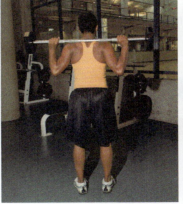

A

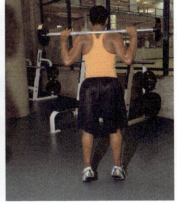

B

© Fitness & Wellness, Inc.

Strength-Training Exercises with Weights *(continued)*

EXERCISE 22   Leg (Hip) Adduction

ACTION Adjust the pads on the inside of the thighs as far out as the desired range of motion to be accomplished during the exercise (a). Press the legs together until both pads meet at the center (b). Slowly return to the starting position.

MUSCLES DEVELOPED Hip adductors (pectineus, gracilis, adductor magnus, adductor longus, and adductor brevis)

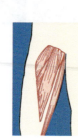

Front

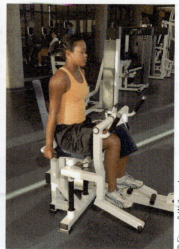

A   B

© Fitness & Wellness, Inc.

EXERCISE 23   Leg (Hip) Abduction

ACTION Place your knees together with the pads directly outside the knees (a). Press the legs laterally out as far as possible (b). Slowly return to the starting position.

MUSCLES DEVELOPED Hip abductors (rectus femoris, sartori, gluteus medius and minimus)

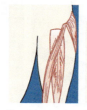

Front   Back

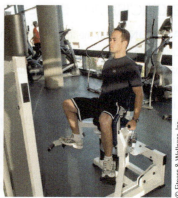

A   B

© Fitness & Wellness, Inc.

EXERCISE 24   Lat Pull-Down

ACTION Starting from a sitting position, hold the exercise bar with a wide grip (a). Pull the bar down in front of you until it reaches the upper chest (b), then return to the starting position.

MUSCLES DEVELOPED Latissimus dorsi, pectoralis major, and biceps

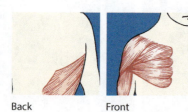

Back   Front

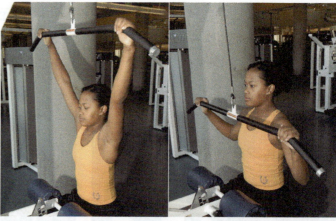

A   B

© Fitness & Wellness, Inc.

Strength-Training Exercises with Weights *(continued)*

EXERCISE 25
Rotary Torso

MACHINE: Face the machine and kneel on the pad provided with the equipment (a). Slowly rotate the hips in a controlled manner as far as possible to the left (b). At the end of the range of motion gradually return to the starting position. Repeat the exercise to the right side.

FREE WEIGHTS Stand with your feet slightly apart. Place a barbell across your shoulders and upper back, holding on to the sides of the barbell. Now gently, and in a controlled manner, twist your torso to one side as far as possible and then do so in the opposite direction.

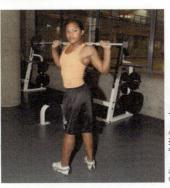

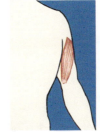

Front

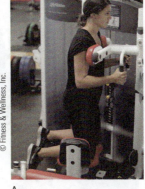

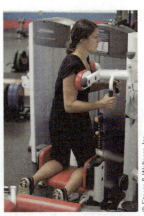

A

B

MUSCLES DEVELOPED Internal and external obliques (abdominal muscles)

....

EXERCISE 26 Triceps Extension

MUSCLES DEVELOPED Triceps

MACHINE Sit in an upright position and grasp the bar behind the shoulders (a). Fully extend the arms (b), then return to the original position.

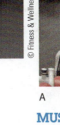

Back

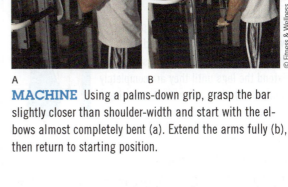

A

B

MACHINE Using a palms-down grip, grasp the bar slightly closer than shoulder-width and start with the elbows almost completely bent (a). Extend the arms fully (b), then return to starting position.

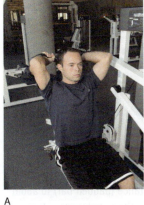

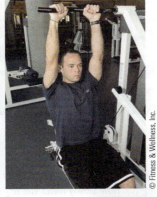

A

B

FREE WEIGHTS In a standing position, hold a barbell with both hands overhead and with the arms in full extension (a). Slowly lower the barbell behind your head (b), then return it to the starting position.

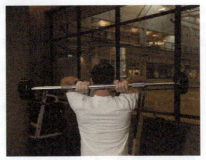

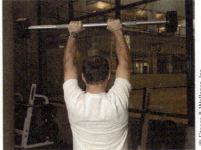

A

B

Strength-Training Exercises with Weights *(continued)*

EXERCISE 27   Arm Curl

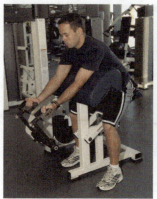
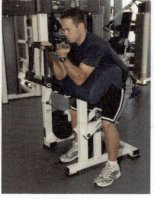

A   B

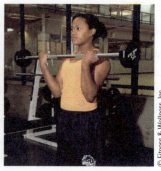
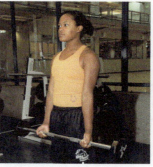

A   B

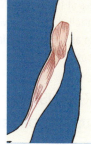

Front

MACHINE Using a supinated (palms-up) grip, start with the arms almost completely extended (a). Curl up as far as possible (b), then return to the starting position.

FREE WEIGHTS Standing upright, hold a barbell in front of you at about shoulder width with arms extended and the hands in a thumbs-out position (supinated grip) (a). Raise the barbell to your shoulders (b) and slowly return it to the starting position.

MUSCLES DEVELOPED Biceps, brachioradialis, and brachialis

EXERCISE 28A   Knee Extension

ACTION Sit in an upright position with the feet under the padded bar and grasp the handles at the sides (a). Extend the legs until they are completely straight (b), then return to the starting position.

MUSCLES DEVELOPED Quadriceps

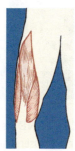

Front

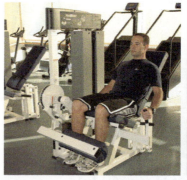
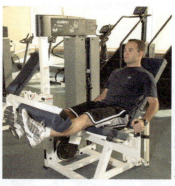

A   B

EXERCISE 28B   Unilateral Eccentric Knee Flexion

ACTION Using a *moderate resistance*, raise the padded bar by extending both knees (see Exercise 28A, a and b). Next, remove the left foot from the padded bar while holding the bar in place with the right leg (c). Now slowly lower the resistance (padded bar) to about 45 degrees (d). Return the left foot to the padded bar and once again press the bar up to full knee extension. Alternate legs by releasing the right foot next and lower the resistance with the left foot. Repeat the exercise about 10 times with each leg. **THIS EXERCISE IS *QUITE HELPFUL* TO STRENGTHEN WEAK KNEES AND PREVENT POTENTIAL FUTURE KNEE PROBLEMS.**

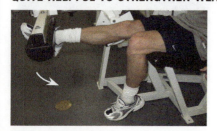
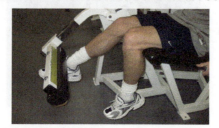
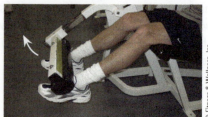

C   D   E

Strength-Training Exercises with Weights *(continued)*

EXERCISE 29 Shoulder Press

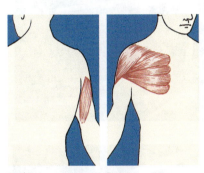

Back   Front

MUSCLES DEVELOPED Triceps, deltoid, and pectoralis major

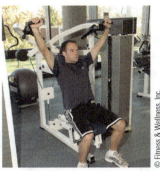

A   B

MACHINE Sit in an upright position and grasp the bar wider than shoulder width (a). Press the bar all the way up until the arms are fully extended (b), then return to the initial position.

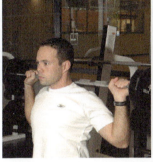

A   B

FREE WEIGHTS Place a barbell on your shoulders (a). Press the weight overhead until complete extension of the arms is achieved (b). Return the weight to the original position. Be sure not to arch the back or lean back during this exercise.

EXERCISE 30 Chest Fly

ACTION Start with the arms out to the side, and grasp the handle bars with the arms straight (a). Press the movement arms forward until they are completely in front of you (b). Slowly return to the starting position.

MUSCLES DEVELOPED Pectoralis major and deltoid

Front

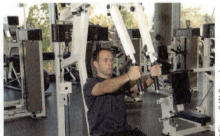

A   B

FREE WEIGHTS **Bent Arm Fly** Lie down on your back on a bench and hold a dumbbell in each hand directly overhead (a). Keeping your elbows slightly bent, lower the weights laterally to a horizontal position (b), then bring them back up to the starting position.

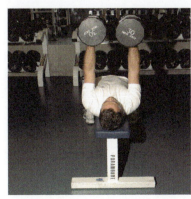

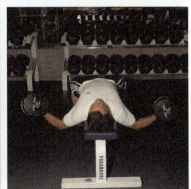

A   B

Strength-Training Exercises with Weights *(continued)*

EXERCISE 31 Squat

MACHINE Place the shoulders under the pads and grasp the bars by the sides of the shoulders (a). Slowly bend the knees to between 90 and 120 degrees (b). Return to the starting position.

MUSCLES DEVELOPED Quadriceps, gluteus maximus, erector spinae

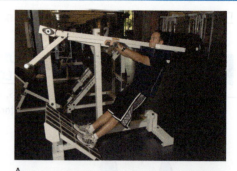

A

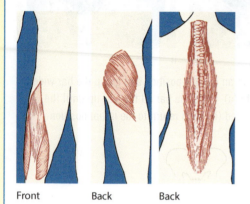

Front   Back   Back

B

© Fitness & Wellness, Inc.

FREE WEIGHTS From a standing position, and with a spotter to each side, support a barbell over your shoulders and upper back (a). Keeping your head up and back straight, bend at the knees and the hips until you achieve an approximate 120-degree angle at the knees (b). Return to the starting position. *Do not perform this exercise alone.* If no spotters are available, use a squat rack to ensure that you will not get trapped under a heavy weight.

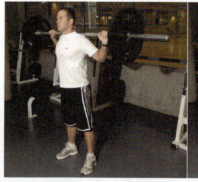

A   B

© Fitness & Wellness, Inc.

Strength-Training Exercises with Weights *(continued)*

EXERCISE 32   Upright Rowing

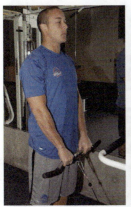
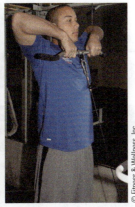

A   B

MACHINE Start with the arms extended and grip the handles with the palms down (a). Pull all the way up to the chin (b), then return to the starting position.

FREE WEIGHTS Hold a barbell in front of you, with the arms fully extended and hands in a thumbs-in (pronated) grip less than shoulder-width apart (a). Pull the barbell up until it reaches shoulder level (b) and then slowly return it to the starting position.

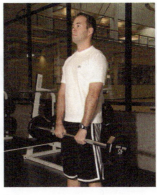
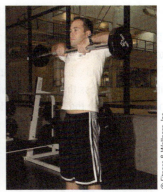

A   B

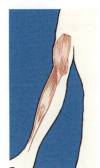
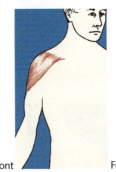
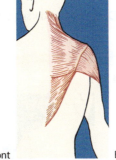

Front   Front   Back

MUSCLES DEVELOPED Biceps, brachioradialis, brachialis, deltoid, and trapezius

---

EXERCISE 33   Seated Leg Curl

ACTION Sit in the unit and place the strap over the upper thighs. With legs extended, place the back of the feet over the padded rollers (a). Flex the knees until you reach a 90- to 100-degree angle (b). Slowly return to the starting position.

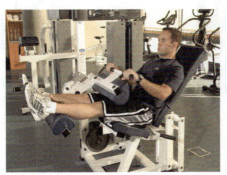

A   B

MUSCLES DEVELOPED
Hamstrings

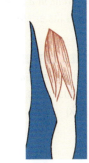

Back

© Fitness & Wellness, Inc.

Strength-Training Exercises with Weights *(continued)*

EXERCISE 34   Bent-Arm Pullover

MACHINE Sit back into the chair and grasp the bar behind your head (a). Pull the bar over your head all the way down to your abdomen (b) and slowly return to the original position.

FREE WEIGHTS Lie on your back on an exercise bench with your head over the edge of the bench. Hold a barbell over your chest with the hands less than shoulder-width apart (c). Keeping the elbows shoulder-width

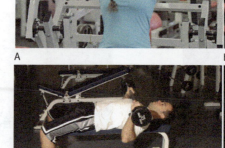
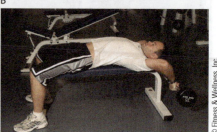

A   B

C   D

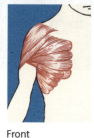

Back   Front

apart, lower the weight over your head until your shoulders are completely extended (d). Slowly return the weight to the starting position.

MUSCLES DEVELOPED Latissimus dorsi, pectoral muscles, deltoid, and serratus anterior

EXERCISE 35   Dip

ACTION Start with the elbows flexed (a), then extend the arms fully (b), and return slowly to the initial position.

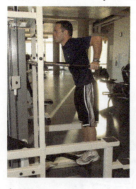
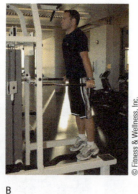
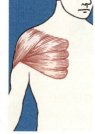

A   B

Back   Front

MUSCLES DEVELOPED Triceps, deltoid, and pectoralis major

EXERCISE 36   Back Extension

ACTION Place your feet under the ankle rollers and the hips over the padded seat. Start with the trunk in a flexed position and the arms crossed over the chest (a). Slowly extend the trunk to a horizontal position (b), hold the extension for 2 to 5 seconds, and then slowly flex (lower) the trunk to the original position.

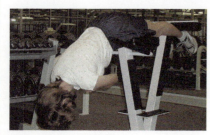
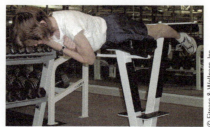
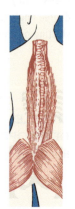

A   B

MUSCLES DEVELOPED Erector spinae, gluteus maximus, and quadratus lumborum (lower back)

Back

Strength-Training Exercises with Weights *(continued)*

EXERCISE 37   Lateral Trunk Flexion

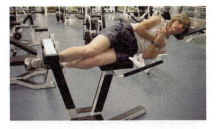
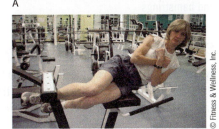

ACTION Lie sideways on the padded seat with the right foot under the right side of the padded ankle pad (right knee slightly bent) and the left foot stabilized on the vertical bar. Cross the arms over the abdomen or chest and start with the body in a straight line. Raise (flex) your upper body about 30 to 40 degrees and then slowly return to the starting position.

MUSCLES DEVELOPED Erector spinae, rectus abdominus, internal and external abdominal obliques, quadratus lumborum, gluteal muscles

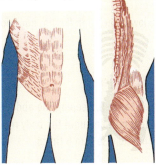

Front   Back

A

B

© Fitness & Wellness, Inc.

Stability Ball Exercises

EXERCISE 38   The Plank

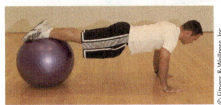

ACTION Place your knees or feet (increased difficulty) on the ball and raise your body off the floor to a horizontal position. Pull the abdominal muscles in and hold the body in a straight line for 5 to 10 seconds. Repeat the exercise 3 to 5 times.

MUSCLES INVOLVED Abdominals, erector spinae, lower back, hip flexors, gluteal, quadriceps, hamstrings, chest, shoulder, and triceps

© Fitness & Wellness, Inc.

EXERCISE 39   Abdominal Crunches

ACTION On your back and with the feet slightly separated, lie with the ball under your back and shoulder blades. Cross the arms over your chest (a). Press your lower back into the ball and crunch up 20 to 30 degrees. Keep your neck and shoulders in line with your trunk (b). Repeat the exercise 10 to 20 times (you may also do an oblique crunch by rotating the ribcage to the opposite hip at the end of the crunch [c]).

MUSCLES INVOLVED Rectus abdominus, internal and external abdominal obliques

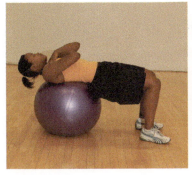
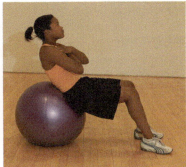
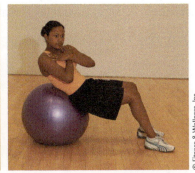

A   B   C

© Fitness & Wellness, Inc.

Stability Ball Exercises *(continued)*

EXERCISE 40   Supine Bridge

ACTION With the feet slightly separated and knees bent, lie with your neck and upper back on the ball; hands placed on the abdomen. Gently squeeze the gluteal muscles while raising your hips off the floor until the upper legs and trunk reach a straight line. Hold this position for 5 to 10 seconds. Repeat the exercise 3 to 5 times.

MUSCLES INVOLVED Gluteal, abdominals, lower back, hip flexors, quadriceps, and hamstrings

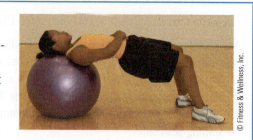

EXERCISE 41   Reverse Supine Bridge

ACTION Lie face up on the floor with the heels on the ball. Keeping the abdominal muscles tight, slowly lift the hips off the floor and squeeze the gluteal muscles until the body reaches a straight line. Hold the position for 5 to 10 seconds. Repeat the exercise 3 to 5 times.

MUSCLES INVOLVED Gluteal, abdominals, lower back, erector spinae, hip flexors, quadriceps, and hamstring

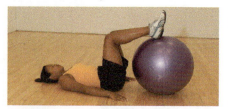
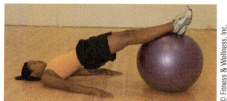

A   B

EXERCISE 42   Push-Ups

ACTION Place the front of your thighs (knees or feet—more difficult) over the ball with the body straight, the arms extended, and the hands under your shoulders. Now bend the elbows and lower the upper body as far as possible. Return to the original position. Repeat the exercise 10 times.

MUSCLES INVOLVED Triceps, chest, shoulder, abdominals, erector spinae, lower back, hip flexors, quadriceps, and hamstrings

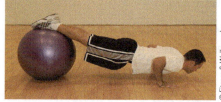

EXERCISE 43   Back Extension

ACTION Lie face down with the hips over the ball. Keep the legs straight with the toes on the floor and slightly separated (a). Keep your arms to the sides and extend the trunk until the body reaches a straight position (b). Repeat the exercise 10 times.

MUSCLES INVOLVED Erector spinae, abdominals, and lower back

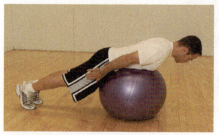
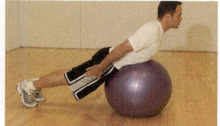

A   B

Stability Ball Exercises *(continued)*

EXERCISE 44   Wall Squat

ACTION Stand upright and position the ball between your lower back and a wall. Place your feet slightly in front of you, about a foot apart (a). Lean into the ball and lower your body by bending the knees until the thighs are parallel to the ground (b). (To avoid excessive strain on the knees, it is not recommended that you go beyond this point.) Return to the starting position. Repeat the exercise 10 to 20 times.

MUSCLES INVOLVED Quadriceps, hip flexors, hamstrings, abdominals, erector spinae, lower back, gastrocnemius, and soleus

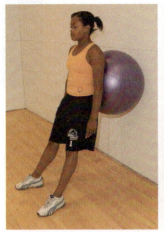
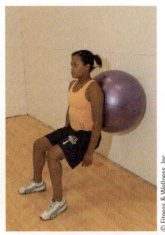

A   B

EXERCISE 45   Jackknives

ACTION Lie face down with the hips on the ball and walk forward with your hands until the thighs are over the ball. Keep the arms fully extended, hands on floor, and the body straight (a). Now, pull the ball forward with your legs by bending at the knees and raising your hips while keeping the abdominal muscles tight (b). Repeat the exercise 10 times.

MUSCLES INVOLVED Hip flexors, abdominals, erector spinae, lower back, quadriceps, hamstrings, chest, and shoulder

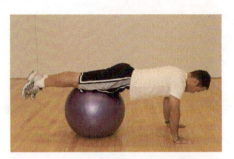

A

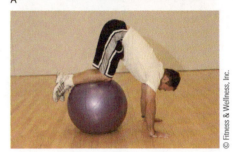

B

EXERCISE 46   Hamstring Roll

ACTION Lie on your back with your knees bent and the heels on the ball. Raise your hips off the floor, while keeping the knees bent (a). Tighten the abdominal muscles and roll the ball out with your feet to extend the legs (b). Now roll the ball back into the original position. Repeat the exercise 10 times.

MUSCLES INVOLVED Hamstrings, abdominals, erector spinae, lower back, hip flexors, quadriceps, and chest

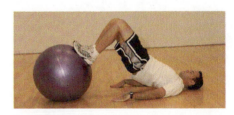

A

B

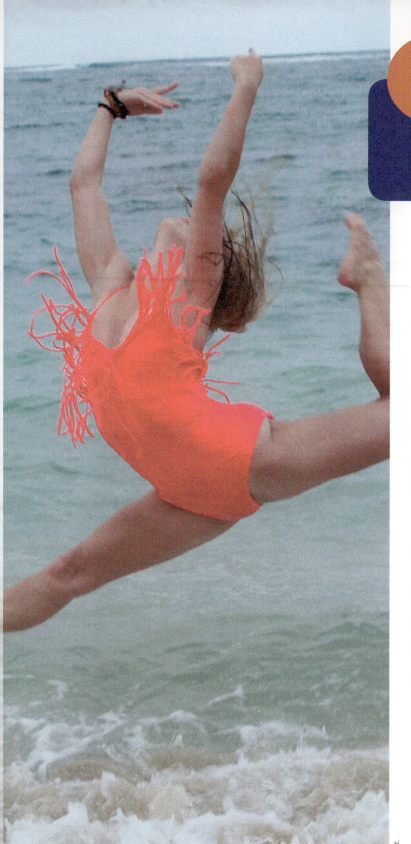

© Fitness & Wellness, Inc.

8

Muscular Flexibility

"Regrettably, most people neglect flexibility training, limiting freedom of movement, physical and mental relaxation, release of muscle tension and soreness, and injury prevention."
—American Council on Exercise (ACE)

Objectives

8.1 Explain the importance of muscular flexibility to adequate fitness.

8.2 Identify the factors that affect muscular flexibility.

8.3 Explain the health-fitness benefits of stretching.

8.4 Become familiar with a battery of tests to assess overall body flexibility (Modified Sit-and -Reach Test, Total Body Rotation Test, and Shoulder Rotation Test).

8.5 Interpret flexibility test results according to health-fitness and physical-fitness standards.

8.6 Learn the principles that govern development of muscular flexibility.

8.7 List some exercises that may cause injury.

8.8 Become familiar with a program for preventing and rehabilitating low back pain.

8.9 Create your own personal flexibility program.

FAQ

Will stretching before exercise prevent injuries?

The research on this subject is controversial. Some data suggest that intense stretching prior to physical activity modestly increases the risk for injuries and leads to a temporary decrease in muscle contraction velocity, strength, and power. Other studies, however, show no changes and even some improvement with intense pre-exercise stretching. The most important factor prior to vigorous exercise is to gradually increase the exercise intensity through mild calisthenics and light- to moderate-intensity aerobic exercise.

To prevent injuries while participating in activities that require flexibility, the American College of Sports Medicine recommends stretching following an appropriate warm-up phase. For activities that do not require much flexibility, you can perform the flexibility program following the aerobic and/or strength-training phase of your training.

Does strength-training limit flexibility?

A popular myth is that individuals with large musculature, frequently referred to as "muscle-bound," are inflexible. Data show that strength-training exercises, when performed through a full range of motion, do not limit flexibility. With few exceptions, most strength-training exercises can be performed from complete extension to complete flexion. Body builders and gymnasts, who train heavily with weights, have better-than-average flexibility.

Will stretching exercises help me lose weight?

The energy (caloric) expenditure of stretching exercises is extremely low. In 30 minutes of aerobic exercise you can easily burn an additional 250 to 300 calories as compared with 30 minutes of stretching. Flexibility exercises help develop overall health-related fitness but do not contribute much to weight loss or weight maintenance.

How much should stretching "hurt" to gain flexibility?

Proper stretching should not cause undue pain. Pain is an indication that you are stretching too aggressively. Stretching exercises should be performed to the point of "mild tension" or "limits of discomfort." It is best to decrease the degree of stretch to mild tension and hold the final position for a longer period of time (10 to 30 seconds).

REAL LIFE STORY | Maria's Experience

I have suffered from really bad back pain over the last couple years. When I moved out of my parents' house to an apartment with a friend, the only bed I could afford was an old, hand-me-down mattress from my older sister. The mattress was fairly soft and sagged a little, so it did not give good support. I started waking up most mornings with an aching back. I was also not very active. Sometimes when I was studying, I would sit hunched over my computer for hours and hours at a time, and between the stress and the sitting in one position for so long, by the time I went to bed my whole back and shoulders would be in intense pain. I went on this way for a long time, having daily back pain. I just assumed it was something I had to live with. It wasn't until I read the *Lifetime Physical Fitness and Wellness* text for school that I learned about the steps you can take to prevent back pain. I learned that my posture when sitting, standing, and sleeping was mostly incorrect, so I tried to pay attention to fixing it. I got a foot rest for when I sit at my desk, and I started sleeping with a pillow supporting my knees when I lie on my back. I also finally saved enough money to buy a new bed with a firmer mattress, which really

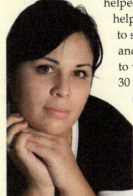
© ARENA Creative/Shutterstock.com

helped. But one of the most helpful changes I made was to start being more active and stretching daily. I like to walk briskly for about 30 minutes, and then do a series of stretches.

I especially like the way the "trunk rotation" and "cat" stretches make my back feel. After stretching, not only does my back feel better, but I also feel less stressed. Thanks to these efforts, my back pain is almost totally gone. I am so glad I learned that I didn't have to live in pain every day.

PERSONAL PROFILE: My Flexibility Health

The following questions will allow you to analyze your knowledge of and commitment to flexibility fitness. If you can't answer all of the questions, the chapter contents will provide the needed information.

I. Have you ever experienced back pain episodes similar to Maria's? ____ Yes ____ No   Can you explain the probable cause of Maria's pain?

II. How would you explain the role of aerobic, strength, and flexibility training on back health?

III. Can you touch your toes without bending your knees while sitting on the floor? ____ Yes ____ No How about the tips of your fingers behind your back with the preferred upper arm (hand) over your shoulder and the other hand coming up from behind your lower back? ____ Yes ____ No

IV. How has your flexibility changed over the last few years?

V. Do you feel that the most important factor affecting your degree of flexibility is your current level of physical activity? ____ Yes ____ No Can you expound on your answer?

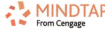
MINDTAP From Cengage   **Complete This Online**
Visit **www.cengagebrain.com** to access MindTap, a complete digital course that includes interactive quizzes, videos, and more.

Very few people take the time to stretch, and only a few of those who stretch do so properly. Though good flexibility in all major muscles groups is an important component of a comprehensive fitness program, its contribution is often overlooked or underestimated. Understanding the benefits of flexibility, factors that affect how flexible a person is, and how to assess flexibility will help you develop a successful stretching program to improve overall fitness and functional mobility throughout life.

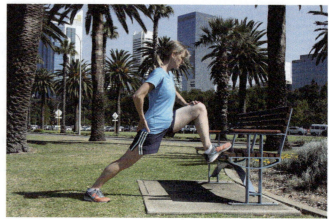
Good flexibility enhances quality of life.

8.1 Benefits of Good Flexibility

Flexibility refers to the achievable **range of motion (ROM)** at a joint or group of joints without causing injury. In daily life, we often have to make rapid or strenuous movements we are not accustomed to making. Abruptly forcing a tight muscle beyond its achievable range of motion may lead to injury. Good flexibility can help avoid strain or injury by improving elasticity of muscles and connective tissue around joints. Improved range of motion in the joints enables greater freedom of movement and increases the individual's ability to participate in many types of sports and recreational activities. Too much flexibility, however, leads to unstable and loose joints, which may increase the injury rate, and may result in joint **subluxation** and dislocation. As long as you are careful not to overstretch joints, participating in a regular flexibility program will enhance your quality of life, making activities of daily living such as turning, lifting, and bending much easier to perform.

Maintains Healthy Muscles and Joints

Taking part in a regular **stretching** program has the primary benefit of maintaining muscle and joint health. When joints are not regularly moved through their entire range of motion, muscles and ligaments shorten in time and flexibility decreases. Repetitive movement through regular or structured exercise—such as with running, cycling, or aerobics—without proper stretching also causes muscles and ligaments to tighten. Dynamic stretching exercises in particular help improve circulation and range of motion in targeted muscles and joints: the boost in heart rate and body temperature increases blood flow to the muscles being stretched and facilitates greater freedom of movement.

Improves Mental Health

Regular stretching also improves mental health. Psychological stress built up over time causes muscles to contract, contributing to tension and anxiety. The subsequent aches and pains that manifest in the body can become uncomfortable and debilitating. Flexibility exercises counter the negative effects of psychological stress by loosening tight muscles, slowing your breathing rate, and releasing endorphins that improve mood and promote relaxation.

Relieves Muscle Cramps

Stretching also helps relieve muscle cramps encountered during or after participation in exercise. Mild stretching exercises in conjunction with calisthenics are helpful in warm-up routines to gradually increase body temperature and blood flow to prepare for more vigorous aerobic or strength-training exercises. In cool-down routines, stretching following exercise facilitates the return to a normal resting state. Fatigued muscles tend to contract to a shorter-than-average resting length, and stretching exercises help fatigued muscles reestablish their normal resting length.

Improves Posture and Prevents Low Back Pain

Incorrect posture and poor mechanics, such as prolonged static postures, repetitive bending and pushing, twisting a loaded spine, and prolonged (more than an hour) sitting with little movement increase strain on the lower back and many other bones, joints, muscles, and ligaments. A good stretching program, particularly when combined with core-strengthening exercises, prevents low back and other spinal column problems by improving and maintaining good postural alignment and helping condition spine stabilizing muscles. Correct posture also promotes proper and graceful body movement and improves personal appearance and self-image.

Relieves Chronic Pain

Flexibility exercises have been prescribed successfully to treat **dysmenorrhea**[1] (painful menstruation), general neuromuscular tension (stress), and knots (trigger points) in muscles and fascia. Physicians often recommend stretching to help relieve arthritis pain and improve range of motion affected by joint damage.

8.2 What Factors Affect Flexibility?

Range of motion around a joint is influenced by joint structure (the shape of the bones), joint cartilage, ligaments, tendons, muscles, skin, tissue injury, and adipose tissue (fat). Muscle elasticity and genetics, body temperature, age, gender, and level of physical activity also affect flexibility.

Joint Structure

Each joint's total range of motion is highly specific: it varies from one joint to another (hip, trunk, shoulder, etc.) and depends mostly on the structure of that joint. For example, the ball and socket structure of the hip joint facilitates ample movement forward and backward and side to side, while the hinge-type joints of the elbow and knee have a more limited range of motion of mostly forward and backward movement. A regular stretching program that includes each joint and muscle group helps maintain range of motion around a joint and can help improve it as well.

Adipose Tissue

The amount of adipose (fat) tissue in and around joints and muscle tissue can also influence flexibility. Excess adipose tissue increases resistance to movement, and the added bulk also hampers joint mobility because of the contact between body surfaces.

Muscular Elasticity and Genetics

Muscular elasticity differs from one individual to the next and is primarily influenced by genetic factors. The propensity toward higher or lower levels of flexibility is often an inherited trait. Despite genetic variables, greater range of motion can be attained in individual muscle groups through plastic and elastic elongation. **Plastic elongation** is the permanent lengthening of soft tissue. Even though joint capsules, ligaments, and tendons are basically non-elastic, they can undergo plastic elongation. This permanent lengthening, accompanied by increased range of motion, is best attained through proper stretching exercises.

Elastic elongation is the temporary lengthening of soft tissue. Muscle tissue has elastic properties and responds to stretching exercises by undergoing elastic or temporary lengthening. Elastic elongation increases extensibility, the ability to stretch the muscles.

Body Temperature

Changes in muscle temperature can also increase or decrease flexibility. Individuals who warm up properly have better flexibility than people who do not. Cool temperatures have the opposite effect, impeding range of motion. Because of the effects of temperature on muscular flexibility, many people prefer to do their stretching exercises after the aerobic

---

GLOSSARY

Flexibility The achievable range of motion at a joint or group of joints without causing injury.

Range of motion (ROM) Entire arc of movement of a given joint.

Subluxation Partial dislocation of a joint.

Stretching Moving the joints beyond the accustomed range of motion.

Dysmenorrhea Painful menstruation.

Plastic elongation Permanent lengthening of soft tissue.

Elastic elongation Temporary lengthening of soft tissue.

Flexibility in Older Adults

Similar to muscular strength, good range of motion is critical in later life (see "Exercise and Aging" in Chapter 9, p. 368). Physical activity and exercise can be hampered severely by lack of good range of motion, and unfortunately, muscle elasticity and bone strength tend to decline as people age. Because of decreased flexibility, older adults lose mobility and may be unable to perform simple daily tasks such as bending forward or turning. Many older adults cannot turn their head or rotate their trunk to look over their shoulder; rather, they must step around 90 to 180 degrees to see behind them. Adequate flexibility is also important in driving. Individuals who lose range of motion with age are unable to look over their shoulder to switch lanes or to parallel park, which increases the risk for automobile accidents.

Because of the pain during activity, older people who have tight hip flexors (muscles) cannot jog or walk very far. A vicious cycle ensues because the condition usually worsens with further inactivity. Lack of flexibility also affects proper balance, which may be a cause of falls and subsequent injury in older adults. The good news is that a simple stretching program can alleviate or prevent this problem and help people return to an exercise program. Physical activities that include both flexibility and neuromotor exercises that improve balance and agility (e.g., tai chi and yoga) are particularly beneficial to reduce the risk of falls and the fear of falling in older adults.[2]

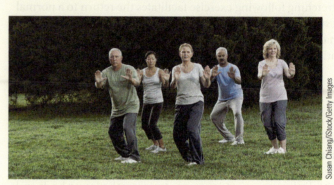

Participation in flexibility-based activities helps maintain functional fitness as people age.

Susan Chiang/iStock/Getty Images

---

phase of their workout. Aerobic activities raise body temperature, facilitating elastic elongation.

Age

Children generally maintain a high level of flexibility until adolescence, when accelerated growth in the bones often bypasses changes in soft tissue, causing a temporary decrease in flexibility. Growth in muscle mass then tends to equalize with skeletal growth in early adulthood, which is why athletes often experience a peak in flexibility in their mid-20s, correlating with the average age of peak sports performance. Aging in later adulthood also decreases the extensibility of soft tissue, resulting in less flexibility in both sexes. Participating in a regular stretching program, however, helps curb that decrease and maintain functional fitness and flexibility throughout older adulthood.

Gender

On average, women have better flexibility than men, and they tend to retain this advantage throughout life. The anatomical differences and hormonal influences that give women greater flexibility primarily exist to facilitate the physiological changes women go through during motherhood. Larger joints in the lower back help expectant mothers maintain stability in pregnancy, and wider hips allow a newborn's head greater ease through the birth canal.

Level of Physical Activity

The most significant contributor to lower flexibility is sedentary living. With less physical activity, muscles lose their elasticity and tendons and ligaments tighten and shorten.

Inactivity also tends to be accompanied by an increase in adipose tissue, which further decreases the range of motion around a joint. Over the years, people who lack adequate flexibility and neglect stretching can expect to see a decline in functional capacity and become more susceptible to injuries. Injury to muscle tissue and tight skin from excessive scar tissue also negatively affect range of motion. Regular stretching increases range of motion not only by increasing muscular elongation, but also by enhancing a person's level of stretch tolerance.

8.3 Assessing Flexibility

Flexibility is joint specific, which means a lot of flexibility in one joint does not necessarily indicate that other joints are just as flexible. Because there is no single flexibility test that can be used to determine overall body flexibility, most health and fitness centers rely strictly on the Sit-and-Reach Test as an indicator of general flexibility. This test measures flexibility of the hamstring muscles (back of the thigh) and, to a lesser extent, the lower back muscles.

To best determine your flexibility profile, the Total Body Rotation Test and the Shoulder Rotation Test—indicators of the ability to perform everyday movements such as reaching, bending, and turning—are also included in this book.

The Sit-and-Reach Test has been modified from the traditional test to take length of arms and legs into consideration in determining the score (Figure 8.1). In the original Sit-and-Reach Test, the 15-inch mark of the yardstick used to measure flexibility is always set at the edge of the box where the feet are placed. This does not take into consideration individual differences in arm length and leg

Figure 8.1 Procedure for the Modified Sit-and-Reach Test.

To perform this test, you will need the Acuflex I* Sit-and-Reach Flexibility Tester, or you may simply place a yardstick on top of a box 12" high.

1. Warm up properly before the first trial.
2. Remove your shoes for the test. Sit on the floor with the hips, back, and head against a wall, the legs fully extended, and the bottom of the feet against the Acuflex I or sit-and-reach box.
3. Place the hands one on top of the other and reach forward as far as possible without letting the head and back come off the wall (the shoulders may be rounded as much as possible, but neither the head nor the back should come off the wall at this time). The technician then can slide the reach indicator on the Acuflex I (or yardstick) along the top of the box until the end of the indicator touches the participant's fingers. The indicator then must be held firmly in place throughout the rest of the test.

4. Now your head and back can come off the wall. Gradually reach forward three times, the third time stretching forward as far as possible on the indicator (or yardstick) and holding the final position for at least 2 seconds. Be sure that during the test you keep the backs of the knees flat against the floor.
5. Record the final number of inches reached to the nearest half inch.

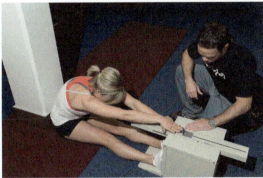

Modified Sit-and-Reach Test.

You are allowed two trials, and an average of the two scores is used as the final test score. The respective percentile ranks and fitness categories for this test are given in Tables 8.1 and 8.4.

*The Acuflex I Flexibility Tester for the Modified Sit-and-Reach Test can be obtained from Figure Finder Collection, Novel Products, P. O. Box 408, Rockton, IL 61072-0408. Phone: 800-323-5143, Fax 815-624-4866.

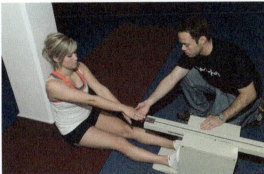

Determining the starting position for the Modified Sit-and-Reach Test.

© Fitness & Wellness, Inc.

length.[3] All other factors being equal, an individual with longer arms, shorter legs, or both receives a better rating because of the structural advantage.

The procedures and norms for the flexibility tests are described in Figure 8.1, Figure 8.2, and Figure 8.3 and Table 8.1, Table 8.2, and Table 8.3. The flexibility test results in these three tables are provided in both inches and centimeters (cm). Be sure to use the proper column to read your percentile score based on your test results. For the flexibility profile, you should take all three tests. You will be able to assess your flexibility profile in Activity 8.1. Because of the specificity of flexibility, pinpointing an "ideal" level of flexibility is difficult. Nevertheless, flexibility is important to health and fitness and independent living, so an assessment will give an indication of your current level of flexibility.

Interpreting Flexibility Test Results

After obtaining your scores and fitness ratings for each test, you can determine the fitness category for each flexibility test using the guidelines given in Table 8.4. You should also look up the number of points assigned for each fitness category in this table. The overall flexibility fitness category is obtained by totaling the number of points from all three tests and using the ratings given in Table 8.5. Record your results in Activity 8.1 and Appendix A.

8.4 Guidelines for Developing Muscular Flexibility

Even though genetics play a crucial role in body flexibility, the range of joint mobility can be increased and maintained through a regular stretching program. Because range of motion is highly specific to each body part, a comprehensive stretching program should include all body parts and follow the basic guidelines for development of flexibility.

The overload and specificity of training principles (discussed in conjunction with strength development in Chapter 7) apply to the development of muscular flexibility. To increase the total range of motion of a joint, the specific muscles surrounding that joint have to be stretched progressively beyond their accustomed length. The ACSM's FITT-VP principles of frequency, intensity, time/repetitions, type, volume, and pattern of exercise can also be applied to flexibility programs.

Types of Stretching Exercises

There are several modes of stretching exercises, and some modes are safer and more effective in terms of helping to increase flexibility:

1. Static (slow-sustained) stretching
2. Ballistic ("bouncing") stretching
3. Dynamic (slow movement) stretching
4. Proprioceptive neuromuscular facilitation (PNF) stretching

Figure 8.2 Procedure for the Total Body Rotation Test

An Acuflex II* Total Body Rotation Flexibility Tester or a measuring scale with a sliding panel is needed to administer this test. The Acuflex II or scale is placed on the wall at shoulder height and should be adjustable to accommodate individual differences in height. If you need to build your own scale, use two measuring tapes and glue them above and below the sliding panel centered at the 15" mark. Each tape should be at least 30" long. If no sliding panel is available, simply tape the measuring tapes onto a wall oriented in opposite directions as shown below. A line also must be drawn on the floor and centered with the 15" mark.

1. Warm up properly before beginning this test.
2. Stand with one side toward the wall, an arm's length away from the wall, with the feet straight ahead, slightly separated, and the toes touching the center line drawn on the floor. Hold out the arm away from the wall horizontally from the body, making a fist with the hand. The Acuflex II measuring scale (or tapes) should be shoulder height at this time.
3. Rotate the trunk, the extended arm going backward (always maintaining a horizontal plane) and making contact with the panel, gradually sliding it forward as far as possible. If no panel is available, slide the fist alongside the tapes as far as possible. Hold the final position at least 2 seconds. Position the hand with the little finger side forward during the entire sliding movement. **Proper hand position is crucial. Many people attempt to open the hand, or push with extended fingers, or slide the panel with the knuckles—none of which is acceptable.** During the test the knees can be bent slightly, but **the feet cannot be moved or rotated**—they must be straight forward. The body must be kept as straight (vertical) as possible.
4. Conduct the test on either the right or the left side of the body. Perform two trials on the selected side. Record the farthest point reached, measured to the nearest half inch and held for at least 2 seconds. Use the average of the two trials as the final test score. Refer to Tables 8.2 and 8.4 to determine the percentile rank and flexibility fitness category for this test.

*The Acuflex II Flexibility Tester for the Total Body Rotation Test can be obtained from Figure Finder Collection, Novel Products, P.O. Box 408, Rockton, IL 61072-0408. Phone: 800-323-5143, Fax 815-624-4866.

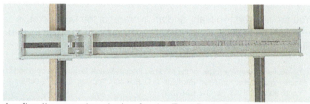

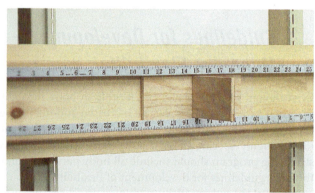

Acuflex II measuring device for the Total Body Rotation Test.

Homemade measuring device for the Total Body Rotation Test.

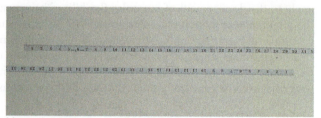

Measuring tapes for the Total Body Rotation Test.

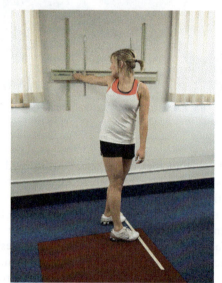

Total Body Rotation Test.

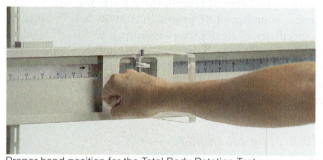

Proper hand position for the Total Body Rotation Test.

© Fitness & Wellness, Inc.

Figure 8.3 Procedure for the Shoulder Rotation Test.

This test can be done using the Acuflex III* Flexibility Tester, which consists of a shoulder caliper and a measuring device for shoulder rotation. If this equipment is unavailable, you can construct your own device quite easily. The caliper can be built with three regular yardsticks. Nail and glue two of the yardsticks at one end at a 90° angle, and use the third one as the sliding end of the caliper. Construct the rotation device by placing a 60" measuring tape on an aluminum or wood stick, starting at about 6" or 7" from the end of the stick.

1. Warm up before the test.
2. Using the shoulder caliper, measure the biacromial width to the nearest fourth of an inch (use the top scale on the Acuflex III). Measure biacromial width between the lateral edges of the acromion processes of the shoulders.
3. Place the Acuflex III or homemade device behind the back and use a reverse grip (thumbs out) to hold on to the device. Place the index finger of the right hand next to the zero point of the scale or tape (lower scale on the Acuflex III) and hold it firmly in place throughout the test. Place the left hand on the other end of the measuring device wherever comfortable.

4. Standing straight up and extending both arms to full length, with elbows locked, slowly bring the measuring device over the head until it is just within your peripheral vision. For subsequent trials, depending on the resistance encountered when rotating the shoulders, move the left grip a half inch to one inch at a time, and repeat the task until you no longer can rotate the shoulders without undue strain or starting to bend the elbows. Always keep the right-hand grip against the zero point of the scale. Measure the last successful trial to the nearest half inch. Take this measurement at the inner edge of the left hand on the side of the little finger.
5. Determine the final score for this test by subtracting the biacromial width from the best score (shortest distance) between both hands on the rotation test. For example, if the best score is 35" and the biacromial width is 15", the final score is 20" (35 − 15 = 20). Using Tables 8.3 and 8.4, determine the percentile rank and flexibility fitness category for this test.

*The Acuflex III Flexibility Tester for the Shoulder Rotation Test can be obtained from Figure Finder Collection, Novel Products, Inc., P. O. Box 408, Rockton, IL 61072-0408. Phone: (800) 323-5143, Fax 815-624-4866.

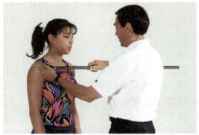
Measuring biacromial width.

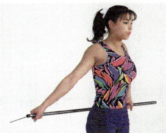
Starting position for the Shoulder Rotation Test (note the reverse grip used for this test).

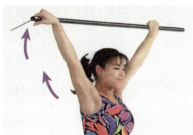
Shoulder Rotation Test.

© Fitness & Wellness, Inc.

Table 8.1 Percentile Ranks for the Modified Sit-and-Reach Test

	Age Category—Men									Age Category—Women								
Percentile Rank	18		19–35		36–49		50		Percentile Rank	18		19–35		36–49		50	
	in.	cm	in.	cm	in.	cm	in.	cm		in.	cm	in.	cm	in.	cm	in.	cm
99	20.8	52.8	20.1	51.1	18.9	48.0	16.2	41.1	99	22.6	57.4	21.0	53.3	19.8	50.3	17.2	43.7
95	19.6	49.8	18.9	48.0	18.2	46.2	15.8	40.1	95	19.5	49.5	19.3	49.0	19.2	48.8	15.7	39.9
90	18.2	46.2	17.2	43.7	16.1	40.9	15.0	38.1	90	18.7	47.5	17.9	45.5	17.4	44.2	15.0	38.1
80	17.8	45.2	17.0	43.2	14.6	37.1	13.3	33.8	80	17.8	45.2	16.7	42.4	16.2	41.1	14.2	36.1
70	16.0	40.6	15.8	40.1	13.9	35.3	12.3	31.2	70	16.5	41.9	16.2	41.1	15.2	38.6	13.6	34.5
60	15.2	38.6	15.0	38.1	13.4	34.0	11.5	29.2	60	16.0	40.6	15.8	40.1	14.5	36.8	12.3	31.2
50	14.5	36.8	14.4	36.6	12.6	32.0	10.2	25.9	50	15.2	38.6	14.8	37.6	13.5	34.3	11.1	28.2
40	14.0	35.6	13.5	34.3	11.6	29.5	9.7	24.6	40	14.5	36.8	14.5	36.8	12.8	32.5	10.1	25.7
30	13.4	34.0	13.0	33.0	10.8	27.4	9.3	23.6	30	13.7	34.8	13.7	34.8	12.2	31.0	9.2	23.4
20	11.8	30.0	11.6	29.5	9.9	25.1	8.8	22.4	20	12.6	32.0	12.6	32.0	11.0	27.9	8.3	21.1
10	9.5	24.1	9.2	23.4	8.3	21.1	7.8	19.8	10	11.4	29.0	10.1	25.7	9.7	24.6	7.5	19.0
05	8.4	21.3	7.9	20.1	7.0	17.8	7.2	18.3	05	9.4	23.9	8.1	20.6	8.5	21.6	3.7	9.4
01	7.2	18.3	7.0	17.8	5.1	13.0	4.0	10.2	01	6.5	16.5	2.6	6.6	2.0	5.1	1.5	3.8

High physical fitness standard

Health fitness standard

Table 8.2 **Percentile Ranks for the Total Body Rotation Test**

	Percentile Rank	Age Category—Left Rotation								Age Category—Right Rotation							
		18		19–35		36–49		50		18		19–35		36–49		50	
		in.	cm	in.	cm	in.	cm	in.	cm	in.	cm	in.	cm	in.	cm	in.	cm
	99	29.1	73.9	28.0	71.1	26.6	67.6	21.0	53.3	28.2	71.6	27.8	70.6	25.2	64.0	22.2	56.4
	95	26.6	67.6	24.8	63.0	24.5	62.2	20.0	50.8	25.5	64.8	25.6	65.0	23.8	60.5	20.7	52.6
	90	25.0	63.5	23.6	59.9	23.0	58.4	17.7	45.0	24.3	61.7	24.1	61.2	22.5	57.1	19.3	49.0
	80	22.0	55.9	22.0	55.9	21.2	53.8	15.5	39.4	22.7	57.7	22.3	56.6	21.0	53.3	16.3	41.4
	70	20.9	53.1	20.3	51.6	20.4	51.8	14.7	37.3	21.3	54.1	20.7	52.6	18.7	47.5	15.7	39.9
	60	19.9	50.5	19.3	49.0	18.7	47.5	13.9	35.3	19.8	50.3	19.0	48.3	17.3	43.9	14.7	37.3
Men	50	18.6	47.2	18.0	45.7	16.7	42.4	12.7	32.3	19.0	48.3	17.2	43.7	16.3	41.4	12.3	31.2
	40	17.0	43.2	16.8	42.7	15.3	38.9	11.7	29.7	17.3	43.9	16.3	41.4	14.7	37.3	11.5	29.2
	30	14.9	37.8	15.0	38.1	14.8	37.6	10.3	26.2	15.1	38.4	15.0	38.1	13.3	33.8	10.7	27.2
	20	13.8	35.1	13.3	33.8	13.7	34.8	9.5	24.1	12.9	32.8	13.3	33.8	11.2	28.4	8.7	22.1
	10	10.8	27.4	10.5	26.7	10.8	27.4	4.3	10.9	10.8	27.4	11.3	28.7	8.0	20.3	2.7	6.9
	05	8.5	21.6	8.9	22.6	8.8	22.4	0.3	0.8	8.1	20.6	8.3	21.1	5.5	14.0	0.3	0.8
	01	3.4	8.6	1.7	4.3	5.1	13.0	0.0	0.0	6.6	16.8	2.9	7.4	2.0	5.1	0.0	0.0
	99	29.3	74.4	28.6	72.6	27.1	68.8	23.0	58.4	29.6	75.2	29.4	74.7	27.1	68.8	21.7	55.1
	95	26.8	68.1	24.8	63.0	25.3	64.3	21.4	54.4	27.6	70.1	25.3	64.3	25.9	65.8	19.7	50.0
	90	25.5	64.8	23.0	58.4	23.4	59.4	20.5	52.1	25.8	65.5	23.0	58.4	21.3	54.1	19.0	48.3
	80	23.8	60.5	21.5	54.6	20.2	51.3	19.1	48.5	23.7	60.2	20.8	52.8	19.6	49.8	17.9	45.5
	70	21.8	55.4	20.5	52.1	18.6	47.2	17.3	43.9	22.0	55.9	19.3	49.0	17.3	43.9	16.8	42.7
	60	20.5	52.1	19.3	49.0	17.7	45.0	16.0	40.6	20.8	52.8	18.0	45.7	16.5	41.9	15.6	39.6
Women	50	19.5	49.5	18.0	45.7	16.4	41.7	14.8	37.6	19.5	49.5	17.3	43.9	14.6	37.1	14.0	35.6
	40	18.5	47.0	17.2	43.7	14.8	37.6	13.7	34.8	18.3	46.5	16.0	40.6	13.1	33.3	12.8	32.5
	30	17.1	43.4	15.7	39.9	13.6	34.5	10.0	25.4	16.3	41.4	15.2	38.6	11.7	29.7	8.5	21.6
	20	16.0	40.6	15.2	38.6	11.6	29.5	6.3	16.0	14.5	36.8	14.0	35.6	9.8	24.9	3.9	9.9
	10	12.8	32.5	13.6	34.5	8.5	21.6	3.0	7.6	12.4	31.5	11.1	28.2	6.1	15.5	2.2	5.6
	05	11.1	28.2	7.3	18.5	6.8	17.3	0.7	1.8	10.2	25.9	8.8	22.4	4.0	10.2	1.1	2.8
	01	8.9	22.6	5.3	13.5	4.3	10.9	0.0	0.0	8.9	22.6	3.2	8.1	2.8	7.1	0.0	0.0

High physical fitness standard
Health fitness standard

Table 8.3 **Percentile Ranks for the Shoulder Rotation Test**

Percentile Rank	Age Category—Men								Percentile Rank	Age Category—Women							
	18		19–35		36–49		50			18		19–35		36–49		50	
	in.	cm	in.	cm	in.	cm	in.	cm		in.	cm	in.	cm	in.	cm	in.	cm
99	2.2	5.6	−1.0	−2.5	18.1	46.0	21.5	54.6	99	2.6	6.6	−2.4	−6.1	11.5	29.2	13.1	33.3
95	15.2	38.6	10.4	26.4	20.4	51.8	27.0	68.6	95	8.0	20.3	6.2	15.7	15.4	39.1	16.5	41.9
90	18.5	47.0	15.5	39.4	20.8	52.8	27.9	70.9	90	10.7	27.2	9.7	24.6	16.8	42.7	20.9	53.1
80	20.7	52.6	18.4	46.7	23.3	59.2	28.5	72.4	80	14.5	36.8	14.5	36.8	19.2	48.8	22.5	57.1
70	23.0	58.4	20.5	52.1	24.7	62.7	29.4	74.7	70	16.1	40.9	17.2	43.7	21.5	54.6	24.3	61.7
60	24.2	61.5	22.9	58.2	26.6	67.6	29.9	75.9	60	19.2	48.8	18.7	47.5	23.1	58.7	25.1	63.8
50	25.4	64.5	24.4	62.0	28.0	71.1	30.5	77.5	50	21.0	53.3	20.0	50.8	23.5	59.7	26.2	66.5
40	26.3	66.8	25.7	65.3	30.0	76.2	31.0	78.7	40	22.2	56.4	21.4	54.4	24.4	62.0	28.1	71.4
30	28.2	71.6	27.3	69.3	31.9	81.0	31.7	80.5	30	23.2	58.9	24.0	61.0	25.9	65.8	29.9	75.9
20	30.0	76.2	30.1	76.5	33.3	84.6	33.1	84.1	20	25.0	63.5	25.9	65.8	29.8	75.7	31.5	80.0
10	33.5	85.1	31.8	80.8	36.1	91.7	37.2	94.5	10	27.2	69.1	29.1	73.9	31.1	79.0	33.1	84.1
05	34.7	88.1	33.5	85.1	37.8	96.0	38.7	98.3	05	28.0	71.1	31.3	79.5	33.4	84.8	34.1	86.6
01	40.8	103.6	42.6	108.2	43.0	109.2	44.1	112.0	01	32.5	82.5	37.1	94.2	34.9	88.6	35.4	89.9

High physical fitness standard
Health fitness standard

Table 8.4 Flexibility Fitness Categories According to Percentile Ranks

Percentile Rank	Fitness Category	Points
≥90	Excellent	5
70–80	Good	4
50–60	Average	3
30–40	Fair	2
≤20	Poor	1

Table 8.5 Overall Flexibility Fitness Category

Total Points	Flexibility Category
≥13	Excellent
10–12	Good
7–9	Average
4–6	Fair
≤3	Poor

Static (Slow-Sustained) Stretching

With **static stretching** or slow-sustained stretching, muscles are lengthened gradually through a joint's complete range of motion and the final position is held for a few seconds. A slow-sustained stretch causes the muscles to relax and thereby achieve greater length. This type of stretch causes little pain and has a low risk for injury. In flexibility-development programs, slow-sustained stretching exercises are the most frequently used and recommended. Static stretching can be active or passive. In an **active static stretch**, the position is held by the strength of the muscle being stretched, as is performed in many yoga poses. Although similar to active static stretching, in a **passive static stretch** the muscles are relaxed (i.e., they are in a passive state), and an external force, provided by another person or apparatus (e.g., a ballet barre or an elastic band), is applied to increase the range of motion.

Ballistic ("Bouncing") Stretching

Ballistic stretching uses the momentum of a moving body or body part to produce the stretch. This type of stretching requires a fast and repetitive bouncing motion to achieve a greater degree of stretch, which sometimes forces joints beyond the normal range of motion. An example would be repeatedly bouncing down and up to touch the toes. Ballistic stretching is the least recommended form of stretching because of the risk of strain or injury to muscles and nerves. This form of stretching should never be performed without a previous aerobic warm-up.

Dynamic (Slow Movement) Stretching

Speed of movement, momentum, and active muscular effort are used in **dynamic stretching** to increase the range of motion around a joint or group of joints. Unlike ballistic stretching, it does not require bouncing motions, but rather uses the slow transition between body positions to increase range of motion with each repetition. Exaggerating a kicking action, walking lunges, and arm circles are all examples of dynamic stretching. Research indicates that dynamic stretches are preferable to static stretches before athletic competition because dynamic stretching does not seem to have a negative effect on the athlete's strength and power.

Proprioceptive Neuromuscular Facilitation (PNF)

Proprioceptive neuromuscular facilitation (PNF) stretching is based on a "contract-and-relax" method and requires the assistance of another person. The procedure is as follows:

1. The person assisting with the exercise provides initial force by pushing slowly in the direction of the desired stretch (assisted stretch). This initial stretch does not cover the entire range of motion.
2. The person being stretched then applies force in the opposite direction of the stretch, against the assistant, who tries to hold the initial degree of stretch as close as possible. This results in an isometric contraction at the angle of the stretch. The force of the isometric contraction can be anywhere from 20 to 75 percent of the person's maximum contraction.
3. After 3 to 6 seconds of isometric contraction, the person being stretched relaxes the target muscle(s) completely. The assistant then increases the degree of stretch slowly to a greater angle, and for the PNF technique, the stretch is held for 10 to 30 seconds.

GLOSSARY

Static (slow-sustained) stretching Exercises in which the muscles are lengthened gradually through a joint's complete range of motion.

Active static stretch Stretching exercise wherein the position is held by the strength of the muscle being stretched.

Passive static stretch Stretching exercise performed with the aid of an external force applied by either another individual or an external apparatus.

Ballistic ("bouncing") stretching Stretching exercises performed with jerky, rapid, and bouncy movements.

Dynamic (slow movement) stretching Stretching exercises that require speed of movement, momentum, and active muscular effort to help increase the range of motion around a joint or group of joints.

Proprioceptive neuromuscular facilitation (PNF) A mode of stretching that uses reflexes and neuromuscular principles to relax the muscles being stretched.

4. If a greater degree of stretch is achievable, the isometric contraction is repeated for another 3 or 6 seconds, after which the degree of stretch is slowly increased again and held for 10 to 30 seconds.

If a progressive degree of stretch is used, steps 1 through 4 can be repeated up to five times. Each isometric contraction is held for 3 to 6 seconds. The progressive stretches are held for about 10 seconds—until the last trial, when the final stretched position is held for up to 30 seconds.

Theoretically, with the PNF technique, the isometric contraction helps relax the muscle being stretched, which results in lengthening of the muscle. Some research indicates that PNF stretching yields greater gains in range of motion than the other forms of stretching.[4] Another benefit of PNF is an increase in strength of the muscle(s) being stretched. Research has shown increases in absolute strength and muscular endurance with PNF stretching. These increases are attributed to the isometric contractions performed during PNF. Disadvantages of PNF are (1) more pain, (2) the need for a second person to assist, and (3) the need for more time to conduct each session.

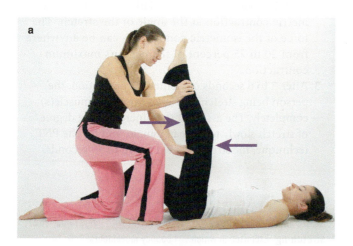

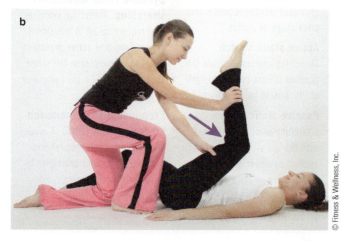

PNF stretching technique: (a) isometric phase, (b) stretching phase.

Physiological Response to Stretching

Located within skeletal muscles are two sensory organs, also known as proprioceptors: the muscle spindle and the Golgi tendon organ. Their function is to protect muscles from injury during stretching.

Muscle spindles are located within the belly of the muscle, and their primary function is to detect changes in muscle length. If overstretched or stretched too fast, the spindles send messages to the central nervous system, and through a feedback loop, motor neurons are activated and cause muscle contraction to resist muscle stretch. This mechanism is known as the stretch reflex. Muscle spindle action explains why injury rates are higher with ballistic stretching. Fast stretching speeds trigger the stretch reflex and cause muscles to contract and develop tension that can lead to injury.

Golgi tendon organs are located at the point where muscle fibers attach to the muscle tendon. When excessive force is generated by a muscle, these organs trigger a response opposite to that of the spindles: an inverse stretch reflex action that inhibits the muscle contraction and leads to muscle relaxation. The Golgi tendon organ prevents injury to the muscle by keeping it from generating too much tension while being stretched. This response explains the effectiveness of the PNF technique in increasing joint range of motion. The isometric contraction following the initial stretch triggers the inverse stretch reflex, thus lessening the tension and allowing the muscle to relax. At this point, the muscle tolerates a greater degree of stretch.

Frequency

Flexibility exercises should be conducted a minimum of 2 or 3 days per week, with stretching daily yielding the most effective results. After 6 to 8 weeks of almost daily stretching, flexibility can be maintained with two or three sessions per week, involving the major muscle and tendon groups of the body. Figure 8.4 summarizes the guidelines for flexibility development.

Figure 8.4 FITT-VP flexibility guidelines.

Frequency:	At least 2 or 3 days per week, with daily being most effective
Intensity:	To the point of feeling tightness or mild discomfort
Time/ Repetitions:	Repeat each exercise 2 to 4 times, holding the final position of a static stretch between 10 and 30 seconds per repetition
Type:	Static, dynamic, or proprioceptive neuromuscular facilitation (PNF) stretching to include all major muscle/tendon groups of the body
Volume:	A target of 60 seconds of total stretching per exercise
Pattern/ When:	Flexibility exercise is most effective when muscles are warmed through light-to-moderate aerobic activity or passively through external methods such as heat packs or hot baths

SOURCE: Adapted from American College of Sports Medicine, *ACSM's Guidelines for Exercise Testing and Prescription* (Philadelphia, PA: Wolters Kluwer/ Lippincott Williams & Wilkins, 10th edition, 2017).

© Fitness & Wellness, Inc.

© Fitness & Wellness, Inc.

Intensity

The **intensity**, or degree of stretch, when doing flexibility exercises should be to only a point of feeling tightness or mild discomfort at the end of the range of motion. Extending a joint past its full range of motion can cause undue pain and may result in tissue damage or injury. If you feel pain, the load is too high; all stretching should be done to slightly below the pain threshold. As participants reach this point, they should try to relax the muscle being stretched as much as possible. After completing the stretch, the body part is brought back gradually to the starting point.

Time/Repetitions

The time required for an exercise session for development of flexibility is based on the number of **repetitions** and the length of time each repetition is held in the final stretched position. As a general recommendation, about 10 minutes of flexibility exercise that includes the major muscle and tendon units of the body should be performed. Two to four repetitions per exercise should be done, holding the final position each time for 10 to 30 seconds.[5]

Generally, research shows that stretching for 10 to 30 seconds is better to increase range of motion than stretching for shorter periods of time and is just as effective as stretching for longer durations. Older adults, however, may derive greater improvements when the final stretched position is held for 30 to 60 seconds. Individuals who are susceptible to flexibility injuries should limit each stretch to 20 seconds. Pilates exercises are recommended for these individuals because they increase joint stability.

Volume

Each exercise should be repeated two to four times with a goal to achieve 60 seconds of total stretching per exercise by adjusting the duration and repetitions. For example, you can perform two 30-second stretches or four 15-second stretches to attain a cumulative time of 60 seconds of stretching for every exercise.

HOEGER KEY TO WELLNESS

To maintain good flexibility, stretch all major muscles and joints to the point of mild discomfort at least 2 to 3 days per week. Repeat each exercise 2 to 4 times, holding the final stretch for 10 to 30 seconds, for a target goal of 60 seconds of total stretching per exercise.

Pattern/When to Stretch?

Unless the activity requires extensive range of motion, the best time to stretch is generally after aerobic or strength-training exercise when muscles are warm. Higher body temperature in itself helps to increase the joint range of motion and facilitate elastic elongation. External methods such as

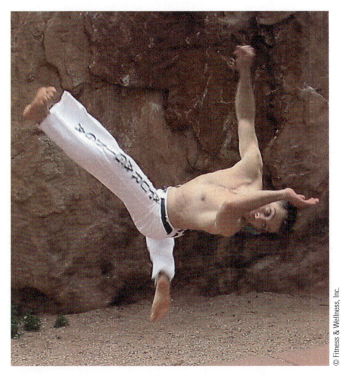

Adequate flexibility helps to develop and maintain sports skill throughout life.

heat packs or hot baths can also be used to warm muscles prior to stretching routines.

A warm-up that progressively increases muscle temperature and mimics movement that will occur during training enhances performance and also serves to warm muscles prior to a stretching routine. For some activities, gentle stretching is recommended in conjunction with warm-up routines. Many people do not differentiate a warm-up from stretching. Warming up means starting a workout slowly with walking, cycling, or slow jogging, followed by gentle stretching (not through the entire range of motion). Stretching implies movement of joints through their full range of motion and holding the final degree of stretch according to recommended guidelines.

Before steady activities (walking, jogging, cycling, etc.), a warm-up of 3 to 5 minutes is recommended. The recommendation is up to 10 minutes before stop-and-go activities (e.g., racquet sports, basketball, and soccer) and athletic participation in general (e.g., football and gymnastics). Activities that require abrupt changes in direction are more likely to cause muscle strains if they are performed without proper warm-up that includes mild stretching.

GLOSSARY

Intensity In flexibility exercise, the degree of stretch.

Repetitions The number of times a given resistance is performed.

Sport-specific or pre-exercise stretching can improve performance in sports that require a greater-than-average range of motion, such as gymnastics, dancing, diving, and figure skating. Intense stretching conducted prior to participating in sports that rely on force and power for peak performance is not recommended, as recent data suggest that acute stretching during warm-up can lead to a temporary short-term (up to 60 minutes) decrease in strength and power. A meta-analysis of over a hundred athletic studies showed that pre-exercise static stretching resulted in a five percent reduction in muscle strength and two percent reduction in explosive power.[6] However, other studies show that short-duration static stretching combined with dynamic stretching does not elicit performance impairments.[7]

Muscles also are fatigued following exercise, and a fatigued muscle tends to shorten, which can lead to soreness and spasms. Stretching exercises help fatigued muscles reestablish their normal resting length and prevent unnecessary pain. Whether performed before or after an exercise, studies show that overall, those who stretch either before or after a workout report a relative decrease in discomfort felt from delayed-onset muscle soreness that typically peaks 24 to 48 hours after physical activity.[8]

HOEGER KEY TO WELLNESS

Intense stretching before participating in sports that rely on explosive force for peak performance is not recommended. Research suggests that it can lead to a temporary (up to an hour) decrease in muscular strength and power.

8.5 *Flexibility Exercises*

To improve body flexibility, each major muscle group should be subjected to at least one stretching exercise during a stretching session. A complete set of exercises for developing muscular flexibility is presented on pages 326–328.

Although you may not be able to hold a final stretched position with some of these exercises (e.g., lateral head tilts and arm circles), you should still perform the exercise through the joint's full range of motion. Depending on the number and length of repetitions, most people can complete flexibility exercises in about 10 minutes.

Exercises that May Cause Injury

Most strength and flexibility exercises are relatively safe to perform, but even safe exercises can be hazardous if they are performed incorrectly. Some exercises may be safe to perform occasionally but when executed repeatedly may cause trauma and injury. Pre-existing muscle or joint conditions (old sprains or injuries) can further increase the risk of harm during certain exercises. As you develop your exercise program, you are encouraged to follow the exercise descriptions and guidelines given in this book.

A few exercises, however, are not recommended because of the potential high risk for injury. These exercises are sometimes done in video workouts and some fitness classes. **Contraindicated exercises** may cause harm because of the excessive strain they place on muscles and joints, in particular, the spine, lower back, knees, neck, or shoulders.

Illustrations of contraindicated exercises are presented in Figure 8.5. Safe alternative exercises are listed below each contraindicated exercise and are illustrated in the exercises for strength (pages 285–294) and flexibility (pages 326–328). In isolated instances, a qualified physical therapist may select one or a few of the contraindicated exercises to treat a specific injury or disability in a carefully supervised setting. Unless you are specifically instructed to use one of these exercises, it is best that you select safe exercises from this book.

Critical Thinking

Carefully consider the relevance of stretching exercises to your personal fitness program. How much importance do you place on these exercises? Have some conditions improved through your stretching program, or have certain exercises contributed to your health and well-being?

8.6 *Preventing and Rehabilitating Low Back Pain*

Few people make it through life without having low back pain at some point. An estimated 60 to 80 percent of the population has been afflicted by back pain or injury. Estimates indicate that more than 75 million Americans suffer from chronic back pain. Nationally, low back pain is the most common cause of work-related disability and the second most common neurological condition (disorder of the nervous system). This backache syndrome costs U.S. industries billions of dollars each year in lost productivity, health services, and worker compensation.

Knowing the most common causes of low back pain can help in prevention and treatment before back pain becomes chronic.

Causes of Low Back Pain

Though low back pain can come as a symptom of chronic illness such as degenerative conditions, bone diseases, or spinal abnormalities, it has been determined that backache syndrome is preventable more than 80 percent of the time and is caused by (a) physical inactivity, (b) excessive body weight,

GLOSSARY

Contraindicated exercises Exercises that are not recommended because they may cause injury to a person.

Figure 8.5 Contraindicated exercises.

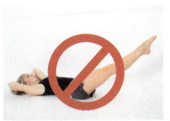
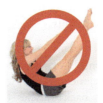
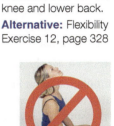

Double-Leg Lift   **Upright Double-Leg Lifts**   **V-Sits**   **Standing Toe Touch**

All three of these exercises cause excessive strain on the spine and may harm discs.

Alternatives: Strength Exercises 4 and 17, pages 286 and 290

Excessive strain on the knee and lower back.

Alternative: Flexibility Exercise 12, page 328

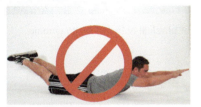
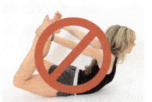
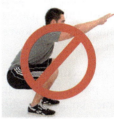

Swan Stretch

Excessive strain on the spine; may harm intervertebral discs.

Alternative: Flexibility Exercise 21, page 329

Cradle

Excessive strain on the spine, knees, and shoulders.

Alternatives: Flexibility Exercises 8 and 21, pages 327 and 329

Full Squat

Excessive strain on the knees.

Alternatives: Flexibility Exercise 8, page 327; Strength Exercises 1, 16, 28A and 28B, pages 285, 290, and 294

Head Rolls

May injure neck discs.

Alternative: Flexibility Exercise 1, page 326

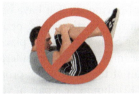
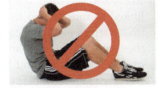

Knee to Chest

(with hands over the shin) Excessive strain on the knee.

Alternative: Flexibility Exercises 15 and 16, page 328

Sit-Ups with Hands Behind the Head

Excessive strain on the neck.

Alternatives: Strength Exercises 4 and 17, pages 286 and 290

Yoga Plow

Excessive strain on the spine, neck, and shoulders.

Alternatives: Flexibility Exercises 12, 15, 16, 18, and 20, pages 328 and 329

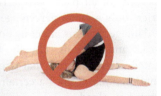

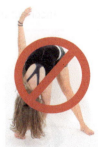

Hurdler Stretch

Excessive strain on the bent knee.

Alternatives: Flexibility Exercises 8 and 12, pages 327 and 328

The Hero

Excessive strain on the knees.

Alternatives: Flexibility Exercises 8 and 14, pages 327 and 328

Windmill

Excessive strain on the spine and knees.

Alternatives: Flexibility Exercises 12 and 20, pages 328 and 329

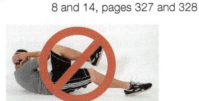
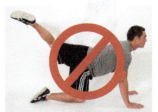

Straight-Leg Sit-Ups   **Alternating Bent-Leg Sit-Ups**

These exercises strain the lower back.

Alternatives: Strength Exercises 4 and 17, pages 286 and 290

Donkey Kicks

Excessive strain on the back, shoulders, and neck.

Alternatives: Flexibility Exercises 1, 14, and 21, pages 326, 328, and 329

© Fitness & Wellness, Inc.

(c) strain and sprain injury to muscles and tissue, (d) psychological stress, and/or (e) poor posture and body mechanics. Research also shows that back injuries are more common among smokers because smoking reduces blood flow to the spine—increasing back pain susceptibility.

Physical Inactivity

The most common reason for chronic low back pain is a lack of physical activity. In particular, a major contributor to back pain is excessive sitting, which causes back muscles to shorten, stiffen, and become weaker. Deterioration or weakening of the abdominal and gluteal muscles, along with tightening of the lower back (erector spinae) muscles, brings about an unnatural forward tilt of the pelvis (Figure 8.6). This tilt puts extra pressure on the spinal vertebrae, causing pain in the lower back.

Excessive Body Weight

Accumulation of fat around the midsection of the body contributes to the forward tilt of the pelvis, further aggravating the pressure on spinal vertebrae. Long-term obesity and weight gain during pregnancy also increase pressure on the spine, contribute to muscular weakness, and cause pelvic misalignment, all of which lead to lower back pain.

Strain and Sprain Injury to Muscles and Tissue

People tend to think of back pain as a problem with the skeleton. Actually, the spine's curvature, alignment, and movement are controlled by surrounding muscles. More than 95 percent of all back pain is related to strain and sprain injuries; only a small percentage is related to intervertebral disk damage. Sprains affect ligaments, whereas strains affect muscles and tendons. Usually, back pain is the result of repeated micro-injuries that occur over an extended time (sometimes years) until a certain movement, activity, or an excessive overload causes a significant injury to the tissues.

Figure 8.6 Incorrect and correct pelvic alignment.

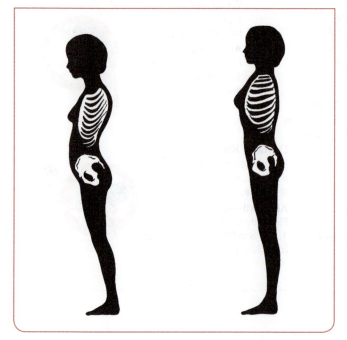

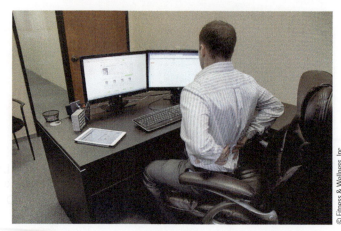

Excessive sitting and lack of physical activity lead to chronic back pain.

© Fitness & Wellness, Inc.

Stress

Psychological stress, too, may lead to back pain. The brain is "hardwired" to the back muscles. Excessive stress causes muscles to contract. Frequent tightening of the back muscles can throw the back out of alignment and constrict blood vessels that supply oxygen and nutrients to the back. Chronic stress also increases the release of hormones that have been linked to muscle and tendon injuries. Furthermore, people under stress tend to forget proper body mechanics, placing themselves at unnecessary risk for injury. If you are undergoing excessive stress and back pain at the same time, proper stress management (see Chapter 12) should be a part of your comprehensive back-care program.

Poor Posture and Body Mechanics

Low back pain is frequently associated with poor posture and improper body mechanics, or body positions. The majority of all low back problems in the United States stem from improper alignment of the vertebral column and pelvic girdle, a direct result of inflexible and weak muscles. Poor posture also strains muscles and ligaments and becomes a risk factor for musculoskeletal problems of the neck, shoulders, and lower back. Evaluating these areas is crucial to preventing and rehabilitating low back pain.

Improving Body Posture

Good posture enhances personal appearance, self-image, and confidence; improves balance and endurance; protects against misalignment-related pains and aches; prevents falls; aids in reducing chronic low back pain; and enhances your overall sense of well-being.[9] The relationships among different body parts are the essence of posture.

Proper body mechanics means using correct positions in all the activities of daily life, including sleeping, sitting, standing, walking, driving, working, and exercising. Because of the high incidence of low back pain, illustrations of proper body mechanics and a series of corrective and preventive exercises are shown in Figure 8.7 and Activity 8.2.

Figure 8.7 **Proper back care.**

Low back pain is caused by (a) physical inactivity, (b) excessive body weight, (c) strain and sprain injury, (d) psychological stress, and/or (e) poor posture and body mechanics. To protect your back and avoid debilitating low back strain, you need to use proper body mechanics and correct improper body posture. Using appropriate body positions and actions in all daily activities is vital for back health. The following guidelines help avoid unnecessary back strain and protect and support your back.

Correct standing position

To learn the correct standing posture, stand a foot away from a wall and place your upper body completely straight against the wall. You will need to tighten the abdominal and gluteal muscles to do so. Next, walk around for a few minutes holding this same position and at the end return to the wall to evaluate how well you maintained the posture.

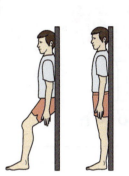

Standing, lifting, and carrying positions

Incorrect: **Correct:**

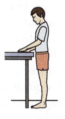 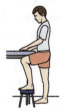

Stand with the aid of a footrest

Always bend at the hips and knees

Hold and carry objects close to the body

 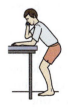

Bend at the knees to lean forward

Correct sitting position

Most people spend many daily hours sitting. Proper sitting and preventing a forward slump is essential for back health. To straighten your back (a) put your head back, (b) pull in your chin toward your chest, (c) tighten your abdominal muscles, and (d) raise your chest. You should always sit in this manner. The following guidelines will also help correct improper sitting throughout the day.

Always use a footrest to keep the knees higher than the hips

Avoid severe rounding of upper back and neck while seated

Sit close to the pedals when driving

To lean forward, bend at the hips and keep the neck and back as straight as possible

Bed posture

A firm mattress is recommended for proper back support. Avoid sleeping flat on your back or face down with large pillows for head support. Lying sideways in a fetal position with a small pillow for head support and a small pillow between the knees, or on your back with the knees supported by a larger pillow, is best.

Incorrect: **Correct:**

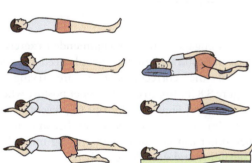

When resting, do it right

When at home resting or relaxing, lie flat on your back with a small pillow under your neck and with pillows under the knees for support. You may also place the lower legs on a chair with your knees bent at 90 degrees. This position is also good to relieve back spasms when suffering from back pain.

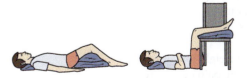

When watching TV or sitting on the floor, do so by lying on a straight-back chair covered with a firm pillow and a second large pillow under the knees.

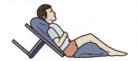

Figure 8.8 Desk ergonomics.

DESK ERGONOMICS
8 Tips for Improving Your Computer Workspace

1 Center your monitor and keyboard in front of you with the top of the monitor at or below eye level. Be sure your monitor viewing distance is at about an arm's length away to prevent eye strain.

2 Rest your feet flat on the floor and position your knees at or below hip height. Use a footrest if your feet don't comfortably reach the floor or lower the keyboard and chair.

3 Adjust the height of your chair so your elbows are at about keyboard level with your wrists positioned straight and in-line with your forearms. Use a wrist rest if needed to ensure minimal bend at the wrists.

4 Place the mouse next to the keyboard to keep your arms and elbows close to your body as you work. Use a mouse pad to protect your hands and forearms from pressing against the hard surface of the desk.

5 Adjust the incline of your chair to provide good support for your lower back. Use a small pillow or lumbar support cushion if needed.

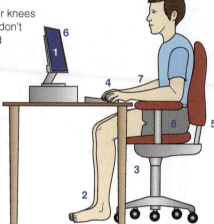

6 Reduce screen glare. Tilt or reposition the monitor as needed, and clean the screen regularly. Set the screen contrast and brightness for comfortable viewing.

7 Take frequent short breaks, 10 minutes per hour of sitting. Breaks can include stretching, walking around, or standing/walking while talking to others.

8 Be mindful to correct your sitting posture often.

Photos © Fitness & Wellness, Inc.

Besides engaging in the recommended exercises to elicit changes in postural alignment, people need to be continually aware of the corrections they are trying to make. See Figure 8.8 for tips to ensure proper posture when working at the desk, and Figure 8.9 for tips to prevent "text neck." As posture improves, you frequently become motivated to change other aspects, such as improving muscular strength and flexibility and decreasing body fat.

When to Call a Physician

In the majority of back injuries, pain is present only with movement and physical activity. According to the National Institutes of Health (NIH), most back pain goes away on its own in a few weeks. A physician should be consulted if any of the following conditions are present:

- Numbness in the legs
- Trouble urinating
- Leg weakness
- Fever
- Unintentional weight loss
- Persistent severe pain even at rest

A physician can rule out any disk damage, arthritis, osteoporosis, slipped vertebrae, spinal stenosis (narrowing of the spinal canal), or other serious condition. For common back pain, the physician may prescribe proper bed rest using several pillows under the knees for leg support (Figure 8.7). This position helps relieve muscle spasms by stretching the muscles involved. Your doctor may also prescribe a muscle relaxant or anti-inflammatory medication (or both) and some type of physical therapy.

In most cases, an X-ray and MRI are not required unless pain lingers for more than 4 to 6 weeks. In the early stages of back pain, tight muscles and muscle spasms tend to compress the vertebrae, squeezing the intervertebral disks and revealing apparent disk problems on an X-ray. In these cases, the real problem is the tight muscles and subsequent muscle spasms. A daily physical activity and stretching program help to decompress the spine, stretch tight muscles, strengthen weak muscles, and increase blood flow (promoting healing) to the back muscles.

Treatment Options

Each year, more than $86 billion is spent in the United States to care for back pain, with limited evidence that increased spending really helps people. Even with severe pain, most people feel better within days or weeks without being treated by health care professionals.[10] Up to 90 percent of people heal on their own. Time is often the best treatment approach. Other treatment options and preventative measures are explored in the sections below.

Pain Medication

To relieve symptoms, you may use over-the-counter pain relievers and hot or cold packs. However, back pain recurs more often in people who rely solely on medication, compared with people who use both medication and exercise therapy to recover.[11]

Figure 8.9 **Looking down at a mobile device increases the effective weight on the neck and spine.**

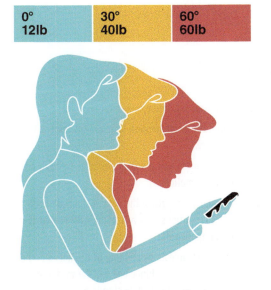

Tips to prevent "text neck"

- Hold smartphones and other mobile devices at eye level whenever possible.
- Look down with your eyes, rather than bending your neck, when browsing social media, reading online, or checking email.
- Use voice recognition features to text and make calls.
- Alter your texting position frequently and take breaks from looking down at mobile devices every 20 minutes.
- Help strengthen neck, back, and core muscles through regular exercise and flexibility exercises (see pages 326–330).

Preventing "text neck"

With more than half of Americans now spending an average of 2 to 4 hours a day hunched over a smartphone or other mobile device, the incidence of tech-related upper body pain is on the rise, particularly among teenagers and young adults. Excessive strain to the neck, shoulders, and back that stems from the overuse of mobile devices has been termed "text neck" and can lead to chronic headaches, injury, or even permanent damage to the spine.

Though an adult's head weighs 10 to 12 pounds, when tipped forward to look down at a mobile device, the effective weight on the neck increases to 40 pounds at a 30-degree angle and 60 pounds at a 60-degree angle. Most smartphone users look down at a device at chest or waist level (a 60-degree angle), increasing the stress load on the muscles and nerves of the neck by 60 pounds for long periods throughout the day. Over time, the effects of poor posture while using mobile devices can cause the shoulders to round forward, the neck muscles to be shortened and tightened, and the natural curvature of the spine to be altered. In young people, the excessive wear and tear on the spine caused by text neck has led to an increased need for regular spinal care to prevent lasting damage as they grow.

The good news is that smartphone users can still enjoy texting and browsing while avoiding upper body strain by practicing improved posture and usage habits.

Exercise Therapy

In terms of alleviating back pain, *exercise is medicine,* but it needs to be the right type of exercise. Aerobic exercise is beneficial because it helps decrease body fat and psychological stress. During an episode of back pain, however, people often avoid activity and cope by getting more rest. In most cases, this restriction on physical activity has been shown in recent studies to be exactly the opposite of what people need to do to reduce low back pain.[12] Patients who continued daily work and physical activity experienced faster recoveries than those treated with bed rest. Rest is recommended if the pain is associated with a herniated disk, but if your physician rules out a serious problem, exercise is a better choice of treatment.

Exercise is the most widely used therapy for low back pain, and controlled rehab programs indicate that for chronic low back pain, exercise is more effective at improving long-term function and pain intensity over traditional nonexercise care.[13] Exercise requires effort by the patient, and it may create discomfort initially, but because exercise helps restore physical function, individuals who start and maintain an aerobic exercise program have back pain less frequently. Individuals who exercise also are less likely to require surgery or other invasive treatments.

You should also stay active to avoid further weakening of the back muscles. Low-impact activities such as walking, swimming, water aerobics, and cycling are recommended. Once you are pain free in the resting state, you need to start correcting the muscular imbalance by stretching the tight muscles and strengthening the weak ones. Stretching exercises are always performed first.

Stretching Exercises

Regular stretching exercises that help the hip and trunk go through a functional range of motion, rather than increasing the range of motion, are recommended. That is, for proper back care, stretching exercises should not be performed to the extreme range of motion. Individuals with a greater spinal range of motion also have a higher incidence of back injury. Spinal stability, instead of mobility, is desirable for back health.

Core-Strengthening Exercises

A strong core musculature is critical for spine and back health and will reduce or completely eliminate pain flare-ups. Spine-stabilizing muscles, referred to as the "core," consist of many distinctive muscles running the length of the torso, including the back, abdominals, hips, chest, and inner and outer thighs. Because having a strong core is the best defense against injury to the spine, a good core-strengthening program can also help reduce back pain or prevent recurring pain.

Behavior Modification Planning

Tips to Prevent Low Back Pain

I PLAN TO   **I DID IT**

- ☐ ☐ Be physically active.
- ☐ ☐ Maintain recommended body weight (excess weight strains the back).
- ☐ ☐ Stretch often using spinal exercises through a functional range of motion.
- ☐ ☐ Regularly strengthen the core of the body using sets of 10 to 12 repetitions to near fatigue with isometric contractions when applicable.
- ☐ ☐ Lift heavy objects by bending at the knees and carry them close to the body. Place one foot forward and keep your knees slightly bent while standing.
- ☐ ☐ Avoid sitting (over 50 minutes) or standing in one position for lengthy periods of time.

- ☐ ☐ Maintain correct posture.
- ☐ ☐ Wear comfortable, low-heeled shoes.
- ☐ ☐ Sleep on your back with a pillow under the knees or on your side with the knees drawn up and a small pillow between the knees.
- ☐ ☐ Try out different mattresses of firm consistency before selecting a mattress.
- ☐ ☐ Warm up properly using mild stretches before engaging in physical activity.
- ☐ ☐ Practice adequate stress management techniques.
- ☐ ☐ Don't smoke (it reduces blood flow to the spine—increasing back pain risk).

Try It

In your class notebook, record how many of the above actions are a regular part of your healthy low back program. If you are not using all of them, what is necessary to incorporate these behaviors into your lifestyle?

MINDTAP From Cengage **Complete This Online**
Visit **www.cengagebrain.com** to access MindTap, a complete digital course that includes interactive quizzes, videos, and more.

HOEGER KEY TO WELLNESS

When it comes to back pain, prevention and treatment through changes in lifestyle are by far the best medicine. Back pain can be prevented more than 80 percent of the time by increasing physical activity, losing weight, correcting posture, engaging in a core-strengthening program, and/or lowering stress levels.

Yoga Exercises

Yoga exercises are particularly beneficial to enhance flexibility and may also help relieve chronic back pain better than conventional medicine. A review of seven studies analyzing the impact of yoga on low back pain and function showed that, overall, yoga was found to significantly reduce pain and increase function in patients suffering from chronic low back pain.[14] **Iyengar yoga** in particular has been shown to relieve chronic low back pain.[15] Following 24 weeks of biweekly classes, yoga participants had greater improvement in functional disability along with a decrease in pain intensity and low back-pain-related depression. These benefits were still present six months after the end of class participation.

Spinal Manipulation

If there is no indication of disease or injury (such as leg numbness or pain), a herniated disk, or fractures, spinal manipulation by a chiropractor or other health care professional can provide pain relief. Spinal manipulation as a treatment

modality for low back pain has been endorsed by the federal Agency for Healthcare Research and Quality (AHRQ). The guidelines suggest that spinal manipulation may help to alleviate discomfort and pain during the first few weeks of an acute episode of low back pain. Generally, benefits are seen in fewer than ten treatments. People who have had chronic pain for more than 6 months should avoid spinal manipulation until they have been thoroughly examined by a physician.

Surgery

Acute or short-term low back pain is most often the result of trauma or injury to the lower back and typically lasts a few days or weeks. Back pain is considered chronic if it persists longer than 3 months. Surgery is seldom the best option, as it often weakens the spine. Scar tissue and surgical alterations also decrease the success rate of a subsequent surgery. Only about 10 percent of people with chronic pain are candidates for surgery. If surgery is recommended, always seek a second opinion. And consider all other options. In many cases, pushing beyond the pain and participating in aggressive physical therapy ("exercise boot camps" for back pain) aimed at strengthening the muscles that support the spine are what's needed to overcome the condition.

GLOSSARY

Iyengar yoga A form of yoga that aims to develop flexibility, strength, balance, and stamina using props (belts, blocks, blankets, and chairs) to aid in the correct performance of asanas, or yoga postures.

Critical Thinking

Consider your own low back health. Have you ever had episodes of low back pain? If so, how long did it take you to recover, and what helped you recover from this condition?

Personal Flexibility and Low Back Conditioning Program

Several exercises for preventing and rehabilitating the backache syndrome are given on pages 328–330. These exercises can be done twice or more daily when a person has back pain. Under normal circumstances, doing these exercises three or four times a week is enough to prevent the syndrome. Using some of the additional core exercises listed in Chapter 7

("Core Strength-Training," page 277) further enhances a low back management program. A strengthening program for a healthy back should be conducted around the endurance threshold—15 or more repetitions to near fatigue. Muscular endurance of the muscles that support the spine is more important than absolute strength because these muscles perform their work during the course of an entire day.

Activity 8.2 allows you to develop your own flexibility and low back conditioning programs. Some exercises that help increase spinal stability and muscular strength and endurance require isometric contractions. The recommendation calls for these contractions to be held for 3 to 30 seconds. The length of the hold depends on your current fitness level and the difficulty of each exercise. For most exercises, you may start with a 3- to 6-second hold. Over the course of several weeks, you can increase the length of the hold up to 30 seconds.

Assess Your Behavior

1. Do you give flexibility exercises the same priority in your fitness program as you do aerobic and strength-training?

2. Are stretching exercises a part of your fitness program at least two times per week?

3. Do you include exercises to strengthen and enhance body alignment in your regular strength and flexibility program?

Assess Your Knowledge

1. Muscular flexibility is defined as the
   a. capacity of joints and muscles to work in a synchronized manner.
   b. achievable range of motion at a joint or group of joints without causing injury.
   c. capability of muscles to stretch beyond their normal resting length without injury to the muscles.
   d. capacity of muscles to return to their proper length following the application of a stretching force.
   e. limitations placed on muscles as the joints move through their normal planes.

2. Good flexibility
   a. promotes healthy muscles and joints.
   b. relieves muscle cramps.
   c. improves posture.
   d. decreases the risk of chronic back pain.
   e. All are correct choices.

3. Plastic elongation is a term used in reference to
   a. permanent lengthening of soft tissue.
   b. increased flexibility achieved through dynamic stretching.
   c. temporary elongation of muscles.
   d. the ability of a muscle to achieve a complete degree of stretch.
   e. lengthening of a muscle against resistance.

4. Which of the following factors affects flexibility?
   a. Age
   b. Gender
   c. Body temperature
   d. Joint structure
   e. All are correct choices.

5. The most significant contributors to loss of flexibility are
   a. sedentary living and lack of physical activity.
   b. weight and power training.
   c. age and injury.
   d. muscular strength and endurance.
   e. excessive body fat and low lean tissue.

6. Which of the following is not a mode of stretching?
   a. PNF
   b. Elastic elongation
   c. Ballistic stretching
   d. Static stretching
   e. All of the choices are modes of stretching.

7. When performing stretching exercises, the intensity, or degree of stretch, should be
   a. through the entire arc of movement.
   b. to about 80 percent of capacity.
   c. to the point of feeling tightness or slight discomfort.
   d. applied until the muscle(s) start shaking.
   e. progressively increased until the desired stretch is attained.

8. The general recommendation when stretching is that the final position reached on each repetition be held for
   a. 1 to 10 seconds.
   b. 10 to 30 seconds.
   c. 30 to 90 seconds.
   d. 1 to 3 minutes.
   e. as long as the person is able to sustain the stretch.

9. The best time to stretch is
   a. before a high-intensity workout.
   b. prior to participating in sports that rely on explosive force and power.
   c. after an adequate warm up or aerobic workout when muscles are warm.
   d. an hour before stop-and-go activities.
   e. None of the choices are correct.

10. Low back pain is associated primarily with
    a. physical inactivity.
    b. poor posture.
    c. excessive body weight.
    d. psychological stress.
    e. All are correct choices.

Correct answers can be found at the back of the book.

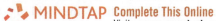

MINDTAP **Complete This Online**
From Cengage   Visit **www.cengagebrain.com** to access MindTap, a complete digital course that includes interactive quizzes, videos, and more.

Activity 8.1   Muscular Flexibility Assessment

Name _____ Date _____

Course _____ Section _____ Gender _____ Age _____

I. Instruction
Conduct the Muscular Flexibility Assessment according to the instructions provided in Figures 8.1, 8.2, and 8.3, pages 307–309. Note your percentile rank from Tables 8.1, 8.2, and 8.3, pages 309–310, and record in the space provided below. Using Table 8.4 (page 311), determine your fitness category and points and record in the spaces below. Total your points for all three assessments to determine your overall flexibility category in Table 8.5, page 311.

II. Test (Table 8.4)

	Percentile Rank	Fitness Category	Points
Modified Sit-and-Reach			
Total Body Rotation ☐ Right ☐ Left			
Shoulder Rotation			

Total Points: (Table 8.5)

Overall Flexibility Category: (Table 8.5)

III. Flexibility Goals

1. Indicate the flexibility category that you would like to achieve by the end of the term.

   _____

2. Describe your feelings about your current body flexibility and any potential implications that your current flexibility levels may have on your health and wellness. Also, briefly state how you plan to achieve your flexibility objective by the end of the term.

   _____
   _____
   _____
   _____
   _____
   _____
   _____
   _____
   _____
   _____

© Fitness & Wellness, Inc.

MINDTAP From Cengage   **Complete This Activity Online**
Visit **www.cengagebrain.com** to access MindTap, a complete digital course that includes interactive quizzes, videos, and more.

Activity 8.2 Flexibility Development and Low Back Conditioning Programs

Name _____ Date _____

Course _____ Section _____ Gender _____ Age _____

I. Stage of Change for Flexibility Training

Using Figure 2.7 (page 73) and Table 2.3 (page 73), identify your current stage of change for participation in a muscular stretching program.

II. Instruction

Perform all of the recommended flexibility exercises given on pages 326–330. Use a combination of slow-sustained and proprioceptive neuromuscular facilitation stretching techniques. Indicate the technique(s) used for each exercise and, where applicable, the number of repetitions performed and the length of time that the final degree of stretch was held.

Stretching Exercises

Exercise	Stretching Technique	Repetitions	Length of Final Stretch (seconds)
Neck Stretches			NA*
Arm circles			NA
Side stretch			
Body rotation			
Chest stretch			
Shoulder hyperextension stretch			
Shoulder rotation stretch			NA
Quad stretch			
Heel cord stretch			
Adductor stretch			
Sitting adductor stretch			
Sit-and-reach stretch			
Triceps stretch			
Hip flexor stretch			
Single-knee-to-chest			
Double-knee-to-chest			
Passive spinal twist			

*Not Applicable

Activity 8.2 **Flexibility Development and Low Back Conditioning Programs** *(continued)*

Stretching Schedule (Indicate days, time, and place where you will stretch):

Flexibility-training days: M ☐   T ☐   W ☐   Th ☐   F ☐   Sa ☐   Su ☐   Time of day: [＿＿]   Place: [＿＿＿]

Low Back Conditioning Program

Perform all of the recommended exercises for the prevention and rehabilitation of low back pain given on pages 328–330. Indicate the number of repetitions performed for each exercise and number of seconds held.

Flexibility Exercises	Repetitions	Seconds Held	Strength/Endurance Exercises	Repetitions	Seconds Held
Hip flexor stretch	☐	☐	Pelvic tilt	☐	☐
Single-knee-to-chest stretch	☐	☐	The cat	☐	☐
Double-knee-to-chest stretch	☐	☐	Abdominal crunch or abdominal curl-up	☐	☐
Passive spinal twist	☐	☐	Reverse crunch	☐	☐
Upper and lower back stretch	☐	☐	Supine plank	☐	☐
Sit-and-reach stretch	☐	☐	Pelvic clock	☐	☐
Gluteal stretch	☐	☐	Lateral bridge	☐	☐
Back extension stretch	☐	☐	Prone bridge	☐	☐
Trunk rotation and lower back stretch	☐	☐	Leg press	☐	☐
			Seated back	☐	☐
			Lat pull-down	☐	☐
			Back extension	☐	☐

Proper Body Mechanics

Perform the following tasks using the proper body mechanics given in Figure 8.7 (page 317). Check off each item as you perform the task:

☐ Standing (carriage) position   ☐ Bed posture

☐ Lifting an object   ☐ Resting position for tired and painful back

☐ Sitting position

Proper Body Mechanics for Back Care

According to the guidelines provided in this chapter and in Figure 8.7 (page 317), indicate below actions that you need to work on to improve posture and body mechanics and prevent low back pain.

_____

_____

_____

_____

_____

_____

© Fitness & Wellness, Inc.

Flexibility Exercises

EXERCISE 1   Neck Stretches

ACTION Slowly and gently tilt the head laterally (a). You may increase the degree of stretch by gently pulling with one hand (b). You may also turn the head about 30 degrees to one side and stretch the neck by raising your head toward the ceiling (see photo c—do not extend your head backward; look straight forward). Now gradually bring the head forward until you feel an adequate stretch in the muscles on the back of the neck (d). Perform the exercises on both the right and left sides. Repeat each exercise several times, and hold the final stretched position for a few seconds.

AREAS STRETCHED Neck flexors and extensors; ligaments of the cervical spine

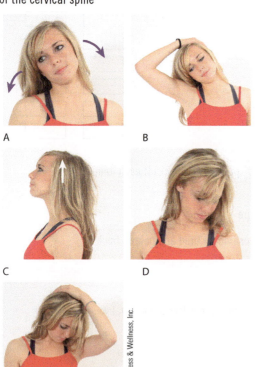

A   B

C   D

E

© Fitness & Wellness, Inc.

EXERCISE 2   Arm Circles

ACTION Gently circle your arms all the way around. Conduct the exercise in both directions.

AREAS STRETCHED
Shoulder muscles and ligaments

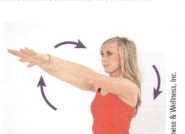

© Fitness & Wellness, Inc.

EXERCISE 3   Side Stretch

ACTION Stand straight up, feet separated to shoulder-width, and place your hands on your waist. Now move the upper body to one side and hold the final stretch for a few seconds. Repeat on the other side.

AREAS STRETCHED Muscles and ligaments in the pelvic region

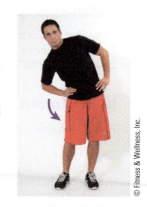

© Fitness & Wellness, Inc.

EXERCISE 4   Body Rotation

ACTION Place your arms slightly away from the body and rotate the trunk as far as possible, holding the final position for several seconds. Conduct the exercise for both the right and left sides of the body. You also can perform this exercise by standing about 2 feet away from the wall (back toward the wall) and then rotating the trunk, placing the hands against the wall.

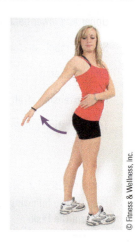

© Fitness & Wellness, Inc.

AREAS STRETCHED Hip, abdominal, chest, back, neck, and shoulder muscles; hip and spinal ligaments

EXERCISE 5   Chest Stretch

ACTION Place your hands on the shoulders of your partner, who in turn will push you down by your shoulders. Hold the final position for a few seconds.

AREAS STRETCHED Chest (pectoral) muscles and shoulder ligaments

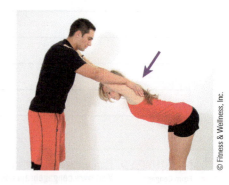

© Fitness & Wellness, Inc.

Flexibility Exercises *(continued)*

EXERCISE 6 Shoulder Hyperextension Stretch

ACTION Have a partner grasp your arms from behind by the wrists and slowly push them upward. Hold the final position for a few seconds.

AREAS STRETCHED Deltoid and pectoral muscles; ligaments of the shoulder joint

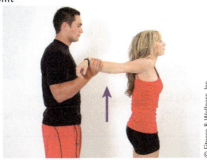

EXERCISE 7 Shoulder Rotation Stretch

ACTION With the aid of surgical tubing or an aluminum or wood stick, place the tubing or stick behind your back and grasp the two ends using a reverse (thumbs-out) grip. Slowly bring the tubing or stick over your head, keeping the elbows straight. Repeat several times (bring the hands closer together for additional stretch).

AREAS STRETCHED Deltoid, latissimus dorsi, and pectoral muscles; shoulder ligaments

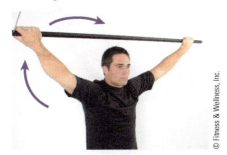

EXERCISE 8 Quad Stretch

ACTION Lie on your side and move one foot back by flexing the knee. Grasp the front of the lower leg and pull the ankle toward the gluteal region. Hold for several seconds. Repeat with the other leg.

AREAS STRETCHED Quadriceps muscle; knee and ankle ligaments

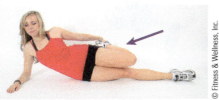

EXERCISE 9 Heel Cord Stretch

ACTION Stand against the wall or at the edge of a step and stretch the heel downward, alternating legs. Hold the stretched position for a few seconds.

AREAS STRETCHED Heel cord (Achilles tendon); gastrocnemius and soleus muscles

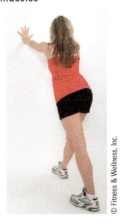

EXERCISE 10 Adductor Stretch

ACTION Stand with your feet about twice shoulder-width apart and place your hands slightly above the knees. Flex one knee and slowly go down as far as possible, holding the final position for a few seconds. Repeat with the other leg.

AREAS STRETCHED Hip adductor muscles

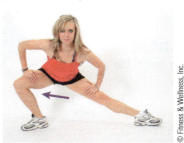

EXERCISE 11 Sitting Adductor Stretch

ACTION Sit on the floor and bring your feet in close to you, allowing the soles of the feet to touch each other. Now place your forearms (or elbows) on the inner part of the thigh and push the legs downward, holding the final stretch for several seconds.

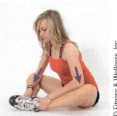

AREAS STRETCHED Hip adductor muscles

Flexibility Exercises *(continued)*

EXERCISE 12   Sit-and-Reach Stretch

ACTION Sit on the floor with legs together and gradually reach forward as far as possible. Hold the final position for a few seconds. This exercise also may be performed with the legs separated, reaching to each side as well as to the middle.

AREAS STRETCHED Hamstrings and lower back muscles; lumbar spine ligaments

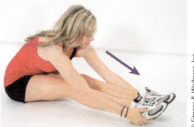

EXERCISE 13   Triceps Stretch

ACTION Place the right hand behind your neck. Grasp the right arm above the elbow with the left hand. Gently pull the elbow backward. Repeat the exercise with the opposite arm.

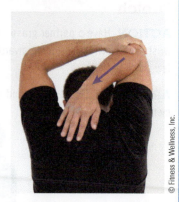

AREAS STRETCHED Back of upper arm (triceps muscle); shoulder joint

NOTE Exercise 14 through Exercise 21 and Exercise 23 are also flexibility exercises and can be added to your stretching program.

Exercises   For the Prevention and Rehabilitation of Low Back Pain

EXERCISE 14   Hip Flexor Stretch

ACTION Kneel down on an exercise mat or a soft surface, or place a towel under your knees. Raise the right knee off the floor and place the right foot about 3 feet in front of you. Place your right hand over your right knee and the left hand over the back of the left hip. Keeping the lower back flat, slowly move forward and downward as you apply gentle pressure over the left hip. Repeat the exercise with the opposite leg forward.

AREAS STRETCHED Flexor muscles in front of the hip joint

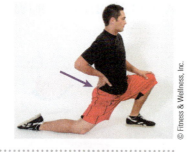

EXERCISE 15   Single-Knee-to-Chest Stretch

ACTION Lie down flat on the floor. Bend one leg at approximately 100 degrees and gradually pull the opposite leg toward your chest. Hold the final stretch for a few seconds. Switch legs and repeat the exercise.

AREAS STRETCHED Lower back and hamstring muscles; lumbar spine ligaments

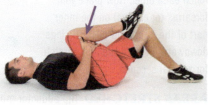

EXERCISE 16   Double-Knee-to-Chest Stretch

ACTION Lie flat on the floor and then curl up slowly into a fetal position. Hold for a few seconds.

AREAS STRETCHED Upper and lower back and hamstring muscles; spinal ligaments

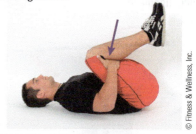

EXERCISE 17   Passive Spinal Twist

ACTION Lie on your back and place your arms flat on the floor laterally out from the sides of the body. Lift your knees into a 90-degree angle. Keeping your head and torso flat and level, slowly lower both knees comfortably to one side. Repeat on the other side.

AREAS STRETCHED Hip and lower back

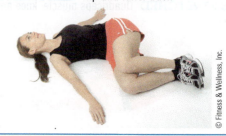

Exercises For the Prevention and Rehabilitation of Low Back Pain *(continued)*

EXERCISE 18   Upper and Lower Back Stretch

ACTION Sit on the floor and bring your feet in close to you, allowing the soles of the feet to touch each other. Holding on to your feet, bring your head and upper chest gently toward your feet.

AREAS STRETCHED Upper and lower back muscles and ligaments

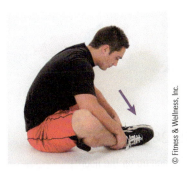

EXERCISE 19   Sit-and-Reach Stretch (See Exercise 12 on page 328)

EXERCISE 20   Gluteal Stretch

ACTION Lie on the floor, bend the right leg, and place your right ankle slightly above the left knee. Grasp behind the left thigh with both hands and gently pull the leg toward the chest. Repeat the exercise with the opposite leg.

AREAS STRETCHED Buttock area (gluteal muscles)

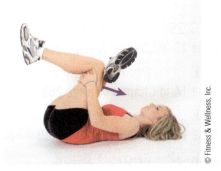

EXERCISE 21   Back Extension Stretch

ACTION Lie face down on the floor with the elbows by the chest, forearms on the floor, and the hands beneath the chin. Gently raise the trunk by extending the elbows until you reach an approximate 90-degree angle at the elbow joint. Be sure the forearms remain in contact with the floor at all times. Do NOT extend the back beyond this point. Hyperextension of the lower back may lead to or aggravate an existing back problem. Hold the stretched position for about 10 seconds.

AREAS STRETCHED Abdominal region

ADDITIONAL BENEFITS Restore lower back curvature

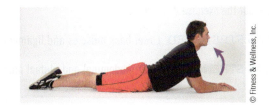

EXERCISE 22   Trunk Rotation and Lower Back Stretch

ACTION Sit on the floor and bend the left leg, placing the right foot on the outside of the left knee. Place the left elbow on the right knee and push against it. At the same time, try to rotate the trunk to the right (clockwise). Hold the final position for a few seconds. Repeat the exercise with the other side.

AREAS STRETCHED Lateral side of the hip and thigh; trunk and lower back

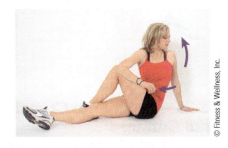

Exercises For the Prevention and Rehabilitation of Low Back Pain *(continued)*

EXERCISE 23 Pelvic Tilt

(See Exercise 12 in Chapter 7, page 288) This is perhaps the most important exercise for the care of the lower back. It should be included as a part of your daily exercise routine and should be performed several times throughout the day when pain in the lower back is present as a result of muscle imbalance.

EXERCISE 24 The Cat

ACTION Kneel on the floor and place your hands in front of you (on the floor) about shoulder-width apart. Relax the trunk and lower back (a). Now arch the spine and pull in your abdomen as far as you can and hold this position for a few seconds (b). Repeat the exercise 4–5 times.

AREAS STRETCHED Lower back muscles and ligaments

AREAS STRENGTHENED Abdominal and gluteal muscles

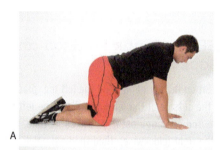
A
B
© Fitness & Wellness, Inc.

EXERCISE 25 Abdominal Crunch or Abdominal Curl-up

(See Exercise 4 in Chapter 7, page 286) It is important that you do not stabilize your feet when performing either of these exercises because doing so decreases the work of the abdominal muscles. Also, remember not to "swing up," but rather to curl up as you perform these exercises.

EXERCISE 26 Reverse Crunch

(See Exercise 11 in Chapter 7, page 288)

EXERCISE 27 Supine Plank

ACTION Lie face up on the floor with the knees bent at about 120°. Do a pelvic tilt (Exercise 12 in Chapter 7, page 288) and maintain the pelvic tilt while you raise the hips off the floor until the upper body and upper legs are in a straight line. Hold this position for several seconds.

AREAS STRENGTHENED Gluteal and abdominal flexor muscles

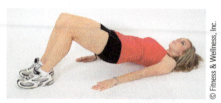
© Fitness & Wellness, Inc.

EXERCISE 28 Pelvic Clock

ACTION Lie face up on the floor with the knees bent at about 120 degrees. Fully extend the hips as in the supine plank (Exercise 27). Now progressively rotate the hips in a clockwise manner (2 o'clock, 4 o'clock, 6 o'clock, 8 o'clock, 10 o'clock, and 12 o'clock), holding each position in an isometric contraction for about 1 second. Repeat the exercise counterclockwise.

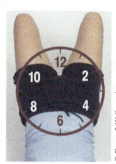
© Fitness & Wellness, Inc.

AREAS STRENGTHENED Gluteal, abdominal, and hip flexor muscles

EXERCISE 29 Lateral Bridge
(See Exercise 13 in Chapter 7, page 288)

EXERCISE 30 Prone Bridge
(See Exercise 14 in Chapter 7, page 289)

EXERCISE 31 Leg Press
(See Exercise 16 in Chapter 7, page 290)

EXERCISE 32 Seated Back
(See Exercise 20 in Chapter 7, page 291)

EXERCISE 33 Lat Pull-Down
(See Exercise 24 in Chapter 7, page 292)

EXERCISE 34 Back Extension
(See Exercise 36 in Chapter 7, page 298)

EXERCISE 35 Lateral Trunk Flex
(See Exercise 37 in Chapter 7, page 299)

9

Personal Fitness Programming

"To give anything less than your best is to sacrifice the gift."
—Steve Prefontaine

Objectives

9.1 **Understand** why a fitness program must fit personal values.

9.2 **Be able to write** a comprehensive fitness program.

9.3 **Dispel** common misconceptions related to physical fitness and wellness.

9.4 **Learn** to properly hydrate and adjust diet to maximize exercise benefits.

9.5 **Become aware** of safety considerations for exercising.

9.6 **Learn** concepts for preventing and treating injuries.

9.7 **Describe** the relationship between fitness and aging.

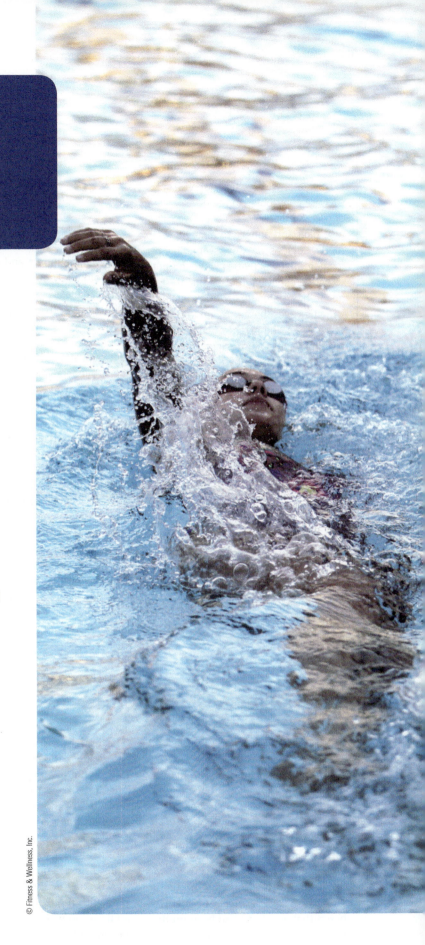

© Fitness & Wellness, Inc.

FAQ

What is the best fitness activity?

No single physical activity, sport, or exercise contributes to the development of overall fitness. Most people who exercise pick and adhere to a single mode, such as walking, swimming, or jogging. Many activities will contribute to cardiorespiratory development. (For a side-by-side comparison of aerobic activities see Chapter 6, Table 6.9, page 247.) The extent of contribution to other fitness components, though, varies among the activities. For total fitness, aerobic activities should be supplemented with strength and flexibility programs. Cross-training—that is, selecting different activities for fitness development and maintenance (jogging, water aerobics, and spinning)—adds enjoyment to the program, decreases the risk of incurring injuries from overuse, and keeps exercise from becoming monotonous. Mixing up a workout routine also helps avoid plateaus in fitness progress. For specific suggestions on incorporating cross-training into a fitness plan, see the topics of "Cross-Training" on page 341 and "Periodization" (and Table 9.1) on pages 344–345 of this chapter.

Are bodyweight exercises like squats and walking lunges considered muscular strength exercises, muscular endurance exercises, or aerobic exercises?

Bodyweight squats and walking lunges are commonly completed in group exercise classes for a minute or longer without rest. In this context, these exercises are considered muscular endurance exercises. They are different than strength exercises done by body builders who are training for muscular hypertrophy and who use relatively short rest intervals between sets and repeatedly work the same muscle groups. Squats and walking lunges have become popular for a good reason: They focus on some of the largest skeletal muscles in the body and, therefore, maximize energy expenditure during a workout. The required muscles also have the potential for large increases in strength, providing a slight boost in the metabolic rate. Squats and lunges also engage core muscles, in addition to leg muscles, thus providing a full-body stability exercise. When performing squats in a class, be sure to complete only as many as you can do with proper form.

When I choose to participate in a sport, can it take the place of my regular aerobic and strength workouts?

The extent to which a sport can deliver the benefits of an aerobic or strength training program depends entirely on the sport. Remember that with most sports, you are not continually increasing intensity or resistance, as you are in a well-designed conditioning program. If your goal is to improve at your sport and reap the most enjoyment from participation, you would do well to add interval training once or twice per week and one to two strength training sessions per week that mimic the actions performed in the sport. Varying your workouts and applying principles of periodization (see pages 344–345 in this chapter) will help you reach peak performance and avoid injury. Proper conditioning during the preseason, followed by sport participation during its season, and general fitness training during the off-season, can be an ideal form of cross-training.

REAL LIFE STORY | Oliver's Experience

As a kid, I always hated gym class. I was not very coordinated and I couldn't hit the ball very far in baseball or score in basketball. I always seemed to be one of the last ones picked for any team. So I told myself I was not meant for sports, and avoided them as much as possible. However, when I got to college, I was feeling out of shape and wanted to find a fun way to get some exercise. I remembered that as a kid I had been pretty good at ping-pong, and that I had sometimes beaten my friends when we would race short distances on foot.

So I thought that even though I wasn't the greatest athlete on the whole, I might have fair speed and agility. Then I searched for a sport that would make use of those advantages, and I decided to try tennis. I took a tennis class, and worked at improving my skills. I made some friends in class that I continue to play with regularly. After a fair amount of practice, I eventually became a halfway decent tennis player! Learning to do well at this one sport has helped me get in

Monkey Business Images/Shutterstock.com

better shape and actually develop the confidence to try other athletic activities, like mountain biking and ultimate Frisbee. I learned that just because I didn't excel at the first few sports I tried, that doesn't mean that I was totally lacking in athletic ability. I am happy that I am able to experience the fun of competing in a sport, and sometimes even winning!

PERSONAL PROFILE: My Lifetime Fitness Program

Based on your experience with your personal fitness program,

I. What is your take-home message from Oliver's experience, and how might it influence your personal fitness program?

II. What is the most efficient type (mode) of exercise that contributes to good health and contributes to lifetime weight management? Can you explain and justify your answer?

III. What exercise prescription principles do you feel you understand well (overload, diminishing return, specificity, rest and recovery, periodization, etc.)? Have you had personal experiences with any of these principles?

IV. Have you ever participated in a HIIT program? ____ Yes ____ No If yes, how did you feel at the end of each training session, and what results did you obtain? If no, what has held you back from trying it?

V. Have you ever been involved in an exercise or sports program that fit well with your personal values at the time? Have you ever felt frustrated about an exercise program because it did not fit well with your values at the time?

VI. Have you ever implemented a successful backup plan when your normal exercise routine was not possible to complete?

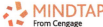 **MINDTAP** From Cengage   **Complete This Online** Visit **www.cengagebrain.com** to access MindTap, a complete digital course that includes interactive quizzes, videos, and more.

Exercise can become a source of interest, accomplishment, and rejuvenation for those who participate in a fitness activity they enjoy. When an exercise session is viewed as a time of personal enjoyment, it brings a sense of satisfaction and is especially helpful in meeting the stressors of daily life. When it is viewed as a chore, an exercise session will still deliver physiological benefits, but may spur the participant toward counterproductive rewards (like unnecessary snacking[1]).

Exercise is also more rewarding when participants find themselves making progress and meeting new challenges. This chapter will help you take a new look at fitness activities you may find rewarding. It will also help you understand exercise prescription so that you are able to avoid injury, break through fitness plateaus, and create your own training programs around your fitness pursuits of choice.

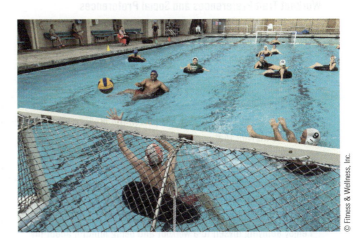

© Fitness & Wellness, Inc.

Choosing activities you enjoy will greatly enhance your adherence to exercise.

9.1 *Choosing an Exercise Program with Your Values in Mind*

The time is now to take advantage of the myriad benefits derived through physical activity and exercise by making physical activity a priority in your daily lifestyle. One of the fun aspects of exercise is being able to choose from many different activities to promote fitness. Use the tools for behavioral change presented in Chapter 2 to reshuffle your schedule and activities to make room for your fitness goals. Eventually you will be able to better align your lifestyle with your fitness priorities. For the best chance at success, balance the other side of the scale as well: Choose exercise that aligns with your values and resources. Select an activity not for its sheer energy expenditure, but for how much you will enjoy the activity itself, how well that activity reflects the rewards you value, and how smoothly the activity will fit the time and resources you have available.

While energy expenditure varies among activities and your intensity of effort (for side-by-side comparisons, see Table 6.9, page 247), the most important factor to promote health and lifetime weight maintenance is regular participation. Choosing activities that you enjoy will greatly enhance your adherence to exercise. People tend to repeat things they enjoy doing. Enjoyment itself is a reward. Reflect on the elements of a fitness program that you value by completing Activity 9.1. For example, an element of fun and social support from family and friends who are willing to join your program may greatly enhance exercise compliance. You may enjoy preparing for a walkathon or 5K (3.1 miles). Or perhaps you enjoy working out under the instruction of a teacher who makes you feel motivated. Maybe you would like to join a hiking group to be outdoors and see the natural beauty in your area. To better enjoy exercise, select a time when you will not be rushed. Keep in mind that exercise sessions should be convenient. A nearby location is recommended. You are not likely to enjoy driving across town to get to the gym, health club, track, or pool. If parking is a problem, you may get discouraged quickly and quit.

| Activity 9.1 | **Personal Reflection on Exercise and Exercise Enjoyment** |

Name _____ Date _____ Grade _____

Instructor _____ Course _____ Section _____

OBJECTIVE

The purpose of this lab is for you to reflect, analyze, and evaluate the meaning of exercise in your life. As you read through the statements posed in this lab, you will be able to better understand your feelings about exercise and write an action plan to help you adopt and adhere to a lifetime exercise program.

I. Rate the following

T = True for all of my workouts
S = True for some of my workouts
O = True for an occasional workout
N = Never true for me

Workout Trait Preferences and Social Preferences

_ I look for exercise that leaves my body feeling stretched, engaged, and rejuvenated.

_ If I am going to spend time exercising, it needs to count. I like exercise that pushes my limits.

_ I am happy with the intensity of a workout when it energizes me and gets my heart pumping.

_ I prefer a workout that science has proven will produce results.

_ I prefer a workout that is not fussy, and I appreciate the simplicity of machines like treadmills, ellipticals, and stationary bicycles.

_ I prefer exercise that allows me time to think.

_ I find that I can workout longer if I can talk with someone, watch or listen to something, or follow an instructor's directions.

_ I enjoy applying myself to a workout and being mindful about my body as I exercise.

_ I enjoy feeling graceful or feeling that I am practicing good form while I exercise.

_ I enjoy the challenge of an activity that takes skill and requires focus and concentration.

_ I am not competitive.

_ I am competitive with myself.

_ I am competitive with others. I am driven by others in a group class or on a team.

_ I enjoy online competitions or programs where I can challenge others.

_ I prefer solo exercise with an ambitious fitness goal.

_ I prefer solo exercise that allows me time to think.

_ I prefer having exercise partners with whom I can talk.

_ I prefer having an exercise partner who is a close friend and a source of support and motivation.

_ I find that a packed workout class energizes me.

_ I love being part of a team or small exercise class.

I. What are your reflections after evaluating your answers to the preceding statements? (What have you learned about your regular workouts? What new workout options would you consider as an occasional exercise solution?)

_____

_____

_____

_____

_____

© Fitness & Wellness, Inc.

Activity 9.1 **Personal Reflection on Exercise and Exercise Enjoyment** *(continued)*

II. Rate the following

T = Always true for me
S = Sometimes true for me
O = Occasionally true
N = Never true for me

Perks and Motivation

_ I am a planner. I love charting my own plan or organizing groups and planning workouts.

_ I have enough to plan in my own life; thus, I enjoy showing up to exercise and having something fun or well-planned waiting for me.

_ I enjoy challenging myself to follow a pre-set program.

_ Once I plan a workout program for myself, or set a goal, I tend to follow through.

_ I find I thrive by having a team or workout group who counts on me to participate regularly.

_ I am motivated by watching an exercise log build up day by day.

_ I enjoy the exhilaration of achievement when I go all out for speed or lift a certain resistance (weight).

_ I appreciate programs with incremental goals that I can confidently master and build upon.

_ I believe that for me it's not about the goal, it's about lifestyle. I want exercise and physical activity to be an interesting and enjoyable part of my life.

_ I find that events or races motivate me.

_ I enjoy conditioning for my sport.

_ I enjoy exercising as a form of networking (tennis, golf, racquetball, etc.).

_ I would love trying a trendy boutique gym.

_ I am driven by a good music playlist.

_ I find that exercise helps me rejuvenate during my busy life. It makes me feel happy and balanced when I go to bed at night.

_ I am motivated by seeing improvements in muscle definition.

_ I am motivated by seeing my weight and body composition at healthy levels.

_ I am motivated by feeling strong, capable, and graceful in everyday life.

_ I love trying a new workout app.

_ I like sharing my workouts on social networks.

_ I like a well-tuned workout that fits my goals. I like to stick to an exercise plan and see the results.

_ I find that changing up fitness activities keeps me interested in my workouts.

_ I am happy to try something new as long as I feel prepared. I like to have an exercise plan properly explained to me by someone with expertise.

_ I enjoy the challenge of stepping into a new sport or activity for the first time.

II. What are your reflections after evaluating your answers to the preceding statements? (What perks can you realistically use to make exercise more enjoyable? What perks do not motivate you?)

_____

_____

_____

_____

_____

_____

III. Rate the following

T = Always true for me
S = Sometimes true for me
O = Occasionally true
N = Never true for me

Scheduling and Setting

_ I am happiest when exercise is scheduled in my weekly agenda and I don't need to worry as to how I will fit in.

_ I know that making exercise a priority makes me feel like my needs are valued and are being met.

_ I like having exercise planned into my day, but prefer wiggle room instead of an exact scheduled time.

_ I am happiest with an open, flexible schedule.

_ I am happy to change my workout plans if it means I can spend time with a friend.

_ I am easily frustrated when I lose fitness gains. Fitness is important to me.

_ If I miss a workout, I become discouraged.

_ I am great at being flexible, and I can make up for a missed workout later in the day or week, even if it is not my ideal workout.

_ I am invigorated by exercising outdoors.

_ I feel safe outdoors in my neighborhood.

_ I find that my motivation levels change depending on the season of the year.

_ I love being in or near the water.

_ I prefer an environment that is familiar and convenient. I am discouraged or impatient when exercise becomes a big hassle because of a new environment.

_ I am comfortable in a gym or exercise studio.

_ I enjoy working out at home where I don't have to worry about what to wear or about what other people are doing.

III. What are your reflections after evaluating your answers to the preceding statements? (What times do you struggle with most? What times are easiest for you? What backup plans are realistic for you when you miss a workout?)

_____

_____

IV. Rate the following

T = Always true for me
S = Sometimes true for me
O = Occasionally true
N = Never true for me

Integrated Exercise

_ I enjoy fitting physical activity into my everyday life, like biking or walking to work; it is a beautiful way to live.

_ I would be completely comfortable if someone walked into my office and found me doing tai chi, squats, or holding a plank position on the floor.

_ I consistently mix up my work schedule or work setting to stand more, take walking breaks, and find other creative ways to be active.

_ I would consider turning down a job or promotion if it meant being totally sedentary during work hours.

IV. What are your reflections after evaluating your answers to the preceding statements? (How can you realistically become more active outside of your exercise routine?)

_____

_____

V. Action Plan: Indicate an overall action plan or specific changes you can implement to help you adopt and adhere to a lifetime program of physical activity and exercise.

_____

_____

Guidelines for Success when Attending a Group Workout Class for the First Time

- *Learn about the class.* If you have the opportunity, ask a gym employee or an experienced student about the class. This will allow you to get a feel for the reputation of the class and give you the opportunity to ask questions you may have. Don't be afraid to be upfront about your fitness level.

- *Ask not only about the class but also about the instructor.* Classes with the same title may vary widely with different instructors.

- *Bring a water bottle, and arrive to the class 5 to 10 minutes early.* If you have the opportunity, introduce yourself to the instructor. Instructors appreciate knowing when they have new students so they can adjust class instruction accordingly. Arriving early will also allow you to choose a position in the middle of the class where you can see the instructor well and also follow experienced class members.

- *If a class requires hand weights, choose light weights at first.* You can always choose a heavier weight once you are familiar with the requirements of the class. Don't be afraid to adapt exercises during the course of the class to fit your fitness level. For example, you may alternate arms when doing bicep curls instead of doing both at the same time. If you can't follow a routine exactly, just keep moving.

- *Be happy with your best effort.* Commend yourself for trying something new.

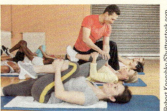
Robert Kneschke/Shutterstock.com

Take a moment also to reflect on the fitness results that are most important to you. You may have a goal to maintain body weight, have more energy, or participate in a sport. This chapter will help you condition for the results you desire.

Being Flexible with Your Exercise Routine

As you implement your exercise program, avoid an all-or-nothing approach. Including exercise in your schedule is a skill that comes with its own learning curve. As you plan your week, visualize ways to fit in exercise. Research has shown that imagining possible obstacles, then visualizing specifically what you will do to overcome them, increases your chance for success. For example, you may have a friend coming to visit and may opt to trade your visit to the gym for a chance to walk and talk or go for a hike with your friend.

As you try new activities, you may be happily surprised by the results. For example, the intensity of hiking over uneven terrain is greater than that of walking. An 8-hour hike can burn as many calories as a 20-mile walk or jog.

HOEGER KEY TO WELLNESS

 Although walking takes longer than jogging, the caloric cost of brisk walking is only about 10 percent lower than that of jogging the same distance.

! Critical Thinking

In your own experience with personal fitness programs throughout the years, what factors have motivated you and helped you the most to stay with a program? What factors have kept you from being physically active, and what can you do to change these factors?

9.2 Keys to Planning Exercise for Health and Fitness

Perhaps you have seen exercise programs that help beginners progress from walking 10 minutes to running a 5K or 10K (6.2 miles) or help beginners train to complete 100 pushups during one workout. Programs like these are based on the same **exercise prescription** principles that you have become familiar with after studying the chapters on cardiorespiratory fitness, muscular fitness, and flexibility. This chapter reviews and builds on what you have already learned and offers the remaining guidelines you need to create a fitness plan based on sound exercise principles. Figure 9.1 (pages 346–347) provides a quick reference guide to help you easily review and apply these principles. Once you are familiar with the concepts of exercise prescription, you will have the ability to create workouts around activities you enjoy.

Basic Exercise Training Principles

As you have seen, the same basic exercise training principles apply to cardiorespiratory endurance, muscular fitness, and flexibility. Now that you are familiar with the way these basic principles work, take a moment to read "A Review of Fundamental Exercise Training Principles" and picture putting them to work in your own exercise program. As you apply these principles in your exercise program, your understanding of them will deepen.

GLOSSARY

Exercise prescription The practice of designing a safe, individualized, and effective exercise program that includes frequency, intensity, time, type, volume, and progression of exercise to improve and/or maintain physical fitness, decrease the risk for chronic diseases, and improve the quality and length of life.

A Review of Fundamental Exercise Training Principles

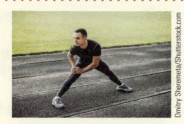

Dmitry Sheremeta/Shutterstock.com

Levels of Fitness and Exercise Exertion

Health fitness standards versus physical fitness standards:
Health fitness standards are the threshold where significant improvements to health and quality of life occur. Physical fitness standards are set higher than health fitness standards: They require more intense exercise and result in improved fitness gains.

Aerobic versus anaerobic: The word *aerobic* comes from the words *air* (aero) and *life* (bio). An exercise is aerobic when it relies on oxygen delivered to tissues throughout the body to continually generate energy. An exercise becomes anaerobic when the intensity of exercise is so high that oxygen cannot be sufficiently delivered to the tissues to generate the required energy to perform the activity. The body, instead, creates energy without oxygen from the small amount of glucose available in the tissue. Such high-intensity activities can only be sustained for 2 to 3 minutes, when glucose supplies are used up. It is important to note that even aerobic workouts sometimes require anaerobic energy production, which supplies immediate energy during any upward change of intensity in activity, until the aerobic system can adjust and supply the required oxygen to meet the new energy demands.

Oxygen uptake (VO_2): The amount of oxygen taken in and used by the body during physical activity is known as oxygen uptake. This amount of oxygen (O_2) is measured in volume (V). The measurement is shown for one minute of exercise. When the volume is measured in liters per minute (L/min) it is referred to as the absolute value of oxygen used. The measurement can be personalized by taking into account how much a person weighs in kilograms. In this case, VO_2max is expressed as volume in milliliters per kilogram of body weight per minute (mL/kg/min) and is referred to as a relative value because the measurement is relative to body weight.

Maximal oxygen uptake (VO_2max): VO_2max is the maximum volume of oxygen a person's body is able to use during maximal effort.

Heart rate reserve (HRR): Heart rate reserve is the difference between the maximal heart rate (MHR),* while you are working your hardest, and the heart rate while you are at rest (RHR). The equation looks like this: HRR = MHR − RHR.

Training intensity (TI) and Physical Activity Perceived Exertion (H-PAPE) scale: Once you know the heart rate reserve, you can decide on training intensity. Training intensity is a way of knowing how hard you are working, and is expressed as a percentage of your HRR. For a light workout, train at a smaller percentage of your HRR, like 30 to 60 percent; for a vigorous workout, train at a larger percentage of your HRR, like 60 to 90 percent.

Individuals may not always want to check their heart rate while exercising. The rate of perceived exertion scale was developed for this purpose. Descriptive words or phrases have been assigned to training intensities. For example, a 40 percent TI is a "light" perceived exertion, whereas a 50 percent TI is a "moderate" perceived exertion.**

Metabolic equivalents (METs): METs are a handy measurement for comparing the intensity of exercise across different types of exercise. The baseline measurement is a single MET. One MET is the amount of oxygen used when a person is at rest (it is the equivalent of a VO_2 of 3.5 mL/kg/min). A 2-MET activity would double the volume of oxygen required at rest. An activity that has the intensity of 3 METs requires three times the amount, and so on. The volume of oxygen required to ride a bike up a steep hill is about 12 times more than the amount utilized when you are at rest, so its intensity would be 12 METs. METs are like VO_2max, in that they indicate the volume of oxygen you are utilizing. And just like VO_2max, they are expressed in mL/kg/min. (See Table 6.9 on page 247 for MET levels of different exercises.)

Muscular strength versus muscular endurance: Muscular strength is the ability to exert maximum force against resistance. It is measured by the maximal amount of weight an individual can lift in a single effort, or 1 RM. Muscular endurance is the ability of a muscle to exert submaximal force repeatedly over time.

Fast twitch versus slow twitch: Slow-twitch fibers have a greater capacity for aerobic work. Fast-twitch fibers have a greater capacity for anaerobic work and are necessary to produce force and power. An individual's ratio of slow-twitch to fast-twitch fibers is genetically determined, but the capacities of both are increased with training. When training for a specific sport, it is important that conditioning match the demands of a sport, as speed and endurance are at opposite sides of the performance spectrum.

FITT-VP: Choosing the Right Amount of Exercise

Four key components of an exercise prescription that are interrelated are frequency, intensity, time, and type (FITT). Changing one aspect may require adjustments in the other three components. For example, increasing intensity requires decreasing time. All four of these aspects combined make up volume (V), which can be increased according to the principle of progression (P)—thus the acronym FITT-VP.

Frequency: The number of times a person exercises in a given time period is referred to as frequency.

Intensity: How hard a person exercises is referred to as intensity. For cardiorespiratory exercise, intensity can be measured by training intensity (TI) and the equivalent Physical Activity Perceived Exertion Scale (H-PAPE), or by metabolic equivalents (METs). Exercising at about 60 percent TI is generally ideal for prolonged exercise. Reaching 80 to 90 percent TI is typical when performing high-intensity interval training (HIIT). Other than in a clinical or laboratory setting, aerobic intensity is

(continued)

generally *not* measured as a percentage of VO₂max because specialized equipment would be required.

In strength-training, intensity refers to the amount of resistance (weight) a person lifts. Lifting about 80 percent of the maximum capacity (one repetition maximum or 1 RM), which works out to be around 8 to 12 repetitions maximum, is a good general recommendation.

Time (duration): The length of an exercise session.

Type (mode): The exercise activity an individual chooses, such as jogging, swimming, cycling, aerobic dance, or climbing, is referred to as the type or mode. In strength-training, there are two specific modes: isometric training and dynamic training. A multi-mode exercise program will mix up the mode of aerobic or strength training either throughout the week or within a single workout.

Volume: Exercise volume is used in cardiorespiratory exercise as a way to measure all types of exercise an individual has done in a day or week. The recommended minimum volume of weekly exercise is 1,000 calories. This type of volume is calculated by multiplying the frequency, intensity (in calories expended per minute), and duration of the exercise session and adding all exercise sessions together for that day or week. The total is expressed in calories expended. For example:

$$5 \text{ days} \times 8 \text{ calories per minute of exercise} \times 30 \text{ minutes}$$
$$= 1,200 \text{ calories}$$

Volume is designed to ensure a person is getting the right quantity of exercise on a weekly basis.

In muscular fitness, volume is perhaps even simpler: it defines all the weight lifted during one strength-training session. The volume of a session is the sum of all repetitions performed multiplied by the resistances used. For example:

$$3 \text{ sets} \times 6 \text{ reps} \times 150 \text{ pounds} = \text{training volume of 2,700 pounds}$$

The volumes of all of the exercises done in one session are then added together. No guidelines have been set as to the appropriate volume of strength training. However, a minimum of two strength training sessions per week involving 8 to 12 different exercises are recommended.

Progression: Your body reaches its maximum potential by adapting gradually to progressive increases in overload. Attempting to overload your muscles or systems too quickly results in injury.

Training Principles

Overload: To improve fitness, the work performed in any activity must be more than the body is typically accustomed to performing.

Individuality: The response to an overload is heterogeneous. This means that every individual responds differently to training, and therefore, the optimum training approach is different for every person. For example, some individuals respond better to intensity and others to endurance. A very small percentage of individuals exhibit minimal or no response to aerobic training (see "Responders versus Nonresponders" in Chapter 6, page 224).

Training effects: As muscles or body systems are consistently overloaded, they will improve in response to the new demands placed on them.

Dose-response: The dose (or amount) of exercise you perform will affect the extent to which your body responds (or adapts). A 20-minute dose of intense exercise will result in greater improvements than a 20-minute dose of moderate exercise. A 20-minute dose of moderate exercise will result in greater improvements than a 10-minute dose of moderate exercise.

Diminishing return: The speed at which fitness improves over time will diminish as an individual nears his or her personal fitness potential.

Specificity: Body systems adapt to the specific demands placed upon them. When training for a specific sport, an individual should choose aerobic/anaerobic, strength, and flexibility exercises that mimic the demands of the sport.

Reversibility: Just as muscles or systems strengthen when they are overloaded, so will they weaken when they cease to be overloaded.

Rest and recovery: Rest and recovery are necessary for proper conditioning. Exercise places stress on body systems. These systems need time to repair and strengthen themselves prior to the next exercise session; otherwise, the systems will be torn down. A hard day of training needs to be followed by a recovery day. Remember a key conditioning principle: Recovery days are recovery days!

Variation: This principle states that one or more aspects of a training program need to be varied over time to maximize training benefits. Minor adjustments and changes in training result in more consistent improvements in performance. Periodization is an application of this principle, allowing for changes in the training program while still progressing towards a specific goal.

Key Methods for Applying the Preceding Principles

Warm-up and cool-down: Exercise sessions should always be preceded by a warm-up of 3 to 5 minutes for steady activities, 10 minutes for stop-and-go activities, or longer prior to a high-intensity effort such as an all-out mile run. A warm-up increases extensibility of muscles and connective tissues, extends joint range of motion, and enhances muscular activity. Following exercise a 10-minute cool-down is recommended because the body relies on muscle contractions to pump excess blood back to the heart. Stopping exercise abruptly causes blood to pool in exercised body parts and allows for less lactic acid removal.

Interval training: Interval training involves cycling through intense efforts of exercise (at 70 to 100 percent TI) and less intense rest periods (30 to 60 percent TI) during a workout. The more intense the effort, the longer the rest period. Interval training produces cardiorespiratory gains faster than training at a moderate-continuous intensity.

High-intensity interval training (HIIT): Interval training that involves intense efforts of 90 percent or higher is referred to as high-intensity interval training. Efforts can surpass 100 percent of the aerobic TI, thus making them an anaerobic effort. These intense efforts last 10 to 60 seconds with recovery periods of complete rest to moderate exercise between. Usually a 1:4 to a 1:1 work-to-rest ratio is used.

Periodization: Periodization breaks up a training regimen into sessions of about 2 to 12 weeks, and changes training goals and

(continued)

variables for each session (such as changing aerobic intensity or alternating between muscular strength and muscular endurance). Periodization divides the season into three cycles (macrocycles, mesocycles, and microcycles). Periodized programs are a way to achieve proper overload and rest. They have been shown to provide faster development and be more effective than nonperiodized programs. Periodization helps avoid fitness plateaus, which can happen in as short as 6 to 8 weeks as the body adapts to the change in training stimuli.

Cross-training: Alternating between a variety of exercise types helps maintain proper overload and prevent overuse injuries. Cross-training also helps people stay interested in and maintain an exercise program. Like periodization, cross-training helps avoid plateaus in progress.

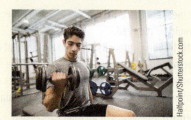

Plyometrics: Rapid/forceful movements, such as jumping on and off a box, with the intent to enhance athletic explosiveness, are known as plyometric training. Exercisers who use plyometrics are advised to warm up properly and take extra precautions to avoid injuries.

* See Chapter 6, page 236, to estimate your MHR and learn to read your RHR.
** See Chapter 6, page 240, to see the full H-PAPE scale.

Interval Training

Faster performance times in aerobic activities (running and cycling) are generated with speed or interval training. People who want to improve their running times often run shorter intervals at faster speeds than the actual racing pace. For example, a person wanting to run a 6-minute mile may run four 440-yard intervals at a speed of 1 minute and 20 seconds per interval. A 440-yard walk/jog can become a recovery interval between fast runs.

High-Intensity Interval Training

High-intensity interval training (HIIT) is a challenging training program that involves high- to very-high-intensity intervals (at least 80 percent of maximal capacity) that usually last 6 to 60 seconds, each followed by a low- to moderate-intensity recovery interval.[2] The HIIT format has been applied to exercises across the workout spectrum, from sprints and cycling for cardiorespiratory fitness; to plyometrics, bodyweight training, and equipment drills with medicine balls and heavy ropes; to power lifting for muscular fitness. By breaking up a workout into smaller segments, HIIT allows the participant to perform a greater training volume at a higher exercise intensity.

Intense efforts can surpass 100 percent of the maximal aerobic capacity, thus making them anaerobic efforts, commonly referred to as supramaximal efforts. For example, one type of HIIT, the Tabata training method, was originally developed for Japanese Olympic speed skaters who performed bursts of efforts on stationary bicycles at 170 percent of the maximal aerobic capacity. The total amount of time spent working at maximum aerobic capacity for the average person typically does not last longer than 2 to 3 minutes during one interval session (trained subjects can do so for about 5 minutes). Maximal aerobic or supramaximal efforts, interspaced by short rest intervals, eventually lead to a drop in work capacity; as a result, the subsequent efforts may become lighter, shorter, or aerobic in nature.

HIIT has been shown to help improve both aerobic and anaerobic fitness at a much faster rate than training at a steady, continuous aerobic intensity. Fitness enthusiasts like HIIT because fitness and weight loss goals are reached faster with this type of training, often with workout sessions of shorter duration, as long as post-exercise caloric intake is carefully monitored and not increased following training.

Boutique gyms that focus on HIIT are a new trend. These gyms tout the benefits of HIIT to their customers, including accelerated fitness results and a boost in metabolic rate for up to 36 hours after workouts. Indeed, when it comes to aerobic improvement, it appears that HIIT speeds gain in aerobic capacity (VO_2max).[3] The metabolic rate also receives a moderate boost even after the HIIT exercise period has ended. Following light- to moderate-intensity aerobic activity, the resting metabolism returns to normal in about 90 minutes. Depending on the volume of training (intensity and number of intervals performed), with HIIT it takes 24 to 72 hours for the body to return to its normal resting metabolic rate. Thus, a greater amount of calories (primarily from fat) are burned up to 3 days following HIIT.

HIIT has a reputation of being a workout for athletes and unsafe for the average fitness enthusiast. On the contrary, high-risk patients facing a variety of chronic illnesses—including chronic obstructive pulmonary disease, Parkinson's disease, and disability from stroke—have successfully carried out and benefited from HIIT under close supervision by a physician. Because a low aerobic capacity is a risk factor for diseases of the cardiovascular system, the medical community is encouraged by this training modality for high-risk patients.

Other benefits of HIIT include increased glucose sensitivity in a matter of weeks, which is encouraging for reversing risk for diabetes. Further, HIIT also decreases blood lipids and appears to accelerate fat loss by changing the body's response to exercise at the cellular level (for more information, see Chapter 5, page 199). For some individuals, a short HIIT workout has been reported to be not only more effective, but also more manageable than a comparable workout of steady exertion.

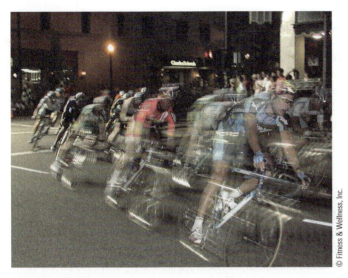

High-intensity interval training promotes fitness, enhances energy expenditure and weight loss, and augments health benefits.

Any individual who is considered medium to high risk, nonetheless, should seek medical clearance and direction from his or her physician prior to attempting a HIIT program.[4]

Four training variables affect HIIT. The acronym DIRT is frequently used to denote these variables:[5]

D = Distance of each speed interval
I = Interval or length of recovery between speed intervals
R = Repetitions or number of speed intervals to be performed
T = Time of each speed interval

Using these four variables, a person can design a practically unlimited number of HIIT sessions.

The intervals consist of a 1:4 to a 1:1 work-to-recovery ratio. The more intense the speed interval, the longer the required recovery interval. For aerobic intervals (lasting longer than 3 minutes), 1:2, 1:1, or even lower ratios are used. For intense supramaximal speed intervals (30 seconds to 3 minutes), recovery intervals that last two to four times as long (1:2 to 1:4) as the work period are required.

A 1:3 ratio, for example, indicates that you'll work at a fairly high intensity for, say, 30 seconds and then spend 90 seconds on light- to moderate-intensity recovery. Be sure to keep moving during the recovery phase. Perform four or five intervals at first, and then gradually progress to 10 intervals. As your fitness improves, you can lengthen the high-intensity proportion of the intervals progressively to 1 minute and/or decrease the total recovery time.

For aerobic sports, HIIT at least once per week improves performance. Though HIIT is most commonly done at a 1:2 or lower work-to-recovery ratio, you also can do a 5- to 10-minute aerobic work interval followed by 1 to 2 minutes of recovery, but the intensity of these longer intervals should not be as high, and only three to five intervals are recommended. Note that the HIIT workouts are not performed in addition to the regular aerobic workouts but, instead, take the place of one of these workouts.

Ultra-Short Workouts

Once HIIT was popularized for a variety of workout types, a new trend of ultra-short high-intensity workouts emerged. These workouts are considered low-volume workouts because the overall amount of time spent exercising is so short that, even at a great level of intensity, the overall volume of exercise remains low. Popular ultra-short circuit-training workouts last for 7 to 10 minutes. Exercisers progress at high intensity through 5 to 12 different body-weight exercises, using alternating muscle groups, that last 30 to 60 seconds with little to no rest between. Participants attempt to work several muscle groups to fatigue while also elevating the heart rate as a result of the intense effort, therefore achieving cardiorespiratory improvement.

Research continues to accumulate in favor of ultra-short workouts,[6] stating that fitness-wise they are as effective as or even more effective than longer steady-intensity workouts (though the total number of calories burned during the ultra-short workout session is lower). Research states that, like HIIT workouts, ultra-short workouts improve aerobic capacity over a shorter number of weeks, boost cardiovascular health, improve metabolism of glucose, and decrease blood lipids and body fat.

In order to achieve the benefits corroborated by research during an ultra-short workout, follow these guidelines:

- Keep intensity high. Like HIIT, all exercises should be done at a minimum of 80 percent of maximal capacity (or "hard" on the H-PAPE scale), meaning the exerciser will perceive it as a difficult workout the entire 7- to 10-minute session.
- Keep rest periods short, up to 15 seconds between exercises, never more.
- Alternate upper-body with lower-body exercises.
- Opt for exercises that engage the core.
- Alternate exercises that demand a sudden boost in heart rate with exercises that allow your heart rate to slow somewhat.
- As with any high-intensity workout, take special care to watch proper exercise form.

Cross-Training

Cross-training combines two or more activities in an exercise program. This type of training is designed to enhance fitness, provide needed rest to tired muscles, and decrease injuries. It can also eliminate the monotony and burnout of single-activity programs and can help avoid plateaus in fitness progress, which can happen in as few as 6 to 8 weeks of a workout as the body becomes efficient at a repeated movement.

GLOSSARY

Cross-training A combination of aerobic activities that contribute to overall fitness.

Sample High-Intensity Interval Training (HIIT) Programs

The following are sample HIIT programs. For intensity levels, you should use the Physical Activity Perceived Exertion Scale (H-PAPE) in Figure 6.9, page 240. Prior to HIIT, be sure to have a sound general aerobic (cardiorespiratory) fitness base—that is, at least 6 weeks of aerobic training, five times per week for 20 to 60 minutes per session. Once you are ready for HIIT, always have a proper 5- to 10-minute aerobic warm-up prior to the first high-intensity interval. Also, in all cases, follow up the final high-intensity interval with a 5- to 10-minute cool-down phase. You can use the same exercise modality (running, cycling, elliptical training, stair climbing, or swimming) for your entire HIIT, or you may use a combination of these activities with some of the following programs, if such is feasible at your facility. Do not perform back-to-back HIIT on consecutive days. Preferably, depending on the intensity and volume of training, allow 2 to 3 days between HIIT sessions.

Five-minute very hard-intensity aerobic intervals: Exercise at a very hard rate (90 percent of maximal capacity) for 5 minutes, followed by 5 to 10 minutes of recovery at a light to moderate intensity. Start with one interval and work up to three by the third to fifth training session. Initially, use a 1:2 work-to-recovery ratio. Gradually decrease the recovery to a 1:1 ratio or even less.

Step-wise intensity interval training: Using 3- to 5-minute intervals, start at a light-intensity rate of perceived exertion and then progressively step up to the very hard-intensity level (light, moderate, somewhat hard, vigorous, hard, and very hard). Start with 3-minute intervals, and as you become more fit, increase to 5 minutes each. As time allows and you develop greater fitness, you can add a step-down approach by progressively stepping down to hard, vigorous, somewhat hard, moderate, and light.

Fartlek training: Fartlek training was developed in 1937 by Swedish coach Gösta Holmér. The word *fartlek* means "speed play" in Swedish. It is an unstructured form of interval training where intensity (speed) and distance of each interval are varied as the participant wishes. There is no set structure, and the individual alternates the intensity (from somewhat hard to very hard) and length of each speed interval, along with the recovery intervals (light to moderate) and length thereof. Total duration of fartlek training is between 20 and 60 minutes.

Tempo training: Although no formal intervals are conducted with tempo training, the intensity of training qualifies it as a HIIT program. Following an appropriate warm-up, tempo runs involve continuous training between vigorous (70%) and hard (80%) for 20 to 60 minutes at a time.

All-out or supramaximal interval training: All-out interval training involves 10 to 20 supramaximal or sprint intervals lasting 30 to 60 seconds each. Because these are supramaximal intervals, they are anaerobic exercise, which means you are working above 100 percent of aerobic capacity. Depending on the level of conditioning and the length of the speed interval, 2 to 5 minutes recovery at a light to moderate level are allowed.

Tabata method: This training modality was named after the researcher who tested a variation of workout-to-recovery ratios with Olympic speed skaters and honed in on a prescription he found particularly effective.[a] The method follows a pattern of 4 minutes of light-intensity exercise followed by 4 minutes of intervals. After a 10-minute warm-up, the participant exercises at or near maximal capacity (90 to 100 percent) for a 20-second burst, followed by 10 seconds of very easy recovery. This 30-second cycle is repeated eight times to complete the 4 minutes of interval training. Always cool down at a very easy pace at the end of the session. When you first attempt this workout, strive for only one 4-minute interval. Gradually build to two and three 4-minute interval training bursts, interspaced with 4 minutes of light-intensity recovery between.

10-20-30 method: This training method was developed by Danish researcher Dr. Thomas Gunnarsson after studying a variety of HIIT workouts using moderately trained runners.[b] After a proper warmup, participants exercise for 10 seconds at maximal effort (100 percent effort), then 20 seconds at a somewhat hard effort (60 percent effort), and then 30 seconds at a light effort (30 percent effort). This cycle is repeated for five minutes.

(continued)

Cardio/resistance training program: You may use a combination of aerobic and resistance training for your HIIT. Following a brief aerobic and strength-training warm-up, select about eight resistance-training exercises that you can alternate with treadmill running, cycling, elliptical training, or rowing. Perform one set of 8 to 20 RM (based on personal preference) on each exercise followed by 90 seconds of aerobic work after each set. You can pace the aerobic intensity according to the preceding strength-training set. For example, you may choose a light-intensity aerobic interval following a 10 RM for the leg press exercise and a vigorous aerobic interval after a 10 RM arm-curl set. Allow no greater recovery time (2 to 5 seconds) between exercise

modes than what it takes to walk from the strength-training exercise to the aerobic station (and vice versa).

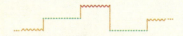

[a] I. Tabata et al., "Effects of Moderate-Intensity Endurance and High-Intensity Intermittent Training on Anaerobic Capacity and VO2max," *Medicine and Science in Sports and Exercise* 28, no. 10 (October 1996): 1327–1330.

[b] T. P. Gunnarsson and J. Bangsbo, "The 10-20-30 Training Concept Improves Performance and Health Profile in Moderately Trained Runners," *Journal of Applied Physiology 113,* no. 1 (July 2012): 16–24.

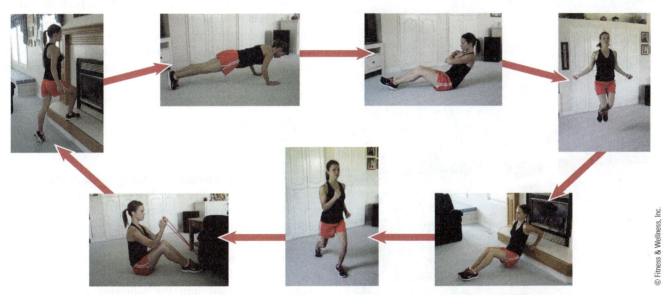

When properly designed and implemented, a person's own body weight can be used to derive both cardiorespiratory endurance and muscular fitness benefits.

Cross-training may combine aerobic and nonaerobic activities such as moderate jogging, speed training, and strength training.

Cross-training can produce better workouts than a single activity. For example, jogging develops the lower body and swimming builds the upper body. Rowing contributes to upper-body development and cycling builds the legs. Combining activities such as these provides good overall conditioning and, at the same time, helps to improve or maintain fitness. As exercisers have become more savvy about achieving results and avoiding injury, cross-training is popping up more often in health-club programs and fitness classes. Combined activity classes are now available and more popular.

Interval training is often coupled with cross-training to improve speed for both anaerobic and aerobic activities. Strength-training, too, compliments cross-training and helps to condition muscles, tendons, and ligaments. Improved strength enhances overall performance in many activities and

sports. For example, road cyclists in one study trained with weights to improve strength. Though the weight training resulted in no improvement in aerobic capacity, the cyclists had a 33 percent improvement in riding time to exhaustion when exercising at 75 percent of their maximal capacity.[7]

Overtraining

Rest is important in any fitness conditioning program. Although the term **overtraining** is associated most frequently with athletic performance, it applies just as well to fitness participants. We all know that hard work improves fitness and

GLOSSARY

Overtraining An emotional, behavioral, and physical condition marked by increased fatigue, decreased performance, persistent muscle soreness, mood disturbances, and feelings of "staleness" or "burnout" as a result of excessive physical training.

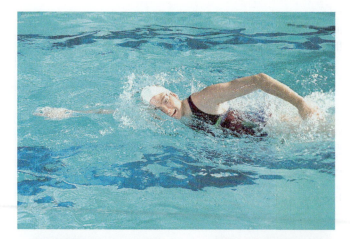

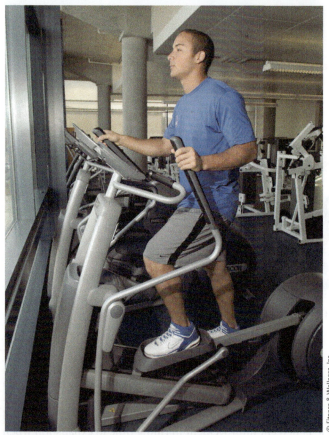

Cross-training enhances fitness, decreases the rate of injuries, and eliminates the monotony of single-activity programs.

© Fitness & Wellness, Inc.

performance. Hard training without adequate recovery, however, breaks down the body and leads to loss of fitness.

Physiological improvements in fitness and conditioning programs occur during the rest periods following training. As a rule, a hard day of training must be followed by a day of light training. Equally, a few weeks of increased training **volume** are to be followed by a few days of light recovery work. During these recovery periods, body systems strengthen and compensate for the training load, leading to a higher level of fitness. If proper recovery is not built into the training routine, overtraining occurs. Decreased performance,

staleness, and injury are frequently seen with overtraining. Tissue damage that leads to injury can begin before symptoms of overtraining have even set in. Thus, to avoid injury and obtain optimal results, training regimens are altered during different phases of the year.

Periodization

Periodization was designed around the premise that the body becomes stronger as a result of training, but if similar workouts are constantly repeated, the body tires and enters a state of staleness and fatigue. Thus, periodization uses variation in intensity and volume to enhance fitness and performance.

Periodization is used most frequently for athletic conditioning. Because athletes cannot maintain peak fitness during an entire season, most athletes seeking peak performance use a periodized training approach. Studies have documented that greater improvements in fitness are achieved by using a variety of training loads. Using the same program and attempting to increase volume and intensity over a prolonged time will result in overtraining.

The periodization training system involves three cycles:

1. Macro cycles
2. Mesocycles
3. Microcycles

These cycles vary in length depending on the requirements of the sport. Typically, the overall training period (season or year) is referred to as a macrocycle. For athletes who need to peak twice a year, such as cross-country and track runners, two macrocycles can be developed within the year.

Macrocycles are divided into smaller weekly or monthly training phases known as mesocycles. A typical season, for example, is divided into the following mesocycles: base fitness conditioning (off-season), preseason or sport-specific conditioning, competition, peak performance, and transition (active recovery from sport-specific training and competition). In turn, mesocycles are divided into smaller weekly or daily microcycles. During microcycles, training follows the general objective of the mesocycle, but the workouts are altered to avoid boredom and fatigue.

The concept behind periodizing can be used in both aerobic and anaerobic sports. In the case of a long-distance runner, for instance, training can start with a general strength-conditioning program and cardiorespiratory endurance cross-training (jogging, cycling, and swimming) during the off-season. In preseason, the volume of strength training is decreased, and the total weekly running mileage, at moderate intensities, is progressively increased. During the competitive season, the athlete maintains a limited strength-training program but now increases the intensity of the runs while decreasing the total weekly mileage. During the peaking phase, volume (miles) of training is reduced even further, while the intensity is maintained at a high level. At the end of the season, a short transition period of 2 to 4 weeks, involving light-to moderate-intensity activities other than running and lifting weights, is recommended.

Behavior Modification Planning

Common Signs and Symptoms of Overtraining

- Decreased fitness
- Decreased sports performance
- Increased fatigue
- Loss of concentration
- Staleness and burnout
- Loss of competitive drive
- Increased resting and exercise heart rate
- Decreased appetite
- Loss of body weight
- Altered sleep patterns
- Decreased sex drive
- Generalized body aches and pains
- Increased susceptibility to illness and injury
- Mood disturbances
- Depression

Try It

If, following several weeks or months of hard training, you experience some of the preceding symptoms, you need to substantially decrease training volume and intensity for a week or two. This recovery phase will allow the body to recover, strengthen, and prepare for the next training phase. In your Behavior Change Tracker or your online journals, modify your training program to allow a light week of training following each 5 to 8 weeks of hard exercise training.

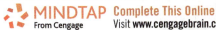

MINDTAP From Cengage **Complete This Online**
Visit **www.cengagebrain.com** to access MindTap, a complete digital course that includes interactive quizzes, videos, and more.

Periodization is frequently used for development of muscular fitness, progressively cycling through the various components (hypertrophy, strength, and power) of strength training. Research indicates that varying the volume and intensity over time is more effective for long-term progression than either single- or multiple-set programs with no variations. Training volume and intensity are typically increased only for large muscle/multi-joint lifts (e.g., bench press, squats, and lat pull-downs). Single-joint lifts (triceps extension, bicep curls, hamstring curls) usually remain in the range of three sets of 8 to 12 repetitions.

A sample sequence—one macrocycle—of periodized training is provided in Table 9.1. The program starts with high volume and light intensity. During subsequent mesocycles (divided among the objectives of hypertrophy, strength, and power), the volume is decreased, and the intensity (resistance) increases. Following each mesocycle, the recommendation is up to 7 days of very light training. This brief resting period allows the body to fully recuperate, preventing overtraining and risk for injury. Other models of periodization are available, but the example provided is the most commonly used.

For aerobic endurance sports, one to three sets of 8 to 12 repetitions to near fatigue performed once or twice a week is recommended. Although strength-training does not enhance maximal oxygen uptake, and strength requirements are not as high with endurance sports, data indicate that strength-training does help the individual sustain submaximal exercise for longer periods of time.

In recent years, the practice of altering or cycling workouts has become popular among fitness participants. Research indicates that periodization is not limited to athletes but has been used successfully by fitness enthusiasts who are preparing for special events such as a 10K run, a triathlon, or a bike race and by those who are simply aiming for higher fitness. Altering training is also recommended for people who progressed nicely in the initial weeks of a fitness program but now feel "stale" and "stagnant." Studies indicate that even among general fitness participants, systematically altering volume and intensity of training is most effective for progress in long-term fitness. Because training phases change continually during a macrocycle, periodization breaks the staleness and the monotony of repeated workouts.

For the nonathlete, a periodization program does not have to account for every detail of the sport. You can periodize workouts by altering mesocycles every 2 to 8 weeks. You can use different exercises, change the number of sets and repetitions, vary the speed of the repetitions, alter recovery time between sets, and even cross-train.

GLOSSARY

Volume (of training) The total amount of training performed in a given work period (day, week, month, or season).

Table 9.1 Periodization Program for Strength

	One Macrocycle			
	Mesocycle 1* Hypertrophy	Mesocycle 2* Strength & Hypertrophy	Mesocycle 3* Strength & Power	Mesocycle 4* Peak Performance
Sets per exercise	3–5	3–5	3–5	1–3
Repetitions	8–12	6–9	1–5	1–3
Intensity (resistance)	Low	Moderate	High	Very high
Volume	High	Moderate	Low	Very low
Weeks (microcycles)	6–8	4–6	3–5	1–2

*Each mesocycle is followed by several days of light training.

© Fitness & Wellness, Inc.

Figure 9.1 Create your own program: Hoeger quick guide to exercise prescription.

Once you adopt a regular pattern of exercise, you can enhance your program by adding elements of strength or aerobic exercise as needed.

If you are just beginning an exercise program, begin by choosing the form of exercise that motivates you most and that best fits with your lifestyle, whether it be aerobic or strength-focused.

cardio

WARM UP
3–5 minutes for steady workouts

10 minutes for stop and go workouts

COOL DOWN
10 minutes for most workouts

STRETCH
The best time to stretch is after a workout when muscles are warm.

BEGIN HERE according to your initial fitness level**

poor/fair begin at week 1

average begin at week 5

active/ excellent begin at week 9

Walking 2–3 mph is equivalent to 30–40% TI.

Week	Duration (min)	Frequency	Training Intensity (TI)
1	15	3	Between 30% and 40%
2	15	4	Between 30% and 40%
3	20	4	Between 30% and 40%
4	20	5	Between 30% and 40%
5	20	4	Between 40% and 60%
6	20	5	Between 40% and 60%
7	30	4	Between 40% and 60%
8	30	5	Between 40% and 60%
9	30	4	Between 60% and 90%
10	30	5	Between 60% and 90%
11	30–40	5	Between 60% and 90%
12	30–40	5	Between 60% and 90%

Allow 4–8 weeks of training as you progress from light to moderate to vigorous.

HEART RATE During the first few weeks of activity, monitor your heart rate and adjust TI accordingly.

exit according to your personal fitness goal

health fitness
significant improvements in health and quality of life

physical fitness
improved quality of life and additional capacity to meet life's demands and sports requirements

sports preparation
contributes to health-related fitness and needed for success in athletics and in lifetime sports and activities

distance training

maintain weight loss

strength

BEGIN HERE by building a basic foundation of strength

The number of reps you can do will vary at different percentages of 1RM, and as the amount of muscle mass increases (muscles with more mass can lift more weight).

FITT GUIDELINES

Frequency: 2–3 days/week on nonconsecutive days is recommended. More frequent training can be done if different muscle groups are exercised on different days. (Allow at least 48 hours between hard strength-training sessions of the same muscle group.)

Intensity (resistance): A good general guideline is to lift at 80% 1 RM, which works out to be sufficient resistance to perform 8–12 reps max for muscular strength, or complete 15–25 reps for muscular endurance. (Older adults and injury prone individuals should use 10–15 reps with moderate resistance of 50–60% of 1 RM.)

Time (sets): 2–4 sets/exercise with 2–3 minutes recovery between sets is recommended for optimal strength development. Complete less than 2 minutes/set if exercises are alternated that require different muscle groups (chest and upper back) or between muscular endurance sets.

Type (mode): Select 8–10 dynamic strenth-training exercises.

The majority of strength gains will be seen in the first 8 weeks of training.

adjust training according to your personal strength goal

general fitness

muscular endurance

maximal strength

body building

sports preparation

maintain weight loss

flexibility

BEGIN HERE

Stretch at least 2-3 days/week, or daily for the best results. Be sure to select flexibility exercises that include all major muscle and tendon groups of the body. Hold the final position of each static stretch for 10 to 30 seconds, and repeat each exercise 2-4 times for a target of 60 seconds of total stretching per exercise.

Stretching is most effective after an aerobic workout, when muscles are warm.

sports preparation

*This guide is designed as a review only of course concepts. For complete discussion of concepts please see each topic in the appropriate chapter.

**Complete the exercise readiness questionnaire on page 39 if you are not currently active. Individuals who are high risk or have chornic disease should undergo a medical examination prior to participating in an exercise program.

Figure 9.1 Create your own program: Hoeger quick guide to exercise prescription *(continued)*

Work at 30–60% training intensity in an activity you enjoy. Aim for a volume of 1000 calories/week by completing a combination of the following: 30 min/day for 5 days/week of moderate physical activity 20 min/day for 3 days/week of vigorous physical activity.

Replace 2 workouts/week with HIIT or vigorous physical activty. Complete additional 2–4 workouts/week at moderate to vigorous intensity.

WHY INCLUDE HIIT?
Increases in VO$_{2max}$ are accelerated when the heart is working around 90 percent TI.

WEEKS 1–6
If unconditioned, complete at least 6 weeeks of base fitness conditioning (aerobic, strength, flexibility) before engaging in sport of choice.

WEEKS 6–10
Adjust aerobic/anaerobic exercise so half of training mimics type of exercise and muscles used in your sport.

WEEKS 10 +
As you begin sports participation continue sport-specific training, and add 1–2 workouts/week of HIIT.

Individuals interested in distance events should include several training sessions where distance is extended beyond race distance but pace is decreased to slightly below race pace. Marathoners are an exception and should max out at about 20 miles three weeks before the race.

Complete a combination of the following: 90 min/day moderate physical activity 5 days/week, 45 min/day vigorous physical activity 3 days/week, 20-30 min of HIIT 2 days/week.

Resistance	Sets	Rest Between Sets*	Frequency (workouts per week)**
8–12 reps max	2–4	2–3 min	2–3
15–25 reps	1–2	1–2 min	2–3
1–6 reps max	2–5	3 min	2–3
8–15 reps near max	3–8	up to 1 min	4–12

PreSeason Sports Conditioning
For weeks 1–6, build a basic foundation of strength. For weeks 6–10 select exercises to match the primary muscles used in your sport.

Sport Season
Maintain strength-conditioning program 2–3 times/week.

Off Season
Perioodize by training for different goals than you train for in conditioning and during the sport season.

Increases in muscle tissue result in increases in the metabolic rate.

Sport-specific stretching can improve performance in sports that require greater-than-average range of motion.

Intense stretching during warm-up in athletic events that rely on force and power for peak performance is not recommended as it may decrease strength and power for up to 60 minutes.

PERIODIZATION AND CROSS TRAINING

The body adapts to a specific exercise program in about 6–8 weeks. Introduce cross training or periodization as you sense you are reaching a fitness plateau.

Vary cardio workouts by
- Increasing intensity.
- Increasing duration.
- Replacing up to 2 workouts with HIIT.
- Changing mode (cross training).

Compare the intensity of various modes of training by comparing METs (see pages xx and xxx).

Vary strength workouts by
- Increasing resistance.
- Increasing reps.
- Increasing or decreasing speed of muscle contractions (concentric and eccentric) speed of eccentric contraction.
- Changing length of rest interval.
- Increasing volume.

Try new strength-training exercises and use a periodized approach as explained on pages xxx–xxx of this chapter.

Aerobic bouts as short at 10 minutes can improve aerobic capacity. Gains in aerobic capacity begin to decrease 48 hours after the most recent training session. For this reason, at least 4 aerobic workouts/week are recommended to maintain or improve aerobic capacity.

FOR FULL DISCUSSION OF CONCEPTS
review the following pages:

FUEL

For guidelines on fueling for aerobic exercise, see pages 360–361.

For guidelines on fueling for muscular fitness, see pages 360–361.

KEYS TO SUCCESS
Remember that for an inactive individual, the greatest health benefits are achieved by initiating moderate physical activity. Beyond that, individuals can achieve greater benefits by participating in more vigorous forms of exercise.

Avoid perfectionism with your workout routine. If you miss a day, do your best to adjust by increasing your physical activity throughout the rest of the day.

Periodization is not for everyone. People who are starting an exercise program, who enjoy a set routine, or who are satisfied with their fitness routine and fitness level do not need to periodize. For new participants, the goal is to start and adhere to exercise long enough to adopt the exercise behavior.

9.3 *Traditional Fitness Activities*

Traditional fitness activities remain popular with good reason (see Figure 9.2). In many cases they are inexpensive and convenient and exercisers often find it easy to join up with others for these traditional workouts.

Walking

Walking at speeds of 4 miles per hour or faster improves cardiorespiratory fitness. From a health-fitness viewpoint, a regular walking program can prolong life. Although walking takes longer than jogging, the caloric cost of brisk walking is only about 10 percent lower than that of jogging the same distance.

Walking is perhaps the best activity to start a conditioning program for the cardiorespiratory system. Inactive people should start with 1-mile walks four or five times per week. Walk times can be increased gradually by 5 minutes each week. Following 3 to 4 weeks of conditioning, a person should be able to walk 2 miles at a 4-mile-per-hour pace, five times per week. Greater aerobic benefits accrue from walking longer and swinging the arms faster than normal. Light hand weights, a backpack (4 to 6 pounds), or walking poles add to the intensity of walking. Because of the additional load on the cardiorespiratory system, extra weights or loads are not recommended for people who have cardiovascular disease.

Figure 9.2 Most popular adult physical activities in the United States.

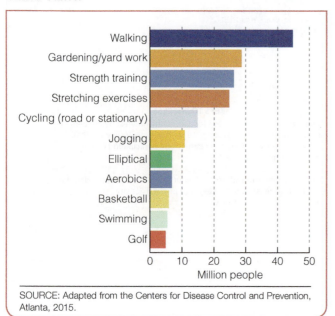

SOURCE: Adapted from the Centers for Disease Control and Prevention, Atlanta, 2015.

Walking in water (chest-deep level) is another excellent form of aerobic activity, particularly for people with leg and back problems. Because of the buoyancy that water provides, individuals submerged in water to armpit level weigh only about 10 to 20 percent of their weight outside the water. The resistance the water creates as a person walks in the pool makes the intensity quite high, providing an excellent cardiorespiratory workout.

Jogging

Jogging three to five times a week is one of the fastest ways to improve cardiorespiratory fitness. The risk of injury, however, especially in beginners, is greater with jogging than walking. For proper conditioning, jogging programs should start with 1 to 2 weeks of walking. As fitness improves, walking and jogging can be combined, gradually increasing the jogging segment until it composes the full 20 to 30 minutes.

A word of caution when it comes to jogging: The risk of injury increases greatly as speed (running instead of jogging) and mileage go up. Jogging approximately 15 miles per week is sufficient to reach an excellent level of cardiorespiratory fitness.

A good pair of shoes is a must for joggers (see the box Choosing Footwear on page 359 in this chapter). Many foot, knee, and leg problems originate from improperly fitting or worn-out shoes. A good pair of shoes should offer good lateral stability and not lean to either side when placed on a flat surface. The shoe also should bend at the ball of the foot, not at midfoot. Worn-out shoes should be replaced. If you suddenly have problems, check your shoes first. It may be time for a new pair.

For safety reasons, joggers should stay away from high-speed roads, not wear headphones, and always run (or walk) against the traffic so that they will be able to see all oncoming traffic. At night, reflective clothing or fluorescent material should be worn on different parts of the body. Carrying a flashlight is even better, because motorists can see the light from a greater distance.

An alternative form of jogging, especially for injured people, those with chronic back problems, and overweight individuals, is deep-water running. This entails running in deep water and is almost as strenuous as jogging on land. The participant usually wears a flotation vest to help maintain the body in an upright position. Many elite athletes train in water to lessen the wear and tear on the body caused by long-distance running. These athletes have been able to maintain high oxygen uptake values through rigorous water running programs.

Hiking

Hiking is an excellent activity for the entire family, especially during the summer and on summer vacations. The intensity of hiking over uneven terrain is greater than that of walking. An hour spent hiking on average is similar to an hour spent playing volleyball or an hour spent biking at 9 or 10 miles per hour. Another benefit of hiking is the relaxing effects of beautiful scenery. A rough day at the office can be forgotten quickly in the peacefulness and beauty of the outdoors.

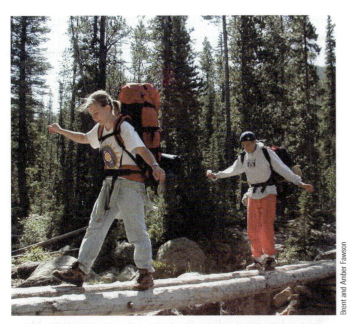

Hiking is an excellent activity to build endurance and relieve stress.

Brent and Amber Fawson

HOEGER KEY TO WELLNESS

The intensity of hiking over uneven terrain is greater than walking. An 8-hour hike can burn as many calories as a 20-mile walk or jog.

Swimming

Swimming is another excellent form of aerobic exercise because it requires the use of almost all of the major muscle groups in the body, thereby providing a good training stimulus for the heart and lungs. Swimming is a great exercise option for individuals who cannot jog or walk for extended periods.

Compared with other activities, the risk of injuries from swimming is low. The aquatic medium helps support the body, taking pressure off bones and joints in the lower extremities and the back.

Maximal heart rates during swimming are approximately 10 to 13 beats per minute (bpm) lower than during running. Cool water temperatures and direct contact with the water seem to help dissipate body heat more efficiently, decreasing the strain on the heart. The horizontal position of the body is also thought to aid blood flow distribution throughout the body, decreasing the demand on the cardiorespiratory system.

Some exercise specialists recommend that this difference in maximal heart rate (10 to 13 bpm) be subtracted prior to determining cardiorespiratory training intensities. For example, the estimated maximal swimming heart rate for a 20-year-old would be approximately 180 bpm [207 − (.7 × 20) − 13]. Studies are inconclusive as to whether this decrease in heart rate in water also occurs at submaximal intensities less than 70 percent of maximal heart rate.

To produce better training benefits during swimming, the swimmer should minimize gliding periods such as those in the breaststroke and side stroke. Achieving proper training intensities with these strokes is difficult. The front crawl is recommended for better aerobic results.

Overweight individuals need to swim fast enough to achieve an adequate training intensity. Excessive body fat makes the body more buoyant, making it easier to spend time floating. This may be good for reducing stress and relaxing, but it does not greatly increase caloric expenditure to aid with weight loss. Walking or jogging in waist- or armpit-deep water is a better choice for overweight individuals who cannot walk or jog on land for very long. If swimming is your main mode of exercise, however, pay particular attention to not overeat following exercise, as cold-water swimming has been shown to stimulate appetite.

Swimming participants also need to remember the principle of specificity of training, which dictates that cardiorespiratory improvements cannot be measured adequately with a land-based walk/jog test. Most of the work with swimming is done by the upper body musculature. Although the heart's ability to pump more blood improves significantly with any type of aerobic activity, the primary increase in the cells' ability to utilize oxygen (VO_2 or oxygen uptake) with swimming occurs in the upper body and not the lower extremities. Therefore, fitness improvements with swimming are best measured through a swim test.

Water Aerobics

The exercises used during water aerobics are designed to elevate the heart rate, which contributes to cardiorespiratory development. In addition, the aquatic medium provides increased resistance for strength improvement with virtually no impact. Because of this resistance to movement, strength gains with water aerobics seem to be better than with land-based aerobic activities.

Another benefit is that water aerobics provides a relatively safe environment for injury-free participation in exercise. The cushioned environment of the water allows patients recovering from leg and back injuries, individuals with joint problems, injured athletes, pregnant women, and obese people to benefit from water aerobics.

As observed with swimming, maximal heart rates achieved during water aerobics are lower than during running. The difference between water aerobics and running is about 10 bpm. Further, research comparing physiologic differences between self-paced treadmill running and self-paced water aerobics exercise showed that even though individuals worked at a lower heart rate in water (163 bpm versus 152 bpm—the equivalent of 85 and 79 percent of maximal heart rate on land, respectively), oxygen uptake level was the same for both exercise modalities (32.4 versus 32.5 ml/kg/min—both 69 percent of land VO_{2max}).[8] Healthy people, nonetheless, can sustain land-based exercise intensities during a water aerobics workout and experience similar fitness benefits as during land aerobics.[9]

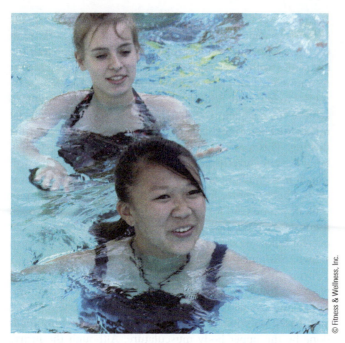

Water aerobics offers fitness, fun, and safety to people of all ages.

Cycling

Because it is a non-weight-bearing activity, cycling is a good exercise modality for people with lower-body or lower-back injuries. Cycling helps to develop the cardiorespiratory system as well as muscular fitness in the lower extremities.

As it is a non-weight-bearing activity, raising the heart rate to the proper training intensity is more difficult with cycling. As the amount of muscle mass involved during aerobic exercise decreases, so does the demand placed on the cardiorespiratory system. The thigh muscles do most of the work in cycling, making it harder to achieve and maintain a high cardiorespiratory training intensity.

Maintaining a continuous pedaling motion and eliminating coasting periods helps the participant achieve a faster heart rate. Exercising for longer periods also helps to compensate for the lower heart rate intensity during cycling.

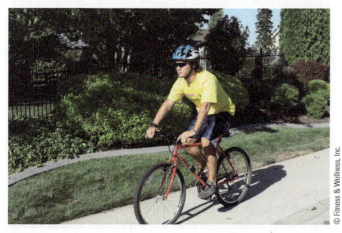

Skill is required for safety and enjoyment of road cycling.

Comparing cycling with jogging, similar aerobic benefits take roughly three times the distance at twice the speed of jogging. Cycling, however, puts less stress on muscles and joints than jogging does, making the former a good exercise modality for people who cannot jog or walk for extended periods of time.

The height of the bike seat should be adjusted so that the knee is flexed at about 30 degrees when the foot is at the bottom of the pedaling cycle. The body should not sway from side to side as the person rides. The cycling cadence also is important for maximal efficiency. Bike tension or gears should be set at a moderate level so that the rider can achieve about 60 to 100 revolutions per minute.

Safety is a key issue in road cycling. According to the CDC, each year about 500,000 emergency room visits in the United States are the result of bicycle-related injuries. These occur most often among children, teens, and males in their early 20s. Three quarters of deaths are a result of head trauma, with one quarter being related to alcohol consumption. Proper equipment and common sense are necessary.

Bike riders must follow the same rules as motorists. Many accidents happen because cyclists run traffic lights and stop signs. Some further suggestions are as follows:

- Select the right bike. Frame size is important. The size is determined by standing flat-footed while straddling the bike. On regular bikes, a one- to two-inch clearance should exist between the groin and the top tube of the frame. For mountain bikes, the clearance should be about three inches. The recommended height of the handlebars is about one inch below the top of the seat. Upright handlebars can also be used by individuals with neck or back problems. Hard/narrow seats on racing bikes tend to be especially uncomfortable for women. To avoid saddle soreness, use wider and more cushioned seats such as gel-filled saddles.
- Use bike hand signals to let the traffic around you know of your intended actions.
- Don't ride side by side with another rider.
- Do ride in pairs or groups whenever possible. Drivers are more likely to notice and take caution around a group of cyclists than a solo cyclist.
- Be aware of turning vehicles and cars backing out of alleys and parking lots; always yield to motorists in these situations, taking special care to stay out of the blind spot of drivers.
- Be on the lookout for storm drains, railroad tracks, and cattle guards, which can cause unpleasant surprises. Front wheels can get caught and riders may be thrown from the bike if they are not crossed at the proper angle (preferably 90 degrees).
- Wear a good helmet, certified by the Snell Memorial Foundation or the American National Standards Institute. Many serious accidents and even deaths have been prevented by use of helmets. Fashion, aesthetics, comfort, or price should not be a factor when selecting and using a helmet for road cycling. Health and life are too precious to give up because of vanity and thriftiness.

- Wear appropriate clothes and shoes. Clothing should be bright, very visible, and lightweight and not restrict movement. Cycling shorts are recommended to prevent skin irritation. For greater comfort, the shorts have extra padding sewn into the seat and crotch areas. They do not tend to wrinkle and they wick away perspiration from the skin. Shorts should be long enough to keep the skin from rubbing against the seat. Experienced cyclists also wear special shoes with a cleat that snaps directly onto the pedal. Take extra warm clothing in a backpack during the winter months in case you have a breakdown and have to walk a long distance for assistance.
- Watch out for ice when it's cold outside. If there is ice on car windows, there will be ice on the road. Be especially careful on bridges as they tend to have ice even when the roads are dry.
- Use the brightest bicycle lights you can when riding in the dark and always keep the batteries well charged. For additional safety, wear reflectors on the upper torso, arms, and legs. Moving bright objects are easier to see by passing motorists. Stay on streets that have good lighting and plenty of room on the side of the road, even if that means riding an extra few minutes to get to your destination.
- Take a cell phone if possible, and let someone else know where you are going and when to expect you back.

Cross-Country Skiing

Cross-country skiing is considered by some to be the ultimate aerobic exercise because it requires vigorous lower and upper body movements. The large amount of muscle mass involved in cross-country skiing makes the intensity of the activity high, yet it places little strain on muscles and joints. One of the highest maximal oxygen uptakes ever measured (85 mL/kg/min) was found in an elite cross-country skier.

Rowing

Rowing is a low-impact activity that provides a complete body workout. It mobilizes most major muscle groups, including those in the arms, legs, hips, abdomen, trunk, and shoulders. Rowing is a good form of aerobic exercise and, because of the nature of the activity (constant pushing and pulling against resistance), also promotes total strength development.

To accommodate different fitness levels, workloads can be regulated on most rowing machines. Stationary rowing, however, is not among the most popular forms of aerobic exercise. People should try the activity for a few weeks before purchasing a unit.

Elliptical Training and Stair Climbing

If sustained for at least 20 minutes, elliptical training and stair climbing are very efficient forms of aerobic exercise. Precisely because of the high intensity of stair climbing, many people stay away from stairs and instead take escalators and elevators. Many people dislike living in two-story homes because they have to climb the stairs frequently.

Elliptical training and stair climbing are relatively safe exercise modalities. Because the feet never leave the climbing surface, they are considered low-impact activities. Joints and ligaments are not strained during climbing. The intensity of exercise is controlled easily because the equipment can be programmed to regulate the workload, making them suitable for participants at all fitness levels as well as a great option for performing HIIT.

Racquet Sports

In racquet sports such as tennis, racquetball, squash, and badminton, the aerobic benefits are dictated by players' skill, the intensity of the game, and how long a given game lasts. Skill is necessary to participate effectively in these sports and also is crucial to sustain continuous play. Frequent pauses during play do not allow people to maintain the heart rate in the appropriate target zone to stimulate cardiorespiratory development.

Many people who participate in racquet sports do so for enjoyment, social fulfillment, and relaxation. For cardiorespiratory fitness development, these people supplement the sport with other forms of aerobic exercise such as jogging, cycling, or swimming.

9.4 Sport-Specific Conditioning

A person wishing to improve in a specific sport will need not only a sound fitness base, but also to train with movements that closely match the demands of the chosen sport. The principle of specificity of training applies to skill-related components just as it does to health-related fitness components. The development of agility, balance, coordination, and reaction time is highly task specific. That is, to develop a certain task or skill, the individual must practice that same task many times. There seems to be very little crossover learning effect.

For instance, properly practicing a handstand (balance) eventually leads to successfully performing the skill, but complete mastery of this skill does not ensure that the person will have immediate success when attempting to perform other static-balance positions in gymnastics. In contrast, power and speed may improve with a specific strength-training program, frequent repetition of the specific task to be improved, or both.

Critical Thinking

Sports participation is a good predictor of adherence to exercise later in life. What previous experiences have you had with participation in sports? Were these experiences positive? What effect do they have on your current physical activity patterns?

Fitness Activities and Trends

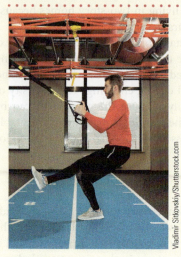

Vladimir Sirkovskiy/Shutterstock.com

Core Training

The "core" of the body consists of the muscles that stabilize the trunk (spine) and pelvis. Core training emphasizes conditioning of all the muscles around the abdomen, pelvis, lower back, and hips, usually by engaging as many muscles as possible during each exercise. These muscles enhance body stability, activities of daily living, and sport performance and support the lower back. Because core exercises have been successful at improving overall fitness and one's ability to meet the demands of daily living, they have remained popular. When the plank core exercise became popular, for example, abdominal crunches fell out of favor. Crunches isolate a limited number of trunk muscles instead of engaging all core muscles, and crunches mimic an action of bending forward that is typically risky for back health, whereas the plank conditions the core for proper stabilization. Core conditioning often incorporates the use of stability balls, foam rollers, and wobble boards, among other pieces of equipment. Further information on core strength training is provided in Chapter 7 (page 277).

Suspension Training

Suspension training, or TRX® training, uses a system of hanging straps or webs that allow participants to juxtapose their body-weight while completing exercises. Exercisers hold the handles of the straps with their feet on the ground or put their feet through the handles with their hands on the ground and adjust the angle of their body position to increase or decrease resistance. Suspension training allows participants to complete traditional strength training exercises like bicep curls, chest presses, and triceps extensions while exercising their full core at the same time.

Pilates Exercise System

The Pilates training system was originally developed in the 1920s by German physical therapist Joseph Pilates. He designed the exercises to help strengthen the body's core by developing pelvic stability and abdominal control, coupled with focused breathing patterns. Previously, Pilates training was used primarily by dancers, but now this exercise modality is embraced by a large number of fitness participants and rehab patients.

Pilates exercises are performed either on a mat (floor) or with specialized equipment to help increase strength and flexibility of deep postural muscles. The intent is to improve muscle tone and length (a limber body), instead of increasing muscle size (hypertrophy). Pilates mat classes focus on body stability and proper body mechanics. The exercises are performed in a slow, controlled,

precise manner. When performed properly, these exercises require intense concentration. Initially, Pilates training should be conducted under the supervision of certified instructors with extensive Pilates teaching experience.

Group Personal Training

Personal trainers are increasingly working with small groups of two to three exercisers to continue providing individualized instruction while keeping costs reasonable. Participants appreciate the accountability they have to the trainer and the group, as well as the sense of belonging that comes from small-group settings. A trainer who understands and can make the most of a group dynamic can also enhance the experience. New technology like web-based workout programs and wearable monitors are growing in popularity and are likely to assist personal trainers in their task of supporting exercisers through a lifestyle change.

Fitness Boot Camp

Fitness boot camp is a vigorous-intensity outdoor/indoor group exercise program that combines traditional calisthenics, running, interval training, bodyweight training (using exercises such as push-ups, lunges, pull-ups, burpees, and squats), plyometrics (see Chapter 7, pages 275–276), and competitive games to develop cardiorespiratory fitness, muscular fitness, and muscular flexibility and lose body fat. This program is based on military-style training and also aims at developing camaraderie and team effort. The program (camp) typically lasts 4 to 8 weeks. Fitness boot camps are challenging, but the group dynamic helps to motivate participants.

Bodyweight Training

Bodyweight training has been around as a strength-training modality for centuries, but fitness enthusiasts are now embracing the concept as they seek to "return to basics." Bodyweight training participants use their own body weight as resistance to develop fitness. Bodyweight exercises are ideal for individuals interested in fitness who do not have access to equipment or facilities. Because bodyweight provides the only source of resistance, a training session can be conducted anywhere. Exercise examples include pull-ups, push-ups, modified dips, curl-ups, step-ups, prone and lateral planks, and pelvic tilts. Some of these exercises are provided in the "Strength-Training Exercises without Weights" section on pages 285–289. As discussed next under "Circuit Training," bodyweight training can be used to develop both cardiorespiratory endurance and muscular fitness.

Circuit Training

Circuit training has also been around for decades. It was often used to condition elite athletes and military personnel in the middle of the 20th century. Circuit training involves a combination of 6 to 12 aerobic and bodyweight-training (strength) exercises performed in rapid sequence one after the other, with very limited rest between exercise stations. Each exercise is performed for a given period of

(continued)

time (10 to 30 seconds) or a specified number of repetitions (10 to 20 repetitions), typically interspaced by short rest periods of 10 to 30 seconds between exercises. Early on, you may use a moderate intensity level (less time or repetitions per exercise) and allow longer rest (30 seconds) between exercises. Over the course of several weeks, you can gradually increase the intensity (time and/or repetitions) and decrease the rest interval between exercises. The exercise sequence is set in an order that allows for opposing muscle groups to alternate between exercise stations. For instance, push-ups can be followed by step-ups and abdominal crunches. The circuit training format can make use of strength-training equipment but also lends itself well to the bodyweight training approach where the person's own body weight provides the resistance rather than using free weights or resistance training machines. Bodyweight circuit training is an effective and low-cost way to begin and maintain a fitness regime. For best results, all major muscle groups of the body should be used in each circuit.

Because of the high intensity and limited rest intervals used with this type of training, the exercise modality is often referred to as high-intensity circuit training, or HICT.[a] The combination of high-intensity aerobic and bodyweight strength-training, with limited rest between exercises, can elicit similar or greater health and fitness benefits in a much shorter period of time than the traditional 20- to 60-minute sessions. A HICT session involving 12 different exercises can be performed in less than 10 minutes per circuit. One to three circuits with 2 to 3 minutes' rest between circuits can be performed per training session. When time is of the essence and a traditional training session is not realistic, a HICT session is recommended.

Cross-Fit

CrossFit® is so named because it aims to take the concept of cross-training to its ultimate level by using constant variation in exercise to develop overall fitness. Participants use weights, bodyweight, and functional equipment like heavy rope or kettlebells to complete a set of daily exercises. The workout is completed at high intensity in an atmosphere that is competitive and includes peer support.

Skill and proper technique are required to perform many of the strength-training exercises, powerlifts, and gymnastics movements. Complex movements that require an all-out/high-level force production to exhaustion can result in poor form that leads to injuries. Attempting to maintain full intensity for arbitrary periods of time in a competitive environment can also lead people to ignore signals from their body, resulting in overtraining. Extreme conditioning programs may sometimes disregard proper recovery intervals between exercises.

Beginners are cautioned to start slowly, learn correct exercise techniques, and gradually progress into the high-intensity workouts. Stretching exercises in addition to those conducted during CrossFit training are encouraged to further develop flexibility fitness. Exercisers who are considering CrossFit are encouraged to investigate a few gyms to find a program that best fits their needs. Gyms will vary in their competitive atmosphere, in whether they approach CrossFit as a way of life or simply as a workout, and in whether they adjust the CrossFit modality to include traditional exercise concepts like completing exercises in repeated sets.

Functional Fitness

Functional fitness involves primarily weight-bearing exercises to develop balance, coordination, good posture, muscular fitness, and muscular flexibility to enhance a person's ability to perform activities of daily living (walking, climbing stairs, lifting, bending) with ease and with minimal risk for injuries. With its roots in physical therapy, functional fitness seeks to correct misalignment, use muscles that specialize in stability, and improve cooperation between physical and neural input and responses. The program's goal is to "train people for real life," rather than a specific fitness component or a given event. Functional fitness training often requires use of fitness equipment such as stability balls, foam blocks, and balancing cushions. Fitness trainers plan classes to target specific everyday activities, even focusing movement around a theme. One class, for example, targeted all the movements used for an evening out to the theater—from side stepping down the aisle to sitting in and rising from the seat to climbing stairs for balcony seating.

Spinning

Spinning is a low-impact aerobic activity performed on specially designed Spinner stationary bicycles in a room or studio with motivational music and under the direction of a certified instructor. Spinning bikes feature racing handlebars, pedals with clips, adjustable seats, and a resistance knob to control workout intensity. Five workout stages, also known as "energy zones," are used to simulate actual cycling training and racing. The workouts are divided into endurance, all-terrain, strength, recovery, and advanced training. New approaches to spinning continue to develop, with cross-discipline classes like spin and swim. New companies are providing online social media support by allowing exercisers to challenge one another to virtual races and to see who is signing up for classes at their gym. Whatever the format, spinning provides a challenging workout for people of all ages and fitness levels.

Yoga

Yoga consists of a system of exercises designed to help align the musculoskeletal system and develop flexibility, muscular fitness, and balance. Yoga is also used as a relaxation technique for stress management. The exercises involve a combination of postures (known as "asanas") along with diaphragmatic breathing, relaxation, and meditation techniques. Classes and instructors vary widely in how much they focus on asanas and proper physical technique versus meditation and philosophy that teaches self-awareness and actualization. Yoga continues to reinvent itself through both new and traditional forms that pop up in studios and gyms across the country. Variations of yoga include anuara, ashtanga, bikram, integral, iyengar, kripalu, kundalini, sivananda, and vinyasa, as well as cross-discipline options like yogalates and yogarobics.

Dance Fitness

Gym-goers are embracing a range of dance-inspired group classes that hone in on different fitness goals. A sustained and upbeat cardio workout is the common feature in Zumba classes, which incorporate Latin

(continued)

and international music (cumbia, salsa, merengue, reggaeton, tango, and rock and roll, among others) with dance to develop fitness and make exercise fun. More recently gaining popularity are barre workouts, based on ballet-inspired movements that offer progressions through flexibility exercises to isometric postures and strength exercises. Barre classes also include exercises not based on traditional dance but that

makes use of the waist-height barre by having participants hold on and juxtapose their bodyweight for strength exercises. Other classes are taking their cues from popular hip-hop dance trends, tribal dance, and India-inspired routines.

[a] B. Klika and C. Jordan, "High-Intensity Circuit Training Using Body Weight: Maximum Results with Minimal Investment," *ACSM's Health & Fitness Journal* 17, no. 3 (2013): 8–13.

Improving Form with an Instructor, Trainer, or an App

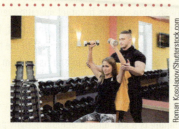

Practicing correct form during exercise is critical to avoiding injury and improving performance, but for the casual exerciser, it often becomes a last priority. It is important to look for opportunities to receive feedback about your form. Try to take advantage of any offer by your gym for time with a personal trainer. Many gyms offer a free hour with initial membership. If you are a runner, you may ask for a trainer who will watch you run on the treadmill and offer suggestions. If you attend a group workout class, consider introducing yourself to the teacher before class and mentioning that you appreciate suggestions for improving form. You may consider a digital solution as well. Apps are available that allow you to film a part of your workout (like a squat) or sport skill (like a tennis serve) and play it back side-by-side with a video of a person practicing correct form. While an app will never be as effective as a live coach, it may help you become more aware and mindful of your form.

The rate of learning in **skill-related fitness** varies from person to person, mainly because these components seem to be determined to a large extent by genetics. Individuals with good skill-related fitness tend to do better and learn faster when performing a wide variety of skills. Nevertheless, few individuals enjoy complete success in all skill-related components. Furthermore, though skill-related fitness can be enhanced with practice, improvements in reaction time and speed are limited and seem to be related to genetic endowment.

Preparing for Sports Participation

To enhance your participation in sports, keep in mind that in most cases it is better to get fit before playing sports rather than play sports to get fit.[10] A good preseason training program will help make the season more enjoyable and prevent exercise-related injuries.

Properly conditioned individuals can participate safely in sports and enjoy the activities to their fullest with few or no

limitations. Unfortunately, sports injuries are often the result of poor fitness and a lack of sport-specific conditioning. Many injuries occur when fatigue sets in following overexertion by unconditioned individuals.

Base Fitness Conditioning

Preactivity screening that includes a health history (see "PAR-Q and Health History Questionnaire," page 39) and/or a medical evaluation appropriate to your sport selection is recommended. Once cleared for exercise, start by building a base of general athletic fitness that includes the four health-related fitness components: cardiorespiratory fitness, muscular fitness, flexibility, and recommended body composition. The base fitness conditioning program should last a minimum of 6 weeks.

As explained earlier and in Chapter 6, for cardiorespiratory fitness select an activity that you enjoy (such as walking, jogging, cycling, step aerobics, cross-country skiing, or elliptical training), and train three to five times per week at a minimum of 20 minutes of continuous activity per session. Exercise at between 60 percent and 80 percent intensity for adequate conditioning. You should feel as though you are training "somewhat hard" to "hard" at these intensity levels.

Strength (resistance) training helps maintain and increase muscular fitness. Following the guidelines provided in Chapter 7, select 10 to 12 exercises that involve the major muscle groups, and train two or three times per week on nonconsecutive days. Select a resistance (weight) that allows you to do 8 to 12 repetitions to near fatigue (8 to 12 RM [repetition maximum] zone based on your fitness goals—see Chapter 7). That is, the resistance will be heavy enough so that when you perform one set of an exercise, you will not be able to do more than the predetermined number of repetitions at that weight. Begin your program slowly and perform between one and three sets of each exercise. Recommended exercises include the bench press, lat pull-down, leg press, leg curl, triceps extension, arm curl, rowing torso, heel raise, abdominal crunch, and back extension.

Flexibility is important in sports participation to enhance the range of motion in the joints. Using the guidelines from Chapter 8, schedule flexibility training 2 or 3 days per week. Perform each stretching exercise four times, and hold each stretch for 15 to 30 seconds. Examples of stretching exercises include the side body stretch, body rotation, chest stretch, shoulder stretch, sit-and-reach stretch, adductor stretch, quad stretch, heel cord stretch, and knee-to-chest stretch.

Guidelines for Success when Learning a New Sport

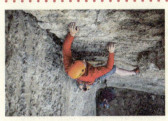

Learn the rules and culture of the sport. Completing a few minutes of online research or having a conversation with a participant can provide helpful information about the sport itself and the culture that surrounds it. It will also give you the chance to become familiar with the sport's terms, equipment needs, and so on.

Exercise to achieve base fitness. If you already exercise regularly, you are in a good position to try a new sport when the opportunity arises.

Begin by getting a general feel for the sport. Try the sport a few times in a noncompetitive environment and allow your body to acclimate to the respective sport movements.

Seek out an instructor who understands form and technique. Even if only for an initial session or two, having personalized feedback or guidance on skill technique will increase success and enjoyment in a new sport. Instructor feedback is a worthwhile invest-ment, allowing you to enjoy and progress as you participate in your new activity.

Begin sport-specific conditioning. Look for ways to make your workout more specific to the demands of your sport. For example, anaerobic conditioning that matches the length of time and power demands of your sport will help the body adapt at the cellular level to generate anaerobic energy under those conditions.

Make time for skill practice. In addition to fitness conditioning and time spent participating in the sport, take the time to repetitively practice the necessary skills. This will allow you to learn the correct form, making good technique automatic during participation. Focus on just one or two skills at a time. Mentally practicing skills has also been shown to improve performance.

Participate in a competitive environment only after 4 to 8 weeks of sport-specific conditioning. The advantage of a competitive environment is that it pushes individuals to work harder to meet the sport and competitive demands than they would otherwise. This benefit, however, becomes a disadvantage for underconditioned participants and can set the stage for overuse injuries.

In terms of body composition, excess body fat hinders sports performance and increases the risk for injuries. Depending on the nature of the activity, fitness goals for body composition range from 12 percent to 20 percent body fat for men and 17 percent to 25 percent for most women.

Sport-Specific Conditioning

Once you have achieved the general fitness base, continue with the program but make adjustments to add sport-specific training. This training should match the sport's requirements for aerobic/anaerobic capabilities, muscular strength and/or endurance, and range of motion.

During the sport-specific training, about half of your aerobic/anaerobic training should involve the same muscles used during your sport. Ideally, allocate 4 weeks of sport-specific training before you start participating in the sport. Then continue the sport-specific training on a more limited basis throughout the season. Depending on the nature of the sport (aerobic versus anaerobic), once the season starts, sports participation itself can take the place of some or all of your aerobic workouts.

The next step is to look at the demands of the sport. For example, soccer, bicycle racing, cross-country skiing, and snowshoeing are aerobic activities, whereas basketball, racquetball, alpine skiing, snowboarding, and ice hockey are stop-and-go sports that require a combination of aerobic and anaerobic activity. Consequently, aerobic training may be appropriate for cross-country skiing, but it will do little to prepare your muscles for the high-intensity requirements of combined aerobic and anaerobic sports.

High-intensity interval training, performed twice per week, is added to the program at this time. For aerobic sports, HIIT at least once per week improves performance. Though HIIT is most commonly done at a 1:2 or lower work-to-recovery ratio, you also can do a 5- to 10-minute aerobic work interval followed by 1 to 2 minutes of recovery, but the intensity of these longer intervals should not be as high, and only three to five intervals are recommended. For anaerobic sports, HIIT up to three times per week is recommended. Note that the HIIT workouts are not performed in addition to the regular aerobic workouts but, instead, take the place of one of these workouts.

Consider sport-specific strength requirements as well. Look at the primary muscles used in your sport, and make sure your choice of exercises works those muscles. Try to perform your strength training through a range of motion similar to that used in your sport. Aerobic/anaerobic sports require greater strength; during the season, the recommendation is three sets of 8 to 12 repetitions to near fatigue, two or three times per week. For aerobic endurance sports, the recommendation is a minimum of one set of 8 to 12 repetitions to near fatigue, once or twice per week during the season.

Stop-and-go sports (basketball, racquetball, and soccer) require greater strength than pure endurance sports (triathlon, long-distance running, and cross-country skiing). For example, recreational participants during the sport-specific

---

GLOSSARY

Skill-related fitness Fitness components important for success in skillful activities and athletic events; encompasses agility, balance, coordination, power, reaction time, and speed.

Natural High During Exercise

Do people get a physical high during aerobic exercise? Exercisers often report feeling like they are "running on a cloud" during and following a challenging endurance workout. This feeling is often referred to as a runner's high and has been the subject of scientific study and debate. As our understanding of the phenomenon emerges, researchers are attributing the euphoria to two different biological reactions.

During vigorous exercise, **endorphins** are released from the pituitary gland in the brain as a response to physical discomfort. Endorphins can create feelings of euphoria and natural well-being. Higher levels of endorphins often result from aerobic endurance activities and may remain elevated for as long as 30 to 60 minutes after exercise.

Endorphin levels also have been shown to increase during pregnancy and childbirth. Endorphins act as painkillers. The higher levels could explain a woman's greater tolerance for the pain and discomfort of natural childbirth and her pleasant feelings shortly after the baby's birth. Several reports have indicated that well-conditioned women have

shorter and easier labor. These women may attain higher endorphin levels during delivery, making childbirth less traumatic than it is for untrained women.

As a response to prolonged stress, the brain also releases endocannabinoids (a natural biological version of marijuana, including a dose that is similar). While endorphins are created only by specialized neurons, endocannabinoids can be created by any body cell, and are believed to induce a feeling of calmness.

Though a runner's high is a common experience for some and elusive to others, researchers agree on the kind of effort most likely to produce the effect: a workout that is challenging (but not painful) and lasts between 30 minutes and 2 hours, depending on the individual's personal physiological makeup.

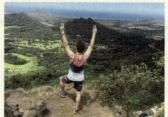
© Fitness & Wellness, Inc.

---

training phase for stop-and-go sports perform three sets of 8 to 12 repetitions to near fatigue, two to three times per week. Competitive athletes and those desiring greater strength gains typically conduct three to five sets of 4 to 12 repetitions to near fatigue three times per week.

For some winter sports, such as alpine skiing and snowboarding, gravity supplies most of the propulsion, and the body acts more as a shock absorber. Muscles in the hips, knees, and trunk are used to control the forces on the body and equipment. Multi-joint exercises, such as the leg press, squats, and lunges, are suggested for these activities.

Before the season starts, make sure that your equipment is in proper working condition. For example, alpine skiers' bindings should be cleaned and adjusted properly so that they will release as needed. This is one of the most important things you can do to help prevent knee injuries. A good pair of bindings is cheaper than knee surgery.

The first few times you participate in the sport of your choice, go easy, practice technique, and do not continue once you are fatigued. Gradually increase the length and intensity of your workouts. Consider taking a lesson to have someone watch your technique and help correct flaws early in the season. Even Olympic athletes have coaches watching them. Proper conditioning allows for a more enjoyable and healthier season.

Training for Distance

Muscles adapt with specific responses to training sessions of extended length. For this reason, athletes who are interested in distance events should include several training sessions when distance is extended beyond race length, but pace is slightly decreased. For example, runners training competitively for a 5K can complete several 7-mile training runs at slower than racing pace. Marathoners (a distance of 26.2 miles) are an

exception, as a 20-mile run appears to be an adequate training distance for necessary adaptations to take place.

Sport-Specific Flexibility Training

Flexibility is key to sports performance and injury prevention and is, therefore, part of any complete sport-conditioning program. Athletes may combine static, dynamic, proprioceptive neuromuscular facilitation (PNF), and controlled ballistic stretches through the range of motion needed for a sport. A baseball player or golfer may proceed back and forth rhythmically through a swing, for example; or a soccer player through a kick.

9.5 General Exercise Considerations

Exercise can and should be enjoyed in a variety of climates and situations, but there are some basic precautions you should know to keep yourself healthy and safe. The following guidelines will help you judge wisely.

Time of Day for Exercise

What time of the day is best for exercise? You can do intense exercise almost any time of the day, with the exception of about 2 hours following a heavy meal or the midday and early afternoon hours on hot, humid days. Moderate exercise seems to be beneficial shortly after a meal because exercise enhances the **thermogenic response**. A walk shortly after a meal burns more calories than a walk several hours after a meal.

Many people enjoy exercising early in the morning because it gives them a boost to start the day. People who exercise in the morning also seem to stick with it more than others because the chances of putting off the exercise session for other reasons are minimized. Some prefer the lunch hour for weight-control reasons. By exercising at noon, they do not eat as big a lunch, which helps keep down the daily caloric intake. Highly stressed people seem to like the evening hours because of the relaxing effects of exercise.

Exercise in Heat and Humidity

Exercising in hot and humid conditions is unsafe. When a person exercises, only 20 to 30 percent of the energy the body produces is used for mechanical work or movement. The rest of the energy (60 to 70 percent) is converted into heat. If this heat cannot be dissipated properly because the weather is too hot or the relative humidity is too high, body temperature increases, and in extreme cases, it can result in death.

The specific heat of body tissue (the heat required to raise the temperature of the body by 1°C) is .38 calorie per pound of body weight (.38 cal/lb). This indicates that if no body heat is dissipated, a 150-pound person has to burn only 57 calories (150 × .38) to increase total body temperature by 1°C. If this person were to conduct an exercise session requiring 300 calories (e.g., running about 3 miles) without any dissipation of heat, the inner body temperature would increase by 5.3°C (300 ÷ 57), which is the equivalent of going from 98.6°F to 108.1°F

This example illustrates clearly the need for caution when exercising in hot or humid weather. If the relative humidity is too high, body heat cannot be lost through evaporation because the atmosphere already is saturated with water vapor. In one instance, a football casualty occurred when the temperature was only 64°F, but the relative humidity was 100 percent. People must be cautious when air temperature is greater than 90°F and the relative humidity is greater than 60 percent.

The American College of Sports Medicine (ACSM) recommends avoiding strenuous physical activity when the readings of a wet-bulb globe thermometer exceed 82.4°F. With this type of thermometer, the wet bulb is cooled by evaporation, and on dry days it shows a lower temperature than the regular (dry) thermometer. On humid days, the cooling effect is less because of less evaporation; hence, the difference between the wet and dry readings is not as great.

When exercising in the heat, avoid the hottest time of the day, between 11:00 a.m. and 5:00 p.m. Surfaces such as asphalt, concrete, and artificial turf absorb heat, which then radiates to the body. Therefore, these surfaces are not recommended.

Following are descriptions of, and first-aid measures for, the three major signs of heat illness, heat cramps, heat exhaustion, and heat stroke:

- **Heat cramps.** Symptoms include cramps; spasms; and muscle twitching in the legs, arms, and abdomen. To relieve heat cramps, stop exercising, get out of the heat, massage the painful area, stretch slowly, and drink plenty of fluids (water, fruit drinks, or electrolyte beverages).
- **Heat exhaustion.** Symptoms include fainting, dizziness, profuse sweating, cold and clammy skin, weakness, headache, and a rapid, weak pulse. If you incur any of these symptoms, stop and find a cool place to rest. If conscious, drink cool water. Do not give water to an unconscious person. Loosen or remove clothing and rub your body with a cool, wet towel or apply ice packs. Place yourself in a supine position with the legs elevated 8 to 12 inches. If you are not fully recovered in 30 minutes, seek immediate medical attention.
- **Heat stroke.** Symptoms include serious disorientation; warm, dry skin; no sweating; rapid, full pulse; vomiting; diarrhea; unconsciousness; and high body temperature. As the body temperature climbs, unexplained anxiety sets in. When the body temperature reaches 104°F to 105°F, the individual may feel a cold sensation in the trunk of the body, goose bumps, nausea, throbbing in the temples, and numbness in the extremities. Most people become incoherent after this stage.

When body temperature reaches 105°F to 107°F, disorientation, loss of fine-motor control, and muscular

---

Symptoms of Heat Illness

If any of these symptoms occur, stop physical activity, get out of the sun, and start drinking fluids.
- Decreased perspiration
- Cramping
- Weakness
- Flushed skin
- Throbbing head
- Nausea/vomiting
- Diarrhea
- Numbness in the extremities
- Blurred vision
- Unsteadiness
- Disorientation
- Incoherency

GLOSSARY

Endorphins Morphinelike substances released from the pituitary gland (in the brain) during prolonged aerobic exercise and thought to induce feelings of euphoria and natural well-being.

Thermogenic response The amount of energy required to digest food.

Heat cramps Muscle spasms caused by heat-induced changes in electrolyte balance in muscle cells.

Heat exhaustion Heat-related fatigue.

Heat stroke An emergency situation resulting from the body being subjected to high atmospheric temperatures.

Choosing Exercise Clothing

Wearing the right type of clothing facilitates your workout rather than hinders it. In general, clothing should fit comfortably and allow free movement of the various body parts. Select clothing according to air temperature, humidity, and exercise intensity.

Avoid nylon and rubberized materials and tight clothes that interfere with the cooling mechanism of the human body or obstruct normal blood flow. Cotton is not an ideal choice either. While it may feel comfortable at the beginning of your workout, 100 percent cotton will absorb and hold moisture throughout your workout (think of the weight of a pair of wet jeans). A cotton-synthetic blend will perform better. Ideally, choose fabrics made of Capilene, Thermax, or any synthetic that draws (wicks) moisture away from the skin. The fibers of these synthetic fabrics, like plastic, are nonabsorbent. The moisture moves along the fibers to disperse and evaporate, enhancing cooling of the body. Polypropylene is another moisture wicking synthetic, but it requires special care to remove odors. Be sure to consider exercise intensity because the harder a person exercises, the more heat the body produces.

Only a minimal amount of clothing is necessary during exercise in the heat to allow for maximal evaporation. Clothing should be lightweight, light-colored, loose-fitting, airy, and absorbent. Examples of commercially available products that can be used during exercise in the heat are CoolMax and Nike's Dri-FIT. (For other important precautions see "Exercise in Heat and Humidity" on page 357 and "Exercise in Cold Weather" below.)

When it comes to caring for your exercise wardrobe, a few tips will help extend the life of your clothing. If you are not going to wash workout clothes immediately, allow them to air out before you throw them in the hamper. To remove any odor-causing bacteria, presoak clothing in water and white vinegar

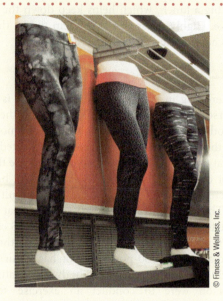

© Fitness & Wellness, Inc.

or in a detergent that contains enzymes. Also, following washing, opt to hang dry workout clothing or lie them flat to dry, as the clothes dryer can reduce elasticity and functionality of activewear over time.

---

weakness set in. If the temperature exceeds 106°F, serious neurological injury and death may be imminent.

Heat stroke requires immediate emergency medical attention. Request help and get out of the sun and into a cool, humidity-controlled environment. While you are waiting to be taken to the hospital emergency room, you should be placed in a semi-seated position, and your body should be sprayed with cool water and rubbed with cool towels. If possible, cold packs should be placed in areas that receive an abundant blood supply, such as the head, neck, armpits, and groin. Fluids should not be given if you are unconscious. In any case of heat-related illness, if the person refuses water, vomits, or starts to lose consciousness, an ambulance should be summoned immediately. Proper initial treatment of heat stroke is vital.

Exercise in Cold Weather

When exercising in the cold, the two factors to consider are frostbite and **hypothermia**. In contrast to hot and humid conditions, cold weather usually does not threaten health because clothing can be selected for heat conservation, and exercise itself increases the production of body heat.

Initial warning signs of hypothermia include shivering, losing coordination, and having difficulty speaking. With a continued drop in body temperature, shivering stops, the muscles weaken and stiffen, and the person feels elated or

intoxicated and eventually loses consciousness. To prevent hypothermia, use common sense, dress properly, and be aware of environmental conditions.

The popular belief that exercising in cold temperatures (32°F and lower) freezes the lungs is false because the air is warmed properly in the air passages before it reaches the lungs. Cold is not what poses a threat; wind velocity is what increases the chill factor most.

For example, exercising at a temperature of 25°F with adequate clothing is not too cold, but if the wind is blowing at 25 miles per hour, the chill factor makes it feel like the temperature is 15°F. The rate of heat loss depends on the action of the wind on the body's surface. There is an insulating layer of warm air on the body's skin. Moving air disrupts this warm layer and allows cooler air to replace the warm air on the body's surface. The faster the wind speed, the quicker the surface cools. This effect is even worse if a person is wet and exhausted. When the weather is windy, the individual should exercise (jog or cycle) against the wind on the way out and with the wind upon returning.

Most people actually overdress for exercise in the cold. Because exercise increases body temperature, a moderate

---

GLOSSARY

Hypothermia A breakdown in the body's ability to generate heat; a drop in body temperature below 95°F.

Choosing Footwear

For decades, a good pair of shoes has been recommended by most professionals to prevent injuries to lower limbs. Shoes manufactured specifically for the choice of activity have been encouraged. Shoes should have good stability, motion control, and comfortable fit. A comfortable fit will generally do more to prevent injury than any particular new shoe technology or feature.[a] Purchase shoes in the middle of or later in the day when feet have expanded and might be one half size larger. For increased breathability, shoes with nylon or mesh uppers are recommended. Salespeople at reputable athletic shoe stores can help you select a good shoe that fits your needs.

A good pair of shoes is a must for joggers. Many foot, knee, and leg problems originate from improperly fitting or worn-out shoes. Because each runner has his or her own anatomical structure and running biomechanics, there is no ideal shoe that will fit every person. Some general guidelines, nonetheless, apply.

A good pair of shoes should offer good lateral stability and not lean to either side when placed on a flat surface. The shoe also

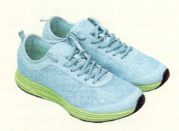

bdstudio/Shutterstock.com

should bend at the ball of the foot, not at midfoot. Worn-out shoes should be replaced. After 500 miles of use, jogging shoes lose about a third of their shock absorption capabilities. If you suddenly have problems, check your shoes first. It may be time for a new pair.

When it comes to choosing socks, the same rationale should be used as is used for choosing exercise clothing. Cotton is not ideal. Double-layer acrylic socks are preferable and help prevent blistering and chafing of the feet.

[a]B.M. Nigg, J. Baltich, S. Hoerzer, and H. Enders, "Running Shoes and Running Injuries: Mythbusting and a Proposal for Two New Paradigms: 'Preferred Movement Path' and 'Comfort Filter,'" *British Journal of Sports Medicine,* published online July 28, 2015, available at http:// bjsm.bmj.com/content/early/2015/07/28/bjsports-2015-095054 .abstract.

Shoeless Running

For most of human history, people ran either barefoot or with minimal shoes. As in walking, the modern running shoe with its bulky padded heel cushion allows runners to land on the heel and roll forward toward the ball of the foot. The impact-collision force while running is often more than three times the person's body weight. Researchers have observed that joggers and runners who don't wear shoes, or who use minimal footwear, land on the front (ball) or middle of the foot. This motion induces them to flex the ankle as contact is made with the ground, resulting in smaller impact forces than ankle-strike runners. Such running mechanics are thought by some to decrease impact-related repetitive stress injuries.

Some experts believe that both the spring in the arch of the foot and the Achilles tendon diminish ground-impact forces. A good illustration is to compare the impact forces generated by landing a jump on the heels versus on the toes.

Shoeless-running proponents believe that wearing cushioned shoes with arch supports alters natural foot-landing actions, weakening muscles and ligaments and rendering feet, ankles, and knees more susceptible to injuries. They recommend wearing a flexible shoe without a heel cushion or arch support. This recommendation has led to the development of barefoot running "shoes." These shoes feature a thin, abrasion-resistant stretch nylon with breathable mesh upper material that wraps around the entire foot to keep rocks and dirt out. At present, the verdict is still out. Data are insufficient to support

either recommendation (shod versus shoeless running). Research is being conducted to determine the best type of footwear to use with repetitive-impact activities.

On the opposite side of the spectrum, many major shoe manufacturers have re-

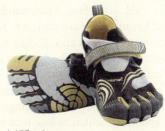

davidf/Getty Images

sponded by creating maximalist running shoes in an effort to mimic the shock-absorbing effect of running on soft surfaces. These shoes may help minimize the impact of some conditions (like previous stress fractures or plantar fasciitis) while aggravating others (such as back, hip, or knee pain). Debate has begun as to whether maximalist shoes now encourage a more careless running stride. If this type of shoe appeals to you, visit a reputable running shoe store and speak with an experienced salesperson.

Any time you transition to a running shoe that is notably different from what you have been wearing, make the transition slowly. Start with shorter runs or complete just a part of your workout in the new shoes. If you decide to give shoeless running a try, allow a minimum of 10 weeks to build back up to your current mileage in the new footwear, with time for recovery and stretching between runs. Otherwise, you may end up with a challenging or severe injury (including foot fractures).

workout on a cold day makes a person feel that the temperature is 20 to 30 degrees warmer than it actually is. Overdressing for exercise can make the clothes damp from excessive perspiration. The risk for hypothermia increases when a person is wet or after exercise stops, when the person is not moving around sufficiently to increase (or maintain) body heat. The focus when dressing for cold weather exercise is to stay warm and dry. Dressing in layers will allow you to shed layers when you begin to get warm and will help you keep moisture from sweat to a minimum.

It is preferable to wear several layers of lightweight clothing instead of one single, thick layer because warm air is trapped between layers of clothes, enabling greater heat conservation when needed. As body temperature increases, remove layers as necessary.

The first layer of clothes should wick moisture away from the skin. Capilene, Thermax, and polypropylene are recommended materials. Avoid cotton next to the skin because once cotton gets wet—whether from perspiration, rain, or snow—it loses its insulating properties. Next, a layer of wool, Dacron, or polyester fleece insulates well even when wet. Lycra tights or sweatpants help protect the legs. The outer layer should be waterproof, wind resistant, and breathable. A synthetic material such as Gore-Tex is best so moisture can still escape from the body. A ski mask or face mask helps protect the face. In extremely cold conditions, exposed skin, such as the nose, cheeks, and around the eyes, can be insulated with petroleum jelly.

Even though the lungs are under no risk when you exercise in the cold, your face, head, hands, and feet should be protected because they are subject to frostbite. Watch for signs of frostbite: numbness and discoloration. In cold temperatures, as much as half of the body's heat can be lost through an unprotected head and neck. A wool or synthetic cap, hood, or hat will help to hold in body heat. Mittens are better than gloves because they keep the fingers together so that the surface area from which to lose heat is less.

For lengthy or long-distance workouts (cross-country skiing or long runs), take a small backpack to carry the clothing you remove. You also can carry extra warm and dry clothes in case you stop exercising away from shelter. If you remain outdoors following exercise, added clothing and continuous body movement are essential to maintain body temperature and avoid hypothermia.

Exercising with the Cold or Flu

When trying to decide whether to exercise when you have a cold or the flu, the most important consideration is to use common sense and pay attention to your symptoms. Usually, you may continue to exercise if your symptoms include a runny nose, sneezing, or a scratchy throat. But, if your symptoms include fever, muscle ache, vomiting, diarrhea, or a hacking cough, you should avoid exercise. After an illness, be sure to ease back gradually into your program. Do not attempt to return at the same intensity and duration that you were used to prior to your illness.

9.6 Nutrition and Hydration during Exercise

Proper nutrition and hydration practices are a critical part of any training program. Disregarding them will slow down fitness improvements and speed the onset of overtraining. Furthermore, properly observing good nutrition and hydration will help keep you safe and allow your body to make the most of recovery time.

Fluid Replacement during Exercise

Especially for prolonged aerobic exercise, make sure you are well hydrated before you begin. Exercise performance is impaired when an individual is dehydrated by as little as 2 percent of body weight. Dehydration at 5 percent of body weight decreases performance by about 30 percent.

Thirst is not an adequate indicator of hydration because feelings of thirst indicate that dehydration has already begun. In preparation for prolonged exercise, the recommendation is to drink plenty of fluids the day before the activity, 16 to 20 ounces about 4 hours prior to exercise, and another 8 to 12 ounces 15 minutes before the start of the activity.

The main objective of fluid replacement during prolonged aerobic exercise is to maintain the blood volume so circulation and sweating can continue at normal levels. Adequate water replacement is the most important factor in preventing heat disorders. Drinking about 6 to 8 ounces of cool water every 15 to 20 minutes during exercise is recommended to prevent dehydration. Cold fluids seem to be absorbed more rapidly from the stomach.

Other relevant points follow:

- Drinking commercially prepared sports drinks is recommended when exercise will be strenuous and carried out for more than an hour. For exercise lasting less than an hour, water is just as effective in replacing lost fluid. The sports drinks you select may be based on your personal preference. Try different drinks at 6 to 8 percent glucose concentration to see which drink you tolerate best and which suits your tastes as well.
- Commercial fluid-replacement solutions (such as Powerade® and Gatorade®) contain about 6 to 8 percent glucose, which seems to be optimal for fluid absorption and performance. Sugar does not become available to the muscles until about 30 minutes after consumption of a glucose solution.
- Drinks high in fructose or with a glucose concentration greater than 8 percent are not recommended because they slow water absorption during exercise in the heat.
- Most sodas (both cola and noncola) contain between 10 and 12 percent glucose, which is too high for proper rehydration during exercise in the heat.
- Do not overhydrate with just water during a very- or ultra-long-distance event, as such can lead to

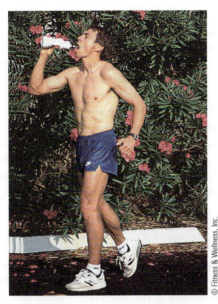

Fluid and carbohydrate replacement are essential when exercising in the heat or for a prolonged period.

hyponatremia (see also "Hyponatremia" in Chapter 3, pages 128–129), or low sodium concentration in the blood. When water loss through sweat during prolonged exercise is replaced by water alone, blood sodium is diluted to the point where it creates serious health problems, including seizures and coma in severe cases.

Meal Timing during Exercise

After a full meal, it is generally advised to wait before exercising. The length of time to wait depends on the amount of food eaten. On the average, after a regular meal, you should wait about 2 hours before participating in strenuous physical activity. But a walk or some other light physical activity is fine following a meal because it helps burn extra calories and stabilize blood sugar and may help the body metabolize fats more efficiently.

When it comes to a pre-workout snack, however, research indicates that eating some food, liquid or solid, prior to physical activity provides energy and nutrients that improve endurance and exercise performance. Of course, how long before exercise, how much food, and what type of food you eat depends on the intensity of exercise and your stomach's tolerance to pre-exercise food. The primary fuel for exercise is provided by carbohydrates, which the body converts to glucose and stores as glycogen. Some protein, along with carbohydrates, is recommended.

Aim to consume 1 gram of carbohydrate per kilogram of body weight (.5 gram of carbohydrate per pound of body weight) within the hour prior to exercise. Solid foods (e.g., granola bars, energy bars, bagels, sugar wafers, or crackers) or semiliquid solid foods (e.g., yogurt, gelatin, or pudding) are acceptable for light-intensity aerobic exercise or strength training. Even a snack consumed a few minutes before exercise helps, as long as you exercise longer than 30 minutes. Through trial and error, you will learn which sport snacks best suit your stomach without interfering with exercise performance.

For intense workouts, consuming carbohydrates with some protein appears to help optimize development and recovery. A combination of these nutrients is recommended prior to and immediately following high-intensity aerobic or strength-training exercise. A small snack or a protein-containing sports drink 30 to 60 minutes before intense exercise is beneficial. For high-intensity aerobic activities, sports drinks consumed 30 to 60 minutes prior to exercise are best because they are rapidly absorbed by the body. Intense exercise causes microtears in muscle tissue, and the presence of amino acids (the building blocks of proteins) in the blood contributes to the healing process and subsequent development and strengthening of the muscle fibers. Post-exercise protein consumption, along with carbohydrates, also accelerates glycogen replenishment in the body after intense or prolonged exercise. Thus, carbohydrates provide energy for exercise and replenishment of glycogen stores after exercise, while protein optimizes muscle repair, growth, glycogen replenishment, and recovery following exercise. Although muscles absorb a greater amount of amino acids up to 48 hours following intense exercise, consumption of the carbohydrate/protein snack immediately following intense exercise, and an hour thereafter, appears to be most beneficial. Aim for a ratio of 4:1 grams of carbohydrates to protein. For example, you may consume a snack that contains 40 grams of carbohydrates (160 calories) and 10 grams of protein (40 calories). To optimize development, make sure you consume some protein with snacks or meals for the next 48 hours as well. Examples of good recovery foods include milk and cereal, a tuna fish sandwich, a peanut butter and jelly sandwich, and pasta with turkey meat sauce. Commercial sports drinks and snacks with a 4:1 ratio are now also readily available.

> **HOEGER KEY TO WELLNESS**
>
> Following an injury, cold should be applied three to five times a day for 15 minutes at a time during the first 36 to 48 hours.

9.7 Exercise-Related Injuries

Surveys indicate that more than half of all new participants incur injuries during the first 6 months of the conditioning program. To enjoy and maintain physical fitness, preventing injury during a conditioning program is essential.

> **HOEGER KEY TO WELLNESS**
>
> A carbohydrate/protein snack immediately following intense exercise, and an hour thereafter, appears to be most beneficial. Aim for a ratio of 4:1 grams of carbohydrates to protein.

The four most common causes of injuries are:

1. High-impact activities
2. Rapid conditioning programs (doing too much too quickly)
3. Improper shoes or training surfaces
4. Anatomical predisposition (i.e., body propensity)

High-impact activities and a significant increase in quantity (duration) of activities are by far the most common causes of injuries. The body requires time to adapt to more intense activities. Most of these injuries can be prevented through a more gradual and correct conditioning (low-impact) program.

Softer training surfaces, such as artificial turf, grass, or dirt, produce less trauma than wood, asphalt, or concrete.

Because few people have perfect body alignment, injuries associated with overtraining may occur eventually. In case of injury, proper treatment can avert a lengthy recovery process. A summary of common exercise-related injuries and how to manage them follows.

Muscle Soreness and Stiffness

Individuals who begin an exercise program or participate after a long layoff from exercise often develop muscle soreness and stiffness. The acute soreness that sets in in the first few hours after exercise is thought to be related to general fatigue of the exercised muscles.

Delayed muscle soreness that appears several hours after exercise (usually about 12 hours later) and lasts 2 to 4 days may be related to actual microtears in muscle tissue, muscle spasms that increase fluid retention (stimulating the pain nerve endings), and overstretching or tearing of connective tissue in and around muscles and joints.

Mild stretching before and adequate stretching after exercise help to prevent soreness and stiffness. Gradually progressing into an exercise program is important, too. A person should not attempt to do too much too quickly. To relieve pain, mild stretching, light-intensity exercise to stimulate blood flow, and a warm bath are recommended.

Exercise Intolerance

When starting an exercise program, participants should stay within safe limits. The best method to determine whether you are exercising too strenuously is to check your heart rate and make sure that it does not exceed the limits of your target zone. Exercising above this target zone may not be safe for unconditioned or high-risk individuals. You do not have to exercise beyond your target zone to gain the desired cardiorespiratory benefits.

Several physical signs will tell you when you are exceeding your functional limitations—that is, experiencing **exercise intolerance**. Signs of intolerance include rapid or irregular heart rate, difficult breathing, nausea, vomiting, lightheadedness, headache, dizziness, unusually flushed or pale skin, extreme weakness, lack of energy, shakiness, sore muscles, cramps, and tightness in the chest. Take time to listen to your body. If you notice any of these symptoms, seek medical attention before continuing your exercise program.

Recovery heart rate is another indicator of overexertion. To a certain extent, recovery heart rate is related to fitness level. The higher your cardiorespiratory fitness level, the faster your heart rate will decrease following exercise. As a rule, heart rate should be below 120 bpm (beats per minute) 5 minutes into recovery. If your heart rate is above 120, you most likely have overexerted yourself or possibly could have some other cardiac abnormality. If you lower the intensity or the duration of exercise, or both, and you still have a fast heart rate five minutes into recovery, you should consult your physician.

HOEGER KEY TO WELLNESS

The higher your cardiorespiratory fitness level, the faster your heart rate will decrease following exercise. As a rule, heart rate should be below 120 bpm 5 minutes into recovery. If your heart rate is above 120, you most likely have overexerted yourself.

Side Stitch

Side stitch is a cramp-like pain in the ribcage that can develop in the early stages of participation in exercise. It occurs primarily in unconditioned beginners and in trained individuals when they exercise at higher intensities than usual. As one's physical condition improves, this condition tends to disappear unless training is intensified.

The exact cause is unknown. Some experts suggest that it could relate to a lack of blood flow to the respiratory muscles during strenuous physical exertion. Some people encounter side stitch during downhill running. If you experience side stitch during exercise, slow down. If it persists, stop altogether. Lying down on your back and gently bringing both knees to the chest and holding that position for 30 to 60 seconds also helps.

Some people get side stitch if they drink juice or eat anything shortly before exercise. Drinking only water 1 to 2 hours prior to exercise sometimes prevents side stitch. Other individuals have problems with commercially available sports drinks during vigorous-intensity exercise. Unless carbohydrate replacement is crucial to complete a long-distance event (more than 60 minutes, such as road cycling, a marathon, or a triathlon), drink cool water for fluid replacement or try a different carbohydrate solution.

Shin Splints

Shin splints, one of the most common injuries to the lower limbs, usually results from one or more of the following: (a) lack of proper and gradual conditioning, (b) doing physical activities on hard surfaces (wooden floors, hard tracks, cement, or asphalt), (c) fallen arches, (d) chronic overuse, (e) muscle fatigue, (f) faulty posture, (g) improper shoes, or (h) participating in weight-bearing activities when excessively overweight.

To manage shin splints:

1. Remove or reduce the cause (exercise on softer surfaces, wear better shoes or arch supports, or completely stop exercise until the shin splints heal).
2. Do stretching exercises before and after physical activity.
3. Use ice massage for 10 to 20 minutes before and after exercise.
4. Apply active heat (whirlpool and hot baths) for 15 minutes, two to three times a day.
5. Use supportive taping during physical activity (a qualified athletic trainer can teach you the proper taping technique).

Muscle Cramps

Muscle cramps are caused by the body's depletion of essential electrolytes or a breakdown in the coordination between opposing muscle groups. If you have a muscle cramp, you should first attempt to stretch the muscles involved. In the case of the calf muscle, for example, pull your toes up toward the knees. After stretching the muscle, rub it down gently, and, finally, do some mild exercises requiring the use of that muscle.

In pregnant and lactating women, muscle cramps often are related to a lack of calcium. If women get cramps during these times, calcium supplements usually relieve the problem. Tight clothing also can cause cramps by decreasing blood flow to active muscle tissue.

Acute Sports Injuries

The best treatment always has been prevention. If an activity causes unusual discomfort or chronic irritation, you need to treat the cause by decreasing the intensity, switching activities, substituting equipment, or upgrading clothing (such as buying proper-fitting shoes).

In cases of acute injury, the standard treatment is rest, cold application, compression or splinting (or both), and elevation of the affected body part. This is commonly referred to as **RICE:**

R = rest
I = ice (cold) application
C = compression
E = elevation

Cold should be applied three to five times a day for 15 minutes at a time during the first 36 to 48 hours by submerging the injured area in cold water, using an ice bag, or applying ice massage to the affected part. An elastic bandage or wrap can be used for compression. Elevating the body part decreases blood flow (and therefore swelling) in that body part.

The purpose of these treatment modalities is to minimize swelling in the area and thus hasten recovery time. After the first 36 to 48 hours, heat can be used if the injury shows no further swelling or inflammation. If you have doubts as to the nature or seriousness of the injury (such as suspected fracture), you should seek a medical evaluation.

Obvious deformities (exhibited by fractures, dislocations, or partial dislocations, as examples) call for splinting, cold application with an ice bag, and medical attention. Do not try to reset any of these conditions by yourself because you could further damage muscles, ligaments, and nerves. Treatment of these injuries should always be left to specialized medical personnel. A quick reference guide for the signs or symptoms and treatment of exercise-related problems is provided in Table 9.2.

9.8 Tailoring Exercise to Health Circumstances

Creating an exercise program is a highly personalized process. Adjusting exercise to meet specific health needs is simply an extension of the need for personalization. If necessary, a participant should work under the care of a physician to take advantage of the benefits of exercise and physical activity.

Asthma and Exercise

Asthma, a condition that causes difficult breathing, is characterized by coughing, wheezing, and shortness of breath induced by narrowing of the airway passages because of contraction (bronchospasm) of the airway muscles, swelling of the mucous membrane, and excessive secretion of mucus. In a few people, asthma can be triggered by exercise itself, particularly in cool and dry environments. This condition is referred to as exercise-induced asthma (EIA).

People with asthma need to obtain proper medication from a physician prior to initiating an exercise program. A regular program is best because random exercise bouts are more likely to trigger asthma attacks. In the initial stages of exercise, an intermittent program (with frequent rest periods during the exercise session) is recommended. Gradual warm-up and cool-down are essential to reduce the risk of an acute attack. Furthermore, exercising in warm and humid conditions (such as swimming) is better because it helps to moisten the airways and thereby minimizes the asthmatic response. For land-based activities (such as walking and aerobics), drinking water before, during, and after exercise helps to keep the airways moist, decreasing the risk of an attack. During the winter months, wearing an exercise mask is recommended to increase the warmth and humidity of inhaled air. People with asthma should not exercise alone and should always carry their medication with them during workouts.

GLOSSARY

Exercise intolerance The inability to function during exercise because of excessive fatigue or extreme feelings of discomfort.

Side stitch A sharp pain in the side of the abdomen.

Shin splints Injury to the lower leg characterized by pain and irritation in the shin region of the leg.

RICE An acronym used to describe the standard treatment procedure for acute sports injuries: rest, ice (cold application), compression, and elevation.

Table 9.2 Reference Guide for Exercise-Related Problems

Injury	Signs/Symptoms	Treatment*
Bruise (contusion)	Pain, swelling, discoloration	Cold application, compression, rest
Dislocations/fracture	Pain, swelling, deformity	Splinting, cold application, seek medical attention
Heat cramp	Cramps, spasms, and muscle twitching in the legs, arms, and abdomen	Stop activity, get out of the heat, stretch, massage the painful area, drink plenty of fluids
Heat exhaustion	Fainting, profuse sweating, cold/clammy skin, weak/rapid pulse, weakness, headache	Stop activity, rest in a cool place, loosen clothing, rub body with cool/wet towel, drink plenty of fluids, stay out of heat for 2–3 days
Heat stroke	Hot/dry skin, no sweating, serious disorientation, rapid/full pulse, vomiting, diarrhea, unconsciousness, high body temperature	Seek immediate medical attention, request help and get out of the sun, bathe in cold water/spray with cold water/rub body with cold towels, drink plenty of cold fluids
Joint sprains	Pain, tenderness, swelling, loss of use, discoloration	Cold application, compression, elevation, rest; heat after 36–48 hours (if no further swelling)
Muscle cramps	Pain, spasm	Stretch muscle(s), use mild exercises for involved area
Muscle soreness and stiffness	Tenderness, pain	Mild stretching, low-intensity exercise, warm bath
Muscle strains	Pain, tenderness, swelling, loss of use	Cold application, compression, elevation, rest; heat after 36–48 hours (if no further swelling)
Shin splints	Pain, tenderness	Cold application prior to and following any physical activity, rest; heat (if no activity is carried out)
Side stitch	Pain on the side of the abdomen below the rib cage	Decrease level of physical activity or stop altogether, gradually increase level of fitness
Tendonitis	Pain, tenderness, loss of use	Rest, cold application, heat after 48 hours

*Cold should be applied three to five times a day for 15 minutes. Heat can be applied three times a day for 15 to 20 minutes.
© Fitness & Wellness, Inc.

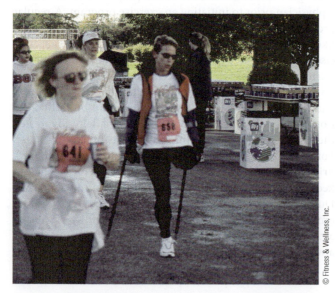

Physically challenged people can participate in and derive health and fitness benefits from a high-intensity exercise program.

Arthritis and Exercise

Individuals who have arthritis should participate in a combined stretching, aerobic, and strength-training program. The participant should do mild stretching prior to aerobic exercise to relax tight muscles. A regular flexibility program following aerobic exercise is encouraged to help maintain good joint mobility. During the aerobic portion of the exercise program, individuals with arthritis should avoid high-impact activities because these may cause greater trauma to arthritic joints. Low-impact activities such as swimming, water aerobics, and cycling are recommended. A complete strength-training program also is recommended, with special emphasis on exercises that will support the arthritic joint(s). As with any other program, individuals with arthritis should start with light-intensity or resistance exercises and build up gradually to a higher fitness level.

Diabetes and Exercise

There are almost 30 million people with diabetes in the United States, with more than 1 million new cases being diagnosed each year. Estimates also indicate that 86 million adult Americans (more than one out of every three) have prediabetes. Type 2 diabetes has been linked to premature mortality and morbidity from cardiovascular disease and to kidney and nerve disease, blindness, and amputation.

There are two types of diabetes: type 1, or insulin-dependent diabetes mellitus (IDDM); and type 2, or non-insulin-dependent diabetes mellitus (NIDDM). In type 1, an autoimmune-related disease found primarily in young people, the pancreas produces little or no insulin. Like everyone else, people with type 1 diabetes benefit from physical activity, but it does not prevent or cure the disease.

Physical activity helps in the prevention and treatment of type 2 diabetes. With type 2, the pancreas may not produce enough insulin or the cells may become insulin resistant, thereby keeping glucose from entering the cell. Type 2 accounts for more than 90 percent of all cases of diabetes, and it occurs mainly in overweight people. (A more thorough discussion of the types of diabetes is given in Chapter 11 page 412).

If you have diabetes, consult your physician before you start exercising. You may not be able to begin until the diabetes is under control. Never exercise alone, and always wear a bracelet that identifies your condition. If you take insulin, the amount and timing of each dose may have to be regulated with your physician. If you inject insulin, do so over a muscle that won't be exercised, then wait an hour before exercising.

Both types of diabetes improve with exercise, although the results are more notable in patients with type 2 diabetes. Exercise usually lowers blood sugar and helps the body use food more effectively. The extent to which the blood glucose level can be controlled in overweight people with NIDDM seems to be related directly to how long and how hard a person exercises. Normal or near-normal blood glucose levels can be achieved through a proper exercise program.

As with any fitness program, the exercise must be done regularly to be effective against diabetes. The benefits of a single exercise bout on blood glucose are highest between 12 and 24 hours following exercise. These benefits are completely lost within 72 hours after exercise. Thus, regular participation is crucial to derive ongoing benefits. In terms of fitness, all diabetic patients can achieve higher fitness levels, including reductions in weight, blood pressure, and total cholesterol and triglycerides.

HOEGER KEY TO WELLNESS

The benefits of a single exercise bout on blood glucose are highest between 12 and 24 hours following exercise. These benefits are completely lost within 72 hours after exercise.

The biggest concern for people with diabetes is exercise-induced hypoglycemia during, following, or even a day after the exercise session. Common symptoms of hypoglycemia include weakness, confusion, shakiness, anxiousness, tiredness, hunger, increased perspiration, headaches, and even loss of consciousness. Physical activity increases insulin sensitivity and muscle glucose uptake, thus lowering blood glucose, an effect that lasts up to 72 hours after exercise. With enhanced insulin sensitivity, a unit of insulin lowers blood glucose to a much greater extent during and following exercise than under nonexercise conditions. Typically, the longer and more intense the exercise bout, the greater the effect on insulin sensitivity.

Both aerobic exercise and strength training are recommended for individuals with type 2 diabetes. According to the ACSM and the American Diabetes Association,[11] patients with type 2 diabetes should adhere to the following guidelines to make their exercise program safe and derive the most benefit:

Aerobic Exercise

- *Intensity.* Exercise at a moderate intensity (40 to 60 percent VO_2max). Additional benefits, however, are gained through a vigorous-intensity program. Insulin sensitivity has been shown to improve by up to 58 percent with HIIT training regimens.[12] The research indicates better blood glucose control by increasing intensity rather than exercise volume. Start your program with 10 to 15 minutes per session, on at least three nonconsecutive days, but preferably exercise 5 days per week.
- *Time (duration).* Aerobic activity duration should be no less than 150 minutes per week or the equivalent of 30 minutes per day at least 5 days per week. As a minimum, each aerobic exercise bout should be at least 10 minutes long and spread throughout the week. Diabetic individuals with a weight problem should build up daily physical activity to 60 minutes per session.
- *Type (mode).* Any type of aerobic activity or preferably a combination of aerobic activities that involves large muscle groups and increases oxygen uptake (VO_2) is recommended. Choose activities that you enjoy doing, and stay with them. As you select your activities, be aware of your condition. For example, if you have lost sensation in your feet, swimming or stationary cycling is better than walking or jogging to minimize the risk for injury.
- *Frequency.* Exercise aerobically at least three times per week, and do not allow more than two consecutive days between exercise sessions. Five days per week are strongly encouraged.
- *Rate of progression.* A gradual increase in exercise to at least 150 weekly minutes in both intensity and volume (duration and frequency) is strongly encouraged. Progression up to 7 hours per week (420 minutes) has been reported by individuals who have successfully been able to maintain a substantial amount of weight loss.

Strength Training

- *Intensity (resistance).* For optimal insulin action, resistance training should be conducted between 50 and 80 percent of the maximal capacity (1 RM) for each exercise, either on free weights or resistance machines.
- *Sets.* A minimum of one set performed to near fatigue of 5 to 10 exercises involving the body's major muscle groups (upper body, core, and lower body). Initially, each set should consist of 10 to 15 repetitions maximum (RM).
- *Frequency.* A minimum of twice per week, but preferably three times per week on nonconsecutive days.
- *Rate of progression.* Progression of intensity, sets, and frequency (in that order) are recommended. Type 2 diabetics are encouraged to gradually increase the resistance and aim to work with 8 to 10 RM. Next, sets can progressively be increased up to four sets per exercise. Finally, frequency may be increased from twice weekly to three times per week.

Additional Exercise Guidelines

- Check your blood glucose levels before and after exercise. Do not exercise if your blood glucose is greater than 300 mg/dL or fasting blood glucose is greater than 250 mg/dL and you have ketones in your urine. If your blood glucose is less than 100 mg/dL, eat a small carbohydrate snack before exercise.
- If you are on insulin or diabetes medication, monitor your blood glucose regularly, and check it at least twice within 30 minutes of starting exercise.
- Schedule your exercise 1 to 3 hours after a meal, and avoid exercise when your insulin is peaking. If you are going to exercise 1 to 2 hours following a meal, you may have to reduce your insulin or blood glucose-reducing medication.
- To prevent hypoglycemia, consume between .15 and .20 gram of carbohydrates per pound of body weight for each hour of moderate-intensity activity. This amount, however, should be adjusted based on your blood glucose monitoring. Up to .25 gram of carbohydrates per pound of body weight may be required for vigorous exercise. Your goal should be to regulate carbohydrate intake and medication dosage so as to maintain blood glucose level between 100 and 200 mg/dL. With physical activity and exercise, you will probably need to reduce your insulin or oral medication, increase carbohydrate consumption, or both.
- Be ready to treat low blood sugar with a fast-acting source of sugar, such as juice, raisins, or another source recommended by your doctor.
- If you feel that a reaction is about to occur, discontinue exercise immediately. Check your blood glucose level and treat the condition as needed.
- When you exercise outdoors, always do so with someone who knows what to do in a diabetes-related emergency.
- Stay well hydrated. Dehydration can have a negative effect on blood glucose, heart function, and performance. Consume adequate amounts of fluids before and after exercise. Drink about 8 ounces of water before you start each exercise session. If you are going to exercise for longer than an hour, drink 8 ounces (1 cup) of a 6 to 8 percent carbohydrate sports drink every 15 to 20 minutes.

People with type 1 diabetes should ingest 15 to 30 grams of carbohydrates during each 30 minutes of intense exercise and follow it with a carbohydrate snack after exercise.

In addition, strength-training twice per week using 8 to 10 exercises with a minimum of one set of 10 to 15 repetitions to near fatigue is recommended for individuals with diabetes. A complete description of strength-training programs is provided in Chapter 7.

Smoking and Exercise

While physical exercise often motivates a person to stop smoking, it does not offset any ill effects of smoking. Smoking greatly decreases the ability of the blood to transport oxygen to working muscles.

Oxygen is carried in the circulatory system by hemoglobin, the iron-containing pigment of the red blood cells. Carbon monoxide, a by-product of cigarette smoke, has 210 to 250 times greater affinity for hemoglobin over oxygen. Consequently, carbon monoxide combines much faster with hemoglobin, decreasing the oxygen-carrying capacity of the blood.

Chronic smoking also increases airway resistance, requiring the respiratory muscles to work much harder and consume more oxygen just to ventilate a given amount of air. If a person quits smoking, exercise does help increase the functional capacity of the pulmonary system.

A regular exercise program seems to be a powerful incentive to quit smoking. A random survey of 1,250 runners conducted at the 6.2-mile Peachtree Road Race in Atlanta, Georgia, provided impressive results. The survey indicated that of the men and women who smoked cigarettes when they started running, 81 percent and 75 percent, respectively, had quit before the date of the race.

9.9   *Women's Health and Exercise*

Women face unique health issues not only physiologically, but also due to societal pressures. Every woman would do well to keep herself educated about correct exercise principles throughout her lifetime so that she can practice sound and healthy habits. The following topics provide general guidance, which can be added upon by the personal physician.

Menstruation and Exercise

Although, on the average, women have a lower physical capacity during menstruation, medical surveys at the Olympic Games have shown that women have broken Olympic and world records at all stages of the menstrual cycle. Menstruation should not keep a woman from exercising, and it will not necessarily have a negative impact on performance.

In some instances, highly trained athletes develop **amenorrhea** during training and competition. This condition is seen most often in extremely lean women who also engage in sports that require strenuous physical effort over a sustained period of time. It is by no means irreversible. At present, we do not fully understand whether the condition is caused by physical or emotional stress related to high-intensity training, excessively low body fat, an energy deficit (low caloric intake) over long periods of time, or other factors.

The Female Athlete Triad

The female athlete triad results when a female exercises too much and consumes too few calories in pursuit of a low weight or smaller body size. The condition is not uncommon among female athletes. Athletes who tend to demand perfection from themselves, as well as those in sports that emphasize body size, are especially at risk. For example, in sports that emphasize body size, the rates of women whose menstrual cycle stops for at least 6 months can reach 69 percent, versus 2 to 5 percent in the average population.[13] The three interrelated conditions that make up the triad are menstrual dysfunction, decreased bone-mineral density, and low energy availability (often due to an eating disorder). Negative health conditions aggravate one another in an escalating cycle. Faulty nutrition and low energy intake, low body fat, physical and emotional stress, hormonal changes, and inability of the body to properly build bones can cause long-term and irreversible health consequences and, in extreme cases, death. Coaches and parents should take care not to place undue emphasis on leanness. Any female whose menstrual cycles are more than 35 days apart or who misses three menstrual cycles should be evaluated by a physician. A parent or coach who suspects an athlete may be at risk should approach the athlete and, if needed, contact a physician who can intervene and provide guidance and treatment. Diagnosis and treatment can be complicated and involve cooperation between the athlete's physician, coaches, and family.

Exercise and Dysmenorrhea

Although exercise has not been shown to either cure or aggravate **dysmenorrhea**, it has been shown to relieve menstrual cramps because it improves circulation to the uterus. Menstrual cramps also could be alleviated by higher levels of endorphins produced during prolonged physical activity, which may counteract pain. Particularly, stretching exercises of the muscles in the pelvic region seem to reduce and prevent painful menstruation that is not the result of disease.

Exercise during Pregnancy

Exercise is beneficial during pregnancy. According to the American College of Obstetricians and Gynecologists (ACOG), in the absence of contraindications, healthy pregnant women are encouraged to participate in regular, moderate-intensity physical activities to continue to derive health benefits during pregnancy.[14] Pregnant women, however, should consult their physicians to ensure that they have no contraindications to exercise during pregnancy. Overall, women who are physically active either before or during

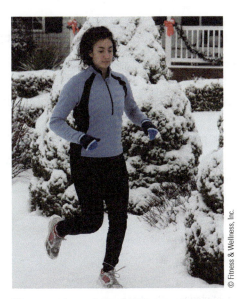

Women and men both should use good judgment to make sure they adhere to sound and healthy exercise habits.

pregnancy are better able to maintain weight gain within the recommended range, and compared with inactive women, they do not deliver large babies. They also have a lower risk for pregnancy-associated diabetes and high blood pressure.

As a general rule, healthy pregnant women can also accumulate 30 minutes of moderate-intensity physical activity on most, if not all, days of the week (a minimum of 150 minutes per week). Physical activity strengthens the body and helps prepare for the challenges of labor and childbirth.

The average labor and delivery lasts 10 to 12 hours. In most cases, labor and delivery are highly intense, with repeated muscular contractions interspersed with short rest periods. Proper conditioning will better prepare the body for childbirth. Moderate exercise during pregnancy also helps to prevent back pain and excessive weight gain, and it speeds recovery following childbirth.

The most common recommendations for exercise during pregnancy for healthy pregnant women with no additional risk factors are as follows:

- Don't start a new or more rigorous exercise program without proper medical clearance.
- Accumulate 30 minutes of moderate-intensity physical activities on most days of the week.
- Instead of using heart rate to monitor intensity, exercise at an intensity level between "low" and "somewhat hard," using the physical activity perceived exertion (H-PAPE) scale in Chapter 6, Figure 6.9 (see page 240).
- Gradually switch from weight-bearing and high-impact activities, such as jogging and aerobics, to

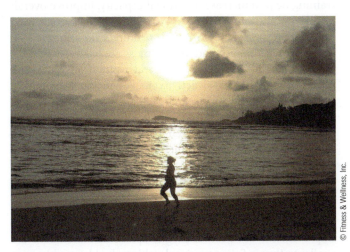

Light- to moderate-intensity exercise is recommended throughout pregnancy.

GLOSSARY

Amenorrhea Cessation of regular menstrual flow.

Dysmenorrhea Painful menstruation.

Contraindications to Exercise During Pregnancy

Stop exercise and seek medical advice if you experience any of the following symptoms:

- Unusual pain or discomfort, especially in the chest or abdominal area
- Cramping, primarily in the pelvic or lower back areas
- Muscle weakness, excessive fatigue, or shortness of breath
- Abnormally high heart rate or a pounding (palpitations) heart rate
- Decreased fetal movement
- Insufficient weight gain
- Amniotic fluid leakage
- Nausea, dizziness, or headaches
- Persistent uterine contractions
- Vaginal bleeding or rupture of the membranes
- Swelling of ankles, calves, hands, or face

non-weight-bearing/lower-impact activities, such as walking, stationary cycling, swimming, and water aerobics. The latter activities minimize the risk of injury and may allow exercise to continue throughout pregnancy.

- Avoid exercising at an altitude above 6,000 feet (1,800 meters), as well as scuba diving because either may compromise the availability of oxygen to the fetus.
- Women who are accustomed to strenuous exercise may continue in the early stages of pregnancy but should gradually decrease the amount, intensity, and exercise mode as pregnancy advances. (Most healthy pregnant women, however, slow down during the first few weeks of pregnancy until morning sickness and fatigue subside.)
- Pay attention to the body's signals of discomfort and distress, and never exercise to exhaustion. When fatigued, slow down or take a day off. Do not stop exercising altogether unless you experience any of the contraindications for exercise listed.
- To prevent fetal injury, avoid activities that involve potential contact or loss of balance or that cause even mild trauma to the abdomen. Examples of these activities are basketball, soccer, volleyball, Nordic or water skiing, ice skating, road cycling, horseback riding, and motorcycle riding.
- During pregnancy, don't exercise for weight loss purposes.
- Get proper nourishment (pregnancy requires between 150 and 300 extra calories per day), and eat a small snack or drink some juice 20 to 30 minutes prior to exercise.
- Prevent dehydration by drinking a cup of fluid 20 to 30 minutes before exercise, and drink 1 cup of liquid every 15 to 20 minutes during exercise.
- During the first 3 months in particular, don't exercise in the heat. Wear clothing that allows for proper

dissipation of heat. A body temperature above 102.6°F (39.2°C) can harm the fetus.

- After the first trimester, avoid exercises that require lying on the back. This position can block blood flow to the uterus and the baby.
- Perform stretching exercises gently because hormonal changes during pregnancy increase the laxity of muscles and connective tissue. Although these changes facilitate delivery, they also make women more susceptible to injuries during exercise.

9.10 Exercise and Aging

The elderly constitute the fastest-growing segment of the population. The number of Americans aged 65 and older increased from 3.1 million in 1900 (4.1 percent of the population) to about 40 million (13 percent) in 2010. By the year 2030, more than 72 million people, or 20 percent of the U.S. population, are expected to be older than 65.

Benefits of Lifelong Exercise

The main objectives of fitness programs for older adults should be to help them improve their functional status and contribute to healthy aging. This implies the ability to maintain independent living status and to avoid disability. A fitness program delivers results with gains in physical and mental capacity—even small efforts bring measurable rewards. Older adults are encouraged to participate in programs that will help develop cardiorespiratory endurance, muscular fitness, muscular flexibility, agility, balance, and motor coordination.

The physical and psychological benefits of regular physical activity for older adults make an impressive list. Physical activity decreases the risk for cardiovascular disease, stroke, hypertension, type 2 diabetes, osteoporosis, obesity, colon cancer, breast cancer, cognitive impairment, anxiety, and depression, and even dementia and Alzheimer's.[15] Physical activity also improves self-confidence and self-esteem. Furthermore, both cardiorespiratory endurance and strength-training help to increase functional capacity, improve overall health status, improve memory and mental acumen, and increase life expectancy. Strength-training also decreases the rate at which strength and muscle mass are lost.

The trainability of older men and women alike and the effectiveness of physical activity in enhancing health have been demonstrated in research. Older adults who increase their physical activity experience significant changes in cardiorespiratory endurance, strength, and flexibility. The extent of the changes depends on their initial fitness level and the types of activities they select for their training (walking, cycling, strength training, and so on).

Exercise Training for Seniors

Improvements in maximal oxygen uptake in older adults are similar to those of younger people, although older people seem to require a longer training period to achieve these changes.

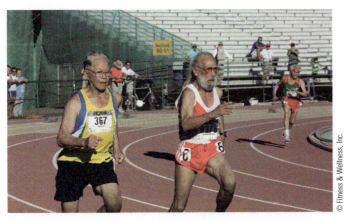

Older adults who exercise enjoy better health, functional capacity, and quality of life and live longer than physically inactive adults.

Table 9.3 Effects of Physical Activity and Inactivity on Older Men

	Exercisers	Nonexercisers
Age (yr)	68.0	69.8
Weight (lb)	160.3	186.3
Resting heart rate (bpm)	55.8	66.0
Maximal heart rate (bpm)	157.0	146.0
Heart rate reserve* (bpm)	101.2	80.0
Blood pressure (mm Hg)	120/78	150/90
Maximal oxygen uptake (mL/kg/min)	38.6	20.3

*Heart rate reserve = maximal heart rate − resting heart rate.

Data from F. W. Kash, J. L. Boyer, S. P. Van Camp, L. S. Verity, and J. P. Wallace, "The Effect of Physical Activity on Aerobic Power in Older Men (A Longitudinal Study)," *The Physician and Sports Medicine* 18, no. 4 (1990): 73–83.

Declines in maximal oxygen uptake average about 1 percent per year between ages 25 and 75. A slower rate of decline is seen in people who maintain a lifetime aerobic exercise program.

Results of research on the effects of aging on the cardiorespiratory system of male exercisers versus nonexercisers showed that the maximal oxygen uptake of regular exercisers was almost twice that of the nonexercisers (see Table 9.3).[16] The study revealed a decline in maximal oxygen uptake between ages 50 and 68 of only 13 percent in the active group, compared with 41 percent in the inactive group. These changes indicate that about one-third of the loss in maximal oxygen uptake results from aging, and two-thirds of the loss comes from inactivity. Blood pressure, heart rate, and body weight also were remarkably better in the exercising group. Aerobic training seems to decrease high blood pressure in older patients at the same rate as in young hypertensive people.

In terms of aging, muscle strength declines by 10 to 20 percent between ages 20 and 50; but between ages 50 and 70, it drops by another 25 to 30 percent. Through strength-training, frail adults in their 80s or 90s can double or triple their strength in just a few months. The amount of muscle hypertrophy achieved, however, decreases with age. Strength gains close to 200 percent have been found in previously inactive adults over age 90. In fact, research has shown that regular strength-training improves balance, gait, speed, **functional independence**, morale, depression symptoms, and energy intake.[17] Strength-trained older adults are 30 percent to 50 percent stronger than their sedentary counterparts.

Although muscle flexibility drops by about 5 percent per decade of life, 10 minutes of stretching every other day can prevent most of this loss as a person ages. Improved flexibility also enhances mobility skills. The latter promotes independence because it helps older adults successfully perform activities of daily living.

Body Composition in Seniors

In terms of body composition, lean body mass typically declines by 2 to 3 percent per decade starting at age 30. Muscle mass starts to decrease at age 40 and accelerates after age 65, with the legs losing muscle mass at a faster rate. Sedentary adults gain about 20 pounds of body weight between ages 18 and 55. As a result, body fat continues to increase through adult life, with a greater tendency toward visceral fat accumulation (especially in men), leading to further increases in risk for chronic disease. Regular aerobic activity and strength-training have been shown to help older adults properly manage body weight and significantly reduce visceral fat.

Exercise and Mental Health in Seniors

A slight decline in memory is also typically associated with aging. Part of this is due to reduction in the size of the hippocampus, the region of the brain primarily responsible for memory. This region begins to decrease in mass by .5 percent each year beginning as early as age 40. Recent studies, however, have shown promise in this area that has surpassed the hopes of researchers. Regular physical activity, aerobic exercise, and strength-training all have been shown to increase the size of the hippocampus and decrease the rate of brain shrinkage. Maintaining a high level of physical fitness in mid-life can reduce a person's chances of developing Alzheimer's by half and dementia by 60 percent.[18] Even becoming physically active later in life has been shown to produce measurable gains in the weight of the hippocampus following just a few months of training.

Older adults who wish to initiate an exercise program are strongly encouraged to have a complete medical evaluation. Particularly for aging adults, any physical activity program needs to be highly personalized to accommodate health needs and highly varying levels of fitness. Recommended activities for older adults include calisthenics, walking, jogging, swimming, cycling, and water aerobics. Strength-training is particularly important for bone health in the absence of weight-bearing aerobic activities.

GLOSSARY

Functional independence The ability to carry out activities of daily living without assistance from other individuals.

Exercise Recommendations for Seniors

Older people should avoid isometric and very high-intensity strength-training exercises (see Chapter 7). Activities that require all-out effort or that require participants to hold their breath tend to lessen blood flow to the heart, cause a significant increase in blood pressure, and increase the load placed on the heart. Older adults should participate in activities that require continuous and rhythmic muscular activity (about 40 to 60 percent of heart rate reserve). These activities do not cause large increases in blood pressure or overload the heart.

Mind-body activities like tai chi offer a particular boon in overall mental and physical health. While providing the same cardiorespiratory workout as a moderate-paced walk, tai chi also improves posture and strength, promotes healthy breathing habits, trains the body in balance, and can improve sensitivity in the soles of the feet, which helps with balance and increases walking speed.

9.11 You Can Get It Done

Once they understand the proper exercise, nutrition, and behavior modification guidelines, people find that implementing a fitness lifestyle program is not as difficult as they thought. With adequate preparation and a personal behavioral analysis, you are now ready to design, implement, evaluate, and adhere to a lifetime fitness program that can enhance your functional capacity and zest for life.

Using the concepts provided thus far in this book and the exercise prescription principles that you have learned, you should now update your personal fitness program in Activity 9.2. You also have an opportunity to revise your current stage of change, fitness category for each health-related component of physical fitness, and number of daily steps taken. You have the tools—the rest is up to you!

Personal Fitness Programming: An Example

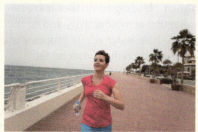
dotshock/Shutterstock.com

Now that you understand the principles of fitness assessment and exercise prescription given in Chapters 6, 7, and 8 and this chapter, you can review this program to cross-check and improve the design of your own fitness program. Let's look at an example.

Mary is 20 years old and 5 feet 6 inches tall. She participated in organized sports on and off throughout high school. During the last 2 years, however, she has participated only minimally in physical activity. She was not taught the principles for exercise prescription and has not participated in regular exercise to improve and maintain the various health-related components of fitness.

Mary became interested in fitness and contemplated signing up for a fitness and wellness course. As she was preparing her class schedule for the semester, she noted a Lifetime Fitness and Wellness course. In registering for the course, Mary anticipated some type of structured aerobic exercise. She knew that good fitness was important to health and weight management, but she didn't quite know how to plan and implement a program.

Once the new course started, she and her classmates received the Stages of Change Questionnaire. Mary learned that she was in the preparation stage for cardiorespiratory endurance, the precontemplation stage for muscular fitness, the maintenance stage for flexibility, and the preparation stage for body composition (see the "The Transtheoretical Model of Change" section in Chapter 2, pages 63–69). Various fitness assessments determined that her cardiorespiratory endurance level was fair, her muscular fitness was poor, her flexibility was good, and her percent body fat was 25 (moderate category).

Cardiorespiratory Endurance

At the beginning of the semester, the instructor informed the students that the course would require self-monitored participation in activities outside the regularly scheduled class hours. Mary was in the preparation stage for cardiorespiratory endurance. Thus, she knew she would be starting exercise in the next couple of weeks.

While in this preparation stage, Mary chose three processes of change to help her implement her program (see Table 2.1, page 65). She thought she could adopt an aerobic exercise program (the positive outlook process of change) and set a realistic goal to reach the good category for cardiorespiratory endurance by the end of the semester (goal setting). By staying in this course, she committed to go through with exercise (commitment). She prepared a 12-week Personalized Cardiorespiratory Exercise Prescription (see Activity 6.3, page 238), wrote down her goal, signed the prescription (now a contract), and shared the program with her instructor and roommates.

As her exercise modalities, Mary selected walking/jogging and aerobics. Initially, she walked or jogged twice a week and did aerobics once a week. By the 10th week of the program, she was jogging three times per week and participating in aerobics twice a week. She also selected techniques for monitoring, self-reevaluation, and countering her processes of change (see Table 2.2, page 72). Using the exercise log in Activity 6.4 (page 248), she monitored her exercise program. At the end of 6 weeks, she scheduled a follow-up cardiorespiratory assessment test (self-reevaluation process of change), and she replaced her evening television hour with aerobic training (countering).

Mary also decided to increase her daily physical activity. She chose to walk 10 minutes to and from school, take the stairs instead of elevators whenever possible, and add 5-minute walks every hour during study time. On Saturdays, she cleaned her apartment and went to a school-sponsored dance at night. On Sundays, she opted to walk to and from church and took a 30-minute leisurely walk after the dinner meal. Mary now was fully in the action stage of change for cardiorespiratory endurance.

(continued)

Figure 9.3 Sample starting muscular strength and endurance periodization program.

	Learning Lifting Technique	Muscular Strength	Muscular Endurance	Muscular Strength
Sets per exercise	1–2	2	2	3
Repetitions	10	12	18–20	8–12 (RM)
Intensity (resistance)	Very low	Moderate	Low	High
Volume	Low	Moderate	Moderate	High
Sessions per week	2	2	2	3
Weeks	2	3	2	3

Selected exercises: Bench press, leg press, leg curl, lat pull-down, rowing torso, rotary torso, seated back, and abdominal crunch.

Training days: ☐ M ☑ T ☐ W ☐ Th ☑ F ☐ S ☐ S

Training time: 3:00PM

Signature: *Mary Johnson*

Goal: Good   Date: 1/12/2018

© Fitness & Wellness, Inc.

Muscular Fitness

After Mary started her fitness and wellness course, she wasn't yet convinced that she wanted to strength-train. Still, she contemplated strength-training because a small part of her grade depended on it. When she read the information on the effect of lean body mass on basal metabolic rate and weight maintenance (consciousness-raising process of change), she thought that perhaps it would be good to add strength-training to her program. She also was contemplating the long-term consequences of loss of lean body mass, its effect on her personal appearance, and the potential for decreased independence and quality of life (emotional arousal process of change).

Mary visited her course instructor for additional guidance. Following this meeting, Mary committed herself to strength-train. While in the preparation stage, she outlined a 10-week periodized training program (Figure 9.3) and opted to aim for the good strength category by the end of the program.

Because this was the first time Mary had lifted weights, the course instructor introduced her to two other students who were already lifting (helping relationships process of change). She also monitored her program with the form provided in Activity 7.3 (page 000). Mary promised herself a movie and dinner out if she completed the first 5 weeks of strength training and a new blouse if she made it through 10 weeks (rewards process technique of change).

Muscular Flexibility

Good flexibility is not a problem for Mary because she regularly stretched 15 to 30 minutes while watching the evening news on television. She had developed this habit the last 2 years of high school to maintain flexibility as a member of the dance-drill team (environment control—as a team member, she needed good flexibility).

Because Mary had been stretching regularly for more than 3 years, she was in the maintenance stage for flexibility. The flexibility fitness tests revealed that she had good flexibility. These results allowed her to pursue her stretching program, because she thought she would be excellent for this fitness component (self-evaluation process of change).

To gain greater improvements in flexibility, Mary chose slow-sustained stretching and proprioceptive neuromuscular facilitation (PNF). She would need help carrying out the PNF technique. She spoke to one of her lifting classmates; together, they decided to allocate 20 minutes at the end of strength-training to stretching (helping relationships process of change), and they chose the sequence of exercises presented in Chapter 8, Activity 8.2 (consciousness-raising and goal setting).

Body Composition

One of the motivational factors to enroll in a fitness course was Mary's desire to learn how to better manage her weight. She had gained a few pounds since entering college. To prevent further weight gain, she thought it was time to learn sound principles for weight management (behavior analysis process of change). She was in the preparation stage of change because she was planning to start a diet and exercise program but wasn't sure how to get it done. All Mary needed was a little consciousness-raising to get her into the action stage.

With the knowledge she had now gained, Mary planned her program. At 25 percent body fat and 140 pounds, she decided to aim for 23 percent body fat so that she would be in the good category for body composition (goal setting). This meant that she would have to lose about 4 pounds (see Activity 4.1, page 159).

Mary's daily estimated energy requirement was about 2,027 calories (see Table 5.3, page 188). Mary also figured out that she was expending an additional 400 calories per day through her newly adopted exercise program and increased level of daily physical activity. Thus, her total daily energy intake would be around 2,427 calories (2,027 + 400).

To lose weight, Mary could decrease her caloric intake by 700 calories per day (body weight × 5; see Activity 5.1, page 189), yielding a target daily intake of 1,727 calories. By decreasing the intake by 700 calories daily, Mary should achieve her target weight in about 20 days (4 pounds of fat × 3,500 calories per pound of fat ÷ 700 fewer calories per day = 20 days). Mary picked the 1,800-calorie diet and eliminated one daily serving of grains (80 calories) to avoid exceeding her target 1,727 daily caloric intake.

The processes of change that helped Mary in the action stage for weight management are goal setting, countering (exercising instead of watching television), monitoring, environment control, and rewards. To monitor her daily caloric intake, Mary used the 1,800-calorie diet plan in Activity 5.3 (page 208). To further exert control over her environment, she gave away all of her junk food. She determined that she would not eat out while on the diet, and she bought only low- to moderate-fat, complex carbohydrate foods during the 3 weeks. As her reward, she achieved her target body weight of 136 pounds.

Assess Your Behavior

1. Do you participate in recreational sports as a means to further improve your fitness and add enjoyment to training?
2. Have you been able to meet your cardiorespiratory endurance, muscular fitness, muscular flexibility, and recommended body composition goals?
3. Are you able to incorporate a variety of activities into your fitness program, and do you vary exercise intensity and duration from time to time in your training?

Assess Your Knowledge

1. Volume of cardiorespiratory exercise is measured as
   a. frequency × intensity (in calories per minute) × duration of exercise, for one full week of exercise.
   b. METS × calories expended, for one workout.
   c. total number of minutes of cardiorespiratory exercise over one week.
   d. minutes of activity vs. minutes of rest per exercise session.
   e. total number of calories burned in relation to total number of calories consumed within an hour of the workout.

2. The intensity of exercise during the HIIT phase of a workout should be
   a. 50 to 80 percent of maximal aerobic capacity.
   b. about 60 percent of maximal aerobic capacity.
   c. 60 to 75 percent of maximal aerobic capacity.
   d. 70 percent of maximal aerobic capacity interspaced with efforts that surpass 100 percent.
   e. at least 80 percent of maximal aerobic capacity to efforts that surpass 100 percent of the maximal aerobic capacity.

3. Using a combination of aerobic activities to develop overall fitness is known as
   a. health-related fitness.
   b. circuit training.
   c. plyometric exercises.
   d. cross-training.
   e. skill-related fitness.

4. How much of your aerobic/anaerobic training should involve the same muscles used in your choice of sport during the sport-specific training phase of your conditioning program?
   a. A negligent amount
   b. 10 percent
   c. 50 percent
   d. 90 percent
   e. All

5. When a person exercises, approximately what percent of energy production by the body is converted into heat?
   a. 5
   b. 15 to 20
   c. 30
   d. 60 to 70
   e. 100

6. Recommended heat stroke treatment includes
   a. seeking immediate emergency medical attention.
   b. getting into a cool, humidity-controlled environment.
   c. placing cold packs on areas where blood supply is abundant.
   d. waiting for emergency help in a semi-seated position.
   e. all of the above.

7. When exercising in the heat, drinking about a cup of cool water every _____ minutes seems to be ideal to prevent dehydration.
   a. 5
   b. 15 to 20
   c. 30
   d. 30 to 45
   e. 60

8. One of the most common causes of activity-related injuries is
   a. high impact.
   b. low level of fitness.
   c. exercising without stretching.
   d. improper warm-up.
   e. All choices cause about an equal number of injuries.

9. Improvements in maximal oxygen uptake in older adults (as compared with younger adults) as a result of cardiorespiratory endurance training are
   a. lower.
   b. higher.
   c. difficult to determine.
   d. nonexistent.
   e. similar.

10. Periodization is a training approach that
    a. uses a systematic variation in intensity and volume.
    b. helps enhance fitness and performance.
    c. is commonly used by athletes.
    d. helps prevent staleness and overtraining.
    e. All are correct choices.

Correct answers can be found at the back of the book.

MINDTAP **Complete This Online**
From Cengage
Visit **www.cengagebrain.com** to access MindTap, a complete digital course that includes interactive quizzes, videos, and more.

Activity 9.2 Personal Fitness Plan

Name _____ Date _____

Course _____ Section _____ Gender _____ Age _____

Instructions
Update your personal fitness plan according to the ACSM guidelines provided in Chapters 6–8 and define your stage of change according to the stages of change model in Chapter 2. Also, reevaluate your fitness goals and write down your new goal to achieve by the end of the term. This activity should be carried out as a homework assignment to be completed over the next seven days.

I. Exercise Clearance
Is it safe for you to participate in an exercise program?   ☐ Yes   ☐ No

II. Fitness Evaluation

Component	Current		Fitness Category Goal		
	Test Results	Fitness Category	Training Frequency per Week	Stage of Change	Fitness Goal
Cardiorespiratory endurance					
Muscular fitness (strength and endurance)					
Muscular flexibility					
Body composition			NA		

© Fitness & Wellness, Inc.

III. Cardiorespiratory Endurance

Outline your cardiorespiratory endurance program according to ACSM guidelines. Include intensity, frequency, duration, aerobic activities, time of day for training, facility where you perform the training, and reward for accomplishing your goal.

_____

_____

_____

_____

IV. Muscular Fitness (Strength and Endurance)

Using ACSM guidelines, outline your muscular fitness (strength and endurance) training program. List the exercises used, sets and repetitions, amount of resistance used, frequency per week, training facility, and reward for accomplishing your goal.

_____

_____

_____

_____

V. Muscular Flexibility

Design your flexibility training program to include the selected exercises, technique used, number of repetitions for each exercise, length of final hold, site for training, and reward for accomplishing your goal.

_____

_____

_____

_____

VI. Recreational Activities

List any other sports or recreational activities in which you participate and include how often and how long you participate. Indicate also the primary reason for participation in these activities (physical activity, fitness, competition, skill development, recreation, stress management) and your future goals for these activities.

_____

_____

_____

_____

Activity 9.2 **Personal Fitness Plan** *(continued)*

VII. Daily Physical Activity

Indicate the efforts that you are making to increase daily physical activity, your feelings about your choice of activities, and what future goals you have regarding daily physical activities.

_____

_____

_____

_____

Total number of daily steps: [   ]

VIII. Body Composition and Fitness Benefits

List all of the activities in which you participate regularly and rate the respective contribution to body composition and other fitness components. Use the following rating scale: 1 = low, 2 = fair, 3 = average, 4 = good, and 5 = excellent.

Activity	Body Composition	Cardiorespiratory	Musc. Fitness	Musc. Flexibility
Example: Jogging	5	5	2	1

Activity 9.2 **Personal Fitness Plan** *(continued)*

IX. Contract

I hereby commit to carry out the above described fitness plan and complete my goals by [ ].

Upon completion of all my fitness goals I will present my results to [ ] and will

reward myself with [ ].

[ ]
My signature

[ ]
Date

[ ]
Witness signature

[ ]
Date

MINDTAP From Cengage **Complete This Online**
Visit **www.cengagebrain.com** to access MindTap, a complete digital course that includes interactive quizzes, videos, and more.

Preventing Cardiovascular Disease

"Exercise can be used as a vaccine to prevent disease and a medication to treat disease. If there were a drug with the same benefits as exercise, it would instantly be the standard of care."
—Robert Sallis

Objectives

10.1 **Define** cardiovascular disease and coronary heart disease.

10.2 **Explain** the importance of a healthy lifestyle in preventing cardiovascular disease.

10.3 **Become familiar** with the major risk factors that lead to the development of coronary heart disease, including physical inactivity, an abnormal cholesterol profile, hypertension, elevated homocysteine and C-reactive protein, inflammation, diabetes, and tobacco use.

10.4 **Assess** your own risk for developing coronary heart disease.

10.5 **Outline** a comprehensive program for reducing the risk for coronary heart disease and managing the overall risk for cardiovascular disease.

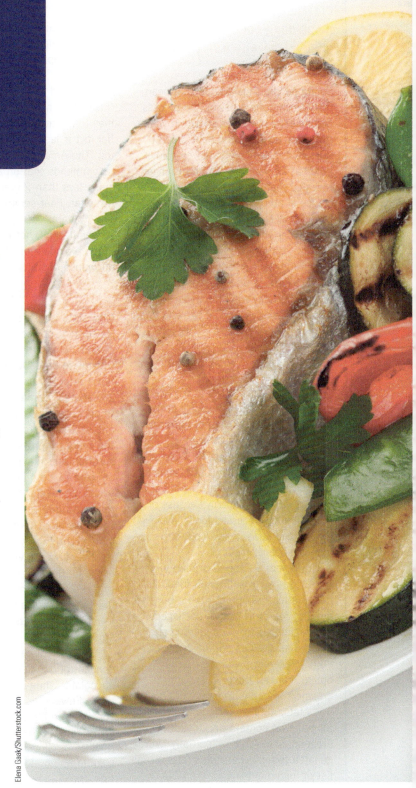

Elena Gaak/Shutterstock.com

FAQ

As a young college student, why should I have to worry about heart disease?

Young people should know that heart disease can affect them. The process begins early in life, as shown in young American soldiers who have died in wars. Autopsies conducted on soldiers killed at 22 years of age and younger revealed that more than half had early stages of atherosclerosis. Elevated blood cholesterol levels are found in children as young as 10 years old. Overall, risk factor management and positive lifestyle habits are the best ways to prevent disease. The choices you make today will affect your health and well-being in middle age and later.

Trans fat has been debated extensively lately. What foods are most likely to contain trans fat?

With extensive media coverage of their harmfulness, the amount of trans fats in foods is decreasing significantly. According to the Centers for Disease Control and Prevention (CDC), trans fats have decreased by about 60 percent in the last decade, primarily because of its removal from processed foods. Although this is good news, many foods still contain significant amounts.

Trans fats are found primarily in fried foods such as French fries, doughnuts, and apple fritters, but they are also found in baked, packaged, and processed foods, including stick margarine, cookies and pastries, biscuits, crackers, pie crusts, pizza dough, canned frosting, and coffee creamer. To decrease consumption of trans fats, always read the food label for trans fat content and look for "hydrogenated fat/oil" or "partially hydrogenated fat/oil" (i.e., trans fats) on the list of ingredients.

Trans fats increase the risk for heart disease and stroke not only by increasing low-density lipoprotein (LDL, or "bad") cholesterol but also by decreasing cardioprotective high-density lipoprotein (HDL, or "good") cholesterol.

The Food and Drug Administration (FDA) does not require food companies to list trans fat content on the label if it is less than .5 gram per serving. The American Heart Association recommends that on average we consume less than 2 grams per day of trans fat. Four servings of a product that contains .49 gram of partially hydrogenated oil, not listed on the food label, provide almost the entire daily allowance of trans fats.

Is chocolate heart healthy?

Chocolate is heart healthy because of its content of cocoa antioxidant polyphenol compounds called flavonoids. Chocolate helps lower the risk for heart attacks, strokes, and even type 2 diabetes. Some of the ingredients in chocolate help reduce LDL (bad) cholesterol, increase blood flow to the brain, improve blood sugar absorption and insulin sensitivity, discourage blood clots, and increase nitric oxide levels. Nitric oxide helps relax and dilate arteries and keep them flexible, lowering blood pressure slightly in hypertensive and prehypertensive individuals. Even modest reductions in blood pressure (two to three points on both systolic and diastolic pressure scales) significantly lower coronary artery disease and stroke mortality.

Dark chocolate has a much higher concentration of flavonoids than milk chocolate, while white chocolate has none. Flavonoids enhance activity of special proteins called sterol regulatory element-binding proteins (SREBPs), which are involved in cholesterol metabolism. Activated SREBPs bind to genes on DNA that increase a protein called apolipoprotein A1 in the liver, which is the major protein component of the "good" HDL cholesterol. Flavonoids also decrease liver production of another protein, apolipoprotein B, which is the major protein component of the "bad" LDL cholesterol, and increase activity of LDL receptors that induce more cholesterol removal from the bloodstream. Flavonoids may also fight atherosclerosis (plaque buildup) in the arteries by decreasing the amount of oxidized LDL cholesterol, a major contributor to atherosclerosis.

Dark chocolate with at least 70 percent cocoa content provides the healthiest compounds. The darker the chocolate, the less room for sugar. Milk chocolate contains about twice as much sugar as the darkest chocolate. And although chocolate has saturated fat, it is primarily stearic acid, which has a neutral effect on cholesterol. Unfortunately, the chocolate Americans love most is loaded with sugar, fat, and calories. Do not consume chocolate made with palm, coconut, hydrogenated, or partially hydrogenated oils, and avoid chewy, caramel, marshmallow, or cream-covered chocolates.

High-quality dark chocolate is not a food to be eaten liberally, but it's a health food to be enjoyed in moderation. Keep in mind that chocolate is calorie dense. Eat too much of any type of chocolate, and you will gain weight. Overweightness and obesity are major health problems, with corresponding negative effects on morbidity and mortality.

As little as .25 ounce of daily dark chocolate has been shown to provide health benefits. The equivalent of one (26 calories, .6 ounce) to two daily dark-chocolate Hershey's Kisses is all that is needed. Unsweetened cocoa powder with skim or fat-free milk and a touch of sweetener is an even better choice. Chocolate should be viewed as a treat—not a health food. Fruits and vegetables are still better sources of flavonoids.

REAL LIFE STORY | Peter's Experience

My father died at the age of 42 of a heart attack. One of my grandfathers also died from heart disease in his fifties. It was a great tragedy for my family to lose my dad and grandpa at such early ages, but it never occurred to me that this was something that could happen to me. However, last year at the age of 25 I found myself weighing almost 240 pounds on a 6-foot frame. I loved high-fat foods like bacon, cheese, and especially baked goods such as muffins or donuts. I have now learned these foods are high in saturated fats, trans fats, and processed carbohydrates. Eating this way caused me to carry a "spare tire" of extra weight around my middle. I knew my habits weren't

healthy, but I didn't give it a lot of thought because I figured, "I'm still young. I can start eating healthier when I get older." However, when I went to see my doctor, I learned that my cholesterol was high: 220. This was a wake-up call for me and I realized that if I didn't change things I could be heading down the same path that led to the deaths of my father and grandfather. I immediately started an exercise program of walking or biking four to five days a week. I drastically cut down on high-fat foods,

most red meats, and refined sugars. I started trying to get 25 grams or more of fiber a day, eating whole grains, fruits, and vegetables. At first the new diet tasted very boring to me, but after a while I developed a taste for healthy foods. I also limited my portion sizes. Over the course of a little over a year, I lost 60 pounds. People I hadn't seen for a while sometimes didn't recognize me at first! When I went back to my doctor recently, I learned that my cholesterol had dropped to 182. I feel like I have given myself and my heart a whole new lease on life.

Felix Mizioznikov/Shutterstock.com

PERSONAL PROFILE: My Cardiovascular Disease Risk

I. Do you try to incorporate as much physical activity as possible throughout every day of the week and avoid excessive sitting? ___ Yes ___ No

II. Do you accumulate a minimum of 30 minutes of moderate-intensity physical activity five times per week or at least 20 minutes of vigorous-intensity exercise three times per week? ___ Yes ___ No

III. Does your diet include fish, poultry, legumes, nontropical oils, and ample amounts of whole grains, fruits, and vegetables, and do you limit the intake of red meats, processed meats, salt, whole-milk products, simple carbohydrates, sweets, sugar-sweetened beverages, and processed foods? ___ Yes ___ No

IV. Are you aware of the most significant risk factors that lead to coronary heart disease and the factors that you have control over by the way you choose to live your life? ___ Yes ___ No

V. Have you ever had a blood lipid analysis test done? ___ Yes ___ No. What do the results of this test tell you about your current lifestyle, genetics, and potential risk for cardiovascular disease?

VI. Are you familiar with the effects of low-grade inflammation on heart disease and lifestyle factors that increase C-reactive protein levels? ___ Yes ___ No

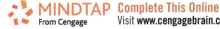 **MINDTAP** From Cengage   **Complete This Online**
Visit **www.cengagebrain.com** to access MindTap, a complete digital course that includes interactive quizzes, videos, and more.

10.1 *Cardiovascular Disease*

About 28.5 percent of all deaths in the United States are attributable to **cardiovascular disease (CVD),** the most prevalent degenerative condition in the United states (Figure 10.1).[1] CVD is a blanket term used to describe diseases and conditions of the heart and blood vessels, including **coronary heart disease (CHD), stroke, peripheral vascular disease,** congenital heart disease, rheumatic heart disease, atherosclerosis, high blood pressure, and congestive heart failure. More than a third of the adult population in the United States has some form of heart and blood vessel disease.

> ─GLOSSARY─
>
> **Cardiovascular disease (CVD)** The array of conditions that affect the heart and the blood vessels.
>
> **Coronary heart disease (CHD)** A condition in which the arteries that supply the heart muscle with oxygen and nutrients are narrowed by fatty deposits, such as cholesterol and triglycerides.
>
> **Stroke** A condition in which the blood supply to part of the brain is blocked or severely restricted, depriving brain tissue of oxygen and nutrients.
>
> **Peripheral vascular disease** Narrowing of the peripheral blood vessels.

Figure 10.1 Incidence of cardiovascular disease in the United States for selected years: 1900–2014.

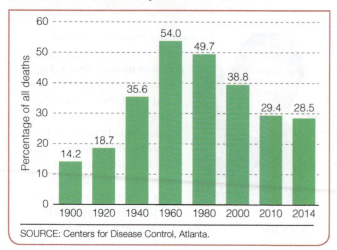

SOURCE: Centers for Disease Control, Atlanta.

According to the CDC, about 60 percent of deaths from heart disease are sudden and unexpected, with no previous symptoms of the disease. Almost half of these deaths occur outside of the hospital, most likely because the individuals failed to recognize early warning symptoms of a heart attack.

About 1.5 million people have new or recurrent heart attacks and strokes each year, and more than 40 percent of them die as a result, including some 375,000 deaths from heart disease and close to 130,000 stroke deaths. More than half of these deaths occur within 1 hour of the onset of symptoms, before the person reaches the hospital.

Although heart and blood vessel disease is still the number-one health problem in the United States, the incidence declined by more than 47 percent between 1960 and 2014 (Figure 10.1), largely because of health education. People now are aware of the risk factors for CVD and are leading a lifestyle that lowers the risk for these diseases. Data from 2014 indicate that most of the risk-factor improvement is associated with better blood pressure control, increased statin use (cholesterol medications), lower smoking rates, and improved medical treatment following a cardiovascular event.

10.2 Most Prevalent Forms of Cardiovascular Disease

Of the many forms of CVD, coronary heart disease (CHD) and stroke are responsible for the most deaths from CVD in the United States. Coronary heart disease is a term used to describe the buildup of plaque in the heart's arteries that can lead to a heart attack. A heart attack occurs when an artery is blocked, depriving the heart muscle of necessary oxygen. A stroke, in turn, is sometimes described as a "brain attack" that occurs when blood flow to the brain is cut off, causing brain cells to die from the lack of oxygen.

10.3 Stroke

About 800,000 new or recurrent strokes are reported each year in the United States. The effects of a stroke can be large or small, depending on where it occurred in the brain and how much of the area was damaged. Injury to cells in particular areas of the brain can cause functions controlled by that area of the brain to be lost. A small stroke might only cause short-term numbness in part of the body, whereas a large stroke can alter a person's speech capability, cause a loss of muscle control, or cause a person to become permanently paralyzed. More than two-thirds of stroke victims who survive are left with some type of permanent disability. Although stroke is the most significant contributor to mental and physical disability in the United States, it does not draw the same attention as CHD, high blood pressure, diabetes, or cancer.

Similar to those for CHD, most risk factors for stroke are preventable. Table 10.1 lists the major risk factors; the first four factors are unchangeable, and therefore beyond a person's control, whereas the latter seven are fully manageable. Dietary guidelines for stroke prevention include a diet that is low in sodium (less than 2,300 mg per day—or under 1,500 mg per day if you are over 50 and have high blood pressure or diabetes), is high in potassium (five or more daily servings of fresh fruit and vegetables—at least 4,700 mg of potassium per day) and nuts (1 ounce per day), limits or avoids alcohol intake, and maintains a healthy weight (aim for a BMI below 25).

HOEGER KEY TO WELLNESS

Cardiovascular disease is the number one cause of death in the United States, yet most of the risk factors for the disease are preventable and reversible and you have extensive control over lifestyle factors that can prevent its onset.

Table 10.1 Stroke Risk Factors

Unchangeable Factors
Age: Increased risk after age 55
Gender: Higher risk in men
Race: African Americans are at greater risk
Family history

Manageable Factors
Tobacco use: Stop!
Blood pressure: Maintain in normal range
Diet: Decrease saturated fat, trans fat, and sodium consumption and increase intake of potassium, fruits, and vegetables
Activity level: Increase frequency and intensity
Weight: Maintain within recommended range
Cholesterol: Aim for normal levels
Diabetes: Prevent or manage condition

Signs of Heart Attack and Stroke

Time is extremely critical when suffering a heart attack or stroke. Any or all of the following signs may occur during a heart attack or a stroke. **If you experience any of these and they last longer than a few minutes, call 911 and seek medical attention immediately**. Failure to do so may cause irreparable damage and even result in death.

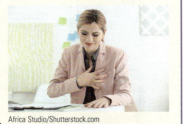

Africa Studio/Shutterstock.com

Warning Signs of a Heart Attack

- Chest pain, discomfort, pressure, or squeezing that lasts for several minutes. These feelings may go away and return later.

- Pain or discomfort in the shoulders, neck, or arms or between the shoulder blades

- Chest discomfort with shortness of breath, lightheadedness, cold sweats, nausea and/or vomiting, a feeling of indigestion, sudden fatigue or weakness, fainting, or sense of impending doom

Warning Signs of Stroke

The acronym **FAST** is commonly used to help recognize and enhance responsiveness for a stroke victim.

- **F**acial drooping. Part of the face is dropping, weak, numb, or hard to move.

- **A**rm weakness. An inability to completely raise one arm.

- **S**peech difficulties. The inability to understand or repeat a simple sentence.

- **T**ime. Time is of the essence when suffering a stroke.

- Other symptoms may include a sudden severe headache, confusion, dizziness, difficulty walking, loss of balance or coordination, or sudden visual difficulty.

Figure 10.2 The heart and its blood vessels.

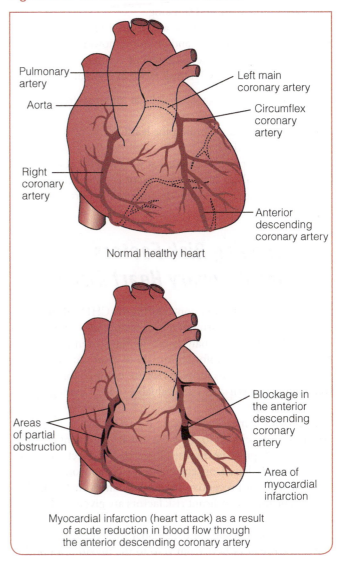

Normal healthy heart

Myocardial infarction (heart attack) as a result of acute reduction in blood flow through the anterior descending coronary artery

10.4 *Coronary Heart Disease*

The most common form of CVD is coronary heart disease (CHD). The heart requires a continual supply of oxygen-rich blood transported through the coronary arteries to function. The heart and the coronary arteries are illustrated in Figure 10.2. CHD occurs when fatty matter, such as cholesterol and triglycerides, builds up to form plaque deposits within the arteries that restrict blood flow. As the passage of flow within the coronary arteries becomes narrower, the blood supply to the heart muscle diminishes, which can precipitate a heart attack.

For decades, CVD has been the leading cause of death in the United States. When CVDs are separated by categories, however, CHD becomes the leading cause of death, accounting for about 20 percent of all deaths and more than half of all deaths from CVD (cancer is the second-leading cause of death, but

more than 100 types of cancer can develop in the human body). CHD is also the leading cause of sudden cardiac deaths. The risk of death is greater in the least-educated segment of the population. Presently, more than 500,000 coronary bypass operations and more than 1 million coronary **angioplasty** procedures are performed in the United States each year.

Coronary Heart Disease Risk Profile

Although genetic inheritance plays a role in CHD, the most important determinant is personal lifestyle. Most of the major **risk factors** for CHD are preventable and reversible. About 50 percent of deaths from CVD among adults 45 to 79 years old

---GLOSSARY---

Angioplasty A procedure in which a balloon-tipped catheter is inserted and then inflated to widen the inner lumen of the artery.

Risk factors Lifestyle and genetic variables that may lead to disease.

are caused by five risk factors: high cholesterol, high blood pressure, obesity, diabetes, and smoking.

CHD risk factor analyses are administered to evaluate whether a person's lifestyle and genetic endowment are potential contributors to the development of coronary disease. The specific objectives of a CHD risk factor analysis are as follows:

- Screen individuals who may be at high risk for the disease.
- Educate people regarding the leading risk factors for developing CHD.
- Implement programs aimed at reducing the risks.
- Use the analysis as a starting point from which to compare changes induced by the intervention program.

10.5 *Leading Risk Factors for Coronary Heart Disease*

The leading risk factors contributing to CHD are listed in Table 10.2. A self-assessment of risk factors for CHD is given in Activity 10.1. This analysis can be done even if you have little or no medical information about your cardiovascular health. The guidelines for zero risk are outlined for each factor, making this self-analysis a valuable tool for managing risk factors for CHD.

To provide a meaningful score for CHD risk, a weighting system was developed to show the impact of leading risk factors on developing the disease (Table 10.2 and Activity 10.1). The system is based on current research and on the work done at leading preventive medical facilities in the United States. The most significant risk factors are given the heaviest numerical weight.

Based on test results and personal lifestyle, a person receives a score anywhere from zero to the maximum number of points for each factor. When the risk points from all of the risk factors are totaled, the final number is used to place an individual in one of five overall risk categories for potential development of CHD (see Activity 10.1).

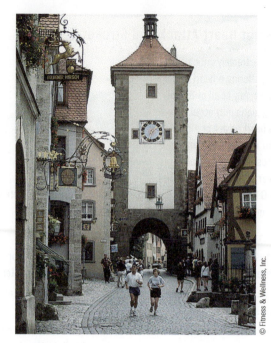

Regular physical activity helps to control most of the major risk factors that lead to heart disease.

The very low CHD risk category designates the group at the lowest risk for developing heart disease based on age and gender. The low category suggests that even though these people are taking good care of their cardiovascular health, they can improve it (unless all risk points come from age and family history). Moderate CHD risk means that people can definitely improve their lifestyle to lower the risk for disease; otherwise, medical treatment may be required. A score in the high or very high CHD risk category points to a strong probability of developing heart disease within the next few years and calls for immediate implementation of a personal risk-reduction program, including professional medical, nutritional, and physical activity intervention.

The leading risk factors for CHD are discussed next, along with the general recommendations for risk reduction.

Physical Inactivity

Physical inactivity is responsible for low levels of cardiorespiratory endurance (the ability of the heart, lungs, and blood vessels to deliver enough oxygen to the cells to meet the demands of prolonged physical activity). The level of cardiorespiratory endurance (or fitness) is given most commonly by the maximal amount of oxygen (in milliliters) that every kilogram (2.2 pounds) of body weight is able to utilize per minute of physical activity (mL/kg/min). As maximal oxygen uptake (VO_{2max}) increases, so does efficiency of the cardiorespiratory system. Improving cardiorespiratory endurance through aerobic exercise and daily physical activity greatly reduces the overall risk for heart disease.

For habitually sedentary people, sudden heavy-duty physical activity, such as shoveling snow or strenuous yard work, can trigger a cardiovascular event. The research shows that

Table 10.2 Weighting System for CHD Risk Factors

Risk Factor	Maximal Risk Points
Unhealthy diet	14
Physical inactivity	8
Tobacco use	8
Body mass index	8
Hypertension	8
Personal history of heart disease	8
Abnormal heart function	8
Diabetes	6
Family history of heart disease	6
Age	4
Tension and stress	3

- Lower blood lipids (cholesterol and triglycerides)
- Decrease low-grade (hidden) inflammation in the body
- Prevent and help control diabetes
- Decrease and control blood pressure
- Reduce body fat
- Motivate toward smoking cessation
- Alleviate tension and stress
- Counteract a personal history of heart disease

Data from the research summarized in Figure 1.7 in Chapter 1 clearly show the tie between physical activity and mortality, regardless of age and other risk factors. A higher level of physical fitness benefits even those who exhibit other risk factors, such as high blood pressure and serum cholesterol, cigarette smoking, and a family history of heart disease. In most cases, less fit people in the study without these risk factors had higher death rates than highly fit people with these same risk factors.

The findings show that the higher the level of cardiorespiratory fitness, the longer the life, but the largest drop in premature death is seen between the "unfit" and the "moderately fit" groups. Even small improvements in cardiorespiratory endurance greatly decrease the risk for cardiovascular mortality. Most adults who engage in a moderate exercise program can attain these fitness levels easily.

The exact amount of physical activity required to decrease the risk for CVD is difficult to establish and most likely varies due to genetics, age, gender, body composition, health status, and personal lifestyle, among other factors. What may be sufficient for a low-risk individual may not be enough for someone else with disease risk factors. For example, an apparently healthy individual at recommended body weight may not need more than 30 daily minutes of accumulated moderate-intensity physical activity. Another person with a weight problem and other risk factors such as high blood pressure, cholesterol abnormalities, and borderline high blood sugar may need a much greater amount of activity to counteract these risk factors.

Scientific studies indicate that, when feasible, vigorous activity is preferable because of greater improvements in aerobic fitness, blood pressure, and glucose control and a larger reduction in CHD risk.[2] Still, do not engage in vigorous exercise without proper clearance and a minimum of 6 weeks of proper conditioning through moderate-intensity activity.

A comprehensive and systematic research review of the effects of physical activity on all-cause mortality that included 80 studies involving more than 1.3 million people concluded that physical activity prolongs life and that premature death risk decreased the most as activity time increased with vigorous exercise.[3] Each weekly hour of light, moderate, or vigorous activity decreased mortality rates by 4, 6, and 9 percent, respectively. Furthermore, for every 1,000 weekly calories expended through exercise, the mortality rate decreased by 11 percent.

In terms of life expectancy, higher levels of physical activity are associated with greater gains in life expectancy. People at the highest level of physical activity gain about 4.5 years in life expectancy, and being active and of normal weight (BMI of 18.5 to 24.9) yields a gain of 7.2 years of life as compared to being inactive and obese.[4]

Healthy Lifestyle Cuts Risk of Sudden Cardiac Death

Sudden cardiac death (SCD) is caused by a sudden, unexpected loss of heart function. It is the largest cause of natural death in the United States, responsible for more than 300,000 to 400,000 adult deaths each year or about half of all heart disease deaths. SCD occurs when the heart's electrical system does not function properly and suddenly becomes very irregular. The

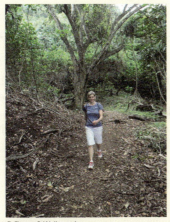
© Fitness & Wellness, Inc.

heart can beat dangerously fast, causing the ventricles to flutter or quiver, and blood is not delivered to the body. The greatest concern is the lack of blood flow to the brain during the initial few minutes, and the person loses consciousness. Death is almost always imminent unless the person receives immediate emergency treatment. SCD can also take place during an attack itself as the heart muscle is damaged because it does not receive sufficient oxygen-rich blood.

Research conducted on more than 81,000 women tracked during 26 years showed that adherence to a "low-risk" lifestyle significantly decreases the risk of SCD. The low-risk lifestyle included the following factors:

- Not smoking
- Being physically active for at least 30 minutes a day
- Not being overweight or obese
- Eating a diet rich in fruits, vegetables, whole grains, nuts, beans, and fish; with considerably more unsaturated than saturated fat; moderate use of alcohol; and low intake of red and processed meats, trans fatty acids, and sugar.

The authors concluded that a low-risk lifestyle could prevent as much as 81 percent of the yearly SCDs in the United States.

SOURCE: S. E. Chiuve, "Adherence to a Low-Risk, Healthy Lifestyle and Risk of Sudden Cardiac Death Among Women," *Journal of the American Medical Association*, 306 (2011): 62–69.

unaccustomed physical exertion increases the risk for a cardiovascular incident 50- to 100-fold.

Although specific recommendations can be followed to improve each risk factor, daily physical activity, avoidance of excessive daily sitting, and a regular aerobic exercise program help to control most of the major risk factors that lead to heart disease. Physical activity and aerobic exercise will:

- Increase cardiorespiratory endurance
- Increase and maintain good heart function, sometimes improving certain electrocardiogram abnormalities
- Improve high-density lipoprotein (HDL) cholesterol

Activity 10.1   Self-Assessment Coronary Heart Disease Risk Factor Analysis

Name _____ Date _____

Course _____ Section _____ Gender _____ Age _____

I. Instructions

The disease process for cardiovascular disease starts early in life, primarily as a result of poor lifestyle habits. Studies have shown beginning stages of atherosclerosis and elevated blood lipids in children as young as 10 years old. Consequently, the purpose of this activity is to establish a baseline coronary heart disease (CHD) risk profile and to point out the "zero-risk" level for each coronary risk factor. When a range is provided for the score (2–8), rate yourself based on how often the episodes occur or how often the statement description applies to you.

Score

1. Physical Activity

Do you get 30 or daily minutes of moderate-intensity physical activity:

Fewer than 3 times per week...8

Between 3 and 4 times per week...3

5 or more times per week...0

2. Abnormal Heart Function

Do you ever feel your heart beat irregularly, skipping beats, fluttering,

or palpitating...2–8

3. Diet (use the highest score if all apply)

Does your regular diet include:

1 or more daily servings of red meat; more than 7 eggs/week; daily butter,
cheese, whole milk, refined carbohydrates (sugar), alcohol, processed foods;
and grilling or cooking meat and poultry at high temperatures..................10–14

3 to 6 servings of red meat/week; 1% or 2% milk; some cheese,
refined carbohydrates, processed foods, and alcohol; some whole grains,
fruits, vegetables, and cold-water fish...4–10

Red meat (<3 oz/serving) or processed meats (<1.5 oz/serving) fewer than 2
times/week; skim milk and skim milk products; limited refined carbohydrates,
processed foods, and alcohol; ample daily amounts of whole-grain products, fruits,
and vegetables; cold-water fish at least 2 times/week.................................0–3

4. Diabetes

Non-diabetic..0

Are you pre-diabetic..3

Are you diabetic..6

5. Blood Pressure

Add scores for both readings
(e.g., 144/88 score = 4)

Systolic		Diastolic		
<120	(0)	<80	(0)	0
121–139	(1)	81–89	(1)	1–2
140–159	(3)	90–99	(3)	3–6
≥160	(4)	≥100	(4)	4–8

6. Body Mass Index (BMI)

<25.0.......................................0

25.0–29.99.............................2

30.0–39.99.............................4

≥40.0.......................................8

Activity 10.1 **Self-Assessment Coronary Heart Disease Risk Factor Analysis** *(continued)*

7. Tobacco	Lifetime non-smoker 0	Smoke 1–9 cigarettes/day 3	
	Ex-smoker more than 1 year 0	Smoke 10–19 cigarettes/day 4	
	Ex-smoker less than 1 year 1	Smoke 20–29 cigarettes/day 5	
	Non-smoker, but live or work in	Smoke 30–39 cigarettes/day 6	
	smoking environment 2	Smoke 40 or more cigarettes/day 8	
	Pipe or cigar smoker, or chew		☐
	tobacco..3		

8. Tension and Stress Are you:	Sometimes tense and stressed 1	
	Often tense and stressed 2	
	Always tense and stressed 3	☐

9. Personal History	Have you ever had a heart attack, stroke, coronary disease, or any known heart problem:	
	During the last year................................ 8 2–5 years ago................................... 3	
	1–2 years ago .... 5 More than 5 years ago 2	
	Never had a heart problem 0	☐

10. Family History	Have any of your blood relatives (parents, uncles, brothers, sisters, grandparents)	
	suffered from cardiovascular disease:	
	One or more before age 51 .... 6 One or more after age 60 2	
	One or more between 51 and 60.............. 4 None had cardiovascular disease..... 0	☐

11. Age	29 or younger 0	
	30–39 1	
	40–49 2	
	50–59 3	
	≥60 4	☐

How to Score

Total Risk Score: ☐

Risk Category...Total Risk Score
Very Low...5 or fewer points
Low .... Between 6 and 15 points
Moderate...Between 16 and 25 points
High..Between 26 and 35 points
Very High..36 or more points

II. Stage of Change for Cardiovascular Disease Prevention

Using Figure 2.7 and Table 2.3 (page 73), identify your current stage of change for participation in a cardiovascular disease risk-reduction program: ☐

III. In a few sentences, using a separate sheet of paper, discuss your family and personal risk for cardiovascular disease. Also, discuss lifestyle changes that you have already implemented in this course, as well as additional changes that you can make to decrease your own risk for cardiovascular disease.

IV. Physical Activity Rating

Number of daily steps at the beginning of the term: ☐   Current number of daily steps: ☐

Current physical activity rating (use Table 1.2, page 13): ☐

© Fitness & Wellness, Inc.

Physical Activity versus Medications

Regular physical activity and exercise have been shown to exceed the benefits of prescription medications in reducing premature mortality in people suffering from heart disease, diabetes, and stroke.[5] Cardiac patients who exercise require less medication, are less likely to have follow-up surgeries or bypasses, and have a much lower risk of dying from a subsequent heart attack than their physically inactive counterparts. Individuals with these chronic conditions should not stop taking their medications, but because of its effectiveness, they should add daily physical activity and regular exercise to their drug-treatment therapy.

Physical Activity and Daily Sitting Time

Also, try to minimize total daily sitting time. The data indicate that excessive daily sitting (commuting to and from work, at a desk, by the computer, and watching television) increases the risk for CVD, obesity, some chronic disorders, and premature mortality. The risk is increased even if you meet the 30 minutes of moderate-intensity physical activity on most days of the week but still spend a large part of the day sitting. If your job (like most nowadays) requires a large portion of the day to be spent in a sitting position, at least get up and take frequent breaks. Small, creative lifestyle changes make a difference, such as always answering the phone standing; walking to the office next door instead of texting, e-mailing, instant messaging, or using the phone; and using stairs instead of riding elevators and escalators. When watching television, make it a point to get up and walk around during each commercial break. Even better, do dips at the edge of the couch or stand up and sit down 20 times to strengthen your thigh muscles.

HOEGER KEY TO WELLNESS

Daily physical activity, including a regular aerobic exercise program, helps to control most of the major risk factors that lead to heart disease.

Physical Activity and Overall Risk Factor Management

While aerobically fit individuals have a lower incidence of CVD, regular physical activity and aerobic exercise by themselves do not guarantee a lifetime free of cardiovascular problems. Overall management of risk factors is the best guideline to lower the risk for CVD. Still, aerobic exercise is one of the most important factors in preventing and reducing cardiovascular problems. Based on the overwhelming amount of scientific data in this area, evidence of the benefits of aerobic exercise in reducing heart disease is far too impressive to be ignored. Low fitness is more dangerous than obesity, smoking, high cholesterol, or diabetes.

As more research studies are conducted, the addition of strength training is increasingly recommended for good heart function. The AHA recommends strength training even for individuals who have had a heart attack or have high blood pressure, as long as they strength train under a physician's advice. Strength training helps control body weight and blood sugar and lowers cholesterol and blood pressure.

Abnormal Electrocardiograms

The **electrocardiogram (ECG or EKG)** is a valuable measure of the heart's function. The ECG provides a record of the electrical impulses that stimulate the heart to contract (Figure 10.3). In reading an ECG, doctors interpret five general areas: heart rate, heart rhythm, axis of the heart, enlargement or hypertrophy of the heart, and myocardial infarction.

During a standard 12-lead ECG, 10 electrodes are placed on the person's chest. From these 10 electrodes, 12 tracings, or "leads," of the electrical impulses as they travel through the heart muscle, or **myocardium,** are studied from 12 different positions. By looking at ECG tracings, medical professionals can identify abnormalities in heart functioning (Figure 10.4). Based on the findings, the ECG may be interpreted as normal, equivocal, or abnormal. An ECG does not always identify

Figure 10.3 Normal electrocardiogram.

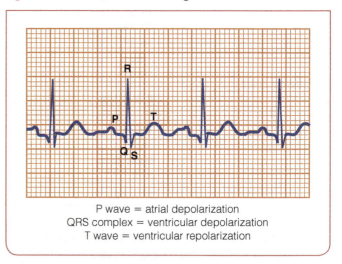

P wave = atrial depolarization
QRS complex = ventricular depolarization
T wave = ventricular repolarization

Figure 10.4 Abnormal electrocardiogram showing a depressed S-T segment.

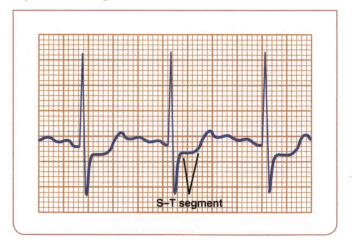

S-T segment

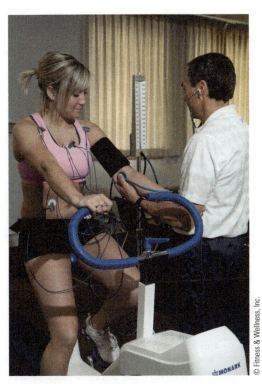

Exercise tolerance test with 12-lead electrocardiograph monitoring (an exercise stress ECG).

response during exercise, and establish actual or functional maximal heart rate for exercise prescription. The recovery ECG is another important diagnostic tool to monitor the return of the heart's activity to normal conditions.

Most adults who wish to start or continue an exercise program don't need a stress ECG. No set of guidelines can cover all cases when a stress ECG is recommended prior to exercise participation. The test, however, is recommended for individuals who are at high risk or are known to have cardiovascular, pulmonary, renal, or metabolic disease. Moreover, people feeling unusually winded in response to normal exertion, unexplained fatigue, or chest pain should have the test done.

At times, the stress ECG has been questioned as a reliable predictor of CHD. Nevertheless, it remains the most practical, inexpensive, noninvasive procedure available to diagnose latent (undiagnosed or unknown) CHD. The test is accurate in diagnosing CHD about 65 percent of the time. The sensitivity of the test increases with the severity of the disease, and more accurate results are seen in people who are at high risk for CVD.

Abnormal Cholesterol Profile

Cholesterol receives much attention because of its direct relationship to heart disease. **Blood lipids** (cholesterol and triglycerides) are carried in the bloodstream by protein molecules of **high-density lipoproteins (HDLs)**, **low-density lipoproteins (LDLs)**, **very low-density lipoproteins (VLDLs)**, and **chylomicrons**. An increased risk for CHD has been established in individuals with high total cholesterol, high LDL cholesterol, and low HDL cholesterol.

An abnormal cholesterol profile contributes to **atherosclerosis**, the buildup of fatty tissue in the walls of the arteries (Figure 10.5). As the plaque builds up, it blocks the blood vessels that supply the myocardium with oxygen and nutrients (the coronary arteries), and these obstructions can trigger a **myocardial infarction**, or heart attack.

Unfortunately, the heart disguises its problems quite well, and typical symptoms of heart disease, such as **angina pectoris**, do not start until the coronary arteries are about

problems, so a normal tracing is not an absolute guarantee. Conversely, an abnormal tracing does not necessarily signal a serious condition.

ECGs are taken at rest, during the stress of exercise, and during recovery. A **stress electrocardiogram** is also known as a graded exercise stress test or a maximal exercise tolerance test. Similar to a high-speed test on a car, a stress ECG reveals the tolerance of the heart to increased physical activity. It is a much better test than a resting ECG to discover CHD.

Stress ECGs also are used to assess cardiorespiratory fitness levels, screen individuals for preventive and cardiac rehabilitation programs, detect abnormal blood pressure

---

GLOSSARY

Electrocardiogram (ECG or EKG) A recording of the electrical activity of the heart.

Myocardium Heart muscle.

Stress electrocardiogram A test also known as a graded exercise stress test during which the workload is increased gradually until the individual reaches maximal fatigue, with blood pressure and 12-lead electrocardiographic monitoring throughout the test.

Cholesterol A waxy substance, technically a steroid alcohol, found only in animal fats and oil and used in making cell membranes, as a building block for some hormones, in the fatty sheath around nerve fibers, and in other necessary substances.

Blood lipids Cholesterol and triglycerides (fats).

High-density lipoproteins (HDLs) Cholesterol-transporting molecules in the blood ("good" cholesterol) that help clear cholesterol from the blood.

Low-density lipoproteins (LDLs) Cholesterol-transporting molecules in the blood ("bad" cholesterol) that tend to release cholesterol. leading to plaque formation (atherosclerosis) in the arteries.

Very low-density lipoproteins (VLDLs) Triglyceride-, cholesterol-, and phospholipid-transporting molecules in the blood.

Chylomicrons Triglyceride-transporting molecules.

Atherosclerosis Fatty or cholesterol deposits in the walls of the arteries leading to formation of plaque.

Myocardial infarction Heart attack; damage to or death of an area of the heart muscle as a result of an obstructed artery to that area.

Angina pectoris Chest pain associated with CHD.

Figure 10.5 Comparison of a normal healthy artery (A) and diseased arteries (B, C, and D).

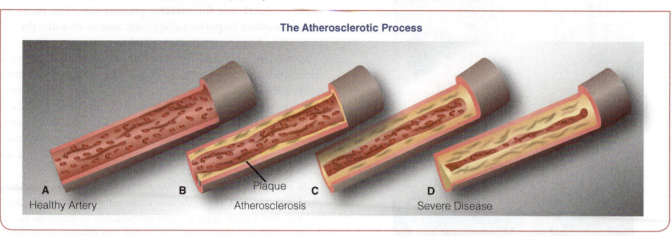

The Atherosclerotic Process

A — Healthy Artery
B — Plaque / Atherosclerosis
C
D — Severe Disease

Heart Disease and Stroke Prevention Guidelines

The American Heart Association (AHA) and the American College of Cardiology have set forth recommendations for heart disease and stroke prevention. These guidelines focus on *cholesterol, lifestyle, obesity,* and *risk assessment.*

In terms of *cholesterol,* the shift is away from focusing on numeric targets, but rather toward a healthy diet pattern like the Mediterranean or the Dietary Approaches to Stop Hypertension (DASH) diets. The emphasis is now on statin (drug) therapy for people who are deemed to be at high risk for cardiovascular disease (CVD). The LDL cholesterol number is no longer the main consideration in treatment. Some experts, however, strongly disagree with these guidelines. They feel that the recommendations will increase the number of people on statin medications and will not be more effective than the previous target-based guidelines (see Table 10.3, page 389). The current recommendations specifically target four high-risk groups for whom statin drugs are recommended:

1. People with preexisting CVD (those who have suffered angina, a heart attack, stroke, or a transient ischemic attack or mini stroke, and anyone who has had a cardiovascular procedure such as angioplasty to widen arteries)

2. Type 2 diabetics between 40 and 75 years of age

3. People with very high LDL cholesterol (190 mg/dL or above)

4. People between 40 and 75 without CVD or diabetes who have a 10-year risk of CVD of at least 7.5 percent based on an *online risk calculator* (see risk assessment in the next column)

Lowering LDL cholesterol, however, is still important. The current guidelines by the AHA encourage people to consume no more than 5 to 6 percent of total daily calories from saturated fat and less than 1 percent from trans fats.

The *healthy lifestyle* guidelines incorporate adequate physical activity, weight management, and dietary patterns that emphasize vegetables, fruits, whole grains, low-fat dairy products, fish, poultry, and nuts. People should limit red meat, processed foods, saturated and trans fats, sodium, and sugary foods and beverages. Physical activity performed on a regular basis, 40 minutes of exercise 3 to 4 days a week, is also encouraged in the guidelines.

Physicians are encouraged to treat *obesity* as a disease and actively work with obese patients to help them lose weight. Telling patients that they need to lose weight is not enough. Physicians should prescribe diets that moderately decrease caloric intake and prescribe a minimum of 2.5 hours of physical activity per week. People need to learn to balance caloric intake and physical activity to achieve and maintain a healthy body weight. All Americans should calculate their BMI at least once a year and keep their BMI under 25. Weight loss surgery may be recommended for extremely obese individuals whose health may be at risk.

A *risk assessment* that calculates the potential 10-year risk for heart attack and stroke is available online at www.heart.org/gglRisk/main_en_US.html. The risk calculator helps health care practitioners evaluate people between the ages of 40 and 79. A prediction equation was developed from community-based populations and includes race, gender, age, total cholesterol, HDL cholesterol, blood pressure, blood pressure medication use, diabetes status, and smoking status. People need to aim for normal blood pressure and blood glucose levels and avoid use of and exposure to tobacco products. If the 10-year risk is 7.5 or higher, the person is encouraged to take a statin. More than 30 million Americans are believed to exceed this rating, including many who have never had any symptoms of CVD. The 7.5 number does not provide an automatic prescription, but rather is a start to the process, not an end.

According to the AHA, "the goal is not to get more people on statins," but to make sure the drugs are used by the people who can benefit from them. *Some health care experts welcome these*

(continued)

recommendations, while others vigorously oppose them because they deemphasize target numbers for the various cholesterol subcategories. Many physicians now use a combination of the two.

Regardless of the effectiveness of statins, medications by themselves cannot replace a healthy lifestyle. A multifaceted healthy lifestyle approach has been proven in research studies to be most effective in managing heart disease and stroke risk. Before you consider taking a statin drug, discuss with your physician steps that you can implement to reduce the risk through a healthier lifestyle.

SOURCE: American Heart Association, "Understanding the New Prevention Guidelines," http://www.heart.org/HEARTORG/Conditions/Understanding-the-New-Guidelines_UCM_458155_article.jsp#.VrEF-Vm3XW4. Also see the Heart Attack Risk Calculator, www.heart.org/gglRisk/main_en_US.html, accessed february 2, 2016.

Table 10.3 Cholesterol Guidelines

	Amount	Rating
Total Cholesterol	<200 mg/dL	Desirable
	200–239 mg/dL	Borderline high
	≥240 mg/dL	High risk
LDL Cholesterol	<100 mg/dL	Optimal
	100–129 mg/dL	Near or greater than optimal
	130–159 mg/dL	Borderline high
	160–189 mg/dL	High
	≥190 mg/dL	Very high
HDL Cholesterol	<40 mg/dL	Low (high risk)
	≥60 mg/dL	High (low risk)

From National Cholesterol Education Program.

75 percent blocked. In many cases, the first symptom is sudden death.

The general recommendation has been to keep the total cholesterol levels at less than 200 mg/dL. A cholesterol level between 200 and 239 mg/dL is borderline high, and levels of 240 mg/dL and above indicate high risk for disease (Table 10.3). Based on 2016 data from the AHA, more than 100 million U.S. adults 20 years of age and older have a total blood cholesterol level at or above 200 mg/dL, with 31 million of them with a level above 240 mg/dL.

Preventive medicine practitioners often recommend a range between 160 and 180 mg/dL for total cholesterol. Furthermore, in the Framingham Heart Study (a 60-year ongoing project in the community of Framingham, Massachusetts), not a single individual with a total cholesterol level of 150 mg/dL or lower has had a heart attack.

As important as it is, total cholesterol is not the best predictor for cardiovascular risk. Many heart attacks occur in people with only slightly elevated total cholesterol. More significant is the way in which cholesterol is carried in the bloodstream. Cholesterol is transported primarily in the form of LDL and HDL.

LDL ("bad") cholesterol tends to release cholesterol, which then may penetrate the lining of the arteries and speed the process of atherosclerosis. The National Cholesterol Education Program (NCEP) guidelines given in Table 10.3 state that an LDL cholesterol value below 100 mg/dL is optimal.

Even when more LDL cholesterol is present than the cells can use, cholesterol seems not to cause a problem until it is oxidized by free radicals (see discussion under "Antioxidants" in Chapter 3, page 118). After cholesterol is oxidized, white blood cells invade the arterial wall, take up the cholesterol, and clog the arteries.

LDL cholesterol particles are of two types: large, or pattern A, and small, or pattern B. Small particles are thought to pass through the inner lining of the coronary arteries more readily, thereby increasing the risk for a heart attack. A predominance of small particles can lead to a sixfold increase in the risk for CHD.

A genetic variation of LDL cholesterol, known as lipoprotein-a or Lp(a), is also noteworthy because a high level of these particles promotes blood clots and earlier development of atherosclerosis. It is thought that certain substances in the arterial wall interact with Lp(a) and lead to premature formation of plaque. About 10 percent of the population has elevated levels of Lp(a). Only medications help decrease Lp(a), and drug options should be discussed with a physician.

Intermediate-density lipoprotein (IDL) is also of concern because these midsize particles are more likely to cause atherosclerosis than a similar amount of LDL cholesterol. For individuals at risk for heart disease, a comprehensive blood lipid profile that includes total cholesterol, HDL cholesterol, LDL cholesterol, Lp(a), IDL, and size pattern (A and B) is recommended.

In a process known as **reverse cholesterol transport**, HDLs act as "scavengers," removing cholesterol from the body and preventing plaque from forming in the arteries. The strength of HDL is in the protein molecules found in its coating. When HDL comes in contact with cholesterol-filled cells, these protein molecules attach to the cells and take their cholesterol.

The belief is that the more HDL ("good") cholesterol, the better. HDL cholesterol is thought to offer some protection against heart disease. The recommended HDL cholesterol value to decrease the risk for CHD is at least 40 mg/dL. An HDL cholesterol level above 60 mg/dL helps lower the risk for CHD.

Fourteen subgroups of HDL particles have been identified, falling into HDL2 and HDL3 categories. HDL2 are larger

GLOSSARY

Reverse cholesterol transport A process in which HDL molecules attract cholesterol and carry it to the liver, where it is changed to bile and eventually excreted in the stool.

particles that carry cholesterol from the arterial wall to the liver for disposal and are more effective in doing so than HDL3 particles. HDL3 particles, however, seem to protect against cholesterol oxidation that results in atherosclerosis.

For the most part, HDL cholesterol is determined genetically. Generally, women have higher levels than men. Because the female sex hormone estrogen tends to raise HDL, premenopausal women have a much lower incidence of heart disease. African American children and adult men have higher HDL values than Caucasians. HDL cholesterol also decreases with age.

Having high HDL cholesterol improves the cholesterol profile and lessens the risk for CHD. Habitual aerobic exercise, a diet high in omega-3 fatty acids, weight loss, no smoking, and modest alcohol intake help raise HDL cholesterol and lower the risk of heart attacks and stroke. Drug therapy may also promote higher HDL cholesterol levels. It is less clear, however, whether increasing HDL with medications is effective as scientific studies have failed to prove that such therapy lowers the risk. Niacin also helps convert HDL3 to HDL2.

Improved HDL cholesterol is clearly related to a regular aerobic exercise program (preferably high intensity, or above 6 metabolic equivalents, for at least 20 minutes three times per week—see Chapter 6). Individual responses to aerobic exercise differ, but generally, the more you exercise, the higher your HDL cholesterol level.

Some evidence questions whether HDL cholesterol truly decreases the risk for CHD. One particular study indicated that people who inherit genes for a higher HDL level do not have less heart disease than those who inherit genes that give them a lower level.[6] The researchers stated that they are not questioning the well-established finding that higher HDL levels are associated with lower heart disease risk. The relationship, however, may not be causative. It is plausible that instead of directly reducing the risk for heart disease, a high HDL level may be a sign that other factors are at play that make heart disease less likely. Another possibility is that some subgroups of HDL molecules do, in fact, protect against heart disease. At present, additional research is required to answer this question.

Counteracting Cholesterol

The average adult in the United States consumes between 400 and 600 mg of dietary cholesterol (cholesterol already in food—see Table 10.4) daily. The body, however, manufactures more than that. Saturated and trans fats raise cholesterol levels more than anything else in the diet. It has been estimated that for every additional 200 mg of dietary cholesterol consumed, blood cholesterol increases by about four points, whereas the average saturated fat consumption in the United States generates approximately 1,000 mg of cholesterol per day.

Dietary cholesterol in foods such as eggs and shrimp is said to be different than the LDL cholesterol in the blood and is no longer viewed as a factor that raises heart disease risk. The exception is people who are "high-responders" to dietary

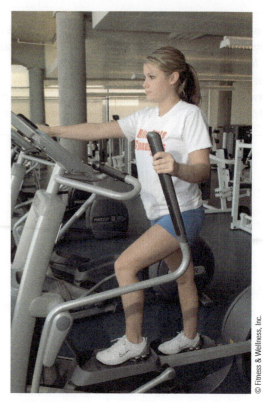

Habitual aerobic exercise helps increase HDL cholesterol ("good" cholesterol).

© Fitness & Wellness, Inc.

cholesterol. Individuals whose LDL cholesterol level is 160 mg/dL or higher, or who have CHD or other risk factors, are encouraged to keep daily dietary cholesterol consumption below 200 mg per day.

There are significant individual differences as to how people handle cholesterol. Some people can have a higher-than-normal intake of saturated and trans fats and still maintain normal levels. Others, who have a lower intake, can have abnormally high levels. As seen in Table 10.4, saturated fats are found mostly in meats and dairy products. Poultry and fish contain less saturated fat than beef does but should be eaten in moderation (about 3 to 6 ounces per day—see Chapter 3).

In a 10-year study of more than 500,000 men and women over the age of 50, those who ate the most red meat (an average of 4.5 ounces per day) had a much higher risk of dying from heart disease and cancer: Men had a 31 percent higher risk of dying during the study period, whereas women had a 50 percent higher risk of dying from heart disease during this time.[7] Cancer risk was about 20 percent higher among men and women who consumed the most red meat.

Unsaturated fats are mainly of plant origin and cannot be converted to cholesterol. Omega-3-rich fish meals (found in salmon, tuna, and mackerel) also help lower **triglycerides** and increase HDL cholesterol.[8] Because of the cardioprotective benefits of omega-3 fatty acids, the AHA recommends eating oily fish at least twice per week. As illustrated in Figure 10.6, baseline blood levels of omega-3 fatty acids are inversely related to the risk of sudden cardiac death.[9]

Table 10.4 Cholesterol and Saturated Fat Content of Selected Foods

Food	Serving Size	Cholesterol (mg)	Sat. Fat (gr)
Bacon	2 slices	30	2.7
Beans (all types)	any	—	—
Beef—lean, fat trimmed off	3 oz	75	6.0
Beef heart (cooked)	3 oz	150	1.6
Beef liver (cooked)	3 oz	255	1.3
Butter	1 tsp	12	0.4
Caviar	1 oz	85	—
Cheese			
American	2 oz	54	11.2
Cheddar	2 oz	60	12.0
Cottage (1% fat)	1 cup	10	0.4
Cottage (4% fat)	1 cup	31	6.0
Cream	2 oz	62	6.0
Muenster	2 oz	54	10.8
Parmesan	2 oz	38	9.3
Swiss	2 oz	52	10.0
Chicken (no skin)	3 oz	45	0.4
Chicken liver	3 oz	472	1.1
Chicken thigh, wing	3 oz	69	3.3
Egg (yolk)	1 lrg	218	1.6
Frankfurter	2	90	11.2
Fruits	any	—	—
Grains (all types)	any	—	—
Halibut, flounder	3 oz	43	0.7
Ice cream	½ cup	27	4.4
Lamb	3 oz	60	7.2
Lard	1 tsp	5	1.9
Lobster	3 oz	170	0.5
Margarine (all vegetable)	1 tsp	—	0.7
Mayonnaise	1 tbsp	10	2.1
Milk			
Skim	1 cup	5	0.3
Low fat (2%)	1 cup	18	2.9
Whole	1 cup	34	5.1
Nuts	1 oz	—	1.0
Oysters	3 oz	42	—
Salmon	3 oz	30	0.8
Scallops	3 oz	29	—
Sherbet	½ cup	7	1.2
Shrimp	3 oz	128	0.1
Trout	3 oz	45	2.1
Tuna (canned—drained)	3 oz	55	—
Turkey, dark meat	3 oz	60	0.6
Turkey, light meat	3 oz	50	0.4
Vegetables (except avocado)	any	—	—

Individuals in the highest quartile of omega-3 fatty acids (mean = 6.87 percent of total fatty acids) have a 90 percent reduction in sudden cardiac death risk as compared with those in the lowest quartile (mean = 3.58 percent of total fatty acids).

Figure 10.6 Relative risk of sudden cardiac death by baseline blood level of omega-3 fatty-acids (FA).

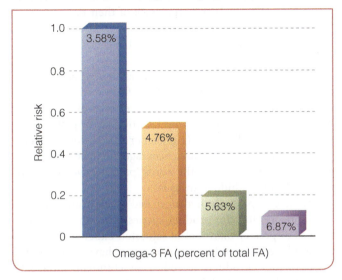

Trans Fat

Foods that contain trans-fatty acids, hydrogenated fat, or partially hydrogenated vegetable oil should be avoided. Studies indicate that these foods elevate LDL cholesterol as much as saturated fats do, but even worse, they lower HDL cholesterol. Trans fat also increases triglycerides, contributes to inflammation, and increases the tendency to form blood clots inside blood vessels. These changes contribute not only to heart disease, but also to gallstone formation. Trans fats are found primarily in fried, baked, packaged, and **processed foods**.

Food companies use trans fat because it is inexpensive to produce, is easy to use, lasts a long time, and adds taste and texture to food. Restaurants and fast-food chains have used oils with trans fat because it can be used repeatedly in commercial fryers.

Hydrogen frequently is added to monounsaturated and polyunsaturated fats to increase shelf life and to solidify them so that they are more spreadable. Hydrogenation can change the position of hydrogen atoms along the carbon chain, transforming the fat into a trans-fatty acid. Margarine and spreads, canned frosting, coffee creamer, chips, commercially produced crackers and cookies, and fast foods can contain trans-fatty acids. Small amounts of trans fat are also found naturally in some meats, dairy products, and other animal-based foods.

The AHA has issued dietary guidelines recommending that people limit trans fat intake to less than 1 percent of total daily caloric intake. This amount represents about 1.5 grams of trans fat a day for a 1,500-calorie diet, 2 grams for 2,000

GLOSSARY

Triglycerides Fats formed by glycerol and three fatty acids.

Processed food A food that has been chemically altered from its natural state through additives such as flavors, flavor enhancers, colors, binders, preservatives, stabilizers, emulsifiers, and fillers or has been manufactured through combination or other methods.

daily calories, and 3 grams for 3,000 daily calories. Because the FDA now requires that all food labels list the trans fat content, people can keep better track of their daily trans fat intake by paying attention to food labels. Additional information on trans fat is found under the "Trans Fatty Acids" section in Chapter 3 (see page 92).

The FDA allows food manufacturers to label any product that has less than half a gram of trans fat per serving as zero. Be aware that if you eat three or four servings of a particular food near a half a gram of trans fat, you may be getting your maximum daily allowance (1 gram per 1,000 calories of daily caloric intake). Thus, you are encouraged to look at the list of ingredients and search for the words "partially hydrogenated" as an indicator of hidden trans fat.

The labels "partially hydrogenated" and "trans-fatty acids" indicate that the product carries a health risk just as high as or greater than that of saturated fat. Now that trans fats are listed on food labels, companies have reformulated many of their products to reduce or eliminate these fats. Some products once high in trans fats now have none or less than half a gram, so they don't have to list them on the label. As a consumer, you are encouraged to check food labels often to obtain current information. Table 10.5 lists the average trans fat content of some foods. These values may vary among brands according to food formulation and ingredients and may change as manufacturers continue to alter food formulations to further decrease or eliminate trans fat content.

Table 10.5 Average Trans Fat Content of Selected Foods*

Food Item	Amount	Grams
Biscuit, breakfast	1	0.5
Bisquick (pancake and baking mix)	⅓ cup mix	1.0
Burrito, steak or ground beef, Taco Bell	1	0.0–1.0
Butter	1 tbsp	0.0–0.3
Country Fried Steak, KFC	1	1.0
Double Quarter Pounder w/cheese, McDonalds	1	2.5
Double Whopper w/cheese, Burger King	1	3.5
Express Taco Salad w/chips	1	1.0
Frosting, canned		0.0–1.5
Margarine, stick	1 tbsp	2.0
Margarine, tub	1 tbsp	0.0–0.5
Milkshakes	1	1.0
Pop Secret Microwave Popcorn	4.5 cups popped	5.0
Tootsie rolls	6 mini	0.5

NOTE: Trans fat intake should be limited to no more than 1 percent of total daily caloric intake or the equivalent of 1 gram per 1,000 calories of energy intake.

*Trans fat content in food items has been decreasing significantly as food manufacturers have decreased or eliminated the content in their products because of FDA regulations that require trans fats to be listed on food labels. Trans fat content also varies between different brands based on food formulation and ingredients. Check food labels regularly to obtain current information.

Lowering LDL Cholesterol

LDL cholesterol levels higher than ideal can be lowered through dietary changes, by losing body fat, by taking medication, and by participating in a regular aerobic exercise program. Research has shown a higher relative risk of mortality in unfit individuals with low cholesterol than fit people with high cholesterol. The lowest mortality rate, of course, is seen in fit people with low total cholesterol levels.

In terms of dietary modifications, a diet lower in saturated fat, trans fats, and refined carbohydrates and high in fiber is recommended. A top priority of the American diet is to replace saturated fat with polyunsaturated and monounsaturated fats because the latter tend to decrease LDL cholesterol and increase HDL cholesterol. Total saturated fat intake should be less than 6 percent of the total daily caloric intake, preferably much lower while on a cholesterol-lowering diet. Trans fat intake should be less than 1 percent of daily caloric intake. Exercise is important because dietary manipulation by itself is not as effective in lowering LDL cholesterol as a combination of diet plus aerobic exercise.

Furthermore, "moderate" fat-intake diets (25 to 35 percent of total caloric intake) are better for heart health (as long as most of it is unsaturated fats) than are low-fat diets or highly refined carbohydrate diets. As you increase the intake of unsaturated fats, be sure to substitute these for some other less healthy foods (red meat, sausages, hamburgers, organ meats, butter, margarines, whole-milk products, etc.); otherwise, weight gain will ensue. Excessive carbohydrate intake, especially refined carbohydrates, raises triglycerides, and as triglycerides go up, HDL cholesterol typically decreases.

HOEGER KEY TO WELLNESS

Dietary recommendations to control blood lipids include a diet that includes polyunsaturated and monounsaturated fats, whole grains, fruits, and vegetables and avoidance of trans fat, saturated fat, and refined/processed carbohydrates (including sugar).

To lower LDL cholesterol significantly, total daily fiber intake must be in the range of 25 to 38 grams per day (see "Fiber" in Chapter 3), and total fat consumption can be in the range of 25 to 35 percent of total daily caloric intake—as long as most of the fat is unsaturated fat and the average cholesterol consumption is lower than 200 mg. Increasing consumption of cholesterol-lowering foods such as plant sterols (added to some spreads and salad dressings), soy protein, nuts (walnuts, almonds, macadamia nuts, peanuts, pecans, and pistachio nuts), vegetables, fruits, whole grains, and foods high in soluble fiber (oats, legumes, and barley) further accelerates the rate of LDL cholesterol reduction. Science also points to a decreased risk of dying from CVD by 31 percent among people who consume seven or more servings of fruits and vegetables per day as compared to those who consume less than one (death rates from all causes were down 42 percent and cancer by 25 percent).[10] Keep in mind that as you add some of these foods to your diet, you have to take other, less healthy foods out.

Among people in the United States, the average fiber intake is less than 15 grams per day. Fiber—in particular, the soluble type—has been shown to lower cholesterol. Soluble fiber dissolves in water and forms a gel-like substance that encloses food particles. This property helps bind and excrete fats from the body. Soluble fibers also bind intestinal bile acids that could be recycled into additional cholesterol. Soluble fibers are found primarily in oats, fruits, barley, legumes, and psyllium. The incidence of heart disease is very low in populations in which daily fiber intake exceeds 30 grams per day, resulting in about a 41 percent reduction in heart attacks.[11]

Psyllium, a grain that is added to some multigrain breakfast cereals, also helps lower LDL cholesterol. As little as 3 grams of psyllium daily can lower LDL cholesterol by 20 percent. Commercially available fiber supplements that contain psyllium (e.g., Metamucil) can be used to increase soluble fiber intake. Three tablespoons daily add about 10 grams of soluble fiber to the diet.

When attempting to lower LDL cholesterol, moderate consumption of healthy fats (polyunsaturated and monounsaturated) is encouraged. A drawback of very low-fat diets (less than 25 percent fat) is that they tend to lower HDL cholesterol and increase triglycerides. If HDL cholesterol is already low, polyunsaturated and monounsaturated fats should be added to the diet. Examples of food items that are high in monounsaturated and polyunsaturated fats are nuts and olive, canola, corn, and soybean oils. The table of nutritive values in Appendix B (available in MindTap at www.cengagebrain.com) can be used to determine food items that are high in monounsaturated and polyunsaturated fats (see also Figure 3.9, page 106).

The NCEP guidelines for people who are trying to decrease LDL cholesterol allow for a diet with up to 35 percent of calories from fat, including 10 percent from polyunsaturated fats and 20 percent from monounsaturated fats. If you are attempting to lower LDL cholesterol, saturated fats should be kept to an absolute minimum.

Margarines and salad dressings that contain stanol ester, a plant-derived compound that interferes with cholesterol absorption in the intestine, are now also on the market. Make sure, however, that they do not contain significant amounts of saturated fat, trans fat, or partially hydrogenated oils. Over the course of several weeks, daily intake of about 3 grams of margarine or 6 tablespoons of salad dressing containing stanol ester lowers LDL cholesterol by more than 10 percent. Dietary guidelines to lower LDL cholesterol levels are provided in the accompanying box on page 395.

The best prescription for controlling blood lipids is the combination of a healthy diet, a sound aerobic exercise program, and weight control. If this does not work, a physician can recommend appropriate drug therapies based upon a blood test to analyze the various subcategories of lipoproteins.

The NCEP guidelines recommend that people consider drug therapy if, after 6 months on a diet low in cholesterol and trans and saturated fats, cholesterol remains unacceptably high. An unacceptable level is an LDL cholesterol above 190 mg/dL for individuals with fewer than two risk factors and no signs of heart disease. For individuals with more than two risk factors and with a history of heart disease, LDL cholesterol above 160 mg/dL is unacceptable.

10 Foods that Promote or Prevent Premature Mortality

Research published in the prestigious *Journal of the American Medical Association* in 2017 suggests that too much intake or substandard intake of 10 specific foods and their respective nutrients contributes to nearly half of all U. S. deaths from heart disease, strokes, and type 2 diabetes.

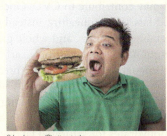

Odua Images/Shutterstock.com

Overeaten foods or nutrients (bad) to eat less of:	Diet-deficient foods and nutrients (good) to eat more of:
1. Salt (sodium) and salty foods	5. Nuts and seeds
2. Processed meats (e.g., hot dogs, sausages, bacon, ham, bologna)	6. Omega-3 fatty acids
3. Sugar-sweetened drinks	7. Vegetables
4. Unprocessed red meats	8. Fruits
	9. Whole grains
	10. Polyunsaturated fats

High sodium intake had the highest correlation with premature mortality, linked to about 10 percent of all deaths. Excessive processed-meat consumption and not eating enough nuts/seeds and seafood were each linked to roughly 8 percent of the deaths.

SOURCE: R. Micha, et al., "Association Between Dietary Factors and Mortality From Heart Disease, Stroke, and Type 2 Diabetes in the United States," *Journal of the American Medical Association* 317 (2017): 912-924.

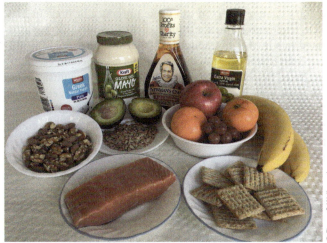

© Fitness & Wellness, Inc.

As long as the number of servings and caloric intake are not increased, substituting high-saturated fat and trans fat products, simple carbohydrates, and refined sugars with unsaturated fat and complex carbohydrate products will significantly decrease the risk for cardiovascular disease.

Saturated Fat Replacement in the Diet

For years people have known that saturated fat raises LDL cholesterol, but researchers have looked at other foods consumed in the American diet that have replaced saturated fat and may contribute to CVD. Once people learned that saturated fats were unhealthy, instead of consuming more fruits, vegetables, legumes, and whole grains, many increased consumption of "low-fat" simple carbohydrates and refined sugars (low-fat varieties of white breads, rolls, cereals, cookies, ice cream, cakes, and desserts). Unknown to most consumers is the fact that desserts are among the top saturated fat contributors in the American diet. Substituting simple/refined carbohydrates for saturated fat doesn't lower LDL cholesterol as effectively as substituting unsaturated fats or even proteins from plant sources with small amounts of fish.

The data show that exchanging refined carbohydrates with high glycemic index values for saturated fat exacerbates blood lipid problems, including higher LDL cholesterol, a reduction in HDL cholesterol, and higher triglycerides. Scientists believe that high-refined-carbohydrate diets increase palmitoleic acid, a minor monounsaturated fatty acid that actually behaves like a saturated fatty acid, increasing LDL cholesterol. Data also indicate that each additional daily serving of sugar-sweetened drinks increases heart disease risk by up to 19 percent.

The evidence shows that people who cut back on saturated fat but increased intake of whole grains and high-fiber fruits and vegetables were 12 percent less likely to have a heart attack with every 5 percent increase in calories from high-fiber foods. On the other hand, those who substituted high-glycemic carbohydrates for saturated fat increased heart attack risk by 33 percent for every 5 percent increase in calories from high-glycemic, low-fiber carbohydrates (such as white bread, pasta, potatoes, and sweets).[12]

The best recommendation is not to limit fat consumption in the diet to the minimum but to maintain a total fat intake of around 25 to 35 percent of total calories, with a primary shift toward polyunsaturated fats. The single most effective dietary change a person can make to reduce or prevent high LDL cholesterol is to substitute polyunsaturated fats for saturated fats in the diet, followed by substituting monounsaturated fats, with the lowest benefit seen in people replacing saturated fat with whole grains.[13] To increase polyunsaturated fat consumption, choose fish, nuts, seeds, and vegetable oils (corn, sunflower, soybean) that are liquid at room temperature (with the exception of tropical oils, including coconut, palm, and palm kernel oils). People with a primarily Mediterranean-style diet have a 50 percent to 70 percent lower risk of suffering or dying from CVD.

At present, it is unknown whether the cardioprotective benefits are the result of limiting saturated fat intake or increasing polyunsaturated fat consumption. Thus, moderate "healthy fat" intake (not low fat)—along with decreased refined carbohydrates and, in most cases, decreased caloric intake—are encouraged. The issue merits further research involving clinical trials (rather than observational studies) before clear answers can be obtained.

Behavior Modification Planning

Blood Chemistry Test Guidelines

People who have never had a blood chemistry test should do so to establish a baseline for future reference. The blood test should include total cholesterol, LDL cholesterol, HDL cholesterol, triglycerides, and blood glucose.

Following an initial normal baseline test at no later than age 20, for a person who adheres to the recommended dietary and exercise guidelines, a blood analysis at least every 5 years prior to age 40 should suffice. A physician may recommend more frequent testing if the person has high cholesterol or is at high risk for heart disease and stroke. After age 40, a blood lipid test is recommended every year in conjunction with a regular preventive medicine physical examination.

A single baseline test is not necessarily a valid measure. Cholesterol levels vary from month to month and sometimes even from day to day. If the initial test reveals cholesterol abnormalities, the test should be repeated within a few weeks to confirm the results.

Try It

Blood chemistry tests are available at many wellness centers on college campuses for under $25 for a comprehensive test that includes total cholesterol, LDL cholesterol, HDL cholesterol, triglycerides, and blood glucose levels. Have you had your blood test done, and are you aware of your blood lipid profile?

Elevated Triglycerides

Triglycerides are the major form of fat stored in the human body. A triglyceride consists of three fatty acid molecules combined with a molecule of glycerol. Triglycerides make up most of the fat in our diet and most of the fat that circulates in the blood. In combination with cholesterol, triglycerides speed up formation of plaque in the arteries. Triglycerides are carried in the bloodstream primarily by VLDLs and chylomicrons. Triglycerides per se don't end up in the atherosclerotic plaque. Chylomicrons are broken down in the blood into fatty acids and remnant-free, cholesterol-rich particles. Fatty acids are stored in muscle or adipose tissue (fat) and scavenger cells that do contribute to atherosclerosis then take up the remnant particles.

Although they are found in poultry skin, lunch meats, and shellfish, these fatty acids are manufactured mainly in the liver from refined sugars, starches, and alcohol. A high intake of alcohol and sugars (honey and fruit juices included) significantly raises triglyceride levels.

To lower triglycerides, avoid pastries, candies, soft drinks, fruit juices, white bread, pasta, and alcohol. In addition, cutting down on overall fat consumption, quitting smoking, reducing weight (if overweight), and doing aerobic exercise are helpful measures. Omega-3 fatty acids also help, but doses higher than those found in fish are required. The AHA recommends 2 to 4

Behavior Modification Planning

Dietary Guidelines to Lower LDL Cholesterol.

I PLAN TO

I DID IT

❑ ❑ Minimize the use of simple and refined carbohydrates (including sugars) and processed foods.

❑ ❑ Consume between 25 and 38 grams of fiber daily, including a minimum of 10 grams of soluble fiber (good sources are oats, fruits, barley, legumes, and psyllium).

❑ ❑ Increase consumption of vegetables, fruits, whole grains, and beans.

❑ ❑ Consume red meats (no more than 3 ounces per serving) fewer than three times per week and limit (less than 1.5 ounces per serving) processed meats to once per week or none at all.

❑ ❑ Do not consume commercially baked foods.

❑ ❑ Avoid foods that contain trans-fatty acids, hydrogenated fat, or partially hydrogenated vegetable oil.

❑ ❑ Increase intake of omega-3 fatty acids (see Chapter 3) by eating two to three omega-3-rich fish meals per week.

❑ ❑ Consume 25 grams of soy protein a day.

❑ ❑ Drink low-fat milk (1 percent or less fat, preferably) and use low-fat dairy products.

❑ ❑ Do not use coconut oil, palm oil, or cocoa butter.

❑ ❑ Consume nuts (1.5 ounces) on a daily basis (almonds, walnuts, peanuts, hazelnuts, or pistachio nuts).

❑ ❑ Limit egg consumption to fewer than three eggs per week if your blood cholesterol is elevated or if your physician tells you that you are a "hyper-responder" to dietary cholesterol (people with normal blood cholesterol may consume an egg on most days of the week).

❑ ❑ Use margarines and salad dressings that contain stanol ester instead of butter and regular margarine.

❑ ❑ Bake, broil, grill, poach, or steam food instead of frying.

❑ ❑ Refrigerate cooked meat before adding to other dishes. Remove fat hardened in the refrigerator before mixing the meat with other foods.

❑ ❑ Avoid fatty sauces made with butter, cream, or cheese.

❑ ❑ Maintain recommended body weight.

Try It

Dietary guidelines for health and wellness were thoroughly discussed in Chapter 3. How have your dietary habits changed since studying these guidelines, and how well do they support the above recommendations to lower LDL cholesterol?

MINDTAP From Cengage   **Complete This Online**
Visit **www.cengagebrain.com** to access MindTap, a complete digital course that includes interactive quizzes, videos, and more.

grams of fish oil daily under a physician's supervision. A group of medications known as fibrates also help lower triglycerides by reducing the liver's production of VLDL and enhancing the removal of triglycerides from the blood.

The desirable blood triglyceride level is less than 150 mg/dL (Table 10.6). For people with cardiovascular problems, this level should be below 100 mg/dL. Levels above 1,000 mg/dL pose an immediate risk for potentially fatal sudden inflammation of the pancreas.

LDL Phenotype B

Some people consistently have slightly elevated triglyceride levels (above 140 mg/dL) and HDL cholesterol levels below

Table 10.6 Triglycerides Guidelines

Amount	Rating
<150 mg/dL	Desirable
150–199 mg/dL	Borderline-high
200–499 mg/dL	High
≥500 mg/dL	Very high

SOURCE: National Heart, Lung and Blood Institute.

35 mg/dL. About 80 percent of these people have a genetic condition called LDL phenotype B. Although the blood lipids may not be notably high, these people are at higher risk for atherosclerosis and CHD.

Critical Thinking

Are you aware of your blood lipid profile? If not, what is keeping you from getting a blood chemistry test? What are the benefits of having it done now rather than later in life?

Cholesterol-Lowering Medications

Effective medications are available to treat elevated cholesterol and triglycerides. Most notable among them are the statins group (Lipitor®, Mevacor®, Crestor®, Livalo®, Pravachol®, Lescol®, Crestor®, and Zocor®), which can lower cholesterol by up to 60 percent in 2 to 3 months. Statins work by inhibiting an enzyme that regulates the amount of cholesterol produced by the liver. They also decrease triglycerides and produce a small increase in HDL levels. The drug Tricor® is commonly used to lower triglycerides.

The guidelines by the American Heart Association and the American College of Cardiology recommend that people at high risk for CVD disease be treated with statin therapy. Unless at high risk, many experts feel that, in general, it is better to lower LDL cholesterol without medication because drugs often cause undesirable side effects. Many people with heart disease must take cholesterol-lowering medication, but medication is best combined with lifestyle changes to augment the cholesterol-lowering effect. For example, when Zocor® was taken alone over 3 months, LDL cholesterol decreased by 30 percent; but when a Mediterranean diet was adopted in combination with Zocor® therapy, LDL cholesterol decreased by 41 percent.[14] In 2012, the FDA added safety alerts to the prescribing information of statins. Although rare among the millions of people who take these medications, the adverse effects include memory loss, cognitive impairment like forgetfulness and confusion, higher blood sugar levels that may lead to a diagnosis of diabetes, and muscle pain. Anyone starting treatment with statin drugs should be aware of these side effects.

Other drugs effective in reducing LDL cholesterol are bile acid sequestrants, which bind the cholesterol found in bile acids. Cholesterol subsequently is excreted in the stools. These drugs often are used in combination with statin drugs.

High dosages (1.5 to 3 grams per day) of nicotinic acid or niacin (a B vitamin) also help lower LDL cholesterol, Lp(a), and triglycerides and increase HDL cholesterol (change HDL3 to HDL2). Niacin in combination with some of the aforementioned drugs also exerts positive effects on IDL and pattern size. A fourth group of drugs, known as fibrates, is used primarily to lower triglycerides.

Elevated Homocysteine

Clinical data indicating that many heart attack and stroke victims have normal cholesterol levels have led researchers to look for other risk factors that may contribute to atherosclerosis. Although it is not a blood lipid, one of these factors is a high concentration of the amino acid **homocysteine** in the blood. It is thought to enhance the formation of plaque and the subsequent blockage of arteries.

The body uses homocysteine to help build proteins and carry out cellular metabolism. It is an intermediate amino acid in the interconversion of two other amino acids—methionine and cysteine. This interconversion requires the B vitamin folate (folic acid) and vitamins B_6 and B_{12}. Typically, homocysteine is metabolized rapidly, so it does not accumulate in the blood or damage the arteries. Still, many people have high blood levels of homocysteine. This might result from either a genetic inability to metabolize homocysteine or a deficiency in the vitamins required for its conversion.

Homocysteine typically is measured in micromoles per liter (μmol/L). Guidelines to interpret homocysteine levels are provided in Table 10.7. Individuals with high homocysteine levels above 15.0 μmol/L have about twice the risk of stroke as compared to individuals whose level is below 9.0 μmol/L. Homocysteine accumulation is theorized to be toxic because it may:

1. Cause damage to the inner lining of the arteries (the initial step in the process of atherosclerosis)

Table 10.7 Homocysteine Guidelines

Level (μmol/L)	Rating
<9.0	Desirable
9–12	Mild elevation
13–15	Elevated
>15	Extreme elevation

Adapted from K. S. McCully, "What You Must Know Now About Homocysteine," *Bottom Line/Health* 18 (January 2004): 7–9.

2. Stimulate the proliferation of cells that contribute to plaque formation
3. Encourage clotting, which could completely obstruct an artery and lead to a heart attack or stroke

Keeping homocysteine from accumulating in the blood seems to be as simple as eating the recommended daily servings of vegetables, fruits, grains, and some meat and legumes. Five servings of fruits and vegetables daily can provide sufficient levels of folate and vitamin B_6 to remove and clear homocysteine from the blood. Vitamin B_{12} is found primarily in animal flesh and animal products. Vitamin B_{12} deficiency is rarely a problem because 1 cup of milk or an egg provides the daily requirement. The body also recycles most of this vitamin; therefore, a deficiency takes years to develop. People who consume five servings

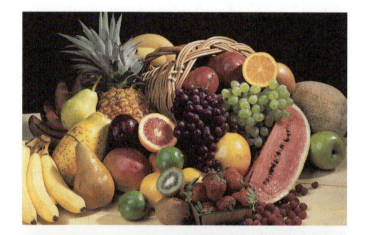

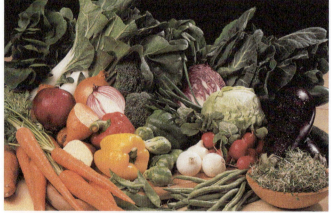

Ample amounts of fruits and vegetables provide the necessary nutrients to keep homocysteine from causing heart disease or stroke.

of fruits and vegetables daily are unlikely to derive extra benefits from a vitamin-B-complex supplement.

Increasing evidence that folate can prevent heart attacks has led to the recommendation that people consume 400 micrograms (mcg) per day—obtainable from five daily servings of fruits and vegetables. Unfortunately, estimates indicate that more than 80 percent of Americans do not get 400 mcg of folate per day (adequate folate intake also is critical for women of childbearing age to prevent birth defects).

Inflammation

In addition to homocysteine, scientists are looking at inflammation as a major risk factor for heart attacks. Sudden inflammation is the body's normal response to injury or infection. Typically, it lasts from a few days to a few weeks. It's the body's protective mechanism as it begins the healing process and sends immune cells and nutrients to areas where they're needed most. Inflammation kills or encapsulates microbes and helps form scar tissue and regenerate damaged tissue.

Short-term inflammation that you can see or feel as a result of a jammed finger, a sore muscle, a sprain, the flu, a fever, a scraped knee, or a cut is beneficial because it indicates that the body is working to fix the damage or respond to invading pathogens. This type of inflammation you can see or feel: a painful ankle, a bruised muscle, arthritis, heartburn, or tender gums.

Chronic low-grade inflammation, however, can occur in a variety of places throughout the body. It leads to continued elevated levels of toxins, and most people are unaware of its existence until damage occurs. Chronic inflammation persists for years or decades in people with unhealthy lifestyles. Physical inactivity, smoking, excessive body weight, a diet high in saturated fat, chronic stress, periodontal disease, and infections that produce no outward symptoms can all cause inflammation.

For years, it has been known that inflammation plays a role in CHD and that inflammation hidden deep in the body is a common trigger of heart attacks, even when cholesterol levels are normal or low and arterial plaque is minimal.

To evaluate ongoing inflammation in the body, physicians have turned to **C-reactive protein (CRP)**, a protein produced in the liver whose levels in the blood increase with injury or irritation (inflammation) anywhere in the body. Individuals with elevated CRP are more prone to cardiovascular events, even in the absence of elevated LDL cholesterol. The evidence shows that CRP blood levels elevate years before a first heart attack or stroke and that individuals with elevated CRP have twice the risk of a heart attack. The risk of a heart attack is even higher in people with both elevated CRP and cholesterol, resulting in an almost ninefold increase in risk (see Figure 10.7).

Because high CRP levels might be a better predictor of future heart attacks than high cholesterol alone, a test known as high-sensitivity CRP (hs-CRP) is used to detect small amounts of CRP in the blood. Results of the hs-CRP test provide a good measure of the probability of plaque rupturing within the arterial wall. The two main types of plaque are soft and hard. Soft plaque is the most likely to rupture. Ruptured plaque releases clots into the bloodstream that can

Figure 10.7 Relationships among CRP, cholesterol, and risk of CVD.

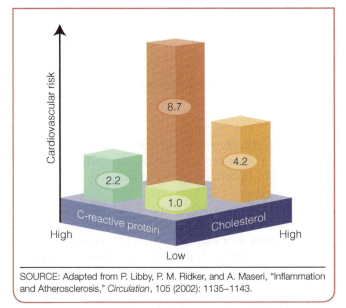

SOURCE: Adapted from P. Libby, P. M. Ridker, and A. Maseri, "Inflammation and Atherosclerosis," *Circulation*, 105 (2002): 1135–1143.

completely block the artery and lead to a heart attack or a stroke. About 75 percent of heart attacks are believed to be caused by plaque rupture. Other evidence has linked high CRP levels to high blood pressure and colon cancer.

Excessive intake of alcohol, hypertension, metabolic syndrome, type 2 diabetes, and very high-protein diets also increase CRP. Evidence further indicates that high-saturated fat fast food and trans fat increase CRP levels for several hours following the meal. And cooking meat and poultry at high temperatures creates damaged proteins called advanced glycation end products, which trigger inflammation. Further, some studies suggest that a high intake of omega-6 fatty acids may cause inflammation (also see Chapter 3, page 90). The current American diet is too high in omega-6 foods. Abdominal obesity (visceral fat) also increases inflammation. With weight loss, CRP levels decrease in proportion to the amount of fat lost.

An hs-CRP test is relatively inexpensive, and it is highly recommended for individuals at risk for heart attack. A level above 2 mg/L appears to be a better predictor of a heart attack than an LDL cholesterol level above 130 mg/dL. General guidelines for hs-CRP levels are given in Table 10.8.

A weakness of the hs-CRP test is that it does not detect differences between acute and chronic inflammation, and results may not be stable from day to day. An acute inflammation, for example, could be the result of a pulled muscle or a

GLOSSARY

Homocysteine An amino acid that, when allowed to accumulate in the blood, may lead to plaque formation and blockage of arteries.

C-reactive protein (CRP) A protein whose blood levels increase with inflammation, at times hidden deep in the body; elevation of this protein is an indicator of potential cardiovascular events.

Table 10.8 High-Sensitivity CRP Guidelines

Amount	Rating
<1 mg/L	Low risk
1–3 mg/L	Average risk
>3 mg/L	High risk

SOURCE: T. A. Pearson et al., "Markers of Inflammation and Cardiovascular Disease," *Circulation* 107 (2003): 499–511.

passing cold. It is chronic inflammation that increases heart disease risk. Thus, a new test that specifically detects chronic inflammation, lipoprotein phospholipase A2 (PAL2), may soon replace the hs-CRP test.

CRP levels decrease with statin drugs, which also lower cholesterol and reduce inflammation. A study on 17,802 apparently healthy men and women with LDL cholesterol below 130 mg/dL but CRP levels above 2.0 mg/L showed that a daily dose of the statin drug Crestor® reduced LDL cholesterol by 50 percent; CRP by 37 percent; and the risk of heart attack, stroke, and death by 54, 48, and 47 percent, respectively.[15]

Exercise, weight loss, proper nutrition, and quitting smoking are helpful in reducing hs-CRP. Omega-3 fatty acids inhibit proteins that cause inflammation. Aspirin therapy also helps by controlling inflammation.

Another newly approved test by the FDA that assesses risk for both CHD and strokes associated with atherosclerosis is the **PLAC blood test**. The test measures the level of Lp-PLA$_2$ (Lipoprotein-associated Phospholipase A$_2$), an enzyme produced inside the plaque when the arteries are inflamed, and indicates risk for plaque rupture. If the Lp-PLA$_2$ level is high, the plaque is more likely to rupture through the inside lining of the artery into the bloodstream where it may cause a clot that could lead to a heart attack or stroke.

Diabetes

Diabetes mellitus is a condition in which blood glucose is unable to enter the cells because the pancreas totally stops producing **insulin**, or it does not produce enough to meet the body's needs, or the cells develop **insulin resistance**. The role of insulin is to "unlock" the cells and escort glucose into the cell.

Almost half of the U.S. population has diabetes or is predisposed to diabetes (prediabetic). In 2017, more than 23 million adults were affected by diabetes, with an estimated 7.6 million undiagnosed cases and another 81.6 million considered to be prediabetics (see Figure 10.8). The rate of diabetes seems to be flattening out and has only increased slightly the last few years, most likely due to a similar slowdown in the increase of obesity. Overall, however, the prevalence has more than doubled the past 20 years. The Centers for Disease Control and Prevention predict that by 2050 one of every three Americans will have diabetes.

The incidence of CVD and death in the diabetic population is quite high. Two of three people with diabetes will die from CVD. People with chronically elevated blood glucose levels may have problems metabolizing fats, which can make

Figure 10.8 Prevalence of diabetes and prediabetes, United States, 2010–2017.

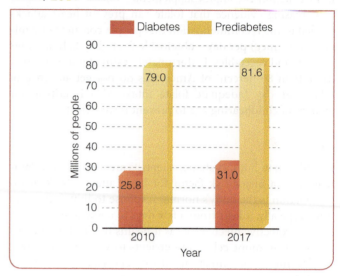

them more susceptible to atherosclerosis, CHD, heart attacks, high blood pressure, and stroke. People with diabetes also have lower HDL cholesterol and higher triglyceride levels.

Furthermore, chronic high blood sugar can lead to stroke, nerve damage, vision loss, kidney damage, sexual dysfunction, and decreased immune function (making people more susceptible to infections). Compared with those who do not have diabetes, diabetic patients are four times more likely to become blind and 20 times more likely to develop kidney failure. Nerve damage in the lower extremities decreases awareness of injury and infection, and a small, untreated sore can result in severe infection and gangrene, which can even lead to an amputation.

An 8-hour fasting blood glucose level above 125 mg/dL on two separate tests confirms a diagnosis of diabetes (Table 10.9). A level of 126 mg/dL or higher should be brought to the attention of a physician.

Types of Diabetes

Diabetes is one of two types: **type 1 diabetes**, or insulin-dependent diabetes mellitus, and **type 2 diabetes**, or non-insulin-dependent diabetes mellitus. Type 1 also has been called "juvenile diabetes" because it is found mainly in young people. With type 1 diabetes, the pancreas produces little or no insulin. With type 2 diabetes, either the pancreas does not produce sufficient insulin or it produces adequate amounts but the cells become insulin resistant, thereby keeping glucose from entering the cell. Type 2 diabetes accounts for 90 to 95 percent of all cases of diabetes.

Table 10.9 Blood Glucose Guidelines

Amount	Rating
≤100 mg/dL	Normal
101–125 mg/dL	Prediabetes
≥126 mg/dL	Diabetes*

*Confirmed by two tests on different days.

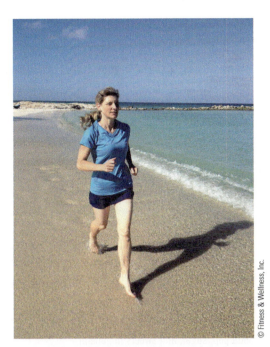

Regular physical activity increases insulin sensitivity and decreases the risk for diabetes.

Presently, more than one in ten American adults have diabetes. Although diabetes has a genetic predisposition, 60 to 80 percent of type 2 diabetes is related closely to overeating, obesity, and lack of physical activity. Type 2 diabetes, once limited primarily to overweight adults, now accounts for almost half of the new cases diagnosed in children. According to the CDC, one in three children born in the United States today will develop diabetes.

More than 80 percent of all people with type 2 diabetes are overweight or have a history of excessive weight. In most cases, this condition can be corrected through regular exercise, a special diet, and weight loss.

Exercise and Diabetes Management

Regular exercise is one of the best ways to lower blood glucose, improve insulin sensitivity, and decrease diabetes-related complications. Aerobic exercise is particularly effective in helping prevent type 2 diabetes. The protective effect is even greater in those with risk factors such as obesity, high blood pressure, and family propensity. The preventive effect is attributed to less body fat and to better sugar and fat metabolism resulting from the regular exercise program. At 3,500 calories of energy expenditure per week through exercise, the risk is cut in half versus that of a sedentary lifestyle.

Both moderate- and vigorous-intensity physical activity are associated with increased insulin sensitivity and decreased risk for diabetes. A single session of exercise makes the cells more sensitive to the effects of insulin for about 24 hours. Even three minutes of light physical activity for every 30 minutes of sitting time has been shown to yield lower blood glucose readings as compared to days when the subjects remained inactive. Thus, the key to increase and maintain proper insulin sensitivity is regularity of the exercise program. Failing to maintain habitual

physical activity voids these benefits. Thus, a simple aerobic exercise program (walking, cycling, or swimming four or five times per week) often is prescribed because it increases the body's sensitivity to insulin. Exercise guidelines for diabetic patients are discussed in detail in Chapter 9.

Strength-training is also increasingly used to help prevent and treat diabetes. During strength-training, muscles use primarily glucose to perform their work. Following a good strength-training workout, muscles will use more glucose during the next 48 hours. And as muscle mass increases with training, so does the body's ability to utilize blood glucose.

New evidence reported in 2016 indicates that low aerobic capacity and muscle strength at age 18 independently increase long-term risk for developing type 2 diabetes, with poor aerobic fitness being a slightly stronger risk factor.[16] Having both low aerobic capacity and muscle strength tripled the risk of future diabetes, even among individuals with normal body weight.

In fact, accumulating evidence indicates that increasing physical activity, losing excess weight, and improving nutrition are more effective to control diabetes and lower CVD risk than relying on drugs to manage the disease.[17] Furthermore, research suggests that diabetic patients are worse off when medications are used to decrease blood sugar levels and blood pressure to *normal or below-normal* levels. Accordingly, diabetic patients are strongly encouraged to adopt healthy lifestyle factors even if glucose levels are controlled with medication.

Stress is another risk factor for diabetes. The stress hormones cortisol and norepinephrine can bind to muscle and fat receptors, altering the way in which they respond. Individuals at risk for type 2 diabetes are encouraged to make stress management a priority of daily life.

Glycemic Index

Although complex carbohydrates are recommended in the diet, people with diabetes need to pay careful attention to the

---

GLOSSARY

PLAC blood test A blood test that measures the level of lipoprotein-associated phospholipase A2, an enzyme produced inside the plaque when the arteries are inflamed, and indicates risk for plaque rupture.

Diabetes mellitus A disease in which the body doesn't produce or utilize insulin properly.

Insulin A hormone secreted by the pancreas; essential for proper metabolism of blood glucose (sugar) and maintenance of blood glucose level.

Insulin resistance The inability of the cells to respond appropriately to insulin.

Type 1 diabetes Insulin-dependent diabetes mellitus, a condition in which the pancreas produces little or no insulin; also known as juvenile diabetes.

Type 2 diabetes Non-insulin-dependent diabetes mellitus, a condition in which insulin is not processed properly; also known as adult-onset diabetes.

Nutritional Guidelines to Prevent and Treat Diabetes

In addition to regular physical activity and proper weight management, a healthy meal plan is widely used to improve blood glucose and prevent and treat diabetes. Weight loss, even if only a 5 to 10 percent reduction in weight, can also make a notable difference in controlling blood sugar. These lifestyle changes (proper nutrition, physical activity, and weight loss) often allow diabetic patients to normalize their blood sugar level without the use of medication.

I PLAN TO   **I DID IT**

Follow an overall healthful dietary pattern that includes:

❑ ❑ A balanced caloric intake to achieve and/or maintain proper body weight.

❑ ❑ Foods that are low on the glycemic index scale.

❑ ❑ Low sugar intake. Cut back on sweet beverages, candy, and sugary desserts. Also, if sugar is listed as one of the top three ingredients on a label, do not consume this food. It is high in sugar.

❑ ❑ Small amounts of lean protein (primarily poultry, fish, or tofu), preferably before consuming any other food. Eating protein-rich foods first blunts the blood sugar spike associated with carbohydrate consumption.

❑ ❑ Complex carbohydrates. Use primarily whole foods, at least three daily servings of whole grains and five to nine servings of legumes, vegetables, and fruits.

❑ ❑ A few small portions of nuts each week.

❑ ❑ Fiber. Water-soluble fiber (found in fruits, vegetables, oats, beans, and psyllium), in particular, helps reduce blood glucose and enhances insulin sensitivity. Aim for at least 15 daily grams of fiber for every 1,000 calories of food intake.

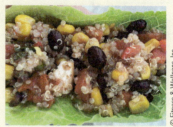
© Fitness & Wellness, Inc.

❑ ❑ Resistant starch (found in unripened bananas, oatmeal, legumes, and cooked and refrigerated potatoes and rice).

❑ ❑ Non-fat dairy products.

Minimize the use of the following foods:

❑ ❑ Processed foods (they often contain added sugar and salt).

❑ ❑ Soda pop, sugar, and sweets in general.

❑ ❑ Fructose in caloric sweeteners, including high-fructose corn syrup, agave, and honey (they contribute to insulin resistance).

❑ ❑ Fruit juices (fruit juices have been linked to increased risk for diabetes because of their high glycemic index, but eating fruit does not negatively affect blood sugar).

❑ ❑ Saturated fats.

❑ ❑ Red meats.

❑ ❑ Processed meats (they pose a greater risk than unprocessed red meat).

❑ ❑ Eggs. Limit egg consumption to less than five eggs per week: Data indicate a greater risk of developing type 2 diabetes in prediabetics and an increased risk of CVD in diabetics.

---

glycemic index (explained in Chapter 5 and detailed in Table 5.1, page 169). Refined and starchy foods (small-particle carbohydrates, which are quickly digested) rank high on the glycemic index, whereas grains, fruits, and vegetables are low-glycemic foods. Refining foods removes the overall content of valuable nutrients, including fiber and many vitamins. Regular consumption of refined carbohydrates, sweets, sugar-sweetened drinks, and even natural fruit juices causes frequent, significant spikes in blood glucose and insulin levels, thus increasing the risk for insulin resistance and subsequent diabetes development.

Foods high on the glycemic index cause a rapid increase in blood sugar. A diet that includes many high-glycemic foods increases the risk for CVD in people with high insulin resistance and **glucose intolerance.** Combining a moderate amount of high-glycemic foods with low-glycemic foods or with some fat and protein, however, can bring down the average index.

Hemoglobin A1c Test

Individuals who have high blood glucose levels should consult a physician to decide on the best treatment. They also might obtain information about the hemoglobin $A1_c$ ($HbA1_c$) test, which measures the amount of glucose that has been in a person's blood over the last 3 months. Blood glucose can become attached to hemoglobin in the red blood cells. Once attached, it remains there for the life of the red blood cell, which is about 3 months. The higher the blood glucose, the higher the concentration of glucose in the red blood cells.

Results of the $A1_c$ test are given in percentages. A normal $A1_c$ level is below 5.7 percent, 5.7 percent to 6.4 percent is viewed as prediabetes, and 6.5 percent or above is diagnosed as diabetes. The $A1_c$ test can actually detect insulin resistance years before the disease progresses to diabetes.

For diabetic patients, the $A1_c$ goal is to keep it under 7 percent. At this level and below, diabetic patients have a lower risk of developing diabetes-related problems of the eyes, kidneys, and nerves. Because the test tells a person how well blood glucose has been controlled over the last 3 months, a change in treatment is almost always recommended if the HbA1$_c$ results are above 8 percent. All people with type 2 diabetes should have an HbA1$_c$ test twice per year.

If you have diabetes and do not know how to control the disease, a certified diabetes educator (CDE) can help you learn how to best manage the disease. A CDE credential requires a minimum of 1,000 hours of diabetes-management training, a certification examination, and continuing education credits to maintain the certification. You can search for a CDE at http://www.NCBDE.org.

Metabolic Syndrome

As the cells resist the actions of insulin, the pancreas releases even more insulin in an attempt to keep blood glucose from rising. A chronic rise in insulin seems to trigger a series of abnormalities referred to as the **metabolic syndrome**. These abnormal conditions include abdominal obesity (see Figure 4.4, page 141), elevated blood pressure, high blood glucose, low HDL cholesterol, high triglycerides, and an increased blood-clotting mechanism. All of these conditions increase the risk for CHD and other diabetes-related conditions (blindness, infection, nerve damage, kidney failure, etc.). Currently, more than 30 percent of Americans 20 years of age and older (about 50 million Americans) have metabolic syndrome. And according to World Health Organization estimates, one-fifth of the world adult population is afflicted by this condition.

People with metabolic syndrome have an abnormal insulin response to carbohydrates—in particular, high-glycemic foods. Research on metabolic syndrome indicates that a low-fat, high-carbohydrate diet may not be the best for preventing CHD and actually could increase the risk for the disease in individuals with high insulin resistance and glucose intolerance. It might be best for these people to distribute daily caloric intake so that 45 percent of the daily calories are derived from carbohydrates (primarily low-glycemic carbohydrates), 35 to 40 percent from fat, and 15 percent from protein.[18] Of the 35 to 40 percent fat calories, most of the fat should come from mono- and polyunsaturated fats and less than 6 percent from saturated fat.

Individuals with metabolic syndrome also benefit from weight loss (if overweight), exercise, and smoking cessation. Insulin resistance drops by about 40 percent in overweight people who lose 20 pounds. A total of 45 minutes of daily aerobic exercise enhances insulin efficiency by 25 percent. Quitting smoking also decreases insulin resistance.

Table 10.10 Blood Pressure Guidelines (expressed in mm Hg)

Rating	Systolic	Diastolic
Normal	<120	<80
Prehypertension	121–139	81–89
Stage 1 hypertension	140–159	90–99
Stage 2 hypertension	≥160	≥100

SOURCE: National High Blood Pressure Education Program.

Hypertension (High Blood Pressure)

Some 60,000 miles of blood vessels run through the human body. As the heart forces the blood through these vessels, the fluid is under pressure. **Blood pressure** is measured in milliliters of mercury (mm Hg), usually expressed in two numbers—**systolic blood pressure** is the higher number, and **diastolic blood pressure** is the lower number. Ideal blood pressure is 120/80 or lower.

Statistical evidence indicates that damage to the arteries starts at blood pressures above 120/80. The risk for CVD doubles with each increment of 20/10, starting with a blood pressure of 115/75.[19] All blood pressures of at least 140/90 are considered to be **hypertension** (Table 10.10). Blood pressures ranging from 120/80 to 139/89 are referred to as prehypertension.

AHA estimates indicate that approximately one in every three adults, or about 86 million American adults, is hypertensive. Two out of three Americans over 60, one out of three between 40 and 60, and one in 14 between 18 and 39 years of age suffer from hypertension. The incidence is higher among African Americans—in fact, it is among the highest in the world.

Diagnosis of Metabolic Syndrome

	Men	Women
Waist circumference	>40 in	>35 in
Blood pressure	>130/85 mm Hg	>130/85 mm Hg
Fasting blood glucose	>100 mg/dL	>100 mg/dL
Fasting HDL cholesterol	<40 mg/dL	<50 mg/dL
Fasting triglycerides	>150 mg/dL	>150 mg/dL

GLOSSARY

Glucose intolerance A condition characterized by slightly elevated blood glucose levels.

Metabolic syndrome An array of metabolic abnormalities that contribute to the development of atherosclerosis triggered by insulin resistance. These conditions include low HDL cholesterol, high triglycerides, high blood pressure, and an increased blood-clotting mechanism.

Blood pressure A measure of the force exerted against the walls of the vessels by the blood flowing through them.

Systolic blood pressure Pressure exerted by the blood against the walls of arteries during forceful contraction (systole) of the heart; the higher of the two numbers in blood pressure readings.

Diastolic blood pressure Pressure exerted by the blood against the walls of arteries during the relaxation phase (diastole) of the heart; the lower of the two numbers in blood pressure readings.

Hypertension Chronically elevated blood pressure.

Almost half of all African American adults are hypertensive and approximately 30 percent and 20 percent of all deaths in men and women in this group, respectively, may be caused by high blood pressure.

Although the threshold for hypertension has been set at 140/90, many experts believe that the lower the blood pressure, the better. Even if the pressure is around 90/50, as long as that person does not have any symptoms of **hypotension**, he or she need not be concerned. Typical symptoms of hypotension are dizziness, lightheadedness, and fainting.

Determining True Resting Blood Pressure

Blood pressure also may fluctuate during a regular day. Many factors affect blood pressure, and one single reading may not be a true indicator of the real pressure. For example, physical activity, emotions, caffeine intake 30 minutes prior to assessment, and stress increase blood pressure; while rest and relaxation decrease blood pressure. Other factors that may increase blood pressure are "white coat hypertension" (nervousness about having blood pressure taken in the doctor's office), talking, sitting with the back unsupported, crossing the legs, having the feet off the ground, or letting the arm hang too low. Consequently, several measurements should be taken before establishing the true resting pressure. A person can also request ambulatory monitoring—that is, using a device that measures and stores the pressure every 20 to 30 minutes for a day or two while the individual engages in all of the daily activities and even while sleeping.

The "Silent Killer"

Based on estimates by the AHA, more than 60,000 Americans die each year as a direct result of high blood pressure. Hypertension is also a contributing factor to many other ailments, and it has been linked to as many as 350,000 annual deaths from all causes. The dramatic increase in hypertension seems to be linked to the obesity epidemic and the aging of the U.S. population. As people age, the arteries become less flexible and as they stiffen, blood pressure rises. Unless appropriate, healthy lifestyle strategies are implemented, people who do not have high blood pressure at age 55 have a 90 percent chance of developing it at some point in their lives.

Hypertension has been referred to as the "silent killer." It does not hurt, it does not make you feel sick, and unless you check it, years may go by before you even realize you have a problem. High blood pressure is a risk factor for CHD, congestive heart failure, stroke, peripheral artery disease, kidney failure, memory and vision loss, erectile dysfunction, and osteoporosis (see Figure 10.9).

All inner walls of arteries are lined by a layer of smooth endothelial cells. Blood lipids cannot penetrate the healthy lining and start to build up on the walls unless the cells are damaged. High blood pressure is thought to be a leading contributor to destruction of this lining. As blood pressure rises, so does the risk for atherosclerosis. The higher the pressure, the greater the damage to the arterial wall, making

Figure 10.9 **Health risks associated with high blood pressure.**

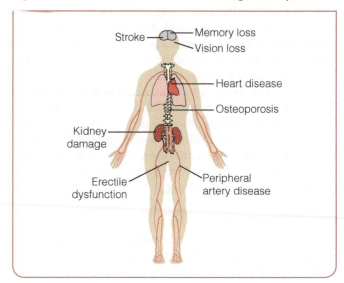

the vessels susceptible to fat deposits, especially if serum cholesterol is also high. Blockage of the coronary vessels decreases blood supply to the heart muscle and can lead to heart attacks. When brain arteries are involved, a stroke may follow.

A clear example of the connection between high blood pressure and atherosclerosis can be seen by comparing blood vessels in the human body. Even when atherosclerosis is present throughout major arteries, fatty plaques rarely are seen in the pulmonary artery, which goes from the right part of the heart to the lungs. The pressure in this artery normally is below 40 mm Hg, and at such a low pressure, significant deposits do not occur. This is one of the reasons that people with low blood pressure have a lower incidence of CVD.

Constantly elevated blood pressure also causes the heart to work much harder. At first the heart does well, but in time, this continual strain produces an enlarged heart, followed by congestive heart failure. Furthermore, high blood pressure

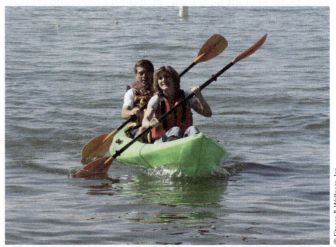

Lifetime physical activity helps maintain healthy blood pressure.

© Fitness & Wellness, Inc.

damages blood vessels to the kidneys and eyes, which can result in kidney failure and loss of vision.

Treating Hypertension

Of all cases of hypertension, 90 percent have no definite cause. Called "essential hypertension," this type of hypertension is treatable. Aerobic exercise, weight reduction, a diet low in salt and fat and high in potassium and calcium, a higher daily protein intake, flaxseed consumption, lower alcohol and caffeine intakes, smoking cessation, stress management, and antihypertensive medication all have been used effectively to treat essential hypertension. Unless it is extremely high, before recommending medication, most sports medicine physicians suggest a combination of the other treatment modalities to lower the blood pressure. In most instances, this treatment brings blood pressure under control.

The remaining 10 percent of hypertensive cases are caused by pathological conditions, such as narrowing of the kidney arteries, glomerulonephritis (a kidney disease), tumors of the adrenal glands, and narrowing of the aortic artery. With this type of hypertension, the pathological cause has to be treated before the blood pressure problem can be corrected..

Critical Thinking

Do you know what your most recent blood pressure reading was, and did you know at the time what the numbers meant? How would you react if your doctor were to instruct you to take blood pressure medication?

Antihypertensive medicines often are the first choice of treatment for these cases, but they produce many side effects. These include lethargy, sleepiness, sexual difficulties, higher blood cholesterol and glucose levels, lower potassium levels, and elevated uric acid levels. A physician may end up treating these side effects as much as the hypertension. Because of the many side effects, about half of the patients stop taking the medication within the first year of treatment. Now a 2015 study has revealed that healthy lifestyle approaches, including a reduction in salt intake and saturated fat consumption, along with increased physical activity, appear to be more effective than taking blood pressure-lowering medication.[20]

Hypertension and Sodium and Potassium Intakes

One of the most significant factors contributing to elevated blood pressure is excessive sodium in the diet (salt, or sodium chloride, contains approximately 40 percent sodium). With a high sodium intake, the body retains more water, which increases the blood volume and, in turn, drives up the pressure. Further, data indicate that a high sodium intake weakens heart and kidney function and makes blood vessels less flexible (increasing blood pressure and worsening atherosclerosis). Excessive sodium also increases calcium excretion in the urine (leading to bone loss and osteoporosis) and may promote stomach and colorectal cancers, contribute to inflammation and asthma, damage blood vessels to the brain (a risk factor for dementia), and interfere with the sympathetic nervous system (the "fight-or-flight" response).

A high intake of potassium seems to regulate water retention by promoting sodium excretion and thus lowering the blood pressure slightly. According to the Institute of Medicine of the National Academy of Sciences, people need to consume at least 4,700 mg of potassium per day. Most Americans get only half that amount. Foods high in potassium include vegetables (especially leafy green ones), citrus fruit, dairy products, fish, beans, and nuts.

HOEGER KEY TO WELLNESS

When it comes to blood pressure, it is better to keep it normal than work to bring it back down once hypertension has developed. Currently, one in every three adults is hypertensive and another 90 percent age 55 and older with normal blood pressure are at risk of developing the disease.

Hypertension and Protein Intake

New studies are also encouraging additional dietary modifications to treat high blood pressure. Data from the well-known Framingham study, published in 2015, indicate that adults consuming more dietary protein from either plant or animal sources have a lower long-term risk of developing hypertension. People in the highest one-third of protein intake (102 grams per day) were at a 40 percent lower risk of developing high blood pressure than those with the lowest intake.[21] The benefits were observed in both normal weight and overweight individuals. Furthermore, high protein intake along with higher fat intake yielded a 59 percent reduction in the risk of developing hypertension.

Physical Activity and Blood Pressure

The relative risk for mortality based on blood pressure and fitness levels is similar to that of physical fitness and cholesterol. In men and women alike, the relative risk for early mortality is lower in fit people with high systolic blood pressure (140 mm Hg or higher) than in unfit people with a healthy systolic blood pressure (120 mm Hg or lower).

Physical activity is critical to maintain healthy body weight. The link between hypertension and obesity seems to be quite strong. Blood volume increases with excess body fat, and each additional pound of fat requires an estimated extra mile of blood vessels to feed this tissue. Furthermore, blood capillaries are constricted by the adipose tissues because these vessels run through them. As a result, the heart muscle must work harder to pump the blood through a longer, constricted network of blood vessels.

GLOSSARY

Hypotension Low blood pressure.

The Hypertension and Salt Connection

Although sodium (salt contains about 40 percent sodium) is essential for normal body functions, the body can function with as little as 200 mg, or a tenth of a teaspoon, daily. Even under strenuous conditions in jobs and sports that incite heavy perspiration, the amount of

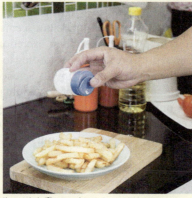

Kungverylucky/Shutterstock.com

sodium required is seldom more than 3,000 mg per day. Yet, sodium intake in the typical U.S. diet is about 4,000 mg per day. The upper limit of sodium intake has been set at 2,300 mg per day, and the 2015-2020 Dietary Guidelines for Americans recommend a daily sodium intake of less than 2,300 mg. Adults over age 51, African Americans, and all individuals with high blood pressure, diabetes, and chronic kidney disease are encouraged to keep daily intake below 1,500 mg. Among Americans, about 95 percent of men and 75 percent of women exceed these guidelines.

Salt-sensitive people, even in the absence of high blood pressure, are encouraged to decrease sodium intake because they have death rates similar to those of people with hypertension. High sodium intake also increases the risk that these people will eventually develop high blood pressure. The AHA has issued guidelines calling for everyone to reduce daily sodium intake to less than 1,500 mg. Science indicates that an intake above 2,000 mg per day harms the human body. Estimates indicate that if Americans were to follow these guidelines, heart attacks and strokes would decrease by 155,000 cases each year.

Two key studies corroborate previous concerns. First, a review of 13 sodium consumption-related studies shows that decreasing sodium intake by about 2,000 mg per day is associated with a 23 and 17 percent reduction in the risk of stroke and CVD, respectively. A second large study projected that reducing sodium intake by 1,200 mg per day would prevent as many as 92,000 deaths a year in the United States. To either prevent or postpone the onset of hypertension and to help some hypertensive people control their blood pressure, consumption of even less sodium than previously recommended is encouraged. Lower sodium intake may also reduce the risk of left ventricular hypertrophy, congestive heart failure, gastric cancer, end-stage kidney disease, osteoporosis, and bloating. Research data support the notion that daily sodium intake should be reduced as much as possible.

Where does all the sodium come from? Part of the answer is given in Table 10.11 (the list does not include salt added at the table). Most of the sodium that people consume, about 75 percent, comes from restaurant, prepared, and processed foods, over whose ingredients the consumer has no control. Restaurant and fast-food items frequently provide between 4,000 and 8,000 mg of sodium per meal, and prepackaged, canned, and frozen foods are often loaded with added salt. Among the worst

Table 10.11 Sodium and Potassium Levels of Selected Foods

Food	Serving Size	Sodium (mg)	Potassium (mg)
Avocado	½	4	680
Banana	1 med	1	440
Beans			
Kidney (canned)	½ cup	436	330
Pinto (cooked)	½ cup	2	398
Refried (canned)	½ cup	377	336
Bologna	3 oz	1,107	133
Bouillon cube	1	960	4
Cantaloupe	¼	17	341
Cheese			
American	2 oz	614	93
Cheddar	2 oz	342	56
Parmesan	2 oz	1,056	53
Chicken, light meat	6 oz	108	700
Frankfurter	1	627	136
Haddock	6 oz	300	594
Ham (honey/smoked)	2 oz	495	91
Hamburger, regular	1	500	321
Marinara pasta sauce	½ cup	527	406
Milk, skim	1 cup	126	406
Pickle, dill	2 oz	550	26
Pizza, cheese—14" diameter	⅛	456	85
Potato	1 med	6	763
Salami	3 oz	1,047	170
Salmon (baked)	4 oz	75	424
Salt	1 tsp	2,132	0
Soups			
Chicken Noodle	1 cup	979	55
Cream of Mushroom	1 cup	955	98
Vegetable Beef	1 cup	1,046	162
Soy sauce	1 tsp	1,123	22
Spaghetti, tomato sauce and cheese	6 oz	648	276
Spinach (cooked, fresh)	1 cup	126	838
Tomato juice	1 cup	680	430
Whopper with cheese	1	1,432	534

SOURCE: Fitness & Wellness, Inc.

offenders are soups, spaghetti sauces, lunch meats, pickled foods, soy sauce, pizza, sandwiches, salad dressings, cheeses, pasta, rice, and crackers.

As a consumer, you need to always read food labels and pick only those items that are low in sodium content. You will do best by downsizing your portion (taking the rest home), sharing the dish with someone else, or trying to find the lower-sodium dishes. You can also retrain your taste buds to enjoy food with less salt.

SOURCES: K. Bibbins-Domingo et al., "Projected Effect of Dietary Salt Reductions on Future Cardiovascular Disease," New England Journal of Medicine 362 (2010): 590–599; J. Buendia et al., "Diets Higher in Protein Predict Lower High Blood Pressure Risk in Framingham Offspring Study Adults," American Journal of Hypertension 28 (2015): 372–379.

Regular physical activity plays a large role in managing blood pressure. On average, fit individuals have lower blood pressure than unfit people. Aerobic exercise of moderate intensity supplemented by strength training is recommended for individuals with high blood pressure.[22]

Aerobic Exercise Comprehensive reviews of the effects of aerobic exercise on blood pressure have found that, in general, people can expect exercise-induced reductions of approximately 4 to 5 mm Hg in resting systolic blood pressure and 3 to 4 mm Hg in resting diastolic blood pressure.[23] Although these reductions do not seem large, a decrease of about 5 mm Hg in resting diastolic blood pressure has been associated with a 40 percent decrease in the risk for stroke and a 15 percent reduction in the risk for CHD.[24] Even in the absence of any decrease in resting blood pressure, hypertensive individuals who exercise have a lower risk for all-cause mortality compared with hypertensive or sedentary individuals. Research data also show that exercise, not weight loss, is the major contributor to the lower blood pressure of exercisers. If they discontinue aerobic exercise, they do not maintain these changes.

Strength-Training Another extensive review of research studies on the effects of at least 4 weeks of strength-training on resting blood pressure yielded similar results.[25] Both systolic and diastolic blood pressures decreased by an average of 3 mm Hg. Participants in these studies, however, were primarily individuals with normal blood pressure. Of greater significance, the results showed that strength-training did not cause an increase in resting blood pressure. More research remains to be done on hypertensive subjects. A key recommendation for strength-training is to never hold your breath during training. Holding your breath while lifting heavy resistances substantially increases blood pressure and can lead to increased arterial stiffness.

Long-Term Benefits of Exercise The effects of long-term participation in exercise are apparently much more remarkable. An 18-year follow-up study on exercising and nonexercising subjects showed much lower blood pressures in the active group.[26] The exercise group had an average resting blood pressure of 120/78 compared with 150/90 for the nonexercise group (Table 10.12). The results of the latter landmark study were corroborated by a 2014 36-year longitudinal study involving almost 14,000 men. Even though average blood pressure rose steadily with age, the increase was significantly less in the fittest participants. The lowest fit men reached a systolic blood pressure of 120 mm Hg by age 46, whereas the fittest men didn't do so until age 54. In terms of diastolic pressure, the results were more remarkable. The lowest fit group exceeded 80 mm Hg at age 42, compared with beyond 90 years of age in the fittest group.[27] The researchers concluded that the potential modifying effect of fitness on blood-pressure trajectory quite clearly delays the development of hypertension.

Aerobic exercise programs for hypertensive patients should be of moderate intensity. Training at 40 to 60 percent intensity seems to have the same effect in lowering blood pressure as training at 70 percent intensity. High-intensity training

Table 10.12 Effects of Long-Term (14–18 years) Aerobic Exercise on Resting Blood Pressure

	Initial	Final
Exercise Group		
Age	44.6	68.0
Blood Pressure	120/79	120/78
Nonexercise Group		
Age	51.6	69.7
Blood Pressure	135/85	150/90

NOTE: The aerobic exercise program consisted of an average four training sessions per week, each 66 minutes long, at about 76 percent of heart rate reserve.

Based on data from F. W. Kash, J. L. Boyer, S. P. Van Camp, L. S. Verity, and J. P. Wallace, "The Effect of Physical Activity on Aerobic Power in Older Men (A Longitudinal Study)," *The Physician and Sports Medicine* 18, no. 4 (1990): 73–83.

(above 70 percent) in hypertensive patients may not lower the blood pressure as much as moderate-intensity exercise. Even so, people may be better off being highly fit and having high blood pressure than being unfit and having low blood pressure. The death rates for unfit individuals with low systolic blood pressure are much higher than those for highly fit people with high systolic blood pressure. Strength-training for hypertensive individuals calls for a minimum of one set of 12 to 15 repetitions that elicit a "somewhat hard" perceived exertion rating, using 8 to 10 multi-joint exercises two or three times per week.

Blood Pressure Management

Most important is a preventive approach. Keeping blood pressure under control is easier than trying to bring it down once it is high. Regardless of your blood pressure history, high or low, you should have it checked routinely. To keep your blood pressure as low as possible, exercise regularly; lose excess weight; eat less sodium-containing food; do not smoke; practice stress management; do not consume more than two alcoholic beverages a day if you are a man or one if you are a woman; and consume more potassium-rich foods, such as potatoes, bananas, orange juice, cantaloupe, tomatoes, and beans. An alcoholic drink is defined as 5 ounces of wine, 12 ounces of beer, 8 ounces of malt liquor, or 1.5 ounces of 80-proof liquor or distilled spirits. The Dietary Approaches to Stop Hypertension (DASH) diet—which emphasizes fruits, vegetables, grains, fish, nuts, low-fat dairy products, fewer sweets, and less saturated fat and cholesterol—lowers systolic and diastolic blood pressure by about 10 and 5 points, respectively (see the box "Guidelines to Stop Hypertension"). The DASH diet has been shown to make blood vessels produce more nitric oxide, a compound that causes blood vessels to relax (decreasing blood pressure). Further, the DASH diet along with a low-sodium diet allows stiff arteries to expand.

Those who are taking medication for hypertension should not stop without the approval of the prescribing physician. If it is not treated properly, high blood pressure can kill. By combining medication with the other treatments, people might eventually reduce or eliminate the need for drug therapy.

Behavior Modification Planning

Guidelines to Stop Hypertension.

I PLAN TO   **I DID IT**

☐ ☐ Participate in a moderate-intensity aerobic exercise program (50% intensity) for 30 to 45 minutes five to seven times per week.

☐ ☐ Participate in a moderate-resistance strength-training program (use 12 to 15 repetitions to near-fatigue on each set) two times per week (seek your physician's approval and advice for this program).

☐ ☐ Lose weight if you are above recommended body weight.

☐ ☐ Limit sodium intake to less than 1,500 mg/day.

☐ ☐ Do not smoke cigarettes or use tobacco in any other form.

☐ ☐ Practice stress management.

☐ ☐ Do not consume more than two alcoholic beverages a day if you are a man or one if you are a woman.

☐ ☐ Consume more potassium-rich foods.

☐ ☐ **Follow the Dietary Approaches to Stop Hypertension (DASH) diet.**

Food Group	Servings
Whole grains	7-8 per day
Fruits and vegetables	8-10 per day
Low-fat or fat-free dairy foods	2-13 per day
Meat, poultry, or fish	2 or less per day
Beans, peas, nuts, or seeds	4-15 per week
Fats and oils	2-3 servings per day
Snacks and sweets	4-5 per week

Try It

In your Online Journal or class notebook, make a comparison of the goals of the DASH diet and Dietary Guidelines for Americans. How do they differ?

Excessive Body Fat

Excessive body fat is an independent risk factor for CHD, but disease risk may actually be augmented by other risk factors that usually accompany excessive body fat. Risk factors such as high blood lipids, hypertension, and type 2 diabetes typically are seen in conjunction with obesity. All of these risk factors usually improve with increased physical activity.

Attaining recommended body composition helps improve several CHD risk factors and helps people reach a better state of health and wellness. While data indicate that a 10 percent weight loss results in significant improvements in CHD risk factors, some studies have shown a reduction in chronic disease risk factors with only a 2 to 3 percent weight loss.[28]

For years, we have known that where people store fat affects risk for disease. People who store body fat in the abdominal area as opposed to in the hips and thighs are at higher risk for disease. Furthermore, when abdominal fat is stored primarily around internal organs (visceral fat—also see Figure 4.4, page 141 and the "Diet, Exercise, and Visceral Fat" box in Chapter 5, page 196), disease risk is greater than when abdominal fat is stored subcutaneously or retroperitoneally.

The best approach to prevent increases in visceral fat is through regular exercise. Men and women who exercise regularly for about 20 minutes per day at a moderate intensity do not gain visceral fat. People who exercise at a vigorous intensity for at least 30 daily minutes actually lose visceral fat, while sedentary individuals continue to increase the visceral fat depot. As little as 6 months of physical inactivity have

been shown to further increase the visceral fat component and the concomitant disease risk.

Data on 21,094 men followed for more than 20 years indicated that an elevated body mass index (BMI) of greater than 25 was associated with an increased risk of heart failure.[29] Furthermore, the data showed that as BMI increased in both active and inactive men, so did the risk for heart failure. The risk for heart failure increased proportionally with increased BMI or decreased physical activity (Table 10.13).

If you have a weight problem and want to get down to recommended weight, you must do the following:

1. Increase daily physical activity up to 90 minutes a day, including aerobic and strength-training programs.

Table 10.13 Relationship between Body Weight, Physical Activity, and Heart Failure Risk

Body Weight and Activity Status	Percent Risk Increase*
Lean** and inactive	19
Overweight and active	49
Overweight and inactive	78
Obese and active	168
Obese and inactive	293

*As compared with lean and active men.

**Lean = BMI < 25, Overweight = BMI ≥25 and ,≤30, Obese = BMI >30.

SOURCE: S. Kenchaiah et al., "Body Mass Index and Vigorous Physical Activity and the Risk of Heart Failure Among Men," *Circulation* 119 (2009): 44–52.

2. Follow a diet lower in fat, refined sugars, and processed foods and high in complex carbohydrates and fiber.
3. Reduce total caloric intake moderately while getting the necessary nutrients to sustain normal body functions.

A comprehensive weight reduction and weight control program is discussed in detail in Chapter 5.

Tobacco Use

An estimated 64 million people in the United States use tobacco products. Of those, more than 52 million smoke cigarettes. Smoking is the single largest preventable cause of illness and premature death in the United States. It has been linked to CVD, cancer, bronchitis, emphysema, and peptic ulcers. In relation to CHD, smoking speeds the process of atherosclerosis and carries a threefold increase in the risk of sudden death after a myocardial infarction.

According to estimates, about 20 percent of all deaths from CVD are attributable to smoking. Smoking prompts the release of nicotine and another 1,200 toxic compounds into the bloodstream. Similar to hypertension, many of these substances are destructive to the inner membrane that protects the walls of the arteries. Once the lining is damaged, cholesterol and triglycerides can be deposited readily in the arterial wall. As the plaque builds up, it obstructs blood flow through the arteries.

Furthermore, smoking encourages the formation of blood clots, which can completely block an artery already narrowed by atherosclerosis. In addition, carbon monoxide, a by-product of cigarette smoke, decreases the blood's oxygen-carrying capacity. A combination of obstructed arteries, less oxygen, and nicotine in the heart muscle heightens the risk for a serious heart problem.

Smoking also increases heart rate, raises blood pressure, and irritates the heart, which can trigger fatal cardiac **arrhythmias**. Another harmful effect is a decrease in HDL cholesterol, the "good" type that helps control blood lipids. Smoking actually presents a much greater risk of death from heart disease than from lung disease.

Pipe and cigar smoking and tobacco chewing also increase the risk for heart disease. Even if the tobacco user inhales no smoke, he or she absorbs toxic substances through the membranes of the mouth, and these end up in the bloodstream. Individuals who use tobacco in any of these three forms also have a much greater risk for cancer of the oral cavity.

The risks for both CVD and cancer start to decrease the moment a person quits smoking. One year after quitting, the risk for CHD decreases by half, and within 15 years, the relative risk of dying from CVD and cancer approaches that of a lifetime nonsmoker. A more thorough discussion of the harmful effects of cigarette smoking, the benefits of quitting, and a complete program for quitting are detailed in Chapter 13.

Tension and Stress

Tension and stress have become part of contemporary life. Everyone has to deal daily with goals, deadlines, responsibilities, and pressures. Almost everything in life (whether positive or negative) can be a source of stress. What creates the health hazard is not the stressor itself but, rather, the individual's response to it.

The human body responds to stress by producing more **catecholamines**, which prepare the body for quick physical action—often called fight or flight. These hormones increase heart rate, blood pressure, and blood glucose levels, enabling the person to take action. If the person actually fights or flees, the higher levels of catecholamines are metabolized and the body can return to a normal state. If, however, a person is under constant stress and unable to take action (as in the death of a close relative or friend, loss of a job, trouble at work, or financial insecurity), the catecholamines remain elevated in the bloodstream.

People who are not able to relax place a constant low-level strain on the cardiovascular system that could manifest as heart disease. Higher levels of the hormones epinephrine and cortisol in highly stressed people raise blood pressure and cholesterol. Even without large amounts of plaque, small deposits on the arterial wall can rupture during stressful events, tearing the blood vessel lining and triggering a clot that causes a heart attack. Chronic stress also causes an increase of the brain chemical neuropeptide Y that promotes storage of visceral fat, further increasing the risk for type 2 diabetes, heart disease, some cancers, and bodywide inflammation. In addition, when people are in a stressful situation, the coronary arteries that feed the heart muscle constrict, reducing the oxygen supply to the heart. If the blood vessels are largely blocked by atherosclerosis, arrhythmias or even a heart attack may follow. The research indicates that people who feel too much stress too often significantly increase their risk for a deadly heart attack.

A little known fact is that the risk of sudden cardiac death is twice as high on Mondays, most likely because of the stress of having to go back to work after the weekend. Heart attacks are also more common in the morning because cortisol levels and stress hormones are highest, on average, at that time of the day.

Anger, anxiety, and hostility also contribute to heart disease by increasing heart rate, blood pressure, blood glucose, cholesterol, and interleukin-6 (a marker for arterial inflammation). Angina risk increases following an outburst of anger and doubles the risk for a heart attack in the first 2 hours thereafter.[30] Depression and isolation have also been linked to higher death rates from heart disease due to an imbalance in the nervous system that increases the risk for arrhythmias.

Weight gain is often the end result of excessive stress. That is because most people tend to eat more when distressed and the choice is typically "comfort foods" that are calorie dense and promote weight gain with the subsequent increased risk for CVD.

GLOSSARY

Arrhythmias Irregular heart rhythms.

Catecholamines Fight-or-flight hormones, including epinephrine and norepinephrine.

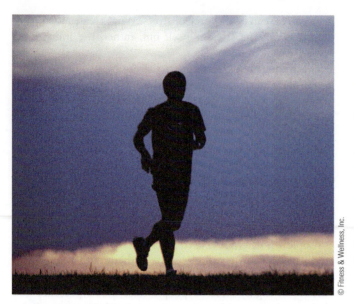

Physical activity is one of the best ways to relieve stress.

Individuals who are under a lot of stress and do not cope well with stress need to take measures to counteract the effects of stress in their lives. One way is to identify the sources of stress and learn how to cope with them. People need to take control of themselves, examine and act upon the things that are most important in their lives, and ignore less meaningful details.

Physical activity is one of the best ways to relieve stress. During exercise, the nervous system shifts from the sympathetic or stress tone to the parasympathetic or rest tone, a benefit that lasts several hours following exercise. When a person takes part in physical activity, the body also metabolizes excess catecholamines and is able to return to a normal state. Exercise steps up muscular activity, which contributes to muscular relaxation after completing the physical activity.

Many executives in large cities are choosing the evening hours for their physical activity programs, stopping after work at the health or fitness club. In doing this, they are able to "burn up" the excess tension accumulated during the day and enjoy the evening hours. This has proved to be one of the best stress management techniques. More information on stress management techniques is presented in Chapter 12.

Personal and Family History

Individuals who have had cardiovascular problems are at higher risk than those who have never had a problem. People with this history should control other risk factors as much as they can. Many of the risk factors are reversible, so this greatly decreases the risk for future problems. The more time that passes after the occurrence of the cardiovascular problem, the lower the risk for recurrence.

A genetic predisposition to heart disease has been demonstrated clearly. All other factors being equal, a person with blood relatives who now have or did have premature heart disease runs a greater risk than someone with no such history. Premature CHD is defined as a heart attack before age 55 in a close male relative or before age 65 in a close female relative. The younger the age at which the relative incurred the cardiovascular incident, the greater the risk for the disease.

In some cases, there is no way of knowing whether the heart problem resulted from a person's genetic predisposition or simply poor lifestyle habits. A person may have been physically inactive, been overweight, smoked, and had bad dietary habits—all of which contributed to a heart attack. Regardless, blood relatives fall in the "family history" category.

For persons with a family history, a series of genetic tests are now available that help identify individuals at risk for heart disease, even though they lead a healthy lifestyle and no other visible signs or symptoms of the disease are present. These include the carotid intima-media thickness or CIMT test (measures plaque thickness inside the arterial wall), 9p21 (two copies of the "heart attack gene"—one inherited from each parent), Apo E (a gene that determines how the body metabolizes nutrients), and the KIF6 (an arginine gene variant). The $A1_c$ test can also detect insulin resistance many years before it progresses to type 2 diabetes. Even if you have a genetic inheritance, lifestyle changes can trump genes in heart disease (and cancer) risk. Data indicate that people with the genetic variant 9p21 who eat a diet high in fruits, vegetables, and nuts have a heart attack risk almost as low as people without this genetic variant.

HOEGER KEY TO WELLNESS

A family history of heart disease is not an indication that you are doomed. A healthy life—free of cardiovascular problems—is something over which you have extensive control by living a wellness-way of life.

A person with a family or personal history is encouraged to watch all risk factors closely and maintain the lowest risk level possible. In addition to living a healthy lifestyle, the person should have a blood chemistry analysis annually to make sure the body is handling blood lipids properly.

Age

Age is a risk factor because of the higher incidence of heart disease as people get older. This tendency may be induced partly by other factors stemming from changes in lifestyle as we get older—less physical activity, poorer nutrition, obesity, and so on.

Although the aging process cannot be stopped, it certainly can be slowed. Physiological age versus chronological age is important in preventing disease. Some individuals in their 60s and older have the body of a 30-year-old. And 30-year-olds often are in such poor condition and health that they almost seem to have the body of a 60-year-old. The best ways to slow the natural aging process are to engage in risk factor management and positive lifestyle habits.

Other Factors Possibly Affecting Coronary Heart Disease Risk

Evidence points to a few other factors that may be linked to coronary heart disease.

Gum Disease

In observational studies, periodontal disease has been linked to CVD, diabetes, respiratory and kidney disease, and certain cancers. The oral bacteria that build up with dental plaque are believed to enter the bloodstream and contribute to inflammation, formation of blood vessel plaque, and blood clotting, and thus increase the risk for heart attack. A tooth abscess, a pus-filled bacterial infection inside the tooth or between the tooth and the gum, can lead to a fatal condition if the infection spreads to the brain or the heart, or causes swelling in the airways that cuts off the air supply to the lungs. Both the American Heart Association and the American Dental Association, however, concur that the observational data do not prove that there is conclusive evidence that gum disease directly contributes to CVD. Most likely, periodontal disease and CHD share common risk factors such as smoking and diabetes. Avoiding sugar-filled sweets and drinks, thoroughly rinsing the mouth with water following food consumption, regular brushing, using an electric toothbrush, daily flossing, scraping the tongue, and irrigating the gums with water are all preventive measures that will help protect you from gum disease.

Sleep

Getting too little, too much, or interrupted sleep have all been linked to high blood pressure, obesity, diabetes, stroke, and heart attacks,

Snoring

Another factor that has been linked to CVD is loud snoring. People who snore heavily may suffer from sleep apnea, a sleep disorder in which the throat closes for a brief moment, causing breathing to stop. Individuals who snore heavily may triple their risk of a heart attack and quadruple their risk of a stroke.

Loneliness

People who live alone are more likely to die from a heart ailment or stroke than those who live with others. Strong social networks are linked to better health and a longer life. The AHA recommends that having a pet can decrease heart disease risk for people who live alone.

Emotional Distress

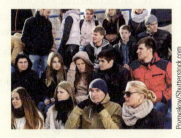
Poznyakov/Shutterstock.com

Sudden emotion-related increases in heart rate often trigger heart problems. For example, the risk of a heart attack is highest on the day of and the first few weeks after receiving unexpected bad news. Sports fans who get overly excited about their team can experience a twofold or higher increase in heart rate. A person with a resting heart rate of 80 to 90 bpm can easily near or reach maximal heart rate in these situations. Heart attacks occur in these cases because the unconditioned heart is unable to sustain the sudden/drastic increase in heart rate.

Extramarital Affairs

An extramarital affair can contribute to a cardiac event. Data indicate that 80 percent of post-sex heart attack deaths occur in people following sex in a hotel room with someone other than their spouse.[a] Researchers believe that such encounters lead to higher levels of arousal, resulting in a sudden and sustained heart rate that an unconditioned heart is unable to tolerate. Sex with your regular partner, however, is not associated with a heart attack. Sexual activity requires no greater energy expenditure than a brisk walk. Contrary to a common belief, data indicate that less than 1 percent of patients recovering from heart attacks suffered the attack within an hour of sexual activity.

Low Birth Weight

Low birth weight, considered to be less than 5.5 pounds, also has been linked to heart disease, hypertension, and diabetes. Individuals with low birth weight should bring this information to the attention of their personal physician and regularly monitor the risk factors for CHD.

Depression

Individuals suffering from depression are at higher risk for heart disease. Depression can worsen heart disease by affecting heart rhythm, blood pressure, blood clotting, and stress hormone levels. Patients with depression who have survived a heart attack are two to three times more likely to die than similar patients without depression. Treating depression, regardless of other health conditions, is essential for a person's well-being.

Lack of Laughter

Laughter has been shown to dilate blood vessels (enhancing blood flow), reduce inflammation, and decrease stress hormones, all of which decrease heart attack and stroke risk.

Excessively-Long Work Schedule

An extra-long weekly work schedule has been linked to CVD, including CHD, hypertension, heart attack, and stroke. And there appears to be a dose-response relationship, that is, the more hours a person works, the higher the risk. As compared to working 45 hours per week, working 55 hours increases the risk by about 16 percent, 65 hours by 50 percent, and 75 hours or more doubles the risk for a cardiovascular problem.

Aspirin Benefits

Aspirin therapy is recommended for some people who have heart disease, but if you have not suffered a heart attack, a daily aspirin is no longer advised. Daily aspirin therapy can cause serious side effects, including ulcers, gastrointestinal bleeding, and kidney failure, among others. For individuals who have had a heart attack or are at moderate risk or higher for heart disease, a physician may recommend an aspirin dosage of about 81 mg per day (the equivalent of a baby aspirin). Such therapy can prevent or dissolve clots that cause a heart attack or stroke. With such daily use, the incidence of a repeated-nonfatal heart attack decreases by about a third. The benefits of daily aspirin therapy, nonetheless, do not outweigh the risk of bleeding in people at low risk for heart disease.

[a]B. A. Franklin, "Sex Can Cause a Heart Attack," *Bottom Line/Health*, 27 (March 2013): 1–3.

10.6 *Cardiovascular Risk Reduction*

Most of the risk factors are reversible and preventable. Having a family history of heart disease and some of the other risk factors because of neglect in lifestyle does not mean you are fated for CVD. A healthier lifestyle—free of cardiovascular problems—is something over which you have extensive control. Be persistent! Willpower and commitment are required to develop patterns that eventually turn into healthy habits and contribute to your total well-being and longevity.

Assess Your Behavior

1. Do you make a conscious effort to increase daily physical activity, are you able to accumulate at least 30 minutes of moderate-intensity activity a minimum of 5 days per week, and do you avoid excessive sitting throughout most days of the week?

2. Is your diet fundamentally low in saturated fat, trans fat, refined carbohydrates, and processed foods; do you meet the daily suggested amounts of fruits, vegetables, and fiber; and do you use primarily unsaturated fats?

3. Have you recently had your blood pressure measured and established your blood lipid profile? Do you know what the results mean, and are you aware of strategies to manage them effectively?

Assess Your Knowledge

1. Coronary heart disease
   a. is the single leading cause of death in the United States.
   b. is the leading cause of sudden cardiac deaths.
   c. is a condition in which the arteries that supply the heart muscle with oxygen and nutrients are narrowed by fatty deposits.
   d. accounts for approximately 20 percent of all deaths in the United States.
   e. All of the choices are correct.

2. The incidence of cardiovascular disease during the past 50 years in the United States has
   a. increased.
   b. decreased.
   c. remained constant.
   d. increased in some years and decreased in others.
   e. fluctuated according to medical technology.

3. Regular aerobic activity helps
   a. lower LDL cholesterol.
   b. lower HDL cholesterol.
   c. increase triglycerides.
   d. decrease insulin sensitivity.
   e. All of the choices are correct.

4. The risk of heart disease increases with
   a. high LDL cholesterol.
   b. low HDL cholesterol.
   c. high concentrations of homocysteine.
   d. high levels of hs-CRP.
   e. All of the choices are correct.

5. An optimal level of LDL cholesterol is
   a. between 200 and 239 mg/dL.
   b. about 200 mg/dL.
   c. between 150 and 200 mg/dL.
   d. between 100 and 150 mg/dL.
   e. below 100 mg/dL.

6. As a part of a CHD prevention program, saturated fat intake should be kept below ___ percent of the total daily caloric intake.
   a. 35
   b. 30
   c. 22
   d. 15
   e. 6

7. Statin drugs
   a. increase the liver's ability to remove blood cholesterol.
   b. decrease LDL cholesterol.
   c. slow cholesterol production.
   d. help reduce inflammation.
   e. All of the choices are correct.

8. Type 2 diabetes is closely related to
   a. overeating.
   b. obesity.
   c. lack of physical activity.
   d. insulin resistance.
   e. All of the choices are correct.

9. Metabolic syndrome is related to
   a. low HDL cholesterol.
   b. high triglycerides.
   c. an increased blood-clotting mechanism.
   d. an abnormal insulin response to carbohydrates.
   e. All of the choices are correct.

10. Comprehensive reviews on the effects of aerobic exercise on blood pressure found that, in general, an individual can expect exercise-induced reductions of approximately
    a. 3 to 5 mm Hg.
    b. 5 to 10 mm Hg.
    c. 10 to 15 mm Hg.
    d. more than 15 mm Hg.
    e. There is no significant change in blood pressure with exercise.

Correct answers can be found at the back of the book.

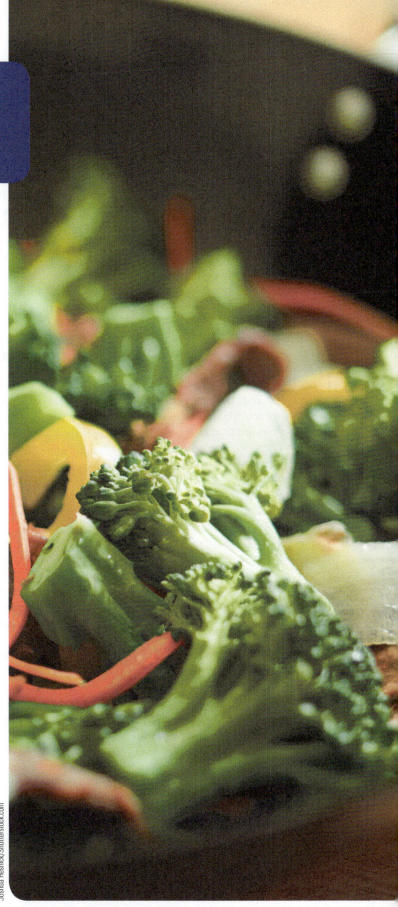

11

Cancer Prevention

"Our science looks at a substance-by-substance exposure and doesn't take into account the multitude of exposures we experience in daily life. If we did, it might change our risk paradigm. The potential risks associated with extremely low-level exposure may be underestimated or missed entirely."
—Heather Logan

Objectives

11.1 **Define** cancer and understand how it starts and spreads.

11.2 **Cite** guidelines for preventing cancer.

11.3 **Delineate** the major risk factors that lead to specific types of cancer.

11.4 **Assess** the risk for developing certain types of cancer.

11.5 **Describe** everyday lifestyle strategies that you can use immediately to decrease overall cancer risk.

Joshua Resnick/Shutterstock.com

FAQ

Can a healthy diet reduce cancer risk?

Ongoing research is under way to examine the effects of foods in preventing and fighting off cancer. Current evidence shows that a healthy diet and maintenance of recommended body weight reduce cancer risk; however, science may never be able to provide conclusive evidence that a certain diet will prevent cancer. Years of research will be required to unravel the role of diet in cancer prevention, and no dietary pattern will ever provide a foolproof solution to reduce your risk. That said, many of the foods that are currently recommended in a cancer-prevention diet are similar to those encouraged to decrease disease risk and enhance health and overall well-being. If you are truly adhering to healthy dietary guidelines (see the Behavior Modification Planning box on page 423), you are most likely eating the right foods to decrease your cancer risk.

Does regular physical activity affect cancer risk?

Regular physical activity and decreased sitting time have been shown to lower the risk for developing some major types of cancer, in particular cancers of the colon, breast, endometrium, lungs, and prostate gland. To date, more than 100 studies have linked increases in physical activity to reduced risk of breast cancer alone. Research shows that as little as 15 minutes of vigorous exercise three times per week decreases breast cancer risk by up to 40 percent in persons of all races and ethnicities.

Other research suggests that strength-training at least twice per week cuts the risk of dying from cancer in men up to 40 percent. Physical activity also prevents type 2 diabetes and obesity. The latter have been linked to colon, pancreatic, gallbladder, ovarian, thyroid, cervical, and possibly other types of cancers. The American Cancer Society recommends that you aim for at least 30 minutes of moderate to vigorous physical activity 5 or more days per week, although 60 to 90 minutes of activity are preferable. For most non-tobacco users, a healthy dietary pattern and regular physical activity are the two most significant lifestyle behaviors that reduce cancer risk.

How does inflammation lead to cancer?

Under normal circumstances, inflammation is a healthy response to injury or infection. The site of injury releases chemicals that direct tissue to grow and rebuild. Once the area is healed, inflammation stops. When inflammation persists after healing is complete, or when inflammation is carried out with no apparent purpose, it is called chronic inflammation. (Many cancers originate from a site of continued irritation and infection.) Chronic inflammation can damage the DNA of normal cells and can help damaged cells survive and divide. Within a tumor, inflammation can recruit new blood vessels that feed the tumor and help it to grow and spread.

Does aspirin therapy protect against cancer?

A landmark study published in the journal *The Lancet* indicated that a regular daily dose of aspirin may decrease cancer risk up to 58 percent in some cases (esophageal cancer) and reduce total cancer deaths by 34 percent after 5 years. Even 15 years later, death rates were still lower by 20 percent among aspirin users, with the biggest drop in cancer deaths seen in esophageal, colorectal, lung, and prostate cancers. Low-dose therapy (75 to 81 mg) was as effective as a larger dose. It is believed that aspirin inhibits the effects of enzymes (COX-2) that promote potential cancer-causing cell damage. Aspirin also decreases low-grade inflammation. Aspirin therapy, however, is not recommended for healthy people because of the small risk of gastrointestinal (GI) bleeding and ulcers. About 50,000 yearly deaths in the United States are attributed to GI bleeding caused partially by aspirin and other nonsteroidal anti-inflammatory drug (NSAID) use. Aspirin therapy damage to the GI tract may not cause any noticeable symptoms, and a fecal occult blood test may be necessary to detect possible bleeding. Hemorrhagic strokes have also been linked to low-dose aspirin therapy. If you are at high risk for cancer, especially colorectal cancer (or cardiovascular disease), you are encouraged to talk to your doctor before starting aspirin therapy. If you take aspirin, do so with warm water, which helps dissolve the tablet faster, making it less likely to cause serious bleeding.

REAL LIFE STORY | Joan's Experience

I was never really that concerned with cancer risk. You hear a lot about how various things cause cancer until it gets to the point where it seems like almost everything causes cancer and it is unavoidable. However, when I took lifetime wellness last year, learning about the key lifestyle factors that decrease cancer risk really motivated me. I liked learning about the positive things someone can do, rather than just the negative things that cause cancer. Also, the lifestyle factors were mostly simple and straightforward things to do. I actually

hung the page from the book with the list of behaviors by my desk as an easy way to remember. After that, I started being more regular about going to the gym, keeping track of whether I was getting enough fiber, and eating a large variety of fruits and vegetables, particularly cruciferous vegetables in salads. I also started drinking cold green tea. It is very good and refreshing. It was fun to try some of the foods that are known to have protective properties. I never

GCRO Images/Shutterstock.com

ate soy before, but I tried soy milk and liked it. I also really enjoy eating blueberries, which are very good for you. I wear sunblock when I know that I will be out in the sun for longer than 15 minutes. I don't smoke, and I avoid secondhand smoke at all costs. I feel happy that I am now doing my best to lessen my chances of getting cancer. All the behaviors that help with that are simple things that make me feel good anyway!

PERSONAL PROFILE: My Cancer-Prevention Program

I. What do you know about your family history of cancer? What do you suspect you might not know?

II. List lifestyle factors that you are aware of in your own daily life that increase cancer risk.

III. List environmental contaminants that you may come in contact with that may cause cancer.

IV. Have you ever felt that tanning and personal appearance are worth the potential risk of developing skin cancer?

V. Are you familiar with cancer prevention self-exams and warning signs to look for in a cancer-prevention program? Do you practice self-exams? Is there a difference between your intentions to practice self-exams and your actual practice of self-exams?

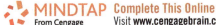

MINDTAP From Cengage   **Complete This Online**
Visit **www.cengagebrain.com** to access MindTap, a complete digital course that includes interactive quizzes, videos, and more.

Cancer is estimated to develop in one of every two men and one of three women in the United States, affecting about three of every four families. Nearly one in four deaths in the United States is due to cancer. Many of these premature deaths could be prevented through a cancer prevention lifestyle that includes abstaining from tobacco, eating a diet with plenty of plant-based foods, avoiding obesity, and being physically active.

To understand why the risk for cancer is influenced by the lifestyle choices we make, we need to first address what cancer is and how it develops. Cancer is not a single disease, but a category of diseases that share similar traits, including gene mutation and uncontrolled cell growth.

11.1 *How Cancer Starts*

An individual starts life with identical DNA in every cell of his or her body. Under normal conditions, the 100 trillion cells in the human body reproduce themselves in an orderly way. Cell growth (cell reproduction) takes place to repair and replace old, worn-out tissue. Cell growth is controlled by **deoxyribonucleic acid (DNA)** and **ribonucleic acid (RNA)**, found in the nucleus of each cell. DNA makes up genes, which are wrapped into coils that form chromosomes in the nucleolus of the cell. A healthy

cell will duplicate, on average, 52 times before it undergoes cell death. Normally, the DNA molecule is duplicated perfectly during cell division. When the DNA molecule is not replicated exactly, specialized enzymes make repairs quickly. Occasionally, however, a cell will divide without being repaired. The two new cells will both carry the resulting defect. Usually, damaged cells are sensed and are instructed to carry out programmed cell death, or PCD, but when conditions allow abnormal cells to survive, they will continue to divide and pass on the defect.

DNA Mutations

Within a person's DNA are three key genes that are involved in cancer development if they become defective: proto-oncogenes, tumor suppressor genes, and DNA repair genes. Proto-oncogenes control the type of cell being created from the DNA instructions (kidney cell, skin cell, and so on) and

┌─ GLOSSARY ─────────────────────────

Deoxyribonucleic acid (DNA) The genetic substance of which genes are made; the molecule that contains a cell's genetic code.

Ribonucleic acid (RNA) The genetic material that guides the formation of cell proteins.

the frequency of cell division. In cell division, these genes act like the gas pedal does in a car, spurring the process on. Tumor suppressor genes slow cell growth during specified points of the cell lifecycle and, therefore, act like the brake pedal in a car. DNA repair genes fix any mistakes that occur during cell division using enzymes they code for this purpose. In a healthy cell, these genes all work together to repair and replace cells. Defects in these genes—whether caused by chance; by external factors such as radiation, chemicals, free radicals, and viruses; or by internal factors such as immune conditions, hormones, and genetic mutations—ultimately allow the cell to grow into a tumor. Mutated **tumor suppressor genes** act like brakes that have gone out, allowing uncontrolled growth. Most tumors have errant copies of more than one of these genes. Proto-oncogenes mutate to become **oncogenes**. (The prefix *onco-* relates to tumors, which is why a doctor who treats cancer is an oncologist.) Oncogenes act like a gas pedal that is stuck down, speeding cell growth. Mutations in oncogenes cannot be inherited, only acquired during a person's lifetime. Mutations in tumor suppressor genes can be inherited, but in most cases are acquired during a person's lifespan. As for mutations in DNA repair genes, they can be either acquired or inherited (as in Lynch syndrome, mentioned in the Cancer Questionnaire on pages 435–436). Mutations in other types of genes are also required for the onset of cancer, such as mutations in cells that recruit a new blood supply to the tumor or target new sites in the body for spreading cancer.

Tumor Formation

The mutations of precancerous cells make them proliferate faster than healthy cells (think of the broken brake pedal or

Stages of Cancer
Stage 0: An abnormal group of cells that are too few to be called a tumor but that may grow into cancer.
Stage 1: A localized tumor that has spread.
Stage 2: A tumor that is large or has spread to the closest lymph nodes.
Stage 3: Cancer that has invaded a significant amount of nearby tissue or spread to several lymph nodes.
Stage 4: Cancer that has metastasized.

gas pedal stuck down). Thus, it becomes more likely that future cell divisions will result in an additional mutation and pass along both mutations. It is not known how many mutations are necessary, but eventually, after several generations of cells have passed on a collection of accumulated mutations, a cancerous cell will develop. Every case of cancer is the result of its own unique history of mutations, which is one reason the disease is so difficult to treat from one case to the next. Two people who have developed breast cancer may have developed it through a varied series of mutations. The cancer in each individual could respond differently to the same medical treatment.

Once a single human cell has become a cancerous cell, that cell will grow and multiply uncontrollably and ultimately form a small tumor (see Figure 11.1). A tumor can be either **benign** or **malignant**. Benign tumors do not invade other tissues and are not cancer. Although they can interfere with normal bodily functions, they rarely cause death.

Figure 11.1 Normal vs. cancerous cell division.

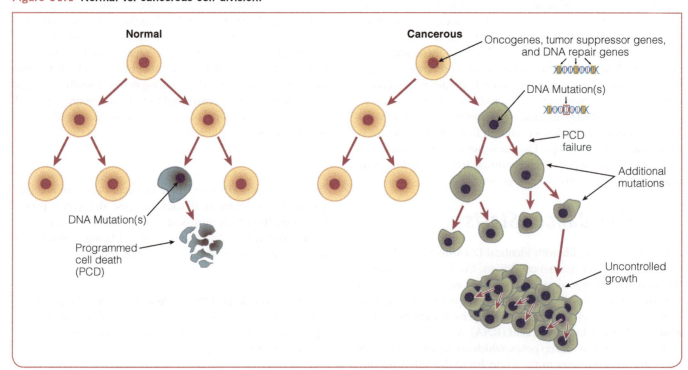

Telomeres, Aging, Cancer, and What You Can Do

The process of abnormal cell division is related indirectly to chromosome segments called **telomeres**. Chromosomes are the threadlike package of DNA in the nucleolus of each cell. Telomeres are protective end caps on chromosomes, similar to the plastic tips on shoelaces. Each time a cell divides, telomeres shorten. After many cell divisions, the telomeres become critically short, and the cell either stops functioning properly or dies.

Research has found that each person is born with varying lengths of telomeres, but only the critically short telomeres are a point of concern. Short telomeres are associated with a variety of diseases and mortality risks. Telomeres shorten naturally as a part of aging. Telomere shortening is accelerated, however, by negative lifestyle factors, including acute stress, obesity, toxins like those that result from smoking, and inflammation, among others. Telomeres are preserved and possibly lengthened by positive lifestyle factors, including stress management, exercise, and good nutrition.

An enzyme known as **telomerase** can restore telomeres after each cell division, so telomeres don't shorten. Most cells in the human body do not have enough telomerase to maintain telomere length. Only a select few cells, such as cells associated with our immune system, use telomerase to allow the division process to continue. Cancer cells are another exception; they maintain their telomeres indefinitely. Almost all cancer cells rely on telomerase for this preservation. As a result, cells continue to reproduce, creating a malignant tumor. Telomeres and telomerase are

a relatively recent discovery. While researchers can use telomere length as an indicator of a person's "real age" and disease risk, scientists are just beginning to understand the complex role telomeres have in the growth of cancerous tumors and their role in the aging process.

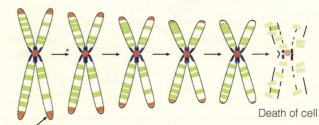

Telomeres   *Successive cell divisions   Death of cell

Erosion of chromosome telomeres in normal cells.

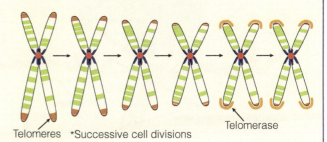

Telomeres   *Successive cell divisions   Telomerase

Action of the enzyme telomerase.

A malignant tumor is a **cancer**. The rate at which cancer cells grow varies from one type to another; some types grow fast, and others take years. A decade or more might pass between the initial mutations (as a result of carcinogenic exposure, chance, or genetics) and the time that cancer is diagnosed. As the tumor continues to grow it invades and destroys normal tissue.

Metastasis

While cancer starts with the abnormal growth of one cell, it can multiply into billions of cancerous cells. When a group of cells are precancerous or are just beginning to multiply, they are said to be "*in situ*," the Latin phrase for "in its place." By definition, cancer at this stage remains encapsulated within the tissue where it developed. The undetected tumor may go for months or years without any significant growth. While it remains encapsulated, it does not pose a serious threat to human health. To grow, however, the tumor requires more oxygen and nutrients.

In time, a few of the cancer cells start producing chemicals that signal the body to start **angiogenesis**, or the growth of a new network of blood vessels and lymphatic vessels that penetrate the tumor and help it grow (*angio*- means relating to blood or lymph vessels and *-genesis* means to originate). These new vessels deliver oxygen and nutrients and carry away waste products. During normal healthy processes,

angiogenesis is limited to a few infrequent functions such as the healing of wounds or the development of the fetus during pregnancy. During cancer, angiogenesis is the precursor of **metastasis**. Through the new blood vessels and lymphatic vessels formed by angiogenesis, cancerous cells now can break away from a malignant tumor and migrate to other parts of the body, where they can cause new cancer (Figure 11.2).

Once a single break-off cancer cell stops in a small blood vessel (capillary) at a new site, it invades the vessel wall and surrounding tissue and grows into a secondary tumor. Any

---

GLOSSARY

Tumor suppressor genes Genes that deactivate the process of cell division.

Oncogenes Genes that initiate cell division.

Benign Noncancerous.

Malignant Cancerous.

Telomeres Strands of molecules at both ends of a chromosome.

Telomerase An enzyme that allows cells to reproduce indefinitely.

Cancer A group of diseases characterized by uncontrolled growth and spread of abnormal cells.

Angiogenesis The formation of blood vessels (capillaries).

Metastasis The movement of cells from one part of the body to another.

Figure 11.2 **How cancer starts and spreads.**

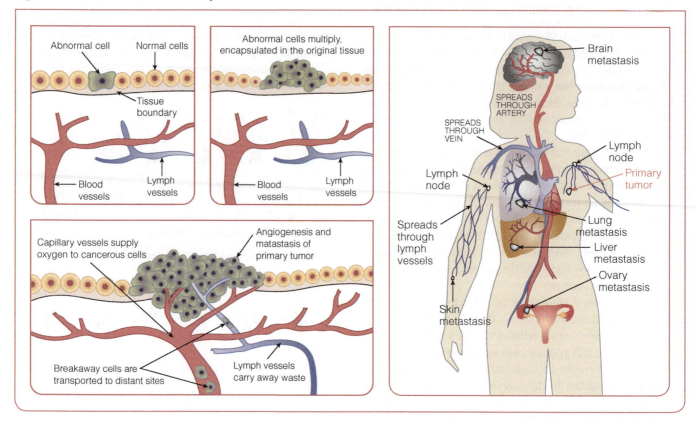

additional tumor that grows will continue to be named after the site of the original tumor. Prostate cancer, for example, that metastasizes and moves to the liver will still be called prostate cancer. Different cancer types vary widely in the way they behave, grow, and spread.

Most adults have precancerous or cancerous cells in their bodies. By middle age, our bodies contain millions of precancerous cells. Adults have had more time to be exposed to **carcinogens** or to occasional accidental mutations during some of the trillions of cell divisions that take place over a person's lifetime.

Once cancer cells metastasize, treatment becomes more difficult. Although therapy can kill most cancer cells, a few cells might become resistant to treatment. These cells then can grow into a new tumor that will not respond to the same treatment.

11.2 *Genetic versus Environmental Risk*

Like coronary heart disease, cancer is largely preventable. Researchers agree that as much as 80 percent of all human cancer is related to lifestyle or environmental factors, and 65 percent of all cases in the United States would have never occurred if Americans followed a healthy diet and avoided obesity and tobacco use. We may never know the precise number of cancer cases that are attributed to genetics or environment because of the complex interplay between our inherited traits and our external environment. In recent years, however, researchers have made great strides in understanding how our genes and environment interact to prevent or trigger cancer.

Genetics play the primary role in susceptibility in about 5 to 10 percent of all cancers. In the majority of cancer cases, cancerous mutations are sporadic and acquired during a person's lifespan. Effects of genetically caused cancer can be seen in the early childhood years or may result in multiple, independent cancers in different sites during a person's lifetime. Some cancers are a combination of genetic and environmental liability, with genetics adding to the environmental risk for certain types of cancers.

Even without environmental effects, genetic risk factors are a complex web of interplaying forces. In many cases, when a family is found to have above average rates of a certain type of cancer, no genetic alteration can be found. Scientists are then left to speculate if the cancer is a result of combined genetic risk factors or environmental exposures the family has had in common.

One person may start accumulating random precancerous gene changes, while family members and neighbors in the same environment do not. When both the affected individual and someone lacking those changes are exposed to a cancer-causing agent in the same environment, the individual who has accumulated these changes will be the only one to develop disease (see Figure 11.3). It is known that the environment works with genetics to trigger precancerous cells. Research is now opening doors in this field of study.

Figure 11.3 **Predisposition for cancer.**

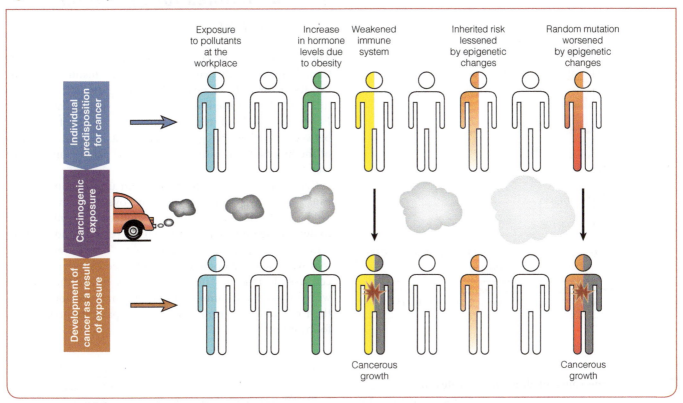

Epigenetics

For most of the 20th century, a person's genetic traits were thought to be unalterable. Once a person inherited risk of disease, it was believed that there was little that could be done to change that risk. The field of **epigenetics** has drastically disrupted our understanding of genetics and has shown that environmental choices change the way our genes work and that certain genes can be turned off and on by lifestyle choices. This happens at the molecular level through one of two processes.

In one process, chemical tags called methyl groups can be added directly to DNA to switch genes off. In a second process, other chemical tags can be added to the proteins (called histones) around which DNA wraps itself, like a spool and thread. These tags then turn genes off by coiling the bundle of protein and DNA tightly so they cannot be reached for transcription or turn genes on by unfurling DNA for transcription. In both processes, tags are added or removed depending on lifestyle choices. Whether the gene is available to be expressed depends on these tags sitting on top of the gene. The word *epigenetics* means "on top of" genetics. A person's genome has been compared to computer hardware, while the epigenome has been compared to computer software, telling the genome how to work.

Epigenetic processes can encourage tumor-friendly changes that do not involve a mutation, or they can help deter tumor development. Epigenetics is already used in some cancer treatments that silence certain genes and reactivate others.

Perhaps even more ground-breaking, researchers have discovered that epigenetic changes acquired from the environment can be passed down from parent to offspring. When parents pass their genetic information on, much of the epigenome is cleared and reset, but some epigenetic tags remain and are passed on to children. While these changes are reversible, they can be detected in offspring two or three generations later. For example, traumatic experiences in one generation may produce fearful associations in offspring. Food choices, in particular, affect our epigenetic code. You may be answering for food choices your grandparents made. Equally, your grandchildren may someday answer for the food choices you make.

11.3 *Incidence of Cancer*

Cancer is the second-leading cause of death in the United States, causing about 23 percent of deaths every year, nearly one in four. It is expected to be the leading cause of death by 2030 and is well on its way: In 2002 only two states had cancer as their number one cause of death, but by 2014 cancer was

---

GLOSSARY

Carcinogens Substances that contribute to the formation of cancers.

Epigenetics The study of differences in an organism caused by changes in gene expression rather than changes in the genome itself.

Figure 11.4 U.S. death rates for major cancer sites, 2014.

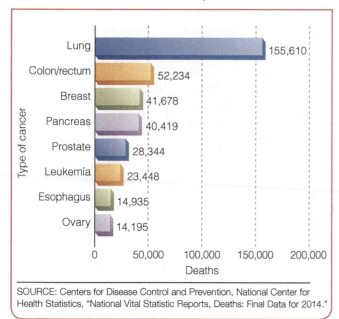

SOURCE: Centers for Disease Control and Prevention, National Center for Health Statistics, "National Vital Statistic Reports, Deaths: Final Data for 2014."

the number one cause of death in 22 states. Breast cancer alone is predicted to affect 50 percent more women in the United States by 2030. The U.S. death rates for the major cancer sites are given in Figure 11.4.

Cancer affects not only adults, but also children. It is the second-leading cause of death in children between ages 1 and 14, after accidents. The major contributor to the increase in incidence of cancer during the last five decades is lung cancer. Tobacco use alone is responsible for 30 percent of all deaths from cancer. Another third of all deaths from cancer are related to unhealthy nutrition, physical inactivity, and excessive body weight (fat).

For the first time, in 2014, cancer was announced as the number-one worldwide cause of death. The global rise in cancer deaths is due primarily to the large increase in tobacco use in developing countries, particularly in India and China, home to 40 percent of the world's smokers. Developing countries face additional affronts because they have higher rates of cancers caused by infections, while still facing growing rates of obesity as they adopt a more sedentary Western lifestyle.

Critical Thinking

Have you ever had, or do you now have, any family members with cancer?

> Can you identify lifestyle or environmental factors as possible contributors to the disease?

> If not, are you concerned about your genetic predisposition, and, if so, are you making lifestyle changes to decrease your risk?

11.4 Guidelines for Preventing Cancer

The biggest factor in fighting cancer today is health education. A survey conducted by the American Institute for Cancer Research (AICR) revealed alarming results about our understanding of the link between lifestyle and cancer risk. Fewer than half of respondents were aware of the link between diets low in vegetables and fruits and cancer risk or of the link between insufficient physical activity and cancer (see Figure 11.5).[1]

Cancer prevention education is an urgent concern because of the real control people have over their own cancer risk. The AICR assessed lifestyle choices of 58,000 people to determine how many of the AICR's recommendations to reduce cancer people were adhering to. The survey showed that with each recommendation adopted by a person, cancer risk decreased. The study results found that people who followed a minimum of five recommendations halved their risk of dying from cancer as compared to people who followed none.[2]

HOEGER KEY TO WELLNESS

Cancer is largely preventable; as much as 80 percent of cancer is related to lifestyle or environmental factors. Genetics play the primary role in only 5 to 10 percent of all cancers.

Cancer prevention education is an urgent concern because people control much of their cancer risk.

Figure 11.5 Percent of public who are aware that the following lifestyle factors affect cancer risk.

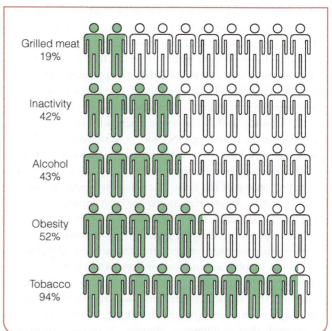

Top Twelve Recommendations for a Cancer Prevention Lifestyle

The American Cancer Society released guidelines on nutrition and physical activity for cancer prevention.[3] These guidelines recommend that people:

1. *Maintain healthy body weight* throughout life.
2. *Adopt a physically active lifestyle*, which should include exercise and limited time spent doing sedentary activities.
3. *Adopt a healthy diet* with emphasis on plant foods.
4. *Limit alcohol consumption.*

Additional existing guidelines that have been established for decades round out a list of top 12 recommendations for a cancer prevention lifestyle:

5. *Abstain from tobacco use* in any form (and limit exposure to secondhand smoke).
6. *Avoid exposure to occupational hazards* (see Figure 11.6) as sometimes encountered by farm, pest-control, gas station, print shop, dry-cleaning, oil refinery, chemical plant, and health care workers; lab technicians (who sterilize equipment); and hair and nail salon employees; among others.
7. *Practice safe sun exposure* and avoid overexposure to ultraviolet light when the sunlight is most intense (see more about sun exposure in Chapter 3, page 122).
8. *Limit the consumption of processed, charred, or well-done meats,* which are high in heterocyclic amines and polyaromatic hydrocarbons. Avoid high-heat cooking and grilling. Do so on rare occasions only.
9. *Have your home periodically tested for radon* (which forms naturally and collects in homes; testing is encouraged even if neighbors have already had their homes tested; see box below).
10. *Have your home periodically tested for arsenic* if you live in a rural community and get your water from a non-public source. State and local EPA offices provide information on radon and arsenic testing.
11. *Be aware of outdoor and indoor air quality* and take necessary precautions. Like many other risk factors, air toxins pose an extremely small but real threat with repeated exposure (to learn about the specific items around you that may be a concern, see "Environmental Red Flags: Contaminants That May Cause Cancer").
12. *Ask your doctor the right questions about Medical Imaging Tests.* Each year x-rays and CT scans save many lives (the cancer risk of having just one of these is miniscule). However, CT scans are being used in higher numbers each year and account for a real, if small, percentage of cancer deaths. Be educated about nonradiation alternatives such as ultrasounds and MRIs, ask about the amount of radiation and number of scans for treatment, and make sure your facility is accredited by the American College of Radiology.

Figure 11.6 **Estimates of the relative role of the major cancer-causing factors.**

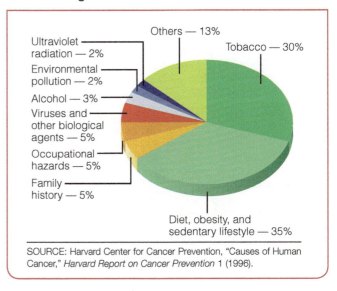

SOURCE: Harvard Center for Cancer Prevention, "Causes of Human Cancer," *Harvard Report on Cancer Prevention* 1 (1996).

How Can I Know Which Substances Cause Cancer?

When following health news, it can seem as if everything you do, touch, or eat is a cause for cancer. You may be surprised to learn the International Agency for Research on Cancer (the IARC, part of the World Health Organization) has created a list of hazards known to cause cancer. Of the millions of chemicals and compounds in the world, only 118 are classified as known to cause cancer (and this list includes not only chemicals but also a variety of risks people face, such as the areca nut, which is chewed in Asia, or hazards, like the profession of being a painter). The IARC has created a series of classifications that go from Group 1, "carcinogenic to humans," down to Group 4, "probably not carcinogenic to humans" (see Figure 11.7). Items that pose risk are classified according to how strong the evidence is that they are, in fact, a cause of cancer. The IARC has added processed meats to Group 1, for example, because evidence is solid that processed meats are known to cause cancer, even though processed meats do not cause nearly as many deaths as tobacco, which is also in Group 1.

Other organizations provide helpful reports and information regarding carcinogens:

- The President's Cancer Panel is a group of three individuals who oversee the National Cancer Institute. (You can read more about this group in the box "Environmental Red Flags: Contaminants That May Cause Cancer," on page 420.)
- The Report on Carcinogens (ROC) is a science-based report that is mandated by the U.S. Congress. (It creates two lists that parallel the IARC's top two groups. The names of the ROC lists are "known to be human carcinogens" and "reasonably anticipated to be human carcinogens.")

Figure 11.7 IARC Classification for agents that may cause cancer and worldwide yearly deaths attributed to selected agents.

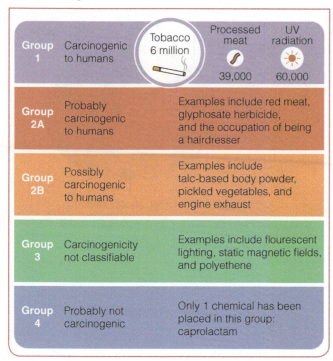

Group 1	Carcinogenic to humans	Tobacco 6 million	Processed meat 39,000	UV radiation 60,000
Group 2A	Probably carcinogenic to humans	Examples include red meat, glyphosate herbicide, and the occupation of being a hairdresser		
Group 2B	Possibly carcinogenic to humans	Examples include talc-based body powder, pickled vegetables, and engine exhaust		
Group 3	Carcinogenicity not classifiable	Examples include flourescent lighting, static magnetic fields, and polyethene		
Group 4	Probably not carcinogenic	Only 1 chemical has been placed in this group: caprolactam		

- The National Institute for Occupational Safety and Health (NIOSH) keeps an updated list of occupational carcinogens.
- The U.S. Department of Health and Human Services keeps a Household Product Database that is easily searchable for substances you may come in contact with daily.

11.5 Adopt Healthy Lifestyle Habits

The most effective way to protect against cancer is to avoid negative lifestyle habits and behaviors. Research sponsored by the American Cancer Society and the National Cancer Institute showed that individuals who have a healthy lifestyle have some of the lowest cancer mortality rates ever reported in scientific studies. In a landmark study, a group of about 10,000 members of the Church of Jesus Christ of Latter-day Saints (commonly referred to as the Mormon church) in California was reported to have only about one-third (men) to one-half (women) the rate of cancer mortality of the general white population[4] (see Figure 11.8). In this study, the investigators looked at three general health habits in the participants: lifetime abstinence from smoking, regular physical activity, and sufficient sleep. Healthy lifestyle guidelines

---

Environmental Red Flags: Contaminants That May Cause Cancer

Since its creation in 1971, the U.S. President's Cancer Panel has monitored exposure by the public to potential environmental cancer risks in daily life. The public remains largely unaware of widespread and underestimated risks, factors that are critical in any cancer prevention efforts. Exposure to environmental contaminants poses a threat to health because contaminants may alter or interfere with a variety of biologic processes. There has been much disagreement about how big a threat environmental toxins pose in cancer risk. Keep in perspective that the most common carcinogenic exposures in the workplace are to tobacco smoke and excessive ultraviolet radiation from sunlight. However, the American Cancer Society estimated that 6 percent of cancer deaths result from environmental toxins and suggests that the majority are lifestyle factors. The President's Cancer Panel, however, called this a gross underestimation considering the number of combined exposures a person experiences in a lifetime, especially during periods of life like puberty when a person may be especially vulnerable. Many cosmetics or self-care products, for example, contain **endocrine disruptors** that interfere with how the body responds to the endocrine system (hormones). Following are several recommendations to minimize environmental toxins exposure, including some released by the presidential panel:

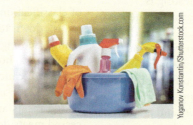

Yuganov Konstantin/Shutterstock.com

1. *Check air-quality indices* such as http://www.AirNow.gov to monitor outdoor pollution. Avoid benzene exposure, which is widespread and found primarily in vehicle exhaust.

2. *Be aware of indoor pollutants,* which are often more pervasive than outdoor pollutants. Limit air fresheners, deodorizers, scented candles, incense, and mothballs. Instead use baking soda, botanical oils, charcoal air filters, or simmer spices on the stovetop. Limit plywood and other manufactured wood products. Avoid exposure to formaldehyde, which is used in particle board, plywood, carpet, draperies, foam insulation, furniture, toiletries, and permanent press fabrics. Exposure is highest when newly installed. Look for labels on manufactured wood that say ULEF—"ultra-low-emitting formaldehyde." Keep a window cracked whenever possible, even in cooler weather, and maintain ventilating systems in any room with a fireplace or range.

3. *Avoid scented cleaning supplies completely,* even those labeled as natural and organic. It may come as a surprise to you that makers of air fresheners and cleaning supplies are not required to disclose harmful chemicals that are in their products. Many contain harmful chemicals that include carcinogens. Dryer sheets may contain limonene (a carcinogen) and other harmful chemicals, and a study

(continued)

by the University of Washington found carcinogens including benzene in a top-selling liquid laundry detergent.[a] Try using a vinegar and water solution for cleaning whenever possible. (Remember to never mix bleach with any acid, including vinegar, because toxic fumes will be produced.) Avoid using traditional dryer sheets. Instead consider using a non-toxic reusable static remover.

4. *Filter tap water* or well water and, whenever possible, use filtered water instead of commercially bottled water.

5. *Properly dispose* of pharmaceuticals, household chemicals, paints, and other products to minimize drinking water and soil contamination.

6. *Eliminate exposure to secondhand smoke* (and tobacco use in general).

7. *Use stainless steel, glass, or BPA-free plastic water bottles.* Look for the recycle category 7 triangle on the bottom of plastic bottles or the letters "PC" for polycarbonate. This indicates that the container may contain BPA (bisphenol A) and should be avoided. BPA is also found in the lining of canned foods (food in glass jars or

cartons is safe), about half of thermal receipts you receive during checkout, and a few other plastic packagings.

8. *Microwave in ceramic or glass* instead of plastic containers.

9. *Remove shoes* before entering a home to avoid bringing in toxic chemicals, including pesticides.

10. *Limit foods grown with pesticides* and meats from animals raised with antibiotics and growth hormones.

11. *Wash your produce.* If you choose to take extra precaution, you may decide to choose a trusted low-pesticide source for purchasing produce items likely to be heavily treated (apples, bell peppers, blueberries, celery, cherries, cherry tomatoes, collard greens, cucumbers, grapes, kale, nectarines, peaches, potatoes, snap peas, spinach, and strawberries). Prewashed produce (indicated on the package) does not have to be washed again.

12. *Use headsets and text, instead of talking on cell phones,* and keep cell phone calls brief to reduce exposure to electromagnetic energy. Although not scientifically proven, there is concern that frequent

exposure to electromagnetic energy from cell phone use increases cancer risk.

13. *Be aware of contaminant exposure in children.* Exposure at a young age is of significant concern because, per pound of body weight, they take in more food, water, air, and other substances than adults do. Their bodies may also be less efficient at removing toxic chemicals, which then remain active longer in their developing brain and organs. Also, cells progress from precancerous to cancerous much faster in children than they do in adults, and tumors metastasize faster than they do in adults. During childhood, cells are constantly dividing so the child can grow. This can result in more copies of a cell that has been mutated due to an environmental toxin. In children, a devastating 80 percent of tumors have metastasized by the time they are diagnosed. Mutations appearing at an early age will also have more years to produce further mutations and develop into cancer.

[a] A. C. Steinemann, I. C. MacGregor, S. M. Gordon, L. G. Gallagher, A. L. Davis, D. S. Ribeiro, and L. A. Wallace, "Fragranced Consumer Products: Chemicals Emitted, Ingredients Unlisted," *Environmental Impact Assessment Review* 31, no. 3 (2011): 328–333.

Figure 11.8 Effects of a healthy lifestyle on cancer mortality rate.

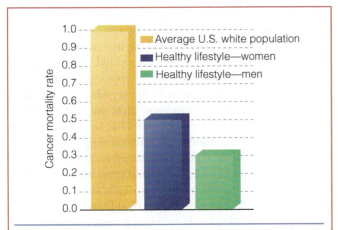

Healthy lifestyle factors include proper nutrition, abstinence from cigarette smoking, regular sleep (7–8 hours per night), and regular physical activity.

SOURCE: J. E. Enstrom, "Health Practices and Cancer Mortality Among Active California Mormons," *Journal of the National Cancer Institute* 81 (1989): 1807–1814.

(encouraged by the church since 1833) include abstaining from all forms of tobacco, alcohol, and drugs, and adhering to a well-balanced diet based on grains, fruits, and vegetables, and moderate amounts of poultry and red meat. Healthy lifestyle factors include proper nutrition, abstinence from cigarette smoking, regular sleep (7–8 hours per night), and regular physical activity.

Additional data from more than 23,000 German participants indicated that people who never smoked, had a body mass index (BMI) of less than 30, exercised at least 3.5 hours per week, and consumed a diet rich in fruits and vegetables and low in meat had a 36 percent lower risk of cancer. The conclusion of the latter two studies is that lifestyle is definitely an important factor in the risk for cancer.[5]

GLOSSARY

Endocrine disruptors Compounds that interfere with the body's endocrine (hormone) system, disturbing the immune system, nervous system, and reproductive system, and causing adverse affects including cancer and birth defects.

11.6 *Consume a Well-Balanced Diet with Ample Amounts of Fruits and Vegetables*

For most Americans who do not use tobacco, increased physical activity and dietary choices are the most important modifiable risk factors. The American Cancer Society estimates that one-third of all cancer incidents in the United States could be related to nutrition and lack of physical activity. A healthy diet, therefore, is crucial to decrease the risk for cancer. The diet should be predominately vegetarian. Dietary fiber, nutrients, and **phytonutrients** appear to work in synergy to prevent and slow cancer development at various stages. **Cruciferous vegetables**, legumes, phytonutrient and antioxidant-rich foods, tea, vitamin D, fiber, calcium, spices, unsaturated fat (including omega-3 fat), and soy products are all encouraged. Processed meat, sugar, and alcohol should be consumed in very limited amounts.

HOEGER KEY TO WELLNESS

Nutrients appear to work in synergy during metabolic processes that prevent cancer and even slow its development at various stages.

Vegetables and Legumes

Vegetables that are thought to protect against cancer include green and dark yellow vegetables, cruciferous vegetables (cauliflower, broccoli, cabbage, kale, Brussels sprouts, and kohlrabi), and beans (legumes). Folate—found naturally in dark green leafy vegetables, dried beans, and orange juice—may reduce the risk for colon and cervical cancers. Brightly colored fruits and vegetables also contain **carotenoids** and vitamin C. Lycopene, one of the many carotenoids (a phytonutrient—see the following discussion), has been linked to lower risk for cancers of the prostate, colon, and cervix.

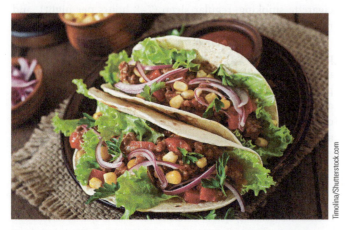

For a cancer-prevention diet, plant foods like whole grains, beans, fruits, and especially vegetables should cover two-thirds or more of your plate.

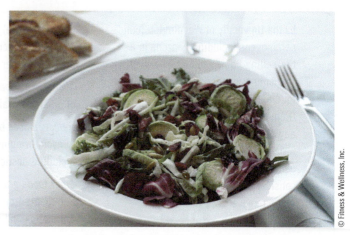

Cruciferous vegetables are recommended in a cancer-prevention diet.

Lycopene is especially abundant in cooked tomato products. A recent study spent a 20-year period testing the blood of 33,000 female nurses and found that the higher the level of carotenoids in the blood, the lower the risk of developing or dying from breast cancer.[6] Frozen fruits and vegetables can be a convenient and nutritious option, particularly because they are picked at their peak, quickly blanched, and immediately frozen. Whether you choose fresh or frozen, keep in mind that cooking with less liquid and with a shorter heating time will preserve the most nutrients.

Phytonutrients

Recall that phytonutrients are compounds in plants that are not essential for survival but have a significant positive effect on human health (they are found in abundance in fruits, vegetables, beans, nuts, and seeds). Most phytonutrients are antioxidants, and therefore prevent cell damage from oxidation. However, phytonutrients are believed to prevent or slow cancer during other stages of growth. For example, they may increase the chance that a mutated cell is destroyed, decrease inflammation, stimulate the immune system, interfere with angiogenesis, or promote cancer-fighting enzymes.

Each plant contains hundreds of phytonutrients. New phytonutrients are continually being discovered, and our understanding of the way combinations of phytonutrients work in synergy with each other and with dietary fiber and nutrients is continually growing. Examples of these nutrients and their impressive effects are found in Table 11.1. To obtain the best possible protection, a minimum of five servings of a variety of fruits and vegetables should be consumed each day. Fruits and vegetables should be consumed several times a day (instead of in one meal) to maintain phytonutrients at effective levels throughout the day. Phytonutrient blood levels drop within 3 hours of consuming foods containing these nutrients.

Antioxidants

Researchers believe that the antioxidant effect of vitamins and the mineral selenium help to prevent cancer. Proteins that require selenium also appear to have a protective effect.

Behavior Modification Planning

Tips for a Healthy Cancer-Fighting Diet

I PLAN TO   I DID IT

I. Increase intake of phytonutrients, fiber, cruciferous vegetables, and antioxidants by

- ❑ ❑ Eating a predominantly vegetarian diet
- ❑ ❑ Eating more fruits and vegetables every day (six to nine servings per day to maximize anticancer benefits)
- ❑ ❑ Increasing the consumption of broccoli, cauliflower, kale, turnips, cabbage, kohlrabi, Brussels sprouts, hot chili peppers, red and green peppers, carrots, sweet potatoes, winter squash, spinach, garlic, onions, dried beans, strawberries, apples, grapes, tomatoes, pineapple, and citrus fruits in my regular diet
- ❑ ❑ Eating vegetables raw or quickly cooked by steaming or stir-frying
- ❑ ❑ Substituting tea and fruit and vegetable juices for coffee and soda

- ❑ ❑ Eating whole-grain breads
- ❑ ❑ Including calcium in the diet (or from a supplement)
- ❑ ❑ Including soy products in the diet
- ❑ ❑ Using whole-wheat flour instead of refined white flour in baking
- ❑ ❑ Using brown (unpolished) rice instead of white (polished) rice

II. Limit saturated and trans fats by

- ❑ ❑ Using primarily unsaturated fats (olive oil, canola oil, nuts, seeds, avocado, fish, flaxseeds, and flaxseed oil)

III. Maintain a healthy weight by

- ❑ ❑ Balancing caloric input with caloric output to maintain recommended body weight

Try It

Make a copy of these "Cancer-Fighting Diet" tips and incorporate two additional dietary behaviors from the list into your lifestyle each week.

MINDTAP From Cengage   **Complete This Online** Visit **www.cengagebrain.com** to access MindTap, a complete digital course that includes interactive quizzes, videos, and more.

Table 11.1 Selected Phytonutrients: Their Effects and Sources

Phytonutrient	Effect	Good Sources
Sulforaphane	Removes carcinogens from cells	Broccoli
PEITC	Keeps carcinogens from binding to DNA	Broccoli
Genistein	Prevents small tumors from accessing capillaries to get oxygen and nutrients	Soybeans
Flavonoids	Helps keep cancer-causing hormones from locking onto cells	Most fruits and vegetables
p-coumaric and chlorogenic acids	Disrupt the chemical combination of cell molecules that can produce carcinogens	Strawberries, green peppers, tomatoes, pineapple
Capsaicin	Keeps carcinogens from binding to DNA	Hot chili peppers

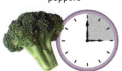

Consume fruits and vegetables several times a day to maintain phytonutrients at effective levels. Phytonutrient blood levels drop a few hours after consuming the source food.

Recall that an antioxidant is a substance that blocks or slows damage to cells caused by oxidation. Antioxidants may come from plant or animal sources. They may be vitamins (organic substances essential for survival), minerals (inorganic substances essential for survival), or phytonutrients. During normal metabolism, most of the oxygen in the human body is converted into stable forms of carbon dioxide and water. A small amount, however, ends up in an unstable form known as oxygen-free radicals, which are thought to attack and damage the cell membrane and DNA, leading to the formation of cancers. Antioxidants are thought to absorb free radicals before they can cause damage and also interrupt the sequence of reactions once damage has begun. Research is still required in this area because a clear link has not been established (for more information about antioxidants, see Chapter 3, page 118). Unless otherwise indicated by a health care practitioner, as with other factors in your diet, antioxidants should be obtained by eating whole foods and not by taking supplements.

GLOSSARY

Phytonutrients Compounds found in fruits and vegetables that block formation of cancerous tumors and disrupt the progress of cancer.

Cruciferous vegetables Plants that produce cross-shaped leaves (cauliflower, broccoli, cabbage, Brussels sprouts, and kohlrabi), which seem to have a protective effect against cancer.

Carotenoids Pigment substances in plants that are often precursors to vitamin A. More than 600 carotenoids are found in nature, about 50 of which are precursors to vitamin A, the most potent one being beta-carotene.

Tea

Polyphenols (a group of phytonutrients) are believed to be cancer-fighting antioxidants found in fresh fruits and vegetables and many grains. Polyphenols are known to block the formation of nitrosamines (see discussion on meat and cancer that follows) and quell the activation of carcinogens. Polyphenols also are thought to fight cancer by shutting off the formation of cancer cells, turning up the body's natural detoxification defenses, and thereby suppressing progression of the disease.

Because tea is a prime source of polyphenols, white, green, and black teas (all produced from the same plant) have been studied as potential agents in cancer protection. Early evidence pointed to certain components in tea that may inhibit cancer at various stages. Some researchers indicated that the antioxidant effect of one of the polyphenols in green tea, epigallocatechin gallate (EGCG), protects cells and DNA from damage that may cause cancer, heart disease, and other diseases associated with free radicals.[7] Observational data on tea-drinking habits in China showed that people who regularly drank green tea had about half the risk for chronic gastritis and stomach cancer, and the risk decreased further as the number of years of drinking green tea increased.[8]

Recent studies, however, have been inconclusive in their attempt to find a connection between green tea consumption and lower cancer risk.[9] A review of more than 20 studies found too much conflicting evidence to recommend drinking tea for cancer prevention purposes.[10] Although there is insufficient evidence to currently recommend it as a cancer-protective food, other studies continue to show many potential benefits of tea, including protection against DNA damage, ultraviolet (UV) radiation, and tumor development.

Vitamin D

The evidence for vitamin D as a protective against cancer continues to be the focus of research. Vitamin D appears to be the most powerful regulator of cell growth and seems to keep cells from becoming malignant. Researchers are still working to understand the cause-and-effect relationship between health and vitamin D levels, but the protective effect of vitamin D appears to be strongest against breast, colon, and prostate cancers and possibly lung and digestive cancers. You should strive for "safe sun" exposure, that is, 10 to 20 minutes of unprotected sun exposure on most days of the week between the hours of 10:00 a.m. and 4:00 p.m. For people living in the northern United States and Canada with limited sun exposure during the winter months, a vitamin D_3 supplement of up to 2,000 IUs per day is strongly recommended. The cancer-protective benefits of this vitamin as well as tips for getting the right level of sun exposure are discussed in detail in Chapter 3 (see "Vitamin D," page 120).

Fiber and Calcium

A high intake of fiber has been linked to decreased risk for colorectal cancer. Observational studies have also linked high levels of dietary fiber with a decreased risk for breast cancer. Fiber is thought to lower estrogen levels and unhealthy insulin levels, protect the intestines by reducing their exposure to toxins, and feed healthy intestinal bacteria that then go on to help fight inflammation throughout the body and improve colon health. Healthy intestinal bacteria are essential, as they breaks down helpful phytonutrients that could not otherwise be absorbed. To benefit from the various types of fiber, obtain fiber from a variety of sources, including different types of grains, vegetables, fruits, and nuts. Daily consumption of 25 (women) to 38 (men) grams of fiber is recommended. Whole grains are high in fiber and contain vitamins and minerals (folate, selenium, and calcium). Calcium may also protect against colon cancer by preventing the rapid growth of cells in the colon, especially in people with colon polyps.

Spices

Although still in the early stages, research is uncovering cancer-fighting phytonutrients in many traditional spices. Turmeric, a member of the ginger family, is an excellent example. In India, where the spice is used in large quantities, incidence of colorectal cancer as well as Alzheimer's and cognitive decline are especially low. The recommended quantity is two-thirds of a teaspoon (or 1,500 milligrams) in a serving for the spice to have its positive effect. Other spices—including ginger, garlic, oregano, curry, pepper, cloves, fennel, rosemary, and black pepper—are all encouraged for use in cooking and at the table.

Monounsaturated and Omega-3 Fats

Although previously viewed as a risk factor, minimal evidence exists that total fat intake affects cancer risk. There is far greater evidence that being overweight or obese increases cancer risk. Excessive caloric intake leads to weight gain, and high-fat foods are typically calorie dense. Thus, indirectly, a high-fat diet can increase cancer risk through excessive body weight.

In any healthy diet, fat intake should be primarily monounsaturated and omega-3 polyunsaturated fats (found in flaxseed and several types of cold-water fish). These types of fat may offer protection against some types of cancers, particularly cancers related to hormone production (like breast cancer) and those linked to chronic inflammation (like colorectal cancer). Omega-3 fats may also inhibit tumor development during various stages of malignant growth.[11]

Soy

Soy has long been valued for its ability to help prevent cancer because of observational studies of Japanese populations, among whom rates of breast and other cancers are low. Soy protein seems to decrease the formation of carcinogens during cooking of meats. Soy foods may help because soy contains chemicals and active compounds that prevent cancer. Among these are isoflavones (phytonutrients), which are structurally similar to estrogen and may prevent breast, prostate, lung, and colon cancers. Isoflavones, frequently referred to as "phytoestrogens" or "plant estrogens," also block angiogenesis. Other phytonutrients and compounds in soy may prevent cancer by regulating cell growth and death, by discouraging metastasis, and by helping at other various stages of cancer development.

One potential drawback of soy was found in studies in which animals who had already developed tumors were given large amounts of soy. The estrogen-like activity of soy isoflavones actually led to the growth of estrogen-dependent tumors. Experts, therefore, caution women with breast cancer or a history of this disease to limit their soy intake. However, observational studies of women's dietary patterns since have not been able to confirm this drawback.

The most current recommendations state that there is not enough evidence to conclude that soy either prevents or promotes breast cancer in American women, though it has protective effects on Japanese women. No specific recommendations are presently available as to the recommended amount of daily soy protein intake to prevent cancer. The Japanese diet includes more than eight times as much soy as the typical American diet. Soy is a part of a person's diet from childhood through adolescence (an important time for development of breast and other tissues) to adulthood. Based on these traditional diets of people in Japan as well as in China, there doesn't seem to be an unsafe natural level of consumption. Soy protein powder supplementation, however, may elevate intake of soy protein to an unnatural (and perhaps unsafe) level. Add soy to your diet with soymilk and whole foods such as tofu, miso, and edamame. It is important to remember the general recommendation to avoid focusing on any single food; instead, obtain the nutrients from a variety of vegetables, nuts, seeds, whole grains, and legumes.

Processed Meat and Protein

For decades, we have known that a diet high in processed and red meats correlates with a greater chance for developing cancer. Salt-cured, smoked, fermented, and nitrite-cured foods have been associated with cancers of the colon, rectum, stomach, and esophagus. Eating substantial amounts of red meat may increase the risk for cancers of the colon, rectum, pancreas, breast, and prostate, as well as renal cancer.

The IARC made big news in 2015 when it added processed meat to its Group 1 classification, meaning it is known to cause cancer in humans. At the same time, red meat was classified as Group 2A, meaning it probably causes cancer in humans (see Figure 11.7). The IARC concluded that a person who regularly eats 50 grams (1.8 oz.) of processed meat per day (the equivalent of a slice and a half of bacon) raises his or her risk of colorectal cancer by 18 percent. The risk goes up as the daily intake of processed meat goes up. For red meat, the risk goes up by 17 percent for every 100 grams (3.5 oz.) eaten per day. While this risk has an undeniable impact on real cancer deaths, it is important to keep the numbers in perspective. Overall lifetime risk of colorectal cancer is 5 percent, which means 1 out of every 20 individuals will be diagnosed with the disease in their lifetime. By adding 18 percent to that overall lifetime risk, a person increases their total lifetime risk to 6 percent.

What Qualifies as Red Meat and Processed Meat?

Red meat is any meat from a mammalian source. This includes beef, pork, and lamb, for example, but does not include poultry or fish. Processed meat is any meat that is not fresh and can include red meat as well as poultry or fish that has been salt-cured, smoked, fermented, or nitrate/nitrite-cured. Before refrigeration was introduced around 1900, and for thousands of years earlier, these methods were used to preserve meat. While these methods were born of necessity, they have continued to be used because people have enjoyed the flavor of processed meat.

Nitrites and Nitrates

Processed meats (hot dogs, ham, bacon, sausage, salami, pepperoni, and lunch meats) should be consumed sparingly and always with vitamin C-rich foods such as orange juice because vitamin C seems to discourage the formation of nitrosamines. These cancer-causing compounds are formed when nitrites and nitrates, which are used to prevent the growth of harmful bacteria in processed meats, combine with other chemicals in the stomach. (Even products that are labeled "no nitrates or nitrites added" carry the risk because these products are made with celery juice, which naturally contains sodium nitrate. Nitrate is a naturally occurring type of salt that, when added to meat, is broken down by bacteria to create nitrite in the meat. As a shortcut, food producers can create nitrite in a lab and use it to quickly cure meat.)

The combination of the heme protein with iron, both found abundantly in red meat, also contributes to the formation of **nitrosamines** in the large intestine, increasing the risk for colorectal cancer.

HCAs and PAHs

Cooking protein at a high temperature should be avoided or done only occasionally. The data suggest that grilling, broiling, or frying meat, poultry, or fish at high temperatures to "medium well" or "well done" leads to the formation of carcinogenic substances known as heterocyclic amines (HCAs) and polycyclic aromatic hydrocarbons (PAHs). These compounds work like other carcinogenic compounds—once these ions enter your body, they seek to bond with organic molecules. DNA is one of those organic molecules they can bond with, and the DNA is destroyed in the process. Individuals who prefer their meat medium well or well done have a much higher risk for colorectal, stomach, breast, and prostate cancers. Cancer risk seems to correlate to the amount of

---

GLOSSARY

Nitrosamines Potentially cancer-causing compounds formed when nitrites and nitrates, which prevent the growth of harmful bacteria in processed meats, combine with other chemicals in the stomach.

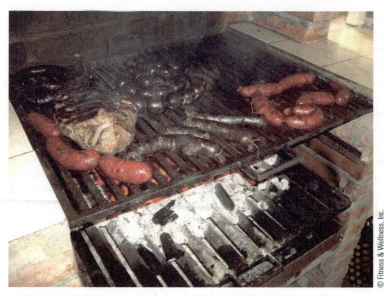

Cooking protein at higher temperature to "medium well" or "well done" should be done only occasionally as such leads to the formation of carcinogenic substances on the surface of meats.

well-done meat an individual consumes, but even small amounts each day add up.

When proteins are cooked at high temperatures, amino acids are changed into HCAs that collect on the surface of meats. Charring meat increases their formation to an even greater extent. PAHs are formed when fat drips onto the rocks or coals of the grill. The subsequent fire flare-up releases smoke that coats the food with PAHs.

An electric contact grill such as a George Foreman grill is preferable when cooking meats because cooking temperatures are easily controlled. The health risks of outdoor grilling can be reduced by following the suggestions outlined below in "Grilling Guidelines to Reduce Cancer Risk."

Recommendations

Every individual should consider personal risk when deciding how much red and processed meat to consume. Red meat should definitely transition away from being the focus of the meal and instead be treated as a side dish. The American Institute for Cancer research recommends consuming less than 18 ounces of cooked red meat per week, or the equivalent of less than 3 ounces on 6 days per week.

Further, nutritional guidelines discourage the excessive intake of animal protein. Too much animal protein appears to decrease blood enzymes that prevent precancerous cells from developing into tumors. An additional benefit of less meat consumption is a healthier environment, as livestock are a major source of methane emission. Livestock also requires a great amount of energy to raise.

Sugar

Recent evidence indicates that frequent consumption of sugar and refined carbohydrates may be associated with greater risk for pancreatic cancer, one of the most deadly forms of cancer.[12] The pancreas produces the hormone insulin to balance blood glucose levels. Another hormone, insulin-like growth factor, which is produced mostly by the liver, assists insulin in regulating blood sugar. Foods with a high glycemic index cause the body to respond by releasing an excessive amount of insulin and insulin-like growth factor. Elevated levels of insulin as well as insulin-like growth factor foster the growth of cancer cells. Researchers also theorize that excessive glucose poisons and kills pancreatic cells, increasing cancer risk. High glucose and high insulin levels also seem to increase the risk of breast, colorectal, and endometrial cancer as well, and certainly increase risk for diabetes. For years we have known that people with diabetes have an increased risk for cancer. Researchers now believe that individuals who are prediabetic also have an increased risk for cancer.

Alcohol Consumption

Alcohol use has been cited as one of the least emphasized causes for increased cancer risk. The National Toxicology Program classifies excessive alcohol consumption in the category "known to be a human carcinogen." Among other cancer-promoting effects, alcohol can damage DNA and proteins while it is being metabolized, the extent of the damage depending on the individual's genetic inheritance.

In the United States, 3.5 percent of all cancer deaths are a result of alcohol consumption, with substantially higher numbers for some cancers. Of breast cancer deaths, 15 percent are attributed to alcohol, with increased risk across all levels of alcohol consumption. Breast cancer risk begins with less than one drink per day and increases by 12 percent with each additional 10 ounces consumed per day (see Figure 11.9).

Figure 11.9 Alcohol and cancer risk.

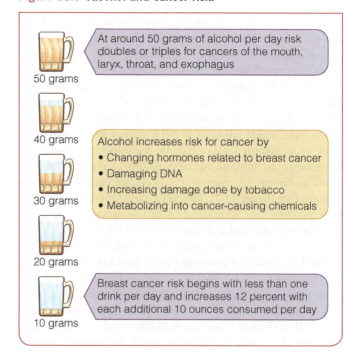

At around 50 grams of alcohol per day risk doubles or triples for cancers of the mouth, laryx, throat, and exophagus

50 grams
40 grams
30 grams

Alcohol increases risk for cancer by
• Changing hormones related to breast cancer
• Damaging DNA
• Increasing damage done by tobacco
• Metabolizing into cancer-causing chemicals

20 grams
10 grams

Breast cancer risk begins with less than one drink per day and increases 12 percent with each additional 10 ounces consumed per day

Grilling Guidelines to Reduce Cancer Risk

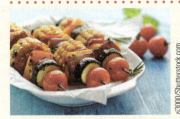

For an occasional outdoor barbecue, what you grill and how you grill are the most important factors. Animal products (both red and white meat) are the culprits, whereas grilling fruit and vegetables does not produce HCAs or PAHs. When grilling meats, the following approach can decrease HCAs and PAHs up to 90 percent.

- Cook meats with natural antioxidants, which decrease or eliminate HCAs and PAHs. Always marinate meat for at least 4 hours using some combination of vinegar, lemon juice, oil (preferably olive oil), and herbs and condiments, including rosemary, red and black pepper, paprika, allspice, garlic, mustard, turmeric, thyme, chives, oregano, basil, sage, or parsley, among others. The marinade is believed to act as a barrier against the heat.

- Keep the meat moist and trim off all excess fat to avoid flare-ups.

- Microwave meat, poultry, and fish for 90 seconds to 2 minutes prior to grilling, which eliminates most of the HCAs.

- Cook at lower heat, less than 350°F, to "medium" rather than "well" or "well done."

- Cook over aluminum foil with small holes cut in the foil so that drippings can pass through.

- Opt for kabobs or smaller cuts of meat that need less time on the grill.

- Turn the meat over frequently, every 3 to 4 minutes.

- Remove all skin before serving.

- Consider grilling on a water-soaked cedar plank or in an aluminum foil packet.

- Add broccoli to your meal. Broccoli has been shown to break down HCAs.

- Keep your grill clean, scrape off all charred remnants, and wash the cooking grid.

- Eat less meat as such increases your risk for cancer.

Should I be concerned about parabens and other chemicals in makeup?

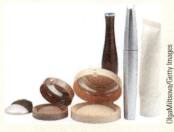

Chemicals in cosmetics and self-care products have been the focus of research and concern in recent years. Some products contain endocrine disruptors (which interfere with how the body responds to hormones) such as parabens and phthalates. Risks are greatest during gestation and infancy, but puberty is also a time of growth and change and therefore increased vulnerability. Teenage girls who use a large number of self-care products are at greater risk. Cosmetics and self-care products are only loosely regulated in the United States, and some ingredients are not required to be listed. In order to lower exposure, look for self-care products that do not list parabens, phthalates, or fragrance in the ingredient list, and consider using phone apps from the Campaign for Safe Cosmetics or the Environmental Working Group Skin Deep database to research products before buying.

to protect against cancer. There is strong evidence that high-dose supplements of certain nutrients increase the risk of certain cancers. The best source of nutrients is a healthy diet.

11.7 Maintain Recommended Body Weight

While nearly all Americans are aware that tobacco causes cancer, only half are aware of any link between obesity and cancer.[13] Furthermore, obese men and women have a more than 50 percent increased risk for dying from any form of

For other forms of cancers, alcohol becomes a serious danger at around 50 grams per day, where risk for cancers of the mouth, larynx, throat, and esophagus double or triple. Excessive alcohol use is also a risk factor for colorectal cancer and a primary cause for liver cancer.

The general recommendation has been that people should consume alcohol in moderation. For women, there may not be a safe level of alcohol consumption in regards to cancer risk.

Nutrient Supplements

An expert panel of the World Cancer Research Fund and the American Institute of Cancer Research stated that unless recommended by your doctor, you should not use supplements

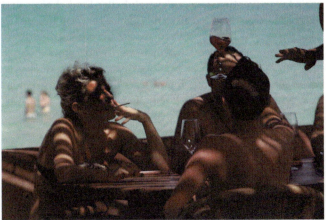

Heavy drinking and smoking greatly increase the risk of oral cancer.

Figure 11.10 U.S. estimated cancer cases preventable by diet, activity, and weight management in the United States per year (for selected sites).

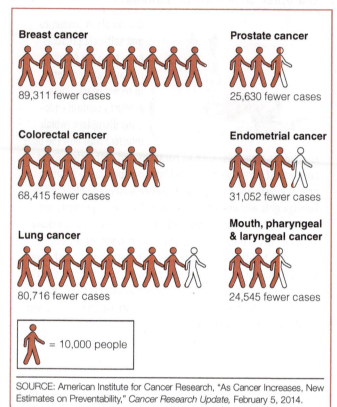

Breast cancer

89,311 fewer cases

Prostate cancer

25,630 fewer cases

Colorectal cancer

68,415 fewer cases

Endometrial cancer

31,052 fewer cases

Lung cancer

80,716 fewer cases

Mouth, pharyngeal & laryngeal cancer

24,545 fewer cases

= 10,000 people

SOURCE: American Institute for Cancer Research, "As Cancer Increases, New Estimates on Preventability," *Cancer Research Update*, February 5, 2014.

cancer, and are more likely to have cancer reoccur after remission.[14] Adult weight gain increases the risk for many cancers, including those of the breast, ovaries, endometrium, colon and rectum, esophagus, pancreas, kidney, liver, prostate, and gallbladder. For each of these types of cancer, the American Institute for Cancer Research has released the number of cases that could be prevented by diet, physical activity, and weight management (see Figure 11.10): 89,311 cases of breast cancer and 68,415 cases of colorectal cancer in the United States never would have occurred.[15] The AICR emphasizes that these numbers are legitimate and reachable goals for preventing cancer through better food choices and weight management. Recall that body fat is an endocrine organ. That is, fat cells create and secrete hormones that direct the body to carry out certain functions. Investigators theorize that too much fat tissue produces excess hormone levels, causes chronic inflammation, affects tumor growth regulators, and increases blood levels of insulin and insulin-like growth factor-1 in the body that stimulate tumor growth.

11.8 *Abstain from Tobacco*

The biggest carcinogenic exposure in the environment—without question—is tobacco use and exposure to secondhand smoke. If we include all related deaths, smoking is responsible for more than 480,000 unnecessary deaths in the

United States each year and 6 million deaths worldwide. That figure is expected to reach 8 million by 2030. Nonsmokers exposed to secondhand smoke represent roughly one in ten deaths from smoking. The average life expectancy for a chronic smoker is about 13 to 14 years shorter than for a nonsmoker.[16]

Of all cancers, at least 30 percent are tied to smoking, and 87 percent of lung cancers are linked to smoking. Cigarette smoking contributes to at least 15 additional types of cancer, including oral, lip, nasal, pharyngeal, laryngeal, esophageal, uterine, stomach, and pancreatic. Use of smokeless tobacco can also lead to nicotine addiction and dependence, as well as increased risk for cancers of the mouth, larynx, throat, and esophagus. If you smoke or use any other tobacco products, STOP NOW! If you do not smoke, DON'T EVER START. If you are ever around people who are smoking, claim your right to clean air or distance yourself from them as much as you possibly can.

11.9 *Avoid Excessive Sun Exposure*

Near-daily "safe sun" exposure—that is, 10 to 20 minutes of unprotected exposure during peak hours of the day—is beneficial to health, but too much exposure to UV radiation is a major contributor to skin cancer. The most common sites of skin cancer are the areas exposed to the sun most often (face, neck, and back of the hands). UV rays are strongest when the sun is high in the sky. Therefore, you should avoid prolonged sun exposure between 10:00 a.m. and 4:00 p.m. Take the shadow test: If your shadow is shorter than you, the UV rays are at their strongest.

There are three main types of skin cancer, each named after the type of cell from which it originates:

1. *Basal cell carcinoma.* Basal cells form the base, or the innermost layer of the epidermis.
2. *Squamous cell carcinoma.* Squamous originates from the word "scale." These flatter cells form the outside layer of the epidermis and shed as new cells form.
3. *Malignant melanoma.* Melanoma originates in cells that create melanin, which gives color to skin.

Basal and squamous cell carcinoma require treatment but in the majority of cases do not spread to other parts of the body. **Melanoma**, the most deadly type of skin cancer, can appear quickly and metastasize in as little as 6 months. In 2016, it caused approximately 10,130 deaths in the United States. That number is expected to double by 2030. About 20 percent of Americans will develop skin cancer in their lifetime. Treatment for nonmelanoma skin cancer increased by more than 75 percent between 1992 and 2006. Melanoma is the number-one cancer killer of young women and increased 800 and 400 percent in young women and young men, respectively, between 1970 and 2009.

How Risky Is the Occasional Sunburn?

One to two blistering sunburns can double the lifetime risk for melanoma, even more so if the sunburn takes place prior

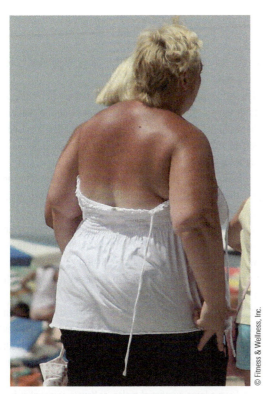

Tanned skin is the body's natural reaction to permanent and irreversible damage—a precursor to severe or fatal skin cancer.

to age 18, when cells divide at a much faster rate than later in life. A person can easily be overexposed during a day in the sun sooner than they expect and not realize until later in the day when the sunburn becomes painful and the damage is already done. Overexposure can be difficult to predict because the strength of the sun exposure varies according to the time of year, a location's latitude and elevation, and the sun's reflection off snow or water, among other factors. Be sure to understand how sun exposure changes by studying the "Sun Exposure" behavior modification planning box in Chapter 3, page 122.

The stinging sunburn comes from **ultraviolet B (UVB) rays**, which are also thought to be the main cause of premature wrinkling and skin aging, roughened/leathery/sagging skin, and skin cancer. Unfortunately, the damage may not become evident until up to 20 years later. By comparison, skin that has not been overexposed to the sun remains smooth and unblemished and, over time, shows less evidence of aging.

How Risky Is Indoor Tanning?

Sun lamps and tanning parlors provide mainly **ultraviolet A (UVA) rays**. Once thought to be safe, they too are now known to be damaging and have been linked to melanoma. As little as 15 to 30 minutes of exposure to UVA rays can be as dangerous as a day spent in the sun. Nothing is healthy about a "healthy tan." Tanning of the skin is the body's natural

reaction to permanent and irreversible damage from too much exposure to the sun. Even small doses of sunlight add up to a greater risk for skin cancer and premature aging. Similar to regular exposure to sun, short-term exposure to recreational tanning at a salon causes DNA alterations that can lead to skin cancer. The tan fades at the end of the summer season, but the underlying skin damage does not disappear.

HOEGER KEY TO WELLNESS

One to two blistering sunburns can double the lifetime risk for melanoma. Take the shadow test: If your shadow is shorter than you, the ultraviolet rays are at their strongest. Limit your exposure to "safe sun" exposure.

11.10 Monitor Estrogen, Radiation Exposure, and Potential Occupational Hazards

Estrogen use has been linked to endometrial and breast cancer in some studies. Estrogen produced by excess fat in women after menopause is of particular concern. Although the exposure to radiation from x-rays increases the risk for cancer, the benefits of x-rays may outweigh the risk involved, and most medical facilities use the lowest dose possible to keep the risk to a minimum. Occupational hazards—such as exposure to asbestos fibers, nickel and uranium dusts, chromium compounds, vinyl chloride, and bischlormethyl ether—increase the risk for cancer. The National Toxicology Program updates a list of environmental exposures every 2 years. The current list includes more than 243 substances, some of which you may be familiar with, while others are more obscure and specific to certain industries. While each carcinogen should be considered individually, it is important to keep in mind that each person will have an individualized reaction to the combined exposures of his or her genetic expression and his or her lifetime environment. Cigarette smoking also magnifies the risk from occupational hazards.

GLOSSARY

Melanoma The most virulent, rapidly spreading form of skin cancer.

Ultraviolet B (UVB) rays Ultraviolet rays that cause sunburn and lead to skin cancers.

Ultraviolet A (UVA) rays Ultraviolet rays that pass deeper into the skin and are believed to cause skin damage and skin cancers.

Protect Yourself from Skin Cancer Risk

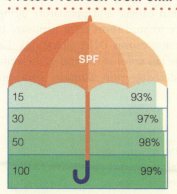

SPF	
15	93%
30	97%
50	98%
100	99%

Nearly 90 percent of the almost 1 million cases of basal cell or squamous cell skin cancers reported yearly in the United States could have been prevented by protecting the skin from excessive sun exposure.

Sunscreen lotion should be applied about 30 minutes before lengthy exposure to the sun because the skin takes that long to absorb the protective ingredients. A **sun protection factor (SPF)** of at least 15 is recommended. SPF 15 means that the skin takes 15 times longer to burn than it would with no lotion. If you ordinarily get a mild sunburn after 20 minutes of noonday sun, an SPF 15 allows you to remain in the sun about 300 minutes before burning. SPF 15 sunscreen lotion blocks 93 percent of UVB rays (the cause of sunburns). Sunscreens with stronger SPF factors are not necessarily better. They should be applied just as often, and they block only an additional 4 to 5 percent of ultraviolet rays. SPF 15 is adequate for most people. An SPF 30, however, is recommended for people with a family history of skin cancer. While SPF refers to blocking UVB rays (the cause of sunburn), it is also important to block UVA rays (more closely associated with causing skin cancer). Select sunscreens labeled "broad spectrum" because these products block both UVA and UVB rays. During peak hours, reapplication is vital. Sunscreen should be reapplied every 2 hours. Dermatologists agree it takes about 1 ounce of sunscreen (picture enough to fill a shot glass) to protect your whole body. For face protection on an average day, it is probably most realistic for the majority of people to apply sunscreen in the morning and then wear a protective hat when outdoors the remainder of the day. Also, do not forget to protect your lips and your eyes.

A lip balm with SPF 30 and sunglasses that block 99 percent to 100 percent of the sun's rays are recommended.

Medical experts are also concerned about hormone-mimicking active ingredients in some sunscreens that are absorbed into the skin and possibly the bloodstream. Under particular scrutiny are the ingredients oxybenzone and retinyl palmitate. Although the jury is still out on any potential harmful health effects of these ingredients, preferably choose a sunscreen that contains zinc oxide, titanium dioxide, or both. These are finely crushed minerals in sunscreens that shield the skin from the sun's ultraviolet rays.

When swimming or sweating, you should reapply sunscreens more often because all sunscreens lose strength when they are diluted. Look for "water resistant" or "very water resistant" sunscreens, which will adhere to the skin for 40 to 80 minutes, respectively, even if the sunscreen promises "continuous protection."

If you plan on being out in the sun for a lengthy period of time, even better than sunscreen is wearing protective clothing, including long-sleeved shirts, long pants, and a hat with a 2- to 3-inch brim all the way around. This sun-protection strategy is even more critical for fair-skinned individuals who burn readily or turn red after only a few minutes of unprotected sun exposure, have a large number of moles, or have a personal or family history of skin cancer risk. Sun-protective fabrics, such as those manufactured by Coolibar® or Sun Precautions®, offer additional protection. You can also use RIT Sun Guard, a laundry additive that when used in washing penetrates the fibers and subsequently absorbs ultraviolet rays during sun exposure. The additive blocks up to 96 percent of UVA and UVB rays.

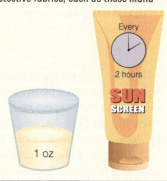

11.11 *Be Physically Active*

An active lifestyle has been shown to have a protective effect against cancer. Physical fitness and cancer mortality in men and women may have a graded and consistent inverse relationship (see Figure 11.11). Leisure-time physical activity alone is associated with a reduced risk of 13 different types of cancer.[17] Physical activity appears to work through a variety of mechanisms to protect against cancer. Exercise releases epinephrine, which helps "natural killer cells" circulate in tumors. Physical activity also reduces insulin levels and leptin levels. High leptin levels promote inflammation and encourage the survival of certain cancers.

A daily 30-minute, moderate-intensity exercise program lowers the risk for colon, breast, and uterine cancers between 20 and 50 percent, and vigorous physical activity may lower the risk of more aggressive and fatal types of prostate cancer.[18] Researchers have found that the activity needs to be of at least moderate intensity to achieve the benefit of reducing overall cancer mortality. Studies have also found that exercise early in life and in mid-life can decrease chances for cancer later in life by up to 40 percent for breast cancer, 55 percent for lung cancer, and 44 percent for colorectal cancer.[19]

HOEGER KEY TO WELLNESS

For most non-tobacco users, a healthy dietary pattern and regular physical activity are the two most significant lifestyle behaviors that reduce cancer risk.

One study spent 35 years following more than 2,000 men and found that at least 30 minutes a day of moderate- to high-intensity physical activity is inversely associated with the risk of premature death from cancer in men.[20] After 10 years, men who switched from low- or medium- to high-intensity physical activity (greater than 5.2 metabolic equivalent task levels) were found

Figure 11.11 Association between physical fitness and cancer mortality.

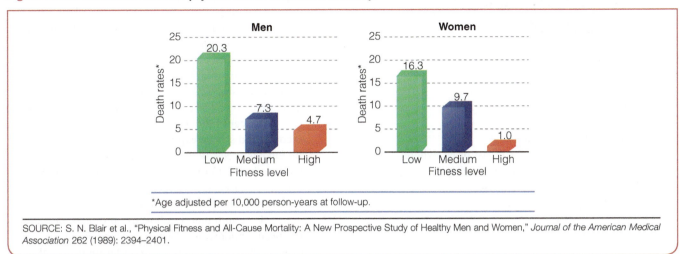

SOURCE: S. N. Blair et al., "Physical Fitness and All-Cause Mortality: A New Prospective Study of Healthy Men and Women," *Journal of the American Medical Association* 262 (1989): 2394–2401.

to have half the risk of dying from cancer. There were no changes in mortality rate when switching from low- to medium-level physical activity. Other data suggest that in men 65 or older, exercising vigorously at least three times per week decreases the risk for advanced or fatal prostate cancer by 70 percent.[21]

Regular strength-training also contributes to lower cancer mortality. A total of 8,677 men between the ages of 20 and 82 were tracked for more than two decades. The data indicated that men who regularly worked out with weights and had the highest muscle strength were up to 40 percent less likely to die from cancer, even among men with a higher waist circumference and BMI.[22]

Growing evidence suggests that the body's autoimmune system may play a role in preventing cancer and that moderate exercise improves the autoimmune system.

11.12 Other Factors

The contributions of many of the other much-publicized factors are not as significant as those just pointed out. Intentional food additives, saccharin, processing agents, pesticides, and packaging materials currently used in the United States and other developed countries seem to have minimal consequences. High levels of tension and stress and poor coping may affect the autoimmune system negatively and render the body less effective in dealing with the various cancers. Chronic stress increases cortisol and inflammatory chemicals that sustain cancer growth.[23]

11.13 Early Detection

Fortunately, many cancers can be controlled or cured through early detection. The real problem comes when cancerous cells spread because they become more difficult to destroy. Therefore, effective prevention, or at least early detection, is crucial. Herein lies the importance of periodic screening. Once a month, women should practice breast self-examination (BSE; see Figure 11.15) and men, testicular self-examination (TSE; see Figure 11.16). Men should pick a regular day each month (e.g., the first day of each month) to practice TSE, and women should perform BSE 2 to 3 days after the menstrual period is over.

GLOSSARY

Sun protection factor (SPF) The degree of protection offered by ingredients in sunscreen lotion; at least SPF 15 is recommended.

Behavior Modification Planning

Cancer Promoters

- Use of or exposure to tobacco products
- Physical inactivity
- Being more than 10 pounds overweight
- Frequent consumption of red meat
- A diet high in fat
- Charred/burned foods
- Frequent consumption of nitrate/nitrite-cured, salt-cured, or smoked foods
- Alcohol consumption

- Excessive sun exposure
- Estrogens
- Methyleugenol (flavoring agent in packaged foods)
- Radon, formaldehyde, and benzene
- Wood dust (high levels)

Try It

In your online journal or class notebook, make a list of cancer promoters around you and note whether you take necessary actions to avoid them. If you do not, note what it would take for you to do so.

11.14 *Nine Warning Signs of Cancer*

Talk to your doctor if you experience any of the following nine warning signs of cancer:

1. Change in bowel or bladder habits
2. Sore that does not heal
3. Unusual bleeding or discharge
4. Thickening or lump in the breast or elsewhere
5. Indigestion or difficulty in swallowing
6. Obvious change in wart or mole
7. Nagging cough or hoarseness
8. Unexplained weight loss
9. Ongoing pain or fatigue

In Activity 11.1, you will be able to determine how well you are doing in terms of a cancer-prevention program. Activity 11.2 provides a questionnaire to alert you to symptoms that may indicate a serious health problem. Although, in most cases, nothing serious will be found, any symptom calls for a physician's attention as soon as possible. Scientific evidence and testing procedures for the prevention and early detection of cancer do change as studies continue to provide new information. The intent of cancer-prevention programs is to educate and guide people toward a lifestyle that will help prevent cancer and enable early detection of malignancy.

Treatment of cancer should always be left to specialized physicians and cancer clinics. Current treatment modalities include surgery, radiation, radioactive substances, chemotherapy, hormones, immunotherapy, and targeted therapies.

11.15 *Cancer: Assessing Your Risks*

Figure 11.12 provides a self-testing questionnaire to help you assess your cancer risk. The factors listed in the questionnaire are the major risk factors for specific cancer sites and by no means represent the only ones that might be involved. Check your status against the factors contained in this questionnaire. Based on the number of risk factors that apply to you, rate yourself on a scale from 1 to 3 (1 for low risk, 2 for moderate risk, and 3 for high risk) for each cancer site. Explanations of the risk factors for the leading types of cancer follow. If you are at higher risk, you are advised to discuss the results with your physician. Record your risk level totals for each cancer site in Activity 11.3.

Risk Factors for Common Sites of Cancer

Lung Cancer

1. *Smoking status.* Tobacco smoke causes nearly nine out of ten cases of lung cancer (includes cigarette, cigar, and pipe smoking). Smoking low-tar or "light"

cigarettes increases lung cancer risk as much as smoking regular cigarettes. The rate for ex-smokers who have not smoked for 10 years is half that of smokers.
2. *Amount and length of time smoked.* The risk increases with the number of cigarettes smoked per day and years the individual has smoked.
3. *Secondhand smoke.* Exposure to secondhand smoke increases lung cancer risk. Some individuals have a greater susceptibility to lung cancer as a result of secondhand smoke exposure.
4. *Radon gas exposure.* Radon, a radioactive gas that tends to build up indoors, is a potential cancer risk. The risk is also much greater for smokers.
5. *Type of industrial work.* Exposure to certain mining materials, uranium and radioactive products, or asbestos has been demonstrated to be associated with lung cancer. Exposure to materials in other industries also carries a higher risk. Smokers who work in these industries have greatly increased risks. Exposure to arsenic, radiation, and air pollution increase the risk for lung cancer.

Colon/Rectum Cancer

1. *Age.* Colon cancer occurs more frequently after 50 years of age.
2. *Family predisposition.* Colon cancer is more common in families that have a previous history of this disease. Also, families who are predisposed to carry hereditary nonpolyposis colon cancer (HNPCC, or Lynch syndrome) are at a higher risk of developing colon cancer. HNPCC also increases the risk for several other cancers, and individuals who are susceptible should talk to their doctor about regular screenings.
3. *Personal history.* Polyps and bowel diseases are associated with colon cancer.
4. *Physical inactivity.*
5. *Race or ethnicity.* African Americans and Jews of Eastern European descent have some of the highest colorectal cancer rates in the world.
6. *Diet.* A diet high in saturated fat, red meat, or both increases your risk for colon cancer, as does a diet low in fiber, fruits and vegetables, and vitamin D and calcium.

Regular screening is an important measure in catching and removing polyps before they can turn into tumors, and is recommended beginning at age 50.

Skin Cancer

1. *UV light exposure.*
2. *Complexion.* Risk factors vary for different types of skin. Individuals with light complexions, with natural blonde or red hair, and who burn easily are at greater risk.
3. *Personal and family history of melanoma and moles.*
4. *Work environment.* Work in mines and around coal tar, radioactive materials, or arsenic (used in some insecticides) can cause cancer of the skin.
5. *Radiation.* Individuals who have undergone radiation treatment run a much higher risk of skin cancer in the treated area.

Activity 11.1   Are You Taking Control of Your Lifestyle to Prevent Cancer?

Name _____ Date _____

Course _____ Section _____ Gender _____ Age _____

Scientists know that most cancers are related to lifestyle and environment—your nutrition, whether you use tobacco in any form, and where you work and play. Thus, you can reduce your cancer risk by taking control of how you live your daily life.

14 Steps to a Healthier Life and Reduced Cancer Risk

Yes   **No**

1. **Are you eating more cruciferous vegetables?**
   They include broccoli, cauliflower, Brussels sprouts, all cabbages, kohlrabi, and kale.

2. **Does your diet include high-fiber foods?**

3. **Do you choose foods with vitamin A?**
   Fresh foods with beta-carotene, including carrots, peaches, apricots, squash, and broccoli are the best source—not vitamin pills.

4. **Are natural sources of Vitamin C included in your diet?**
   You'll find Vitamin C in lots of fruits and vegetables, including grapefruit, cantaloupe, oranges, strawberries, red and green peppers, broccoli, and tomatoes.

5. **Do you eat sufficient selenium-bearing foods?**
   Selenium is found in fish, Brazil nuts (primarily unshelled), and whole grains. Strive to obtain at least 100 mcg of selenium per day—but no more than 400 mcg per day.

6. **Are you physically active for at least 30 minutes, and do you avoid excessive sitting on most days of the week?**
   Total number of daily steps: _____   Total minutes of daily physical activity: _____

7. **Do you maintain healthy weight (a BMI between 18.5 and 24.9)?**

8. **Do you limit barbecuing and cooking meats at high temperatures to the point that they are "medium well" or "well done"?**

9. **Do you limit salt-cured, smoked, and nitrite-cured foods?**
   Choose bacon, ham, hot dogs, or salt-cured fish only occasionally if you like them a lot.

10. **Do you smoke cigarettes or use tobacco in any other form?**

11. **If you drink alcohol at all, is your intake moderate (no more than 2 drinks per day for men, 1 for women, or none at all for women with a family history of breast, esophagus, larynx, rectum, or liver cancers)?**

12. **Do you get almost daily "safe sun" exposure, and yet respect the sun's rays?**
    "Safe sun" exposure means 10 to 20 minutes of unprotected sun exposure (without sunscreen) to the face, arms, and hands during peak daylight hours on most days of the week (10:00 a.m. to 4:00 p.m.), but yet you respect the sun's rays (your skin does not turn pink or red and you do not sunburn). If not, do you take a daily vitamin D_3 supplement?

    Do you protect yourself with sunscreen (at least SPF 15) and wear long sleeves and a hat, especially during midday hours, if you are going to be exposed to the sun for a prolonged period of time?

13. **If you have a family history of cancer of any type, have you brought this to the attention of your personal physician?**

14. **Are you familiar with the seven warning signals for cancer?**

If you answered "yes" to most of these questions, **congratulations**. You are taking control of simple lifestyle factors that will help you feel better and reduce your risk for cancer.

© Fitness & Wellness, Inc.

Activity 11.2 Early Signs of Illness

Name _____ Date _____

Course _____ Section _____ Gender _____ Age _____

Major illnesses often begin with minor symptoms that if recognized early, allow you to control or cure the condition. In many cases, nothing is seriously wrong. Should you experience any of the following symptoms, however, you are strongly encouraged to bring them to the attention of your physician as soon as possible. In the following statements, please check only the conditions that apply.

☐ 1. Persistent unusual fatigue.

☐ 2. Sudden change in sleeping habits or feeling sleepy most of the day.

☐ 3. Sudden unexplained weight gain or loss (about 6 to 10 lb. in 10 weeks).

☐ 4. Pain or discomfort anywhere in the body that is not easily explained.

☐ 5. Severe headaches with no apparent reason.

☐ 6. A sore anywhere in the body that does not heal within a month.

☐ 7. Changes in moles, warts, or a skin blemish that begin to bleed, itch, or change in color, shape, or size.

☐ 8. Difficulty in swallowing, sudden vomiting occurrences, vomiting blood, or blood in coughed-up phlegm.

☐ 9. Shortness of breath or pain in the chest that may radiate to the jaw, shoulders, arms, or between the shoulder blades.

☐ 10. Fainting spells without reason.

☐ 11. Blurred vision or changes in vision such as seeing haloes.

☐ 12. Hoarseness or loss of voice without apparent reason that lasts several days.

☐ 13. A nagging cough that is getting worse.

☐ 14. Excessive thirst.

☐ 15. Swelling in the limbs/ankles or abdomen.

☐ 16. Persistent indigestion or abdominal pain.

☐ 17. A significant change in bowel habits, interchanging attacks of diarrhea and constipation.

☐ 18. Bowel movements that look unusually dark or rectal bleeding.

☐ 19. In men, discomfort/difficulty urinating, cloudy or reddish-looking urine, or discharge from the tip of the penis.

☐ 20. In women, vaginal bleeding or spotting between regular menstrual periods or following menopause.

☐ 21. In women, a lump or unusual thickening in a breast, changes in the shape or size of the breast, dimpling of the skin, "depression" of the nipples, any alteration in the breast noticeable by a change in position of the body, or any clear or bloody discharge after gently squeezing each nipple between your thumb and index finger .

☐ 22. Excessive sweating.

© Fitness & Wellness, Inc.

Figure 11.12 Cancer questionnaire: assessing your risks.

Name:_____ Date:_____

Course:_____ Section:_____ Gender:_____ Age:_____

Assessing Your Risks for Cancer

Read each question concerning each site and its specific risk factors. Be honest in your responses. Your risk increases as you move beyond item 1 for each factor. For example, the risk for breast cancer increases progressively as you age. If none of the answers apply skip to the next question. Based on the number of risk factors that apply to you, rate yourself on a scale from 1 to 3 (1 for low risk, 2 for moderate risk, and 3 for high risk) for each cancer site. Record your results in Activity 11.3.

Lung Cancer
■ Smoking status
1. Nonsmoker
2. Smoker

■ Cigarettes smoked/day
1. NA
2. Less than 1 pack
3. 1–2 packs
4. 2+ packs

■ Years smoked
1. None
2. 1–15
3. 15–25
4. >25

■ Radon gas exposure
1. No
2. Yes
3. Yes and smoker

■ Type of industrial work
1. Mining
2. Uranium and radioactive products
3. Asbestos

Colon/Rectum Cancer
■ Age
1. ≤40
2. 41–60
3. >60

■ Family predisposition
1. No
2. Yes

■ Personal history
1. No
2. Polyps
3. Bowel diseases

■ Physically active
1. Yes
2. No

■ Either African American or a Jew of Eastern European descent
1. No
2. Yes

■ Family history of HNPCC (or Lynch Syndrome)
1. No
2. Yes

■ Diet
1. High in fiber
2. Low in fiber

■ Alcohol
1. No alcohol
2. <1 drink/day
3. 1 drink/day for women, 2 for men
4. >1 drink/day for women, >2 for men

Skin Cancer
■ Practice safe sun exposure
1. Yes
2. No

■ Fair to light complextion
1. No
2. Yes

■ Personal or family history
1. No
2. Yes

■ Work in mines, around coal tar, radioactive materials, or arsenic
1. No
2. Yes

■ Radiation treatment
1. No
2. Yes

■ Abnormal moles or more than 50 moles
1. No
2. Yes

Breast Cancer
■ Age
1. ≤35
2. 36–50
3. ≥51

■ Caucasian
1. No
2. Yes

■ Family history
1. No
2. One family member
3. Two or more family members

■ Personal history of breast or ovarian cancer
1. No
2. Yes

■ Maternity
1. First pregnancy before age 30
2. First child after age 30
3. No children

■ Hormone replacement therapy
1. No
2. Short-term use
3. Long-term use

■ Physically active
1. Yes
2. No

■ Alcohol
1. No alcohol
2. <1 drink/day
3. 1 drink/day
4. >1 drink/day

■ Significantly overweight
1. No
2. Yes and premenopausal
3. Yes and postmenopausal

■ Dense breast tissue
1. No
2. Unknown
3. Yes

Cervical Cancer
■ Human papilloma virus (HPV) infection
1. Never been infected
2. Previously or currently infected

■ Smoking status
1. Nonsmoker
2. Ex-smoker
3. Current smoker

■ HIV and chlamydia infections
1. Neither one
2. HIV
3. Chlamydia
4. Both

■ Fruits and vegetables
1. ≥5 servings/day
2. 3–4 servings/day
3. 1–2 servings/day
4. <1 serving/day

■ Overweight
1. No
2. Yes

■ Using birth control pills
1. No
2. Yes

■ Pregnancy
1. Two or fewer
2. Prior to age 17
3. Multiple pregnancies

■ Family history
1. No
2. Yes

Endometrial Cancer
■ Estrogen therapy
1. No
2. Yes

■ Age
1. ≤40
2. 41–49
3. ≥50

■ Caucasian
1. No
2. Yes

■ Pregnancy
1. Yes
2. No

■ Body weight
1. At recommended weight
2. Overweight
3. Obese

■ Diabetes
1. No
2. Yes

■ Total years of menstrual cycles
1. "Normal"
2. Greater than "normal" (early start and/or late cessation)

■ Hypertensive
1. No
2. Yes

■ Physically active
1. Yes
2. No

■ Family predisposition
1. No
2. Yes

Prostate Cancer
■ Age
1. ≤64
2. ≥65

■ Family history
1. No
2. Yes

■ African American
1. No
2. Yes

■ Diet
1. Low in saturated fat
2. High in saturated fat

■ Physically active
1. Yes
2. No

Testicular Cancer
■ Had an undescended testicle
1. No
2. Yes

■ Abnormal testicular development
1. No
2. Yes

■ Family history of testicular cancer
1. No
2. Yes

■ Caucasian
1. No
2. Yes

Pancreatic Cancer
■ Age
1. ≤55
2. ≥56

(continued)

Figure 11.12 Cancer questionnaire: assessing your risks. *(continued)*

- Tobacco use
1. No
2. Yes

- Sugar intake
1. Low
2. Moderate
3. Excessive

- Obese
1. No
2. Yes

- Now have or have had chronic pancreatitis, cirrhosis, or diabetes
1. No
2. Yes

- Physically active
1. Yes
2. No

- African American
1. No
2. Yes

- Family history
1. No
2. Yes

- Family history of HNPCC (or Lynch Syndrome)
1. No
2. Yes

Kidney and Bladder Cancer

- Smoking history
1. Nonsmoker
2. Ex-smoker
3. Cigarette smoker

- Diagnosed with congenital (inborn) abnormalities of the kidneys or bladder
1. No
2. Yes

- Exposure to aniline dyes, naphthalenes, or benzidines
1. No
2. Yes

- History of schistosomiasis (a parasitic bladder infection)
1. No
2. Yes

- Suffer from frequent urinary tract infections
1. No
2. Yes

- Family predisposition
1. No
2. Yes

- Overweight
1. No
2. Yes

- High blood pressure
1. No
2. Yes

Oral Cancer

- Tobacco use
1. Nonuser
2. Ex-user

3. Pipe, cigar, or smokeless tobacco
4. Cigarettes

- Alcohol
1. No alcohol
2. <1 drink/day
3. 1 drink/day for women, 2 for men
4. >1 drink/day for women, >2 for men

- Practice safe sun exposure
1. Yes
2. No

Esophageal and Stomach Cancer

- Servings of fruits and vegetables do you consume daily
1. >8
2. 5–8
3. 3–5
4. <3

- Frequency that you consume salt-cured, smoked, or nitrate-cured foods
1. Rarely
2. Less than once/week
3. 1–3 times/week
4. >3 times/week

- Have been told you have an imbalance in stomach acid
1. No
2. Yes

- History of pernicious anemia
1. No
2. Yes

- Diagnosed with chronic gastritis or gastric polyps
1. No
2. Yes

- Family history of esophageal or stomach cancer
1. No
2. Yes

- Overweight
1. No
2. Yes

- Use alcohol or tobacco in any form
1. No
2. Yes

Ovarian Cancer

- Age
1. <50
2. 51–60
3. 61–70
4. >70

- Personal history of ovarian problems
1. No
2. Yes

- Have had estrogen postmenopausal hormone therapy
1. No
2. Yes

- Extensive history of menstrual regularities
1. No
2. Yes

- Family history
1. None
2. Colon/Rectum cancer
3. Endometriosis
4. Breast cancer
5. Ovarian cancer

- Personal history of breast cancer
1. No
2. Yes

- Have had a child
1. Yes
2. No

- Body weight
1. Normal
2. 10–50 pounds overweight
3. >50 pounds overweight

- Family history of nonpolyposis colon cancer
1. No
2. Yes

- Family history of HNPCC (or Lynch Syndrome)
1. No
2. Yes

Thyroid Cancer

- Age
1. <35
2. 35–55
3. 56–70
4. >70

- Received radiation therapy to the head and neck region in childhood or adolescence
1. No
2. Yes

- Family history of thyroid cancer
1. No
2. Yes

- Sex
1. Male
2. Female

Liver Cancer

- Family history of cirrhosis of the liver
1. No
2. Yes

- Personal history of hepatitis B or hepatitis C virus
1. No
2. Yes

- Have been exposed to vinyl chloride (industrial gas used in plastics manufacturing)
1. No
2. Yes

- Have been exposed to aflatoxin (natural food contaminant)
1. No
2. Yes

- Alcohol
1. None
2. ≤2 drinks/day
3. ≥3 drinks/day

- Either Asian American or Pacific Islander
1. No
2. Yes

Leukemia

- Family history
1. No
2. Yes

- Suffer from Down syndrome or other genetic abnormalities
1. No
2. Yes

- Have had excessive exposure to ionizing radiation
1. No
2. Yes

- Exposed to environmental chemicals
1. No
2. Yes

Lymphomas

- Physically active
1. Yes
2. No

- Family history of lymphomas
1. No
2. Yes

- Exposed to
1. Herbicides
2. Organic solvents

- Have had an organ transplant
1. No
2. Yes

- Have been diagnosed with any of the following
1. Epstein-Barr virus
2. HIV
3. Human T-cell leukemia/lymphoma virus-1 (HTLV-1) virus

- Age
1. <50
2. 51–60
3. 61–70
4. >70

- Caucasian
1. No
2. Yes

- Radiation treatment
1. No
2. Yes

Figure 11.13 Warning signs of melanoma: ABCDE rule.

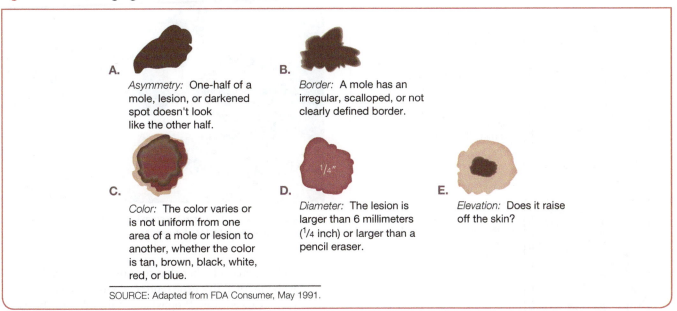

A. *Asymmetry:* One-half of a mole, lesion, or darkened spot doesn't look like the other half.

B. *Border:* A mole has an irregular, scalloped, or not clearly defined border.

C. *Color:* The color varies or is not uniform from one area of a mole or lesion to another, whether the color is tan, brown, black, white, red, or blue.

D. *Diameter:* The lesion is larger than 6 millimeters (¹/₄ inch) or larger than a pencil eraser.

E. *Elevation:* Does it raise off the skin?

SOURCE: Adapted from FDA Consumer, May 1991.

Risks for skin cancer are difficult to state. For instance, a person with a dark complexion can work longer in the sun and be less likely to develop cancer than a light-skinned person. Furthermore, a person wearing a long-sleeved shirt and a wide-brimmed hat who spends hours working in the sun has less risk than a person wearing a swimsuit who sunbathes for only a short time. The risk increases greatly with age, and family history also plays a role. Changes in moles, warts, or skin sores are important and should be evaluated by your doctor (see Figure 11.13).

> ### ! Critical Thinking
>
> What significance does a "healthy tan" have in your social life? Are you a "sun worshiper," or are you concerned about skin damage, premature aging, and potential skin cancer in your future?

Skin Self-Exam One of the easiest and quickest self-exams is a brief survey to detect possible skin cancers (see Figure 11.14). A simple skin self-exam can reduce deaths from melanoma by as much as 63 percent, saving as many as 4,500 lives in the United States each year. Unlike most cancers, a majority of melanoma cases can be visually recognized by the patient before the tumor has the chance to spread. Unfortunately, only a very small number of at-risk individuals perform skin self-exams. This is especially troubling because melanoma is being found in younger patients at escalating rates. Skin self-evaluations are a simple precaution but offer a great chance for early detection.

- Make a drawing of yourself. Include a full frontal view, a full back view, and close-up views of your head (both sides), the front and back of your hands, the tops of your feet, and the soles of your feet (a common site for advanced melanoma because they are often ignored).
- After you get out of the bath or shower, examine yourself closely in a full-length mirror. On your sketch, make note of any moles, warts, darkened skin, or other skin marks you find anywhere on your body. Pay particular attention to areas that are exposed to the sun constantly, such as your face, the tops of your ears, and your hands. But remember that melanoma often develops on parts of the body that receive little sun exposure.
- Briefly describe each mark on your sketch—its size, color, texture, and so on.
- Repeat the exam about once a month. Watch for changes in the size, texture, or color of moles, warts, or other skin marks. If you notice any difference, contact your physician. You also should contact a doctor if you have a sore that does not heal.
- If you find you are not as diligent as you would like to be about regularly checking your own skin, consider scheduling a check up exam with a dermatologist. Make an appointment for a full-body skin exam and ask for advice about how frequently you should schedule follow up exams.

Breast Cancer

1. *Age.* The risk for breast cancer increases significantly after 50 years of age.
2. *Family history.* The risk for breast cancer is higher in women with a family history of breast and ovarian cancers. The risk is even higher if more than one family member has developed these cancers and is further enhanced by the closeness of the relationship (e.g., a mother or sister with breast cancer indicates a higher risk than a cousin with breast cancer).

Figure 11.14 Skin self-examination.

The American Cancer Society recommends you stand in front of a mirror and

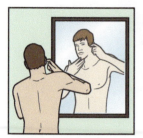

Examine your face (especially the nose, mouth, and lips), front and back of the ears, neck, chest, abdomen, and upper back. Women should also lift their breasts to examine the skin underneath.

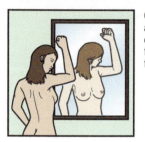

Check both sides of your arms, underarms, both sides of the hands, between the fingers, and under the fingernails.

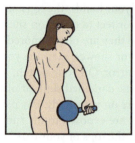

With the aid of a handheld mirror, scan your lower back, buttocks, and genital area.

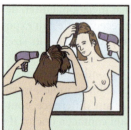

Using a comb, a hair blow dryer, and if possible, the assistance of a friend or family member, thoroughly examine the entire scalp.

Sit down on a chair or bench and

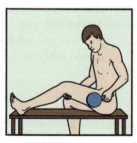

Inspect the front of your thighs, lower legs, the top and soles of your feet, between the toes, and under the toenails. Using a handheld mirror, inspect the back of your thighs and the lower legs.

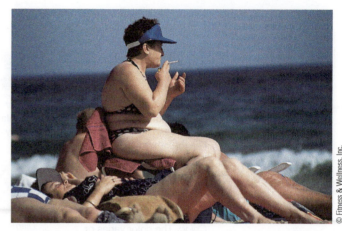

Excessive sun exposure, cigarette smoking, and excessive body weight are major risk factors for cancer.

© Fitness & Wellness, Inc.

and 50 percent higher chance of ovarian cancer. Women who inherited this gene represent 5 to 10 percent of breast cancer cases. Prophylactic removal of the breasts and/or ovaries significantly decreases the risk of breast cancer. Not all women who opt to have the surgery necessarily would develop breast cancer. As this is an extremely emotional and personal decision, women who are contemplating preventive surgery should seek professional counseling prior to undertaking this option.

4. *Personal history.* A previous history of breast or ovarian cancer indicates a higher risk.

5. *Maternity.* The risk is higher in women who have never had children and in women who bear children after 30 years of age. Women are encouraged to breast feed their babies at least up to 6 months as such also reduces the risk for breast cancer.

6. *Physical inactivity.* Regular aerobic exercise has consistently been associated with a lower risk of breast cancer. Some research even indicates that the risk of dying from breast cancer decreases by more than 40 percent in women with high aerobic fitness as compared to less fit women. Vigorous aerobic activity at least three times per week seems most effective. Adding strength-training twice a week is also helpful.

7. *Hormone replacement therapy (HRT).* Long-term use of a combination of progesterone and estrogen increases the risk. The risk seems to apply to current and recent users.

8. *Alcohol.* Even one alcoholic drink per day slightly enhances breast cancer risk in women. Two or more drinks per day clearly enhance the risk.

9. *Obesity.* Adipose tissue increases estrogen levels. Higher estrogen levels, particularly following menopause, increase the risk. Following menopause, it is fat cells and not the ovaries that are the main producer of estrogen. Women with a high BMI have a 39 percent greater risk of developing hormone-induced breast cancer. Women with high BMIs have a 35 percent greater risk of developing a particularly aggressive type of breast cancer that is not induced by hormones, suggesting that obesity works to induce breast cancer in multiple ways.[24]

3. *Genes.* Inherited mutations in genes (breast cancer gene 1, or BRCA1, and breast cancer gene 2, or BRCA2) are found in families with high rates of breast cancer. Of the general population, 1 in every 500 to 1,000 women carry this genetic mutation. These women have as much as an 80 percent greater chance of developing breast cancer

Activity 11.3   **Cancer Risk Profile**

Name _____   Date _____

Course _____ Section _____ Gender _____ Age _____

I. Risk Assessment

Instructions—Read the section "Cancer: Assessing Your Risks" (beginning on page 432) and complete the Cancer Questionnaire: Assessing Your Risks in Figure 11.12 (pages 435–436). Rate yourself on a scale from 1 to 3 (1 = low risk, 2 = moderate risk, 3 = high risk) according to the risk factors provided for each site and write the scores and risk categories in the blanks provided.

Cancer Site	Total Points		Risk Category
	Men	Women	
Lung	☐	☐	☐
Colon-Rectum	☐	☐	☐
Skin	☐	☐	☐
Breast		☐	☐
Cervical		☐	☐
Endometrial		☐	☐
Prostate	☐		
Testicular	☐		
Pancreatic	☐	☐	☐
Kidney and Bladder	☐	☐	☐
Oral	☐	☐	☐
Esophageal and Stomach	☐	☐	☐
Ovarian		☐	
Thyroid	☐	☐	☐
Liver	☐	☐	☐
Leukemia	☐	☐	☐
Lymphomas	☐	☐	☐

© Fitness & Wellness, Inc.

Activity 11.3 Cancer Risk Profile *(continued)*

II. Stage of Change for Cancer Prevention

Using Figure 2.7 and Table 2.3 (page 73), identify your current stage of change for participation in a cancer-prevention program:

III. Personal Interpretation

In the space provided, discuss your results for the various cancer sites. State your feelings about cancer and comment on any experiences that you may have had with cancer patients.

_____

_____

_____

_____

_____

_____

_____

_____

_____

IV. Cancer Prevention: Behavior Modification

Discuss lifestyle habits that you should eliminate and habits that you need to adopt to reduce your own risk of cancer. Also indicate how you can best implement and adhere to these changes.

_____

_____

_____

_____

_____

_____

_____

_____

_____

© Fitness & Wellness, Inc.

About 5 to 10 percent of breast cancers may be related to gene mutations; the most common are BRCA1 and BRCA2. These are tumor suppressor genes. Researchers believe that the majority of breast cancer cases that run in families are a result of environmental influences combined with more common gene mutations that result in only a slight increase in breast cancer risk.

Up until recently, breast cancer occurred slightly more frequently in white women than African American women. The latter, however, were more likely to die from the disease. Sadly, African American women are now equally likely to develop breast cancer as white women and continue to have an increased risk of dying from the disease. The increase in risk is thought to be partially attributed to changes in reproductive age, number of children borne by each mother, and rising rates of obesity. Health disparities related to socioeconomic status also play a role.

Other possible risk factors for breast cancer are high breast-tissue density (a mammographic measure of the amount of glandular breast tissue relative to fatty breast tissue), a long menstrual history (onset of menstruation prior to age 13 and ending later in life), postmenopausal hormone therapy, recent use of oral contraceptives or postmenopausal estrogens, atypical hyperplasia or carcinoma in situ, high saturated fat intake, high refined carbohydrate intake, chronic cystic disease, and ionizing radiation.

Men should not feel immune to breast cancer. Although not common in men, approximately 2,000 men in the United States are diagnosed with breast cancer and 400 die from it each year.

The latest data suggest that 30 percent of breast cancer cases would never have occurred if women kept to a healthy weight, never smoked, drank little to no alcohol, and avoided hormone therapy.[25] To further decrease the risk, increase fiber, folic acid, monounsaturated fat, and vegetable consumption, and increase daily physical activity.

Among women diagnosed with breast cancer, those who walk 2 to 3 miles per hour one to three times per week are 20 percent less likely to die of the disease. Those who walk three to five times per week cut their risk in half.[26] Researchers believe that the decreased levels of circulating ovarian hormones through physical activity decrease breast cancer risk. Physical activity also decreases inflammation and body fat, both risk factors for cancer.

Breast Cancer Screening Breast cancer screening has been a hotly debated topic in recent years, especially **mammogram** screening. The controversy is based on the fact that breast cancer screening is not a precise science, similar to several other types of screening for various cancers. The issue is complex, and guidelines published in recent years have changed to recommend fewer mammograms and beginning them at a later age. Officials creating these guidelines point to concerns for women who are misdiagnosed as possibly having cancer, or overdiagnosed for a small group of precancerous cells. As a result, these women often undergo unnecessary stress and medical intervention. A woman who has an abnormal screening test will undoubtedly experience fear and stress as she continues the process of finding out whether it is cancer. However, women might be better able to deal with screening results if it were widely known that misdiagnosis happens frequently.

Of women who receive mammograms annually, half will experience a false positive result at least once in ten years.[27]

Cost is also a factor. Several organizations and physicians, nonetheless, indicate that mammograms lead to early detection and have contributed to the current 90 percent survival rate. Early detection increases the chance that the cancer can be treated with a lumpectomy instead of more invasive and disfiguring surgery. Dr. Otis Brawley, Chief Medical Officer of the American Cancer Society, stated in 2009, "This is one screening test I recommend unequivocally, and would recommend to any woman 40 and over."[28]

Previously, the American Cancer Society (ACS) recommended yearly mammograms beginning at age 40, and clinical breast exams by a physician every three years for women between ages 20 and 40 and every year for women older than age 40. The organization revised its guidelines in 2015 to recommend yearly mammograms beginning at age 45, and mammograms every other year beginning at age 55. Women should be aware of any change in their breasts and report it to a physician.

Personal risk factors should be considered when determining when to start mammograms, whether to request breast exams from a physician during check-up visits, and how often each should be done. Women with low to moderate risk should consider practicing monthly BSE (see Figure 11.15) and having their breasts examined by a doctor as a part of a cancer-related checkup. They should also receive periodic mammograms. Women at high risk should practice monthly BSE and have their breasts examined regularly by a doctor. See your doctor for the recommended examinations (including mammograms and physical exam of breasts).

Cervical Cancer (Women)

1. *Human papilloma virus (HPV).* The most significant risk factor is infection with the HPV, a group of more than 100 related viruses, some of which can cause cervical cancer. The virus is frequently transmitted through vaginal, anal, or oral sex or simply by skin-to-skin contact with a body area infected with HPV. Most infected women do not develop cervical cancer, but other factors (see the following) can contribute to its development.
2. *Smoking.* The risk doubles in women who smoke. Tobacco by-products are found in cervical mucus of women who smoke.
3. *Infections.* Both human immunodeficiency virus (HIV) and chlamydia (bacterial infection—see Chapter 14) infections increase the risk of cervical cancer.
4. *Diet.* Low consumption of fruits and vegetables has been linked to higher cervical cancer risk.
5. *Excess weight.* Women who are overweight are at higher risk.
6. *Birth control pills.* Long-term use of birth control pills increases the risk. The risk decreases once their use is stopped.

GLOSSARY

Mammogram Low-dose x-rays of the breasts used as a screening technique for the early detection of breast tumors.

Figure 11.15 Breast self-examination.

Looking

Stand in front of a mirror with your upper body unclothed. Look for changes in the shape and size of the breast, and for dimpling of the skin or "pulling in" of the nipples. Any changes in the breast may be made more noticeable by a change in position of the body or arms. Also look for changes in shape from one breast to the other.

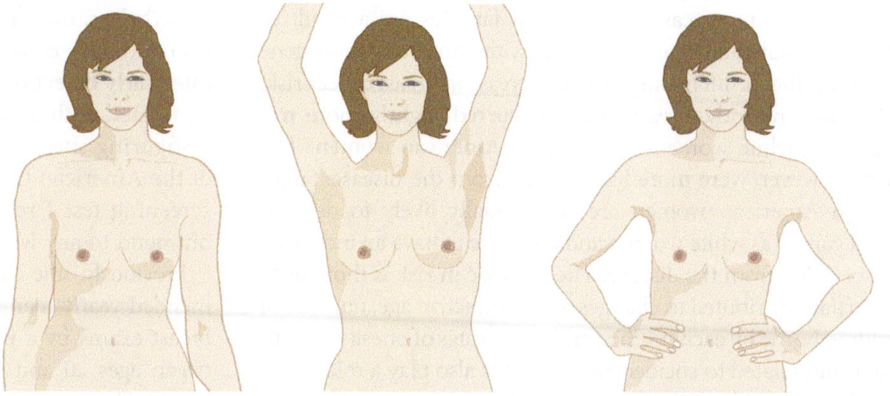

1. Stand with your arms down.

2. Raise your arms overhead.

3. Place your hands on your hips and tighten your chest and arm muscles by pressing firmly.

Feeling

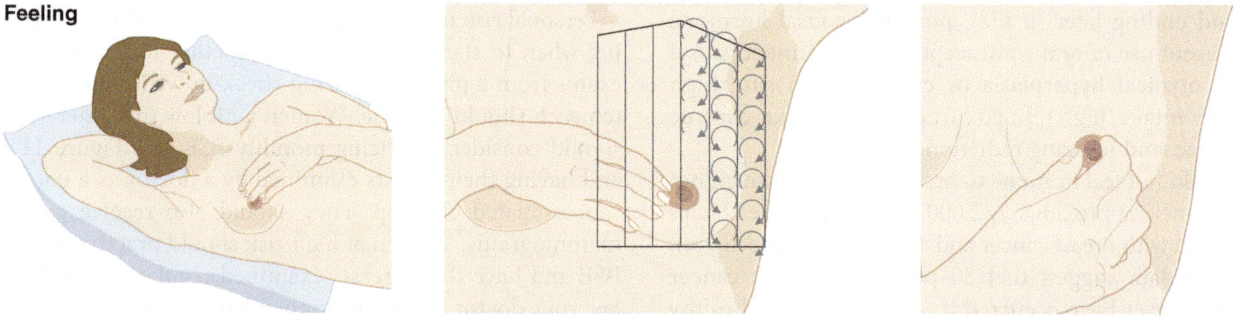

1. Lie flat on your back. Place a pillow or towel under one shoulder, and raise that arm over your head. With the opposite hand, you'll feel with the pads, not the fingertips, of the three middle fingers, for lumps or any change in the texture of the breast or skin.

2. The area you'll examine is from your collarbone to your bra line and from your breastbone to the center of your armpit. Imagine the area divided into vertical strips. Using small circular motions (the size of a dime), move your fingers up and down the strips. Apply light, medium, and deep pressure to examine each spot. Repeat this same process for your other breast.

3. Gently squeeze the nipple of each breast between your thumb and index finger. Any discharge, clear or bloody, should be reported to your doctor immediately.

SOURCE: From D. Hales, *An Invitation to Health,* 11th ed. © 2005. Cengage Learning.

7. *Pregnancies.* Multiple pregnancies (three or more) increase the risk. Pregnancy prior to age 17 also increases the risk.

8. *Family history.* Cervical cancer may run in families because women in these families are less able to fight off the HPV.

Early detection through regular screening is critical for cancer prevention. A Pap test, which screens for precancerous cells, should be done at age 21 and then repeated every three years up to age 65. Starting at age 30, if you choose to do so, an HPV test that looks for the virus that causes cellular changes may be used with the Pap test. When both tests are performed, it is referred to as co-testing. If your test results are normal, your chance of getting cervical cancer in the next few years is very low. Your physician may then inform you that you can wait 5 years prior to your next screening. The Food and Drug Administration may soon recommend a DNA test for women 25 and older to help screen for cervical cancer.

HPV vaccines are available to prevent cervical cancer and other diseases caused by HPV (see Chapter 14, "HPV: Diagnosis and Treatment," page 527). Both vaccines protect against HPV types 16 and 18, which cause most cervical cancers. The vaccines are recommended for women between the ages of 11 and 26. To get the full benefits of the vaccine, women should get vaccinated before they become sexually active.

Endometrial Cancer (Women)

1. *Estrogen use.* Cancer of the endometrium is associated with high cumulative exposure to estrogen. Obesity, a long menstrual history, and hormone replacement therapy all increase estrogen exposure. You should consult your physician before starting or stopping any estrogen therapy.

2. *Age.* Endometrial cancer is seen in older age groups.

3. *Race.* White women have a higher occurrence, but African American women have a higher incidence of death.

4. *Family history.* While the genetic source has not yet been identified, there are families with an increased risk for endometrial cancer. Other women who carry the genetic abnormalities for HNPCC (or Lynch syndrome) have a 40 to 60 percent risk of developing endometrial cancer.

5. *Pregnancy history.* The fewer children the woman has delivered, the greater the risk for endometrial cancer.

6. *Excessive weight.*

7. *Diabetes.*

8. *Total number of menstrual cycles (periods).* The greater the number of lifetime menstrual cycles (periods), the greater the risk.

9. *Hypertension.* Cancer of the endometrium is associated with high blood pressure.

10. *Physical inactivity.* The risk for endometrial cancer is higher among physically inactive women.

Prostate Cancer (Men)

The prostate gland is a cluster of smaller glands that encircle the top section of the urethra (urinary channel) at the point where it leaves the bladder. Although the function of the prostate is not entirely clear, the muscles of these small glands help squeeze prostatic secretions into the urethra.

1. *Age.* The highest incidence of prostate cancer is found in men over age 60 (more than 70 percent of cases).

2. *Family history.* A man with a brother or father who has had prostate cancer has twice the risk of developing the disease than someone who has no family history.

3. *Race.* African American men have the highest rate in the world.

4. *Diet.* A diet high in red meat or high-fat dairy products may increase the risk of developing aggressive prostate cancer. Frequent consumption of processed food or sugary beverages may increase risk by two to three times. Taking folic acid supplements may also increase risk (though obtaining folate by consuming vegetables is safe).

5. *Physical inactivity.* The risk may be greater in physically inactive men.

Prostate cancer is difficult to detect and control because the causes are not known. Death rates can be lowered through early detection and awareness of the warning signs. Detection is done by a digital rectal exam of the gland and a prostate-specific antigen (PSA) blood test once a year after the age of 50. Possible warning signs include difficulties in urination (especially at night), painful urination, blood in the urine, and constant pain in the lower back or hip area. See Figure 11.16 for the self-examination procedure for men.

Factors that may decrease the risk include increasing the consumption of tomato-rich foods and fatty fish in the diet two or three times per week, avoiding a high-fat (especially animal fat) diet, increasing daily consumption of produce, legumes, and grains, and getting sufficient vitamin D. Vigorous exercise such as jogging or swimming has been

Figure 11.16 Testicular self-examination.

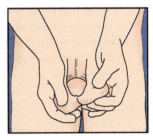
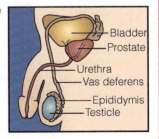

How to Examine the Testicles

You can increase your chances of early detection of testicular cancer by regularly performing a testicular self-examination (TSE). The following procedure is recommended:

- Perform the self-exam once a month. Select an easy day to remember such as the first day or first Sunday of the month.
- Learn how your testicle feels normally so that it will be easier to identify changes. A normal testicle should feel oval, smooth, and uniformly firm, like a hard-boiled egg.
- Perform TSE following a warm shower or bath, when the scrotum is relaxed.
- Gently roll each testicle between your thumb and the first three fingers until you have felt the entire surface. Pay particular attention to any lumps, change in size or texture, pain, or a dragging or heavy sensation since your last self-exam. Do not confuse the epididymis at the rear of the testicle for an abnormality.
- Bring any changes to the attention of your physician. A change does not necessarily indicate a malignancy, but only a physician is able to determine that.

Bladder
Prostate
Urethra
Vas deferens
Epididymis
Testicle

Behavior Modification Planning

Lifestyle Factors That Decrease Cancer Risk

Factor	Function
Physical activity	Controls body weight, may influence hormone levels, and strengthens the immune system.
Fiber	Contains anti-cancer substances, increases stool movement, and blunts insulin secretion.
Fruits and vegetables	Contain phytonutrients and vitamins that thwart cancer.
Recommended weight	Helps control hormones that promote cancer.
Healthy grilling	Prevents formation of heterocyclic amines (HCAs) and polycyclic aromatic hydrocarbons (PAHs), both carcinogenic substances.
Tea	Contains polyphenols that neutralize free radicals, including epigallocatechin gallate (EGCG), which protects cells and the DNA from damage believed to cause cancer.
Spices	Provide phytonutrients and strengthen the immune system.
Vitamin D	Disrupts abnormal cell growth.
Monounsaturated fat	May contribute to cancer cell destruction.

Try It

In your online journal or class notebook, note ways you can incorporate all of these factors into your everyday lifestyle.

shown to lower risk of advanced prostate cancer by as much as 70 percent in older men, and even brisk walking has been shown to halt the cancer's progression.

> **(!) Critical Thinking**
>
> You have learned about many of the risk factors for major cancer sites. How will this information affect your health choices in the future? Will it be valuable to you, or will you quickly forget all you have learned and remain in a contemplation stage at the end of this course?

11.16 *What Can You Do?*

If you are at high risk for any form of cancer, you are advised to discuss this with your physician. An ounce of prevention is worth a pound of cure. Most cancers are lifestyle related, so being aware of the risk factors and following basic recommendations for preventing cancer will greatly decrease your risk for developing it.

Assess Your Behavior

1. Are you physically active on most days of the week?
2. Does your diet include ample amounts of colorful fruits and vegetables and fiber, and is it low in red and processed meats?
3. Are you aware of your family history of cancer?
4. Do you practice monthly breast self-examination (women) or testicular self-examination (men)?

5. Do you respect the sun's rays? Do you use sunscreen lotion or wear protective clothing when you are in the sun for extended periods of time? Do you perform regular skin self-examinations?
6. Are you familiar with the nine warning signs of cancer?

Assess Your Knowledge

1. Cancer can be defined as
   a. a process whereby some cells invade and destroy the immune system.
   b. uncontrolled growth and spread of abnormal cells.
   c. the spread of benign tumors throughout the body.
   d. interference with normal body functions through blood-flow disruption caused by angiogenesis.
   e. All are correct choices.

2. Cancer treatment becomes more difficult when
   a. cancer cells metastasize.
   b. angiogenesis is disrupted.
   c. a tumor is encapsulated.
   d. cells are deficient in telomerase.
   e. cell division has stopped.

3. The leading cause of deaths from cancer in women is
   a. lung cancer.
   b. breast cancer.
   c. ovarian cancer.
   d. skin cancer.
   e. endometrial cancer.

4. Cancer
   a. is primarily a preventable disease.
   b. is often related to tobacco use.
   c. has been linked to dietary habits.
   d. risk increases with obesity.
   e. All are correct choices.

5. About 65 percent of cancers are related to
   a. genetics.
   b. environmental pollutants.
   c. viruses and other biological agents.
   d. ultraviolet radiation.
   e. diet, obesity, and tobacco use.

6. A cancer-prevention diet should include
   a. ample amounts of fruits and vegetables.
   b. cruciferous vegetables.
   c. phytonutrients.
   d. fish one to two times per week instead of red meat.
   e. all of the above.

7. The most common carcinogenic exposures in the workplace are to
   a. asbestos fibers.
   b. cigarette smoke and ultraviolet radiation from sunlight.
   c. biological agents.
   d. nitrosamines.
   e. pesticides.

8. Which of the following is not a warning signal for cancer?
   a. Change in bowel or bladder habits
   b. Nagging cough or hoarseness
   c. A sore that does not heal
   d. Indigestion or difficulty in swallowing
   e. All of the above are warning signs for cancer.

9. The risk for breast cancer is higher in
   a. women younger than age 50.
   b. women with more than one family member with a history of breast cancer.
   c. women who drink no alcohol rather than one glass of red wine per day.
   d. women who had children prior to age 30.
   e. all of the above groups.

10. The risk for prostate cancer can be decreased by
    a. consuming selenium-rich foods.
    b. adding fatty fish to the diet.
    c. avoiding a high-fat diet.
    d. including tomato-rich foods in the diet.
    e. all of the above.

Correct answers can be found at the back of the book.

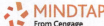

MINDTAP From Cengage **Complete This Online**
Visit **www.cengagebrain.com** to access MindTap, a complete digital course that includes interactive quizzes, videos, and more.

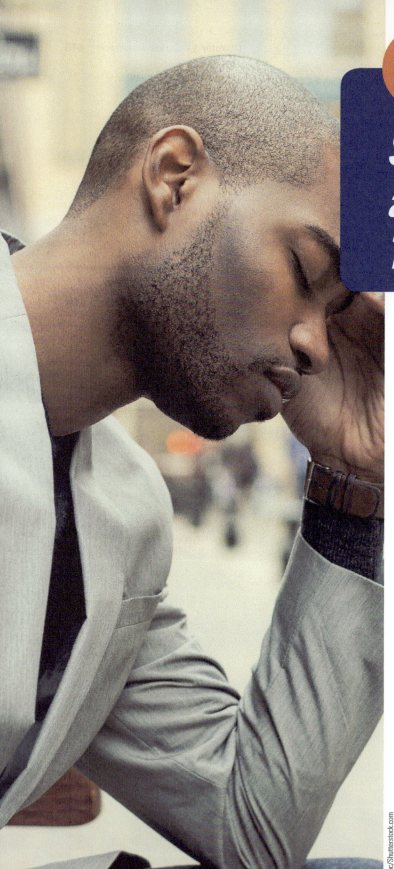

PathDoc/Shutterstock.com

Stress Assessment and Management Techniques

"If we all threw our problems in a pile and saw everyone else's, we'd grab ours back."
—Regina Brett

Objectives

12.1 **Understand** the importance of the mind–body connection in the manifestation of emotions and disease.

12.2 **Learn** the consequences of sleep deprivation on mental and physical health.

12.3 **Define** stress, eustress, and distress.

12.4 **Explain** the role of stress in maintaining health and optimal performance.

12.5 **Identify** the major sources of stress in your life.

12.6 **Define** the two major types of behavior patterns.

12.7 **Learn** to lower your vulnerability to stress.

12.8 **Develop** time-management skills.

12.9 **Define** the role of physical exercise in reducing stress.

12.10 **Describe** and learn to use various stress-management techniques.

12.11 **Learn** how you're affected by stress.

12.12 **Find** out how vulnerable you are to stress.

FAQ

Is all stress detrimental to health and performance?

Living in today's world without encountering stress is nearly impossible. The good news is that stress can be self-controlled. Unfortunately, most people have accepted stress as a normal part of daily life, and even though everyone has to face it, few seem to understand it or know how to cope with it effectively. It is difficult to succeed and have fun in life without "runs, hits, and errors." In fact, stress should not be avoided entirely because a certain amount is necessary for motivation, performance, and optimum health and well-being. When stress levels push people to the limit, however, stress becomes distress and they no longer function effectively.

How can I most effectively deal with distress (negative stress)?

Feelings of stress are the result of the body's instinct to defend itself. If you start to experience mental, social, and physical symptoms such as exhaustion, headaches, sleeplessness, frustration, apathy, loneliness, and changes in appetite, you are most likely under excessive stress and need to take action to overcome the stress-causing event(s). Do not deal with these symptoms through alcohol, drugs, or other compulsive behaviors, which will not get rid of the stressor that is causing the problem. Stress management is best accomplished by maintaining a sense of control when excessive demands are placed on you.

First, recognize when you are feeling stressed. Early warning signs include tension in your shoulders and neck and clenching of your fists or teeth. Now, determine if there is something that you can do to control, change, or remove yourself from the situation. Most importantly, change how you react to stress. Be positive, avoid extreme reactions (anger, hostility, hatred, or depression), try to change the way you see things, work off stress through physical activity, and master one or more stress management techniques to help you in situations in which it is necessary to cope effectively. Finally, take steps to reduce the demands placed on you by prioritizing your activities—"Don't sweat the small stuff." Realize that it is not stress that makes you ill; it is the manner in which you react to stress that leads to illness and disease.

REAL LIFE STORY | Sreevita's Experience

Throughout high school and college, the biggest source of stress for me has been my long habit of procrastination. Whenever I have a project I need to do, I automatically estimate the minimum amount of time it will take, and then wait until there is exactly that amount of time (or less!) before the project is due, and only then do I start. This means that everything is done in a mad rush, on a stress and adrenaline high, worrying that I might not make my deadline. I know this is a bad pattern. Not only does it cause me a lot of stress, but sometimes I underestimate how long something will take, and the amount of time left really isn't enough to finish the job or do it well. But the problem is that I am addicted to the pattern of having a flood of adrenaline carry me through the task, so I am not able to get motivated when the deadline is still far away. In fact, when I think of a task that I need to do, rather than feeling motivated to begin, I will often have thoughts that it will be horrible and hard and that I might fail. These thoughts are so unpleasant that I will try to push the idea of the project out of mind entirely. But one of the strategies I have used recently to try to overcome my procrastination is baby steps. In fact, I will try to break a task down into the smallest pieces possible. For instance, if I have to start writing a report, my first step may be to just turn on the computer. Or to just open up the word-processing program. And then to just write one rough sentence (which doesn't even have to be good). By making each step as simple and unintimidating as possible, I can make a start. I celebrate the accomplishment of each baby step, even if it was just something as simple as turning on the computer. Once I start making progress, I usually find that the project is not as painful as I feared. I have also discovered something else surprising—exercising regularly and taking a yoga class have actually helped me procrastinate less! Since my procrastination is linked to feelings of anxiety about a task, and aerobic exercise and yoga give me a feeling of calm and well-being, when I exercise regularly, I procrastinate less.

Michaeljung/Shutterstock.com

PERSONAL PROFILE: Stress Management Survey

I. Do you experience mostly eustress (positive stress) or distress (negative stress) in your daily life? Explain.

II. Identify a recent life stressor. Can you explain the general adaptation syndrome stage that you are currently experiencing?

III. List significant factors that cause stress in your life, and indicate how you deal with those situations when they arise.

IV. Explain personal time management techniques that you use given the many challenges and responsibilities you face in daily life.

V. Have you ever used relaxation techniques to effectively manage stress? If so, explain the experience.

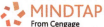 **MINDTAP** From Cengage   **Complete This Activity Online**
Visit **www.cengagebrain.com** to access MindTap, a complete digital course that includes interactive quizzes, videos, and more.

According to a growing body of evidence, virtually every illness known to modern humanity—from arthritis to migraine headaches, from the common cold to cancer—appears to be influenced for good or bad by our emotions. To a profound extent, emotions affect our susceptibility to and our **immunity** from disease. The way we react to the events that come along in life can determine in great measure how our bodies will react to disease-causing organisms. The feelings we have and the way we express them can either boost our immune system or weaken it.

Emotional health is a key part of total wellness. Most emotionally healthy people take care of themselves physically—they eat well, exercise, and get enough rest. They work to develop supportive personal relationships. In contrast, many people who are emotionally unhealthy are self-destructive. For example, they may abuse alcohol and other drugs or may overwork and lack balance in their lives. Emotional health is so important that it affects what we do, who we meet, who we marry, how we look, how we feel, how the course of our lives unfolds, and even how long we live.

12.1 *The Mind–Body Connection*

Emotional and physical health are inseparably connected. Certain parts of the brain are associated with specific emotions and hormone patterns that, when released, can affect the body. In essence, how we think and react can have a helpful or harmful impact on our physical health.

Emotions Can Trigger Physical Responses

Emotions have to be expressed somewhere, somehow. If they are suppressed repeatedly or a person feels conflict about controlling them, they often reveal themselves through harmful physical symptoms.

The brain is the most important part of the nervous system. For the body to survive, the brain must be maintained. When the entire body is under severe stress, all other organs sacrifice to keep the brain alive and functioning.

The brain's powerful influence over the body is brought about via a complex link between the emotions and the immune system. The brain is the cognitive center of the body, the place where ideas are generated, memory is stored, and emotions are experienced. Every time the brain manufactures an emotion, physical reactions accompany it. The brain's natural chemicals form literal communication links among the brain and with the cells of the body, including those of the immune system.

The immune system patrols and guards the body against attackers. This system consists of about a trillion cells called **lymphocytes** (the cells responsible for waging war against disease or infection) and trillions of molecules called **antibodies**. The brain and the immune system are closely linked in a connection that allows the mind to influence both susceptibility and resistance to disease. A number of immune system cells—including those in the thymus gland, spleen, bone marrow, and lymph nodes—interact with the nervous system through neurotransmitters and signaling molecules.

Cells of the immune system are equipped to respond to these chemical signals from the central nervous system. For example, the surface of the lymphocytes contains receptors for a variety of central nervous system chemical messengers (hormones), such as catecholamines, prostaglandins, serotonin, endorphins, sex hormones, the thyroid hormone, and the growth hormone. Certain white blood cells possess the ability to receive messages from the brain.

Because of these receptors on the lymphocytes, physical and psychological stress alter the immune system. Stress causes the body to release several powerful neurohormones that bind with the receptors on the lymphocytes and suppress immune function. Stress also causes the nerves to release a molecule known as neuropeptide Y (NPY) that impairs immune-system cells that fight infection. NPY is also believed to cause excessive eating when under stress.

12.2 *What is Stress?*

Just what is **stress**? Dr. Hans Selye, one of the foremost authorities on stress, defined it as "the nonspecific response of the human organism to any demand that is placed upon it."[1]

Figure 12.1 Relationship between stress and health and performance.

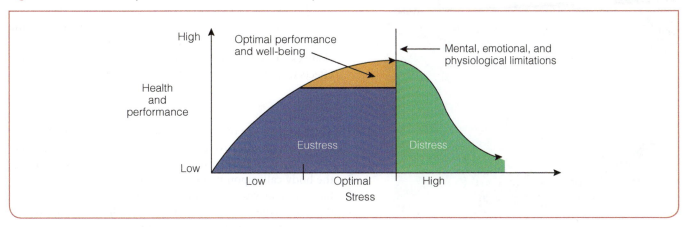

"Nonspecific" indicates that the body reacts in a similar fashion when encountering a stress-causing event, also called a **stressor**. A stressor can be any event that disrupts the body's normal internal state, regardless of the nature of the event. Stressors can come from physical events, like accidents or illness, or emotional events, like anxiety from school and work demands. The instinctive set of psychological and physiological changes the body goes through to prepare a person to cope with a stressor is called the **stress response**. In simpler terms, the stress response is the body's mental, emotional, and physical response to any situation that is new, threatening, frightening, or exciting.

Eustress and Distress

Stress is a fact of modern life, and every person needs an optimal level of stress that is most conducive to adequate health and performance. Whether stress becomes helpful or harmful to health arises from the way people react to stress. Many people thrive under stress; others under similar circumstances are unable to handle it. Their reaction to a stressor determines whether that stress is positive or negative. Dr. Selye defined the ways in which we react to stress as either eustress or distress. In both cases, the nonspecific response is almost the same. In the case of **eustress**, health and performance continue to improve even as stress increases. On the other hand, **distress** refers to the unpleasant or harmful stress under which health and performance begin to deteriorate. When stress levels reach mental, emotional, and physiological limits, stress becomes distress and the person no longer functions effectively. The relationship between stress and performance is illustrated in Figure 12.1.

> **!**
> ### Critical Thinking
> Can you identify sources of eustress and distress in your personal life during this past year? Explain your emotional and physical response to each stressor and how the two differ.

12.3 How the Body Responds and Adapts to Stress

The body continually strives to maintain a constant internal environment. This state of physiological balance, known as **homeostasis**, allows the body to function as effectively as possible. When a stressor triggers a nonspecific response, homeostasis is disrupted. This reaction to stressors, best explained by Dr. Selye through the **general adaptation syndrome (GAS)**, is composed of three stages: alarm reaction, resistance, and exhaustion and recovery.

Alarm Reaction

The alarm reaction is the immediate response to a stressor (whether positive or negative). During the alarm reaction,

---GLOSSARY---

Immunity The function that guards the body from invaders, both internal and external.

Lymphocytes Immune system cells responsible for waging war against disease or infection.

Antibodies Substances produced by the white blood cells in response to an invading agent.

Stress The mental, emotional, and physiological response of the body to any situation that is new, threatening, frightening, or exciting.

Stressor A stress-causing event.

Stress response The instinctive set of psychological and physiological changes the body goes through to prepare a person to cope with a stressor.

Eustress Positive stress; health and performance continue to improve even as stress increases.

Distress Negative stress; unpleasant or harmful stress under which health and performance begin to deteriorate.

Homeostasis A natural state of equilibrium, which the body attempts to maintain by constantly reacting to external forces that attempt to disrupt this fine balance.

General adaptation syndrome (GAS) A theoretical model that explains the body's adaptation to sustained stress. It includes three stages: alarm reaction, resistance, and exhaustion and recovery.

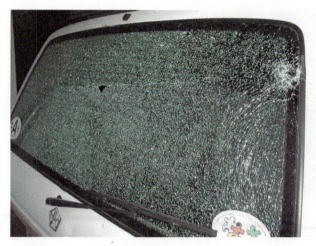

Vandalism causes distress, or negative stress.

© Fitness & Wellness, Inc.

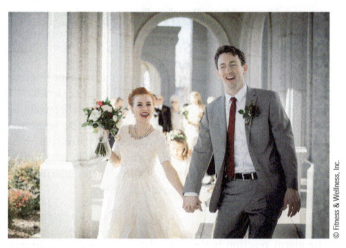

Marriage is an example of positive stress, also known as eustress.

© Fitness & Wellness, Inc.

the body evokes an initial physiological reaction that mobilizes internal systems and processes to minimize the threat to homeostasis. The instant physiological reaction to stress, called the **fight-or-flight mechanism**, prepares an individual to take action by activating the body's vital defense systems. This innate survival mechanism has enabled humans since the beginning of time to react quickly to life-threatening situations: it heightens the senses and fuels vital systems with added energy to prepare the body to fight a threat or flee to safety. This stimulation originates in the hypothalamus and the pituitary gland in the brain. The hypothalamus activates the **sympathetic nervous system**, and the pituitary activates the release of catecholamines (hormones) from the adrenal glands, including cortisol and epinephrine (also known as adrenaline).

When you first perceive a stressor, your brain becomes more alert, your muscles tighten, and your heart and breathing rate quicken to supply your body with increased blood and oxygen (see Figure 12.2). This well-orchestrated and near-instantaneous sequence of psychological and physiological changes brought on by the fight-or-flight mechanism makes up the alarm reaction, the first stage of GAS. Unfortunately,

the same reaction is also activated by any life stressor—life-threatening or not—like traffic jams, college tests, or relationship difficulties. When the reaction is repeated over time in the form of chronic distress, the prolonged physiological changes can take a toll on the body with harmful long-term effects (see "Long-term effects" in Figure 12.2).

Resistance

The second stage of GAS is resistance. When a stressor subsides through effective coping techniques, the body recovers and returns to homeostasis. However, if a stressor persists, the body calls upon its limited reserves to build up its resistance as it strives to maintain homeostasis. For a short while, the body copes effectively and meets the challenge of the stressor until it can be overcome (Figure 12.3).

Exhaustion and Recovery

If stress becomes chronic and intolerable, the body continues to resist, draining its limited reserves. The body then loses its ability to cope and enters the exhaustion and recovery stage. During this third stage of GAS, the body functions at a diminished capacity, suppressing the immune system and vital functions while it recovers from stress. In due time, following an "adequate" recovery period (which varies greatly), the body recuperates and is able to return to homeostasis. If chronic stress persists during the exhaustion stage, however, immune function is compromised, which can damage body systems and lead to disease.

In modern stress research, Dr. Selye's concept of the exhaustion stage has been expanded to include the cumulative long-term wear and tear on the body that results from chronic stress exposure—a concept known as **allostatic load**. Selye's theory blamed depleted energy and adrenal reserves (adrenal fatigue) for negative long-term physiological effects. The primary cause of disease vulnerability during the exhaustion stage is now believed to be the repetition of the stress response itself. [2] Research shows that a high allostatic load raises the risk for many health disorders—among them, coronary heart disease (CHD), hypertension, eating disorders, ulcers, diabetes, asthma, depression, migraine headaches, sleep disorders, and chronic fatigue—and may even play a role in the development of certain types of cancers.

Figure 12.2 illustrates how blood levels of the stress hormone cortisol, inflammatory molecules, and low-density

┌─ GLOSSARY ────────────────────────────────────

Fight-or-flight mechanism The instant physiological reaction of the body to stress that prepares the individual to take action by activating the body's vital defense systems.

Sympathetic nervous system Part of the autonomic nervous

system that activates the fight-or-flight response.

Allostatic load The cumulative long-term wear and tear on the body as a result of chronic stress exposure.

Figure 12.2 **Physiological response to stress: fight-or-flight mechanism and long-term effects of chronic distress.**

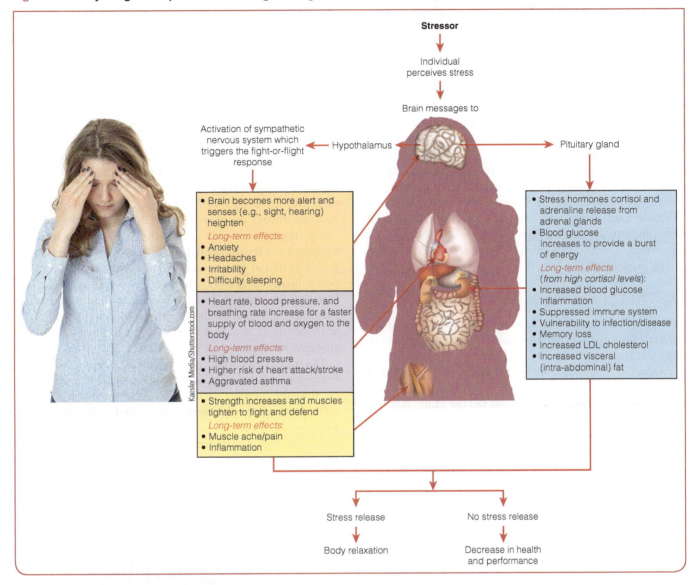

Figure 12.3 **General adaptation syndrome, the body's response to stress that can end in exhaustion, illness, or recovery.**

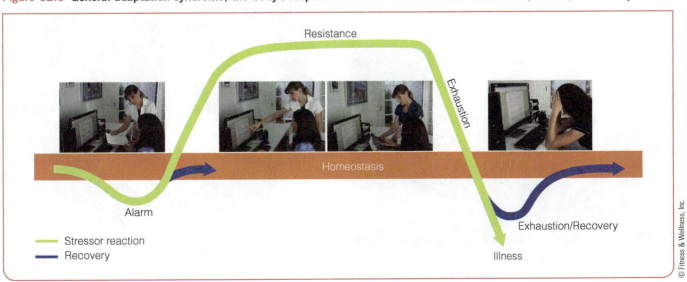

lipoprotein (LDL) cholesterol all increase during the stress response. High cortisol levels have been associated with the buildup of visceral fat (harmful intra-abdominal fat), even among lean individuals[3] (see Chapter 4, page 141). Elevated cortisol levels alone cause inflammation, a condition implicated in many chronic diseases. Inflammatory molecules further promote atherosclerosis and make plaque more likely to rupture, leading to a heart attack or stroke. In a review of studies evaluating the effects of tension on heart health, researchers found that chronic distress can increase the risk of CHD by as much as 27 percent. The findings are significant, suggesting that stress can be as threatening as a 50-point increase in LDL cholesterol, or the equivalent of smoking five extra cigarettes per day.[4] Recognizing the risks of a high allostatic load, individuals can take preventative steps to overcome sources of distress before they lead to long-term illness through effective coping techniques (see "Coping with Stress," page 469).

Examples of General Adaptation Syndrome

An example of the stress response through the GAS can be illustrated in college test performance. As you prepare to take an exam, you experience an initial alarm reaction. If you understand the material, study for the exam, and do well (eustress), the body recovers and stress is dissipated. If, however, you are not adequately prepared and fail the exam, you trigger the resistance stage. You are now concerned about your grade, and you remain in the resistance stage until the next exam. If you prepare and do well, the body recovers. But, if you fail once again and can no longer bring up the grade, exhaustion sets in and physical and emotional breakdowns may occur. Exhaustion may be further aggravated if you are struggling in other courses as well.

The exhaustion stage is also manifested by athletes and the most ardent fitness participants. Staleness is usually a manifestation of overtraining. Peak performance can be sustained for only about 2 to 3 weeks at a time. Any attempts to continue intense training after peaking leads to exhaustion, diminished fitness, and mental and physical problems associated with overtraining (see Chapter 9, page 345). Thus, athletes and some fitness participants also need an active recovery phase following the attainment of peak fitness.

12.4 Sources of Stress

Several instruments have been developed to assess sources of stress in life. A practical instrument to assess stressors is the **stress events scale**, presented in Activity 12.1, which identifies life events within the past 12 months that may have an impact on your physical and psychological well-being. The stress events scale is divided into two sections. Section 1, to be completed by all respondents, contains a list of potential stress-causing life events with four additional blank spaces for other events experienced but not listed in the survey. Section 2 contains additional statements designed for students only (students should fill out both sections). Common stressors in the lives of college students are depicted in Figure 12.4.

The scale requires the testee to rate the extent to which life events had a positive or negative impact on his or her life at the time these events occurred. The ratings are on a 7-point scale. A rating of −3 indicates an extremely undesirable impact (shock). A zero (0) rating indicates neither a positive nor a negative impact (**neustress**, or indifference). A rating of +3 indicates an extremely desirable impact (jubilance).

Figure 12.4 **Stressors in the lives of college students.**

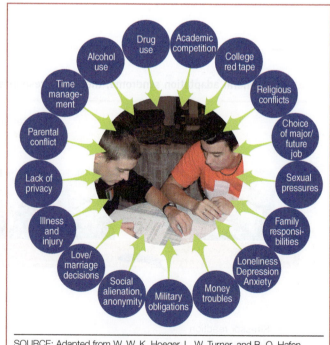

SOURCE: Adapted from W. W. K. Hoeger, L. W. Turner, and B. Q. Hafen, *Wellness Guidelines for a Healthy Lifestyle*, Wadsworth/Thomson Learning, 2007.

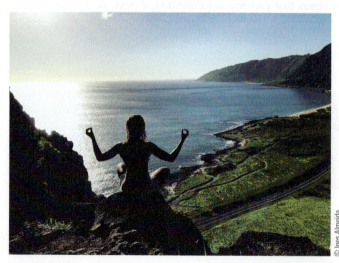

Taking time out during stressful life events is critical for good health and wellness.

© Ines Almeida

After the person evaluates his or her life events, the negative and the positive points are totaled separately. Both scores are expressed as positive numbers (e.g., positive ratings of 2, 1, 3, and 3 = 9 points of positive score; negative ratings of −3, −2, −2, −1, and −2 = 10 points of negative score). A final "total life change" score can be obtained by adding the positive score and the negative score together as positive numbers (total stress events score = 9 + 10 = 19 points).

Because negative and positive changes alike can produce nonspecific responses, the total life change score is a good indicator of total life stress. Most research in this area, however, suggests that the negative change score is a better predictor of potential physical and psychological illness than the total change score. More research is necessary to establish the role of total change and the role of the ratio of positive to negative stress.

12.5 How Perception and Attitude Affect Health

Common life events are not the only source of stress in life. The habitual manner in which people explain the things that happen to them is their **explanatory style**. It is a way of thinking when all other factors are equal and when there are no clear-cut right and wrong answers. The contrasting explanatory styles are pessimism and optimism. People with a pessimistic explanatory style interpret events negatively; people with an optimistic explanatory style interpret events in a positive light— "Every cloud has a silver lining."

A pessimistic explanatory style can delay healing time and worsen the course of illness in several major diseases. For example, it can affect the circulatory system and general outlook for people with CHD. Blood flow actually changes as thoughts, feelings, and attitudes change. People with a pessimistic explanatory style have a higher risk of developing heart disease. Studies of explanatory style verify that a negative explanatory style also compromises immunity. Blood samples taken from people with a negative explanatory style revealed suppressed immune function, a low ratio of helper-to-suppressor T-cells, and fewer lymphocytes.

In contrast, an optimistic style tends to increase the strength of the immune system. An optimistic explanatory style and the positive attitude it fosters can also enhance the ability to resist infections, allergies, autoimmunities, and even cancer. A change in explanatory style can lead to a remarkable change in the course of disease. An optimistic explanatory style and the positive emotions it embraces—such as love, acceptance, and forgiveness—stimulate the body's healing systems.

Self-Esteem

Self-esteem is a way of viewing and assessing yourself. Positive self-esteem is a sense of feeling good about your capabilities, goals, accomplishments, place in the world, and relationship to others. People with high self-esteem respect themselves and take a healthy and productive view of their own limitations. Self-esteem is a powerful determinant of health behavior and, therefore, of health status. Healthy self-esteem is one of the best things people can develop for overall health, both mental and physical. A good, strong sense of self can boost the immune system, protect against disease, and aid in healing.

Whether people get sick—and how long they stay that way—may depend in part on the strength of their self-esteem. For example, low self-esteem worsens chronic pain. The higher the self-esteem, the more rapid the recovery. If people have strong self-esteem, the outlook is improved. If self-esteem is poor, however, their health can decline in direct proportion as their attitude and negative perceptions worsen.

Belief in yourself is one of the most powerful weapons you have to protect your health and live a longer, more satisfying life. It has a dramatic and positive impact on wellness, and you can work to harness it to your advantage.

Fighting Spirit

A **fighting spirit** involves the healthy expression of emotions, whether they are negative or positive. At the other extreme is hopelessness, a surrender to despair. A fighting spirit can play a major role in recovery from disease. People with a fighting spirit accept their disease diagnosis, adopt an optimistic attitude filled with faith, seek information about how to help themselves, and are determined to fight the disease. A fighting spirit makes people take charge.

A fighting spirit may be the underlying factor in what is called **spontaneous remission** from incurable illness. More and more physicians believe that the phenomenon is real and that the patient is the key in spontaneous remission. They believe the patient's attitude, especially the presence of a fighting spirit, is responsible for victory over disease. Fighters are not stronger or more capable than others—they simply do not give up as easily. They enjoy better health and live longer, even when physicians and laboratory tests say they should not. Fighters are intrinsically different from people who give up, and their health status reflects those differences.

GLOSSARY

Stress events scale A questionnaire used to assess sources of stress in life.

Neustress Neutral stress; stress that is neither harmful nor helpful.

Explanatory style The way people perceive the events in their lives, from an optimistic or a pessimistic perspective.

Self-esteem A sense of positive self-regard and self-respect.

Fighting spirit Determination; the open expression of emotions, whether negative or positive.

Spontaneous remission Inexplicable recovery from incurable disease.

Activity 12.1   Stress Events Scale

Name _____ Date _____

Course _____ Section _____ Gender _____ Age _____

Introduction

The list of stress-causing life events below may have potential adverse effects on your physical and psychological well-being. Check only those events that occurred during the past 12 months and rate the event on a 7-point scale ($-3, -2, -1, 0, +1, +2, +3$) using the following guidelines:

Negative Effect	Indifferent	Positive Effect
−3 Shocked	0	+3 Jubilant
−2 Dismayed		+2 Delighted
−1 Dissatisfied		+1 Pleased

Section 1: General

	Life Event	Stress Rating		Life Event	Stress Rating
1. Death of a family member	☐	____	10. Change/status of		
2. Death of a close friend or acquaintance	☐	____	Self esteem	☐	____
3. Substance abuse (addiction to drugs/alcohol)	☐	____	Boyfriend/girlfriend	☐	____
4. Imprisonment	☐	____	Family relationships	☐	____
5. Law violation (including traffic violations)	☐	____	Personal health (illness/disease/injury)	☐	____
6. Marriage	☐	____	Family or friend(s) health status	☐	____
7. Sexual intimacy	☐	____	Fitness level	☐	____
8. Pregnancy	☐	____	Sleeping habits	☐	____
9. Divorce			Nutrition habits	☐	____
Your own	☐	____	Study habits	☐	____
Your parents	☐	____	Friendship(s)	☐	____
Other close relative or friend	☐	____	Peer acceptance	☐	____
			Social activities	☐	____
			Recreational activities	☐	____
			Mode of transportation	☐	____

Activity 12.1 Stress Events Scale *(continued)*

Section 1: General (continued)	Life Event	Stress Rating
11. Ability to laugh and have fun	☐	_____
12. Financial status		
Sufficient for needs	☐	_____
Increase/decrease in income	☐	_____
Mortgage loan	☐	_____
Vehicle loan	☐	_____
Student loan(s)	☐	_____
Other (specify):_____	☐	_____
13. Work responsibilities		
New job	☐	_____
Loss of job	☐	_____
Change in work responsibilities	☐	_____
Change in work hours	☐	_____
Relationship with superior(s)	☐	_____
Relationship with coworkers	☐	_____
14. Time management	☐	_____
15. Exceptional personal accomplishment		
Specify: _____	☐	_____
16. Holidays		
Christmas	☐	_____
Thanksgiving	☐	_____
Other (specify):_____	☐	_____
17. Vacation	☐	_____
18. Ability to recoup from trials, tribulations, and challenges	☐	_____
19. Spirituality	☐	_____
20. Other(s), list: _____	☐	_____
21. _____	☐	_____
22. _____	☐	_____
23. _____	☐	_____

Section 2: Education	Life Event	Stress Rating
24. Choice of school	☐	_____
25. Change in school	☐	_____
26. Starting or stopping school	☐	_____
27. Loneliness	☐	_____
28. Privacy	☐	_____
29. Military obligations	☐	_____
30. Selecting/changing a major or minor	☐	_____
31. School-related activities		
Missed classes	☐	_____
Grade(s)	☐	_____
Academic probation	☐	_____
Course(s)	☐	_____
Exam(s)	☐	_____
Assignment(s)	☐	_____
Academic workload	☐	_____
College instructor(s)	☐	_____
32. Joining a fraternity/sorority	☐	_____
33. Housing		
Satisfied	☐	_____
Relationship with roommates	☐	_____
Changing roommates	☐	_____
Dismissal from dorm or residence	☐	_____
Moving	☐	_____
34. Graduation	☐	_____
35. Career employment	☐	_____
36. Other(s), list: _____	☐	_____
37. _____	☐	_____
38. _____	☐	_____

How to Score

Upon completion of the questionnaire, add all the negative and positive scores separately (e.g., positive ratings: 2, 1, 3, and 3 = 9 points positive score; negative ratings: −3, −2, −2, −1, and −2 = 10 points negative score). A final "total stress score" can be obtained by adding the positive score and the negative score together as positive numbers (total stress score: 9 + 10 = 19 points). Stress ratings based on your score are given below. The negative score is the best indicator of stress (distress or negative stress) in your life.

Score Interpretation

Stress Category	Negative Score	Total Score
Poor	≥15	≥30
Fair	9–14	20–29
Average	6–8	15–19
Good	1–5	6–14
Excellent	0	1–5

Copyright © Fitness & Wellness, Inc., Boise, ID, 2010.

Stress Events Scale Results

	Points	Stress Category
Negative score:	_____	_____
Positive score:	_____	NA
Total score:	_____	_____

© Fitness & Wellness, Inc.

12.6 *How Behavior Patterns Affect Health*

Individuals can also bring on unnecessary stress as a result of their behavior patterns. The two main types of behavior patterns, type A and type B, are based on several observable characteristics.

Several attempts have been made to develop an objective scale to identify type A individuals properly, but these questionnaires are not as valid and reliable as researchers would like them to be. Consequently, the main assessment tool to determine behavioral type is still the **structured interview**, during which a person is asked to reply to several questions that describe type A and type B behavior patterns. The interviewer notes not only the responses to the questions but also the individual's mental, emotional, and physical behaviors as he or she replies to each question.

Based on the answers and the associated behaviors, the interviewer rates the person along a continuum, ranging from type A to type B. Along this continuum, behavioral patterns are classified into five categories: A-1, A-2, X (a mix of type A and type B), B-3, and B-4. The type A-1 person exhibits all type A characteristics, and the B-4 person shows a relative absence of type A behaviors. The type A-2 individual does not exhibit a complete type A pattern, and the type B-3 individual exhibits only a few type A characteristics.

Type A

Type A behavior characterizes a primarily hard-driving, overambitious, aggressive, and at times hostile and overly competitive person. Type A individuals often set their own goals, are self-motivated, try to accomplish many tasks at the same time, are excessively achievement oriented, and have a high degree of time urgency.

Type B

In contrast, **type B** behavior is characteristic of calm, casual, relaxed, and easygoing individuals. Type B people take one thing at a time, do not feel pressured or hurried, and seldom set their own deadlines.

Type C

We also know that many individuals perform well under pressure. They typically are classified as type A but do not demonstrate any of the detrimental effects of stress. Drs. Robert and Marilyn Kriegel came up with the term *type C* to characterize people with these behaviors.[5]

Type C individuals are just as highly stressed as type A personalities but do not seem to be at higher risk for disease than type B. The keys to successful type C performance seem to be commitment, confidence, and control. Type C people are highly committed to what they are doing, have a great deal of confidence in their ability to do their work, and are in constant control of their actions. In addition, they enjoy their work and maintain themselves in top physical condition to be able to meet the mental and physical demands of their work.

Certain Type A Behavior Increases Risk for Disease

Though not all type A behavior is undesirable, individuals who undergo prolonged stress and commonly express anger or hostility increase their risk for CHD and other stress-related disease. Because higher levels of stress are more common in type A behavior, type A individuals have generally been counseled to lower their stress and prevent disease by modifying certain behaviors. Many type A characteristics that are damaging to health are learned behaviors. Consequently, if people can identify sources of stress and make changes in their behavioral responses, they can move along the continuum and respond more like type B individuals.

Next time you feel like getting even with someone for what that person may have done to you, you may want to consider that your anger may be more likely to hurt you. Anger increases heart rate and blood pressure and leads to constriction of blood vessels. Over time, these changes can cause damage to the arteries and eventually lead to a heart attack. Studies indicate that hostile people who get angry often, more intensely, and for longer periods of time have up to a threefold increased risk for CHD and are seven times more likely to suffer a fatal heart attack by age 50.

Many experts also believe that emotional stress is far more likely than physical stress to trigger a heart attack. People who are impatient and readily annoyed when they have to wait for someone or something—an employee, a traffic light, a table in a restaurant—are especially vulnerable.

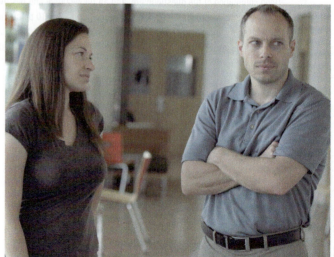

Anger and hostility can increase the risk for disease.

© Fitness & Wellness, Inc.

Behavior Modification Planning

Changing a Type A Personality

I PLAN TO   **I DID IT**

❏ ❏ Make a contract with yourself to slow down and take it easy. Put it in writing. Post it in a conspicuous spot, then stick to the terms you set up. Be specific. Abstractions ("I'm going to be less uptight") don't work.

❏ ❏ Work on only one or two things at a time. Wait until you change one habit before you tackle the next one.

❏ ❏ Eat more slowly and eat only when you are relaxed and sitting down.

❏ ❏ If you smoke, quit.

❏ ❏ Cut down on your caffeine intake because it increases the tendency to become irritated and agitated.

❏ ❏ Take regular breaks throughout the day, even as brief as 5 or 10 minutes, when you totally change what you're doing. Get up, stretch, get a drink of cool water, and walk around for a few minutes.

❏ ❏ Work on fighting your impatience. If you're standing in line at the grocery store, study the interesting things people have in their carts instead of getting upset.

❏ ❏ Work on controlling hostility. Keep a written log. When do you flare up? What causes it? How do you feel at the time? What preceded it? Look for patterns and figure out what sets you off. Then do something about it. Either avoid the situations that cause your hostility or practice reacting to them in different ways.

❏ ❏ Plan some activities just for the fun of it. Load a picnic basket in the car and drive to the country with a friend. After a stressful physics class, stop at a theater and see a good comedy.

❏ ❏ Choose a role model, someone you know and admire who does not have a type A personality. Observe the person carefully; then try out some techniques the person demonstrates.

❏ ❏ Simplify your life so you can learn to relax a little bit. Figure out which activities or commitments you can eliminate right now, then get rid of them.

❏ ❏ If morning is a problem time for you and you get too hurried, set your alarm clock half an hour earlier.

❏ ❏ Take time out during even the most hectic day to do something truly relaxing. Because you won't be used to it, you may have to work at it at first. Begin by listing things you'd really enjoy that would calm you. Include some things that take only a few minutes: Watch a sunset, lie out on the lawn at night and look at the stars, call an old friend and catch up on news, take a nap, sauté a pan of mushrooms and savor them slowly.

❏ ❏ If you're under a deadline, take short breaks. Stop and talk to someone for 5 minutes, take a short walk, or lie down with a cool cloth over your eyes for 10 minutes.

❏ ❏ Pay attention to what your own body clock is saying. You've probably noticed that every 90 minutes or so, you lose the ability to concentrate, get a little sleepy, and have a tendency to daydream. Instead of fighting the urge, put down your work and let your mind wander for a few minutes. Use the time to imagine and let your creativity run free.

❏ ❏ Learn to treasure unplanned surprises: a friend dropping by unannounced, a hummingbird outside your window, a child's tightly clutched bouquet of wildflowers.

❏ ❏ Savor your relationships. Think about the people in your life. Relax with them and give yourself to them. Give up trying to control others and resist the urge to end relationships that don't always go as you'd like them to.

Try It

If type A describes your personality, pick three of these strategies and apply them in your life this week. At the end of each day, determine how well you have done that day and evaluate how you can improve the next day.

12.7 *Vulnerability to Stress*

Researchers have identified a number of factors that can affect the way in which people handle stress. How people deal with these factors can actually increase or decrease vulnerability to stress. The questionnaire provided in Activity 12.2 lists these factors so that you can determine your vulnerability rating. Many of the items on this questionnaire are related to health, social support, self-worth, and nurturance (sense of being needed). All of these factors are crucial to your physical, social, mental, and emotional well-being and are essential

---

GLOSSARY

Structured interview An assessment tool used to determine behavioral patterns that define type A and type B personalities.

Type A The behavior pattern characteristic of a hard-driving, overambitious, aggressive, and at times hostile and overly competitive person.

Type B The behavior pattern characteristic of a calm, casual, relaxed, and easygoing individual.

Type C The behavior pattern of individuals who are just as highly stressed as the type A but do not seem to be at higher risk for disease than the type B individuals.

Behavior Modification Planning

Tips to Manage Anger

I PLAN TO **I DID IT**

☐ ☐ Commit to change and gain control over the behavior.

☐ ☐ Remind yourself that chronic anger leads to illness and disease and may shorten your life.

☐ ☐ Recognize when feelings of anger are developing and ask yourself the following questions:

☐ ☐ • Is the matter really that important?

☐ ☐ • Is the anger justified?

☐ ☐ • Can I change the situation without getting angry?

☐ ☐ • Is it worth risking my health over it?

☐ ☐ Tell yourself, "Stop, my health is worth it" every time you start to feel anger.

☐ ☐ Prepare for a positive response: Ask for an explanation or clarification of the situation, walk away and evaluate the situation, exercise, or use appropriate stress management techniques (breathing, meditation, and imagery) before you become angry and hostile.

☐ ☐ Manage anger at once; do not let it build up.

☐ ☐ Never attack anyone verbally or physically.

☐ ☐ Keep a journal and ponder the situations that cause you to be angry.

☐ ☐ Seek professional help if you are unable to overcome anger by yourself: You are worth it.

Try It

If you and others feel that anger is disrupting your health and relationships, these management strategies are critical to help restore a sense of well-being in your life. In your online journal or class notebook, list all of the strategies on a separate sheet of paper, study them each morning, and then evaluate yourself every night for the next week. If you gain control over the behavior, continue with the exercise until it becomes a healthy behavior. If you still struggle, professional help is recommended.

MINDTAP From Cengage **Complete This Activity Online**
Visit **www.cengagebrain.com** to access MindTap, a complete digital course that includes interactive quizzes, videos, and more.

---

to cope effectively with stressful life events. The more integrated you are in society, the less vulnerable you are to stress and illness.

Positive correlations have been found between social support and health outcomes. People can draw on social support to weather crises. Knowing that someone else cares, that people are there to lean on, and that support is out there is valuable for survival (or growth) in times of need.

The health benefits of physical fitness have already been discussed extensively. The questionnaire in Activity 12.2 will help you identify specific areas in which you can make improvements to help you cope more efficiently.

As you complete Activity 12.2, you will notice that many of the items describe situations and behaviors that are within your control. To make yourself less vulnerable to stress, improve the behaviors that make you more vulnerable to stress. You should start by modifying the behaviors that are easiest to change before undertaking some of the most difficult ones. After completing the questionnaire, record the results in Activity 12.3 and in your fitness and wellness profile in Appendix A.

12.8 Sleep Management

In today's society, sleep is largely undervalued. How few hours of sleep we can "get by on" is sometimes even touted as an achievement. However, researchers continue to find that sleep matters much more than it is often given credit for.

Sleep is a natural state of rest that is vital for good health and wellness. It is an anabolic process that allows the body to restore and heal itself. Though we may feel like we are winding down when we lie down to rest at night, our body—particularly the brain—is doing just the opposite. Getting a good night's rest takes advantage of one of the body's most powerful mechanisms to replenish depleted energy levels and allow the brain, muscles, organs, and various body tissues to repair themselves. Neurons in the brain become highly active during sleep, working to store new information in long-term memory, consolidate older memories, and make creative connections. A regular sleep schedule that provides sufficient and quality sleep each night helps enhance memory, improve concentration, regulate body weight, and maintain the immune system's ability to fight off disease.

How Much Sleep Do I Need?

The exact amount of sleep that each person needs varies among individuals. The National Sleep Foundation recommends adults ages 18 to 64 get between 7 and 9 hours of sleep. Experts believe that the last 2 hours of sleep are the most vital for well-being. That means if average adults need 7 to 9 hours of sleep and routinely get 6, they may be forfeiting the most critical sleep hours for health and wellness. Most people do not address sleep disorders until they start to cause mental and physical damage.

While there is no magic formula to determine how much sleep you need, if you don't need an alarm clock to get up

Activity 12.2   Stress Vulnerability Questionnaire

Name _____ Date _____

Course _____ Section _____ Gender _____ Age _____

I. Stress Vulnerability Questionnaire

Item	Strongly Agree	Mildly Agree	Mildly Disagree	Strongly Disagree
1. I try to incorporate as much physical activity* as possible in my daily schedule.	1	2	3	4
2. I exercise aerobically for 20 minutes or more at least three times per week.	1	2	3	4
3. I regularly sleep 7 to 8 hours per night.	1	2	3	4
4. I take my time eating at least one hot, balanced meal a day.	1	2	3	4
5. I drink fewer than two cups of coffee (or equivalent) per day.	1	2	3	4
6. I am at recommended body weight.	1	2	3	4
7. I enjoy good health.	1	2	3	4
8. I do not use tobacco in any form.	1	2	3	4
9. I limit my alcohol intake to no more than one drink (women) or two (men) per day.	1	2	3	4
10. I do not use hard drugs.	1	2	3	4
11. There is someone I love, trust, and can rely on for help if I have a problem or need to make an essential decision.	1	2	3	4
12. There is love in my family.	1	2	3	4
13. I routinely give and receive affection.	1	2	3	4
14. I have close personal relationships with other people that provide me with a sense of emotional security.	1	2	3	4
15. There are people close by whom I can turn to for guidance in time of stress.	1	2	3	4
16. I can speak openly about feelings, emotions, and problems with people I trust.	1	2	3	4
17. Other people rely on me for help.	1	2	3	4
18. I am able to keep my feelings of anger and hostility under control.	1	2	3	4
19. I have a network of friends who enjoy the same social activities that I do.	1	2	3	4
20. I take time to do something fun at least once a week.	1	2	3	4
21. My religious beliefs provide guidance and strength in my life.	1	2	3	4
22. I often provide service to others.	1	2	3	4
23. I enjoy my job (or major or school).	1	2	3	4
24. I am a competent worker.	1	2	3	4
25. I get along well with coworkers (or students).	1	2	3	4
26. My income is sufficient for my needs.	1	2	3	4
27. I manage time adequately.	1	2	3	4
28. I have learned to say "no" to additional commitments when I already am pressed for time.	1	2	3	4
29. I take daily quiet time for myself.	1	2	3	4
30. I practice stress management as needed.	1	2	3	4

Rating**

Excellent (great stress resistance)	0–30
Good (little vulnerability to stress)	31–40
Average (somewhat vulnerable to stress)	41–50
Fair (vulnerable to stress)	51–60
Poor (very vulnerable to stress)	≥61

Total Points: ☐

*Walk instead of driving, avoid escalators and elevators, or walk to neighboring offices, homes, and stores.
**Record total points and rating in Activity 12.3.

© Fitness & Wellness, Inc.

MINDTAP From Cengage   **Complete This Activity Online**
Visit **www.cengagebrain.com** to access MindTap, a complete digital course that includes interactive quizzes, videos, and more.

Activity 12.3 Stress Profile

Name _____ Date _____

Course _____ Section _____ Gender _____ Age _____

I. Assessments

Date:

Stress Events Scale			
Score (negative points only)			
Stress Rating			
Stress Vulnerability Questionnaire			
Score			
Rating			
Stress Management			
Technique(s) to be used			

II. In your own words, express how life stresses and your personality affect you in daily life.

_____

_____

_____

_____

_____

_____

III. In the space provided below, list, in order of priority, behaviors you would like to change to help you decrease your vulnerability to stress. Also, briefly outline how you intend to accomplish these changes.

Behavior(s)

1._____

2._____

How to accomplish the change(s)

_____

_____

_____

© Fitness & Wellness, Inc.

Stress Coping Strategies

- Balance personal, work, and family needs and obligations.
- Have a sense of control and purpose in life.
- Increase self-efficacy.
- Be optimistic.
- Express your emotions.
- Get adequate sleep.
- Eat well-balanced meals.
- Be physically active every day.
- Do not worry about things that you cannot control (e.g., the weather).
- Actively strive to resolve conflicts with other people.
- Prepare for stressful events the best possible way (public speaking, job interviews, exams).
- Limit or abstain from alcohol intake.
- Do not use tobacco in any form.
- View change as positive and not as a threat.
- Obtain social support from family members and friends.
- Use stress management programs and counselors available through work and school programs.
- Seek help from church leaders.
- Engage in nonstressful activities (reading, sports, hobbies, and social events).
- Get involved in your community.
- Practice stress management techniques.
- Adopt a healthy lifestyle.

every morning, you wake up at about the same time, and you are refreshed and feel alert throughout the day, you most likely have a healthy sleeping habit.

What Happens If I Don't Get Enough Sleep?

The way we live today—always multitasking, overscheduling our days, checking text messages and e-mails every few minutes, and spending late-nights "relaxing" in front of a screen—has become a major factor in people's poor sleep habits. Our fast-paced schedules contribute to a steady production of the stress hormone cortisol that can lead to insomnia and other interruptions in sound sleep. Further, the amount of artificial light Americans encounter from indoor lighting and screen time disrupts the body's internal clock, making natural sleep patterns difficult to sustain. Sleep deprivation in the United States has become such a problem that the CDC has called insufficient sleep a public health epidemic. Up to 70 million adults in the United States suffer from a sleep or wakefulness disorder.[6]

Sleep deprivation weakens the immune system; impairs mental function; and has a negative impact on physical, social, academic, and job performance. Lack of sleep also affects stress levels, mood, memory, behavioral patterns, and cognitive performance. Cumulative long-term consequences include an increase in the risk for cardiovascular disease, high blood pressure, obesity, diabetes, and psychological disorders like depression. People who get less sleep have a threefold increased risk of getting a cold, are more likely to develop CHD earlier in life, have more inflammation in the body, and have higher blood levels of the stress hormone cortisol. What most people notice is a chronic state of fatigue, exhaustion, and confusion.

Stress-wise, getting to bed too late often leads to oversleeping, napping, missing classes, poor grades, and distress. It further increases tension, irritability, intolerance, and confusion, and it may cause depression and life dissatisfaction. Not getting enough sleep can also lead to vehicle accidents with serious or fatal consequences as people fall asleep behind the wheel. More than 6,000 fatal crashes each year may be attributed to sleepy drivers (sleepy drivers are just as dangerous as drunk drivers). Irregular sleep patterns, including sleeping in on weekends, also contribute to many of the aforementioned problems.

Although more than 100 sleep disorders have been identified, they can be classified into four major groups:

1. Problems with falling and staying asleep
2. Difficulties staying awake
3. Difficulties adhering to a regular sleep schedule
4. Sleep-disruptive behaviors (including sleepwalking and sleep terror disorder)

College Students Are Among the Most Sleep-Deprived

College students are some of the most sleep-deprived people of all. On average, they sleep about 6.5 hours per night, and approximately 30 percent report chronic sleep difficulties. Only 8 percent report sleeping 8 or more hours per night. For many students, college is the first time they have complete control of their schedule, including when they go to sleep and how many hours they sleep.

Lack of sleep during school days and pulling all-nighters interfere with the ability to pay attention and to learn, process, and retain new information. You may be able to retain the information in short-term memory, but most likely it will not be there for a cumulative exam or when you need it for adequate job performance. Deep sleep that takes place early in the night and a large portion of the REM (rapid eye movement) dream sleep that occurs near the end of the night have both been linked to learning. The brain has been shown to consolidate new information for long-term memory while you sleep. Convincing sleep-deprived students to get adequate sleep is a real challenge because they often feel overwhelmed by school, work, and family responsibilities. Students who go to sleep early and get about 8 hours of sleep per night are more apt to succeed.

Tips to Sleep Better

To enhance the quality of your sleep, you should do the following:

- Exercise and be physically active, but avoid vigorous exercise 4 hours prior to bedtime.

- Avoid eating a heavy meal or snacking 2 to 3 hours before going to bed (digestion increases your metabolism).

- Limit the amount of time that you spend around artificial light in the evening, including screen time from surfing and socializing on-line, texting, and watching television.

- Go to bed and rise about the same time each day.

- Keep the bedroom cool, quiet, and dark.

- Develop a bedtime ritual (meditation, prayer, or white noise).

- Use your bed for sleeping only (do not watch television, do home-work, or use a laptop in bed).

- Relax and slow down 15 to 30 minutes before bedtime.

- Do not drink coffee or caffeine-containing beverages several hours before going to bed.

- Do not rely on alcohol to fall asleep (alcohol disrupts deep sleep stages).

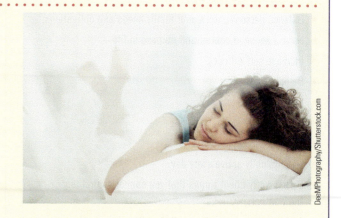

- Avoid long naps (a 20- to 30-minute "power nap" can be beneficial during an afternoon slump without interfering with night-time sleep).

- Have frank and honest conversations with roommates if they have different sleep schedules.

- Evaluate your mattress every 5 to 7 years for comfort and support; if you wake up with aches and pains or you sleep better when you are away from home, it is most likely time for a new mattress.

Does It Help to "Catch Up" on Sleep on Weekends?

Staying up late Friday or Saturday nights and crashing the next day disrupts the circadian rhythm, the biological clock that controls the daily sleep−wake schedule. Such disruption influences quantity and quality of sleep and keeps people from falling asleep and rising at the necessary times for school, work, or other required activities. In essence, the body wants to sleep and be awake at odd times of the 24-hour cycle.

A term used to describe the cumulative effect of needed sleep that you don't get is "sleep debt." Sleeping in on weekends in an attempt to "catch up" on missed sleep during the weekdays doesn't solve the problem and may actually be worse for your health. Though past research has shown modest health benefits from trying to make up for lost sleep, recent studies have found the digression from the body's routine sleep pattern can cause negative effects that may outweigh the benefits. A 2015 study tracking 447 men and women over age 30 found that those who maintained a regular sleep schedule on weekdays but slept in later on weekends had lower HDL (good) cholesterol, higher insulin resistance, higher triglycerides, and higher body mass index. The greater the divergence from regular sleep schedule between weekdays and weekends, the greater the risk for obesity, heart disease, and diabetes.[7]

Planning to make up sleep on weekends after a week's worth of insufficient sleep is much like planning to eat healthier 2 days out of the week to try to counteract 5 days of consuming a poor diet. The better approach is to maintain a regular sleep schedule that provides sufficient sleep each night so that you can consistently be at your best the next day.

To improve your sleep pattern, you need to exercise discipline and avoid staying up late to watch a movie or leaving your homework or studying for an exam until the last minute. As busy as you are, your health and well-being are your most important asset. You only live once. Keeping your health and living life to its fullest potential requires a good night's rest.

12.9 Time Management

According to Benjamin Franklin, "Time is the stuff life is made of." The present hurry-up style of American life is not conducive to wellness. The hassles involved in getting through a routine day often lead to stress-related illnesses. People who do not manage their time properly quickly experience chronic stress, fatigue, despair, discouragement, and illness.

Surveys indicate that most Americans think time moves too fast for them, and more than half of those surveyed think they have to get *everything* done. The younger the respondents, the more they struggled with lack of time. Almost half wished they had more time for exercise and recreation, hobbies, and family. Healthy and successful people are good time managers, able to maintain a pace of life within their comfort zone, and attribute their success to smart work, not necessarily hard work.

Behavior Modification Planning

Common Time Killers

Have you minimized the role of these time killers in your life?

I PLAN TO

I DID IT

I PLAN TO	I DID IT	
❑	❑	Watching television, listening to radio/music
❑	❑	Excessive sleeping
❑	❑	Surfing/socializing online
❑	❑	Unnecessary texting or emailing
❑	❑	Daydreaming
❑	❑	Shopping
❑	❑	Socializing/parties

I PLAN TO	I DID IT	
❑	❑	Excessive recreation
❑	❑	Talking on the telephone
❑	❑	Worrying
❑	❑	Procrastinating
❑	❑	Drop-in visitors
❑	❑	Confusion (unclear goals)
❑	❑	Indecision (what to do next)
❑	❑	Interruptions
❑	❑	Perfectionism (every detail must be done)

Try It

Using Activity 12.4, find the time killers in your life and make the necessary changes as required.

Five Steps to Time Management

Trying to achieve one or more goals in a limited time can create a tremendous amount of stress. Many people just don't seem to have enough hours in the day to accomplish their tasks. The greatest demands on their time, nonetheless, are frequently self-imposed—trying to do too much, too fast, too soon.

Some time killers, such as eating, sleeping, and recreation, are necessary for health and wellness, but in excess, they lead to stress in life. You can follow five basic steps to make better use of your time (also see Activity 12.4):

1. *Find the time killers.* Many people do not know how they spend each part of the day. Keep a 4- to 7-day log and record at half-hour intervals the activities you do. Record the activities as you go through your typical day so that you will remember all of them. At the end of each day, decide when you wasted time. You may be shocked by the amount of time you spent on your phone, online, sleeping (more than 8 hours per night), or watching television.

2. *Set long- and short-range goals.* Setting goals requires some in-depth thinking and helps put your life and daily tasks in perspective. What do I want out of life? Where do I want to be 10 years from now? Next year? Next week? Tomorrow? You can use Activity 12.5 to list these goals.

3. *Identify your immediate goals and prioritize them for today and this week* (use Activity 12.6—make as many copies as necessary). Each day, sit down and determine what you need to accomplish that day and that week. Rank your "today" and "this week" tasks in four categories: (a) top priority, (b) medium priority, (c) low priority, and (d) trash.

   Top-priority tasks are the most important ones. If you were to reap most of your productivity from 30 percent of your activities, which would they be? Medium-priority activities are those that must be done but can wait a day or two. Low-priority activities are those to be done only upon completing all top- and middle-priority activities. Trash activities are not worth your time (e.g., cruising the hallways or channel surfing).

4. *Use a daily planner to help you organize and simplify your day.* New digital tools have made it easier to have daily tasks and calendared items readily accessible for quick reference from laptops, smartphones, or other mobile devices. In this way, you can access your priority list, appointments, notes, phone numbers, and addresses conveniently from your backpack, pocket, or purse. Many individuals think that planning daily and weekly activities is a waste of time. A few minutes to schedule your time each day, however, may pay off in hours saved.

   As you plan your day, be realistic and find your comfort zone. Determine the best way to organize your day. Which is the most productive time for work, study, and errands? Are you a morning person, or are you getting most of your work done when people are quitting for the day? Pick your best hours for top-priority activities. Be sure to schedule enough time for exercise and relaxation. Recreation is not necessarily wasted time. You need to take care of your physical and emotional well-being to ensure a balanced lifestyle.

5. *Conduct nightly audits.* Take 10 minutes each night to figure out how well you accomplished your goals that day. Successful time managers evaluate themselves daily. This simple task helps you see the entire picture. Cross off the goals you accomplished, and carry over to the next day those you did not get done. You may realize that some goals can be moved down to low priority or can be trashed.

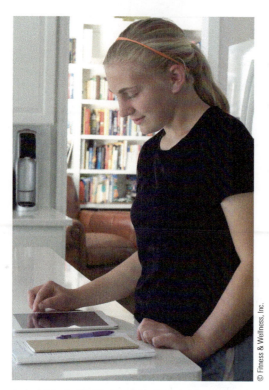

Planning and prioritizing activities simplify your days.

Go through the list of strategies in Activity 12.7 weekly to determine whether you are becoming a good time manager. Provide a "yes" or "no" answer to each statement. If you are able to answer "yes" to most questions, congratulations: you are becoming a good time manager.

HOEGER KEY TO WELLNESS

The present hurry-up style of American life is not conducive to wellness. Most Americans think time moves too fast for them and wish they had more time for exercise and recreation, hobbies, and family. Plan your days wisely and schedule physical activity and time for yourself each day.

12.10 *Managing Technostress*

In today's fast-paced, 24/7 digital world, technology permeates every corner of our environment—not only in our computers, televisions, and handheld devices, but also in our cars, shopping centers, home appliances, and even some shoes and clothing. Students and workers are spending more time at the computer than ever before, and continue to spend downtime

Tips for Better Time Management

In addition to the five major steps, the following can help you make better use of your time:

- *Delegate.* If possible, delegate activities that someone else can do for you. Scheduling with a coworker to cover your work shift so you can adequately prepare for an exam might be well worth the expense and your time.

- *Say "no."* Learn to say "no" to activities that keep you from getting your top priorities done. You can do only so much in a single day. Nobody has enough time to do everything he or she would like to get done. Don't overload either. Many people are afraid to say no because they feel guilty if they do. Think ahead, and think of the consequences. Are you doing it to please others? What will it do to your well-being? Can you handle one more task? At some point, you have to balance your activities and look at life and time realistically.

- *Avoid boredom.* Doing nothing can be a source of stress. People need to feel that they are contributing and that they are productive members of society. It is also good for self-esteem and self-worth. Set realistic goals and work toward them each day.

- *Plan ahead for disruptions.* Even a careful plan of action can be disrupted. An unexpected phone call or visitor can change or impede your schedule. Planning your response ahead of time helps you deal with these setbacks.

- *Get it done.* Select only one task at a time, concentrate on it, and see it through. Many people do a little here, do a little there, and then do something else. In the end, nothing gets done. An exception to working

on just one task at a time is when you are doing a difficult task. Rather than "killing yourself," interchange with another activity that is not as hard.

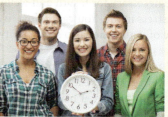

- *Eliminate distractions.* If you have trouble adhering to a set plan, remove distractions and trash activities from your eyesight. Television, radio, the Internet, magazines, open doors, or studying in a park might distract you and become time killers.

- *Set aside "overtimes."* Regularly schedule time that you did not think you would need as overtime to complete unfinished projects. Most people underschedule rather than overschedule time. The result is usually late-night burnout. If you schedule overtimes and get your tasks done, enjoy some leisure time, get ahead on another project, or work on other low-priority activities.

- *Plan time for you.* Set aside special time for yourself daily. Life is not meant to be all work. Use your time to walk, read, or listen to your favorite music.

- *Reward yourself.* As with any other healthy behavior, positive change or a job well done deserves a reward. People often overlook the value of rewards, even if they are self-given. Still, they practice behaviors that are rewarded and discontinue those that are not.

Activity 12.4 Finding Time Killers

Name _____ Date _____

Course _____ Section _____ Gender _____ Age _____

> Keep a 4- to 7-day log and record at half-hour intervals the activities you do (make additional copies of this form as needed). Record the activities as you go through your typical day, so you will remember them all. At the end of each day, decide when you wasted time. Using a highlighter, identify the time killers on this form and plan necessary changes for the next day.

6:00	
6:30	
7:00	
7:30	
8:00	
8:30	
9:00	
9:30	
10:00	
10:30	
11:00	
11:30	
12:00	
12:30	
1:00	
1:30	
2:00	
2:30	
3:00	
3:30	
4:00	
4:30	
5:00	
5:30	
6:00	
6:30	
7:00	
7:30	
8:00	
8:30	
9:00	
9:30	
10:00	
10:30	
11:00	
11:30	
12:00	

© Fitness & Wellness, Inc.

Activity 12.5 Planning Long- and Short-Range Goals

Name _____ **Date** _____

Course _____ **Section** _____ **Gender** _____ **Age** _____

> Below, list your goals as indicated. You may want to keep this form and review it in years to come.

I. List three goals you wish to accomplish in life:

1. _____
2. _____
3. _____

II. List three goals you wish to see accomplished 10 years from now:

1. _____
2. _____
3. _____

III. List three goals you wish to accomplish this year:

1. _____
2. _____
3. _____

IV. List three goals you wish to accomplish this month:

1. _____
2. _____
3. _____

V. List three goals you wish to accomplish this week:

1. _____
2. _____
3. _____

Signature: _____ **Date:** _____

© Fitness & Wellness, Inc.

Activity 12.6   Daily and Weekly Goals and Priorities

Name _____   Date _____

Course _____   Section _____   Gender _____   Age _____

Take a few minutes each Sunday night to write down the goals or tasks you wish to accomplish that week. As with your daily goals, rank them as top, medium, low, or "trash" priorities. (Make as many copies of this form as needed.) At the end of the week, evaluate how well you accomplished your goals. Cross off the goals you accomplished and carry over to the next week those you did not get done.

Week: ___ / ___ to ___ / ___

Top-Priority Goals

1. _____
2. _____
3. _____
4. _____

Medium-Priority Goals

1. _____
2. _____
3. _____
4. _____

Low-Priority Goals

1. _____
2. _____
3. _____
4. _____

Trash (do only after all other goals have been accomplished)

1. _____
2. _____
3. _____
4. _____

Take 10 minutes each morning to write down the goals or tasks you wish to accomplish that day. Rank them as top, medium, low, or "trash" priorities. (Make as many copies of this form as needed.) At the end of the day, evaluate how well you accomplished your tasks for the day. Cross off the goals you accomplished and carry over to the next day those you did not get done.

Date: ___ / ___   Day of the Week: _____

Top-Priority Goals

1. _____
2. _____
3. _____
4. _____

Medium-Priority Goals

1. _____
2. _____
3. _____
4. _____

Low-Priority Goals

1. _____
2. _____
3. _____
4. _____

Trash (do only after all other goals have been accomplished)

1. _____
2. _____
3. _____
4. _____

© Fitness & Wellness, Inc.

Activity 12.7   **Evaluating Time Management Skills**

Name _____ Date _____

Course _____ Section _____ Gender _____ Age _____

Weekly, go through the list of strategies below and write a "yes" or "no" response to each statement. If you are able to answer "yes" to most questions, congratulations, you are becoming a good time manager.

Strategy	Date:													
1. I evaluate my time killers periodically.														
2. I have written down my long-range goals.														
3. I have written down my short-term goals.														
4. I use a daily planner.														
5. I conduct nightly audits.														
6. I conduct weekly audits.														
7. I delegate activities that others can do.														
8. I have learned to say "no" to additional tasks when I'm already in overload.														
9. I plan activities to avoid boredom.														
10. I plan ahead for distractions.														
11. I work on one task at a time until it's done.														
12. I have removed distractions from my work.														
13. I set aside overtimes.														
14. I set aside special time for myself daily.														
15. I reward myself for a job well done.														

© Fitness & Wellness, Inc.

MINDTAP From Cengage   **Complete This Activity Online**
Visit **www.cengagebrain.com** to access MindTap, a complete digital course that includes interactive quizzes, videos, and more.

Tips to Manage Technostress

- **Turn it off.** Turn off your cell phone while at the movies, while enjoying dinner, or when wanting to spend uninterrupted quality time with family members and friends.

- **Slow down your reaction time.** Though technology often seems to run at hyper-speed, it doesn't mean you need to try and keep up at an impractical pace. Utilize e-mail filters, and schedule set times during the day to check texts, e-mails, and phone messages. You don't need to respond as soon as a message pops up on your phone or in your inbox.

- **Remove digital distractions.** Don't let your gadgets distract you from your school and work productivity, particularly in situations that require sustained attention and concentration, like studying for an exam, finishing a project, or writing creatively.

- **Avoid the urge to multitask.** Research has found that multitasking actually lowers overall productivity, and students and employees who constantly switch between tasks are less likely to retain important information and more likely to make mistakes. Instead, practice focusing your energy on one task at a time through completion.

- **Take time to fully unplug.** Don't let technology dominate your life. Schedule regular gadget-free time away from your computer, cell phone, or other handheld devices to allow both your eyes and mind to rest. Take time to exercise outdoors, enjoy a peaceful walk, read a favorite book in paperback, or watch the sunset.

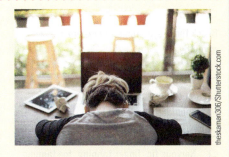

theskaman306/Shutterstock.com

hours surfing the web, video gaming, texting, and socializing online. The average teenager sends and reads more than 3,000 text messages per month! With society's ever-growing dependence on technology, it's rare that an hour passes without most Americans looking at a screen.

Though innovation is meant to help improve the flow of work and daily life, technology has also been associated with feelings of anxiety and irritability, headaches, mental fatigue, lost productivity, and poor job performance. Tech-related stress has been termed **technostress** and, as the name implies, refers to stress caused by the inability to adapt or cope with technology in a healthy way. The technology itself is not the source of stress, but how people handle and react to it. Distraction and lack of focus due to the never-ending interruption of incoming texts, e-mails, phone calls, and social notifications has been called the epidemic of our digital age. People often feel stressed because they don't know how to manage the daily onslaught of resources and information made available on the web, leading to feelings of being overwhelmed with "information overload."

! Critical Thinking

Technological advances provide many benefits to our lives. What positive and negative effects do these advances have upon your daily living activities, and what impact are they having on your stress level?

At school and on the job, working with technology can also cause frustration and a perceived lack of control when faced with errors and unexpected hiccups, including hardware failures, slow computer speeds, lost data, and other tech-related problems. Each new innovation—despite the promise of making work or life more efficient—comes with a learning curve that demands new skills and the ability to adapt to new programs and tools with faster reaction times. As a result, new technology can become a stressor in itself, causing many people to become resistant to technological advances. Constant connectivity, even in digital activities meant to be leisurely, can lead to overstimulation, blurred boundaries between work and play, isolation and/or increased distance in relationships, loss of concentration and attention span, and unhealthy attachment to technological devices. See "Tips to Manage Technostress" to learn ways to help reduce stress associated with modern technology.

12.11 Coping with Stress

The ways in which people perceive and cope with stress seem to be more important in the development of disease than the amount and type of stress. First, the person must recognize the presence of a problem. Many people either do not want to believe that they are under too much stress or they fail to recognize some of the typical symptoms of distress. Noting some of the stress-related symptoms (see the "Common Symptoms of Stress" box) helps a person respond more objectively and initiate an adequate coping response.

GLOSSARY

Technostress Stress resulting from the inability to adapt to or cope with digital technologies in a healthy way.

Behavior Modification Planning

Common Symptoms of Stress

Check those symptoms you experience regularly.

- ❏ Headaches
- ❏ Muscular aches (mainly in neck, shoulders, and back)
- ❏ Grinding teeth
- ❏ Nervous tic, finger tapping, toe tapping
- ❏ Increased sweating
- ❏ Increase in or loss of appetite
- ❏ Insomnia
- ❏ Nightmares
- ❏ Fatigue
- ❏ Dry mouth

- ❏ Stuttering
- ❏ High blood pressure
- ❏ Tightness or pain in the chest
- ❏ Impotence
- ❏ Hives
- ❏ Dizziness
- ❏ Depression
- ❏ Irritation
- ❏ Anger
- ❏ Hostility
- ❏ Fear, panic, anxiety
- ❏ Stomach pain, flutters
- ❏ Nausea
- ❏ Cold, clammy hands

- ❏ Poor concentration
- ❏ Pacing
- ❏ Restlessness
- ❏ Rapid heart rate
- ❏ Low-grade infection
- ❏ Loss of sex drive
- ❏ Rash or acne

Try It

If you regularly experience some of these symptoms, use your online journal or class notebook to keep a log of when these symptoms occur and under what circumstances. You may find out that a pattern emerges when experiencing distress in life.

Identify and Change Stressors Within Your Control

When people have stress-related symptoms, they should first try to identify and change or remove stressors that are within their control when possible. If the cause of stress is unknown, keeping a log of the time and days when the symptoms occur, as well as the events preceding and following the onset of symptoms, may be helpful.

For example, a couple noted that every evening around 6:00 p.m., the wife became nauseated and had abdominal pain. After seeking professional help, both were instructed to keep a log of daily events. It soon became clear that the symptoms did not occur on weekends but always started just before the husband came home from work during the week. Following some personal interviews with the couple, it was determined that the wife felt a lack of attention from her husband and responded subconsciously by becoming ill to the point at which she required personal care and affection from her husband. Once the stressor was identified, appropriate behavior changes were initiated to correct the situation.

Other stressors can be changed or minimized by drawing deliberate personal boundaries. Most of us feel anxiety when a person treats us in a way that does not feel acceptable to us. We may feel used or manipulated to some extent. For example, a person may ask you for a great deal of time and resources or expect you to adopt a belief you are uncomfortable with. Personal boundaries allow you to take control of and responsibility for your own life and who you are. By setting physical or emotional personal boundaries, you are able to live with integrity, to ask that people treat you in the way you feel you should be treated. Be honest and upfront in your associations and relationships. Take ownership of your feelings. When you feel you need to assert your personal boundaries, start your sentence by saying "I feel." And remember that your feelings are valid and that you have unique needs and preferences. You will need to confidently say "no" in some situations. Remember that you are the only person who can truly balance your life and decide what to allow into your life. While you will never be able to control the outcome of a conversation, you can express how you feel you ought to be treated. It is true that friends sacrifice to help one another, but it is also true that no friendship can develop when both sides cannot be upfront about personal boundaries.

Accept and Cope with Stressors Beyond Your Control

In other instances, the circumstances are such that the stressor cannot be removed. Examples of such situations are the death of a close family member, the first year on the job, an intolerable roommate, or a difficult college course. In these situations, accepting that the stressor is beyond your control is often the best way to release symptoms of worry and anxiety. If the stressor continues to be a problem that interferes with optimal health and performance, individuals can call upon the following stress management strategies—including physical activity and relaxation techniques—to cope more effectively.

Physical Activity

Exercise is one of the simplest tools to control stress. The value of exercise in reducing stress is related to several factors, the main one being a decrease in muscular tension. A fatigued muscle is a relaxed muscle. For example, a person can be distressed because he or she has had a miserable 8 hours of work with a difficult boss. To make matters worse, it is late and, on the

Behavior Modification Planning

Thirty-Second Body Scan

This simple 30-second exercise helps you scan the body to raise stress awareness.

- ❑ Am I clenching my teeth?
- ❑ Am I furrowing my brow?
- ❑ Are my shoulders tense?
- ❑ Am I breathing rapidly?
- ❑ Am I tapping my fingers?
- ❑ Do I feel knots in my stomach?
- ❑ Are my arms, thighs, or calves tight?

- ❑ Am I nervously bouncing my leg or foot?
- ❑ Am I curling my toes?
- ❑ Do I feel uneasiness anywhere else in my body?

Try It

A body scan can be performed daily or several times a day to help you learn and recognize when you are distressed. People are often unaware of stress signals and activities that are causing excess stress. Increasing awareness allows you to initiate proper actions to more effectively manage stress. An example would be to breathe deeply for 1 to 3 minutes while doing the body scan and repeating positive affirmations (e.g., "I am at peace" or "I am calm and relaxed").

---

way home, the car in front is going much slower than the speed limit. The fight-or-flight mechanism—already activated during the stressful day—begins again: catecholamines (hormones) rise, heart rate and blood pressure shoot up, breathing quickens and deepens, muscles tense, and all systems say "go." However, no action can be initiated and stress can't be dissipated, because the person cannot just hit the boss or the car in front.

A real remedy would be to take action by "hitting" the swimming pool, the tennis ball, the weight room, or the jogging trail. Engaging in physical activity reduces muscular tension and metabolizes increased catecholamines (which were triggered by the fight-or-flight mechanism and brought about the physiological changes). Furthermore, while the individual is concentrating on the tennis game, there isn't enough time to think about an irrational boss or other undesirable events. Although exercise does not solve problems at work or take care of slow drivers, it certainly helps the person cope with stress and prevents stress from becoming a chronic problem. Family or roommates will likely appreciate a more relaxed homecoming, where work problems can be left behind and where a parent in particular is able to dedicate energy to family activities.

Beyond the short-term benefits of exercise in lessening stress, a regular aerobic exercise program strengthens the cardiovascular system. Because the cardiovascular system seems to be affected seriously by stress, a stronger system should be able to cope more effectively. For instance, good cardiorespiratory endurance has been shown to lower resting heart rate and blood pressure. Because both heart rate and blood pressure rise in stressful situations, initiating the stress response at a lower baseline counteracts some negative effects of stress. Cardiorespiratory-fit individuals can cope more effectively and are less affected by the stresses of daily living.

Research also has shown that physical exercise requiring continuous and rhythmic muscular activity, such as aerobic exercise, stimulates alpha-wave activity in the brain. These are the same wave patterns commonly seen during meditation and relaxation.

Further, during vigorous aerobic exercise lasting 30 minutes or longer, morphine-like substances referred to as **endorphins** are thought to be released from the pituitary gland in the brain. These substances not only act as painkillers, but also seem to induce the soothing, calming effect often associated with aerobic exercise. Research has also shown that moderate-intensity exercise has an immediate effect on a person's mood and the effects last up to 12 hours following activity. Thus, exercise mitigates the daily stress that leads to mood alterations. Exercise is free and easily accessible to everyone. Pick an activity that you enjoy and use it to combat stress, blue moods, anxiety, and depression. Stress management experts often recommend selecting activities like **yoga** and **tai chi** that combine physical activity with additional stress reduction techniques. These activities regularly incorporate meditation, breathing, muscle relaxation, or a combination of these techniques—along with physical activity—to help people dissipate stress.

HOEGER KEY TO WELLNESS

Exercise is one of the simplest tools to control stress. Exercise requiring continuous and rhythmic muscular activity stimulates alpha-wave activity in the brain. These are the same wave patterns seen commonly during meditation and relaxation.

GLOSSARY

Endorphins Morphine-like substances released from the pituitary gland in the brain during prolonged aerobic exercise and thought to induce feelings of euphoria and natural well-being.

Yoga A school of thought in the Hindu religion that seeks to help the individual attain a higher level of spirituality and peace of mind.

Tai chi A self-paced form of exercise often described as "meditation in motion" because it promotes serenity through gentle, balanced, low-impact movements that bring together the mind, body, and emotions.

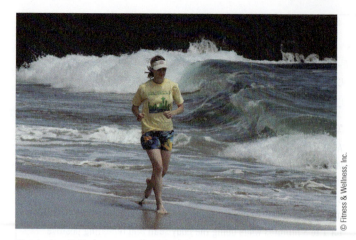

Physical activity is an excellent tool to control stress.

Physical activity can have a long-term impact in preventing stress in every stage of life. Studies show that teens who play sports in the crucial development years of adolescence have fewer symptoms of depression and stress into early adulthood. Participation in sports teams helps youth enjoy better mental health, improved moods, and increased energy—all factors that protect against the incidence of depression, which typically peaks between ages 18 and 29. Another way that exercise helps lower stress is to deliberately divert stress to various body systems. Dr. Selye explains in his book *Stress without Distress* that, when one specific task becomes difficult, a change in activity can be as good as or better than rest itself.[8] For example, if a person is having trouble with a task and does not seem to be getting anywhere, jogging or swimming for a while is better than sitting around and getting frustrated. In this way, the mental strain is diverted to the working muscles, and one system helps the other to relax.

Other psychologists indicate that when muscular tension is removed from emotional strain, the emotional strain disappears. In many cases, the change of activity suddenly clears the mind and helps put the pieces together.

Additional benefits of physical exercise give people a psychological boost because exercise does the following:

- Alleviates insomnia
- Provides an opportunity to meet social needs and develop new friendships
- Allows the person to share common interests and problems
- Develops discipline
- Provides the opportunity to do something constructive

HOEGER KEY TO WELLNESS

Sports help youth enjoy better mental health, improved moods, and increased energy, all factors that protect against the incidence of depression, which typically peaks between ages 18 and 29.

Yoga

Yoga is an excellent stress-coping technique. It is a school of thought in the Hindu religion that seeks to help the individual attain a higher level of spirituality and peace of mind. Although its philosophical roots can be considered spiritual, yoga is based on principles of self-care.

Practitioners of yoga adhere to a specific code of ethics and a system of mental and physical exercises that promote control of the mind and the body. In Western countries, many people are familiar mainly with the exercise portion of yoga. This system of exercises (postures or asanas) can be used as a relaxation technique for stress management. The exercises include a combination of postures, diaphragmatic breathing, muscle relaxation, and meditation that help buffer the biological effects of stress. Although people are unable to avoid all life stressors, they can definitely change emotional response through performing yoga postures, observing and controlling their breathing pattern, and reflecting on the moment, all of which are actions that help calm the mind and the body.

Western interest in yoga exercises developed gradually over the last century, particularly since the 1970s. The practice of yoga exercises helps align the musculoskeletal system and increases muscular flexibility, muscular strength and endurance, and balance. Research also confirms that yoga can help improve mood and cognition and reduce stress.[9] Yoga exercises help to dispel stress by raising self-esteem, clearing the mind, slowing respiration, promoting neuromuscular relaxation, and increasing body awareness. Yoga exercises have also been used to help treat chemical dependency, treat insomnia, and prevent injury. In addition, the exercises help relieve back pain and control involuntary body functions like heart rate, blood pressure, oxygen consumption, and metabolic rate. Because yoga therapy has been shown to be clinically beneficial for rehabilitation after a stroke, yoga is also used in many hospital-based programs for cardiac patients to help manage stress and decrease blood pressure.[10]

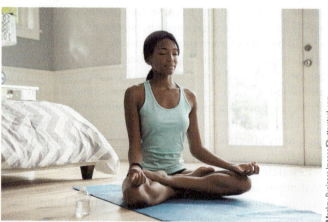

Yoga exercises help induce the relaxation response.

Behavior Modification Planning

Characteristics of Good Stress Managers

Do you have the habits and characteristics of someone who manages stress well?

I PLAN TO
I DID IT

GOOD STRESS MANAGERS...

☐ ☐ are physically active, eat a healthy diet, and get adequate rest every day.

☐ ☐ believe they have control over events in their life (have an internal locus of control).

☐ ☐ understand their own feelings and accept their limitations.

☐ ☐ recognize, anticipate, monitor, and regulate stressors within their capabilities.

☐ ☐ control emotional and physical responses when distressed.

☐ ☐ use appropriate stress management techniques when confronted with stressors.

☐ ☐ recognize warning signs and symptoms of excessive stress.

☐ ☐ schedule daily time to unwind, relax, and evaluate the day's activities.

☐ ☐ control stress when called upon to perform.

☐ ☐ enjoy life despite occasional disappointments and frustrations.

☐ ☐ look success and failure squarely in the face and keep moving along a predetermined course.

☐ ☐ move ahead with optimism and energy and do not spend time and talent worrying about failure.

☐ ☐ learn from previous mistakes and use them as building blocks to prevent similar setbacks in the future.

☐ ☐ give of themselves freely to others.

☐ ☐ find deep meaning in life.

Try It

Change is threatening for many people, but often required. Pick three of these strategies and apply them in your life. After several days, determine the usefulness of these strategies to your physical, mental, social, and emotional well-being.

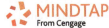 **MINDTAP** From Cengage **Complete This Online**
Visit **www.cengagebrain.com** to access MindTap, a complete digital course that includes interactive quizzes, videos, and more.

Of the many styles of yoga, more than 60 are presently taught in the United States. Classes vary according to their emphasis. Some styles of yoga are athletic, while others are passive in nature.

The most popular variety of yoga in the Western world is **hatha yoga**, which incorporates a series of static-stretching postures performed in specific sequences (asanas) that help induce the relaxation response. The postures are held for several seconds while participants concentrate on breathing patterns, meditation, and body awareness.

Today, most yoga classes are variations of hatha yoga, and many typical stretches used in flexibility exercises have been adapted from hatha yoga. Examples include:

1. *Integral yoga* and *viny yoga*, which focus on gentle and static stretches
2. *Iyengar yoga*, which promotes muscular strength and endurance
3. *Yogalates*, which incorporates Pilates exercises to increase muscular strength
4. *Power yoga* or *yogarobics*, a high-energy form that links many postures together in a dance-like routine to promote cardiorespiratory fitness

As with flexibility exercises, the stretches in hatha yoga should not be performed to the point of discomfort. Instructors should not push participants beyond their physical limitations. Similar to other stress management techniques, yoga exercises are best performed in a quiet place for 15 to 60 minutes per session. Many yoga participants like to perform the exercises daily.

To appreciate yoga exercises, a person has to experience them. The discussion here serves only as an introduction. Although yoga exercises can be practiced with the instruction of a book or video, most participants take classes. Many of the postures are difficult and complex, and few individuals can master the entire sequence in the first few weeks.

Individuals who are interested in yoga exercises should initially pursue them under qualified instruction. Many universities offer yoga courses, and you can check online for a listing of yoga instructors or classes in your area. Yoga courses are also offered at many health clubs and recreation centers. Because instructors and yoga styles vary, you may want to sit in on a class before enrolling. The most important thing is to look for an instructor whose views on wellness parallel your own. Instructors are not subject to national certification standards. If you are new to yoga, you are encouraged to compare a couple of instructors before you select a class.

Tai Chi

Tai chi chuan (full name) originated in China centuries ago and is practiced today for defense training and for physical and mental health benefits. The martial side, however, is no longer the focus of its practice, so the activity can be

---

GLOSSARY

Hatha yoga A form of yoga that incorporates specific sequences of static-stretching postures to help induce the relaxation response.

performed by young, old, and even very old. In tai chi, the muscles and joints are never extended beyond 70 percent of maximum potential—rather, movements are performed with the muscles in a relaxed versus tense state—making it among the safest low-impact forms of exercise. Surveys show that nearly 3 million people in the United States practice tai chi,[11] and many fitness practitioners use it in conjunction with aerobic and strength training.

Tai chi is often described as "meditation in motion" because it is performed with flowing, rhythmic movements that focus heavily on breathing and slow execution. The main objective is to promote tranquility and reflection through postures that combine meditation and dance. The postures are performed in sequences known as "sets" that require concentration, coordination, controlled breathing, muscle relaxation, strength, flexibility, gait, and body balance.

Research has attributed many health benefits to tai chi, including diabetes management, arthritis relief, lower blood pressure, faster recovery from heart disease and injury, improved strength and flexibility, better sleep, and improved physical work capacity. Tai chi has gained prevalence with physicians as a supplementary treatment to help prevent or improve medical conditions associated with aging. Among older adults, improved gait and the capability to perform activities of daily living are frequently reported, and some studies have found tai chi to help maintain bone density in elderly women when practiced regularly over time.[12] Tai chi is frequently used for stress management to relieve tension, stress, and anxiety. The mental aspect of having to concentrate on leading the movement and paying attention to detail through the gentle actions dissipates stress. The activity leaves no room to think or worry about other problems, thus calming and relaxing the mind and body.

To master tai chi, you need initial professional guidance. You are encouraged to join the group or class available at many college campuses or community health clubs. The class should emphasize fitness and health benefits over combat techniques. Once you have mastered many of the sets available, you can practice the activity on your own.

Relaxation Techniques

Relaxation techniques can help cope with stress by slowing down the body and quieting the mind. When the body

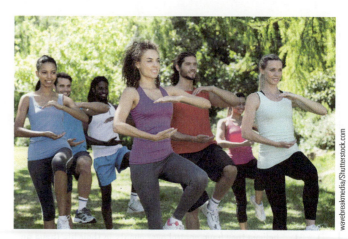

Tai chi's flowing, rhythmic movements help relieve stress and promote tranquility and reflection.

reaches a deep state of relaxation, blood pressure, heart rate, muscle tension, and breathing rate decrease, which lowers stress and brings about feelings of calmness and control. Although benefits are reaped immediately after engaging in any of the several relaxation techniques, several months of regular practice may be necessary for total mastery. The relaxation exercises that follow should not be considered cure-alls. If these exercises do not prove to be effective, more specialized textbooks and professional help are called for. (Some symptoms may not be caused by stress but rather may be related to a medical disorder.)

Biofeedback

Clinical application of **biofeedback** has been used for many years to treat various medical disorders. Besides its successful application in managing stress, it is commonly used to treat medical disorders such as essential hypertension, asthma, heart rhythm and rate disturbances, cardiac neurosis, eczematous dermatitis, fecal incontinence, insomnia, and stuttering. Biofeedback as a treatment modality has been defined as a technique in which a person learns to influence physiological responses that are not typically under voluntary control or responses that normally are regulated but for which regulation has broken down as a result of injury, trauma, or illness.

Behavior Modification Planning

Five-Minute De-stress Technique

The following simple exercise can be used as an effective stress management technique, especially when coming home at the end of the day. De-stress by taking 5 minutes before getting into your evening routine by removing your shoes, lying on the carpet, and placing your feet up on a chair. Use a rolled-up towel at the base of the skull for neck tension or along the middle of the spine for back tension. The lower back should be flat on the floor. Completely relax and practice deep breathing for 5 minutes.

Try It

This simple exercise will help you reduce stress at the end of the day and start your evening right.

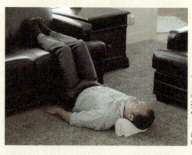

In simpler terms, biofeedback is the interaction with the interior self. This interaction enables a person to learn the relationship between the mind and the biological response. The person can "feel" how thought processes influence biological responses (e.g., heart rate, blood pressure, body temperature, and muscle tension) and how biological responses influence thought processes.

As an illustration of this process, consider the association between a strange noise in the middle of a dark, quiet night and the heart rate response. At first, the heart rate shoots up because of the stress the unknown noise induces. The individual may even feel the heart palpitating in the chest and, while still uncertain about the noise, attempt not to panic to prevent an even faster heart rate. Upon realizing that all is well, the person can take control and influence the heart rate to come down. The mind, now calm, is able to exert almost complete control over the biological response.

Complex electronic instruments are required to conduct biofeedback. The process entails a three-stage, closed-loop feedback system:

1. A biological response to a stressor is detected and amplified.
2. The response is processed.
3. Results of the response are fed back to the individual immediately.

The person uses this new input and attempts to change the physiological response voluntarily—this attempt, in turn, is detected, amplified, and processed. The results then are fed back to the person. The process continues with the intent of teaching the person to reliably influence the physiological response for the better (Figure 12.5). The most common methods used to measure physiological responses are monitoring the heart rate, finger temperature, and blood pressure; electromyograms; and electroencephalograms. The goal of biofeedback training is to transfer the experiences learned in the laboratory to everyday living.

Although biofeedback has significant applications in treating various medical disorders, including stress, it requires adequately trained personnel and, in many cases, costly equipment. Therefore, several alternative methods that yield similar results are frequently substituted for biofeedback. For example, research has shown that exercise and progressive muscle relaxation, used successfully in stress management, seem to be just as effective as biofeedback in treating essential hypertension.

Progressive Muscle Relaxation

Progressive muscle relaxation, developed by Dr. Edmund Jacobsen in the 1930s, enables individuals to relearn the sensation of deep relaxation. The technique involves progressively contracting and relaxing muscle groups throughout the body. Because chronic stress leads to high levels of muscular tension, acute awareness of how progressively tightening and relaxing the muscles feels can release the tension in the muscles and teach the body to relax at will.

Feeling the tension instigated during the exercises also helps the person to be more alert to signs of distress because this tension is similar to that experienced in stressful situations. In everyday life, these feelings then can cue the person to do relaxation exercises.

Relaxation exercises should be done in a quiet, warm, well-ventilated room. The recommended exercises and the duration of the routine vary from one person to the next. Most important is that the individual pay attention to the sensation he or she feels each time the muscles are tensed and relaxed.

The exercises should encompass all muscle groups of the body. Following is an example of a sequence of progressive muscle relaxation exercises. The instructions for these exercises can be read to the person, memorized, or recorded. At least 20 minutes should be set aside to complete the entire sequence. Doing the exercises faster defeats their purpose. Ideally, the sequence should be done twice a day.

The individual performing the exercises stretches out comfortably on the floor, face up, with a pillow under the knees and assumes a passive attitude, allowing the body to relax as much as possible. Each muscle group is to be contracted in sequence, taking care to avoid any strain. Muscles should be tightened to only about 70 percent of the total possible tension to avoid cramping or some type of injury to the muscle.

To produce the relaxation effects, the person must pay attention to the sensation of tensing and relaxing. The person holds each contraction about 5 seconds and then allows the muscles to go totally limp. The person should take enough time to contract and relax each muscle group before going on to the next.

Figure 12.5 Biofeedback mechanism.

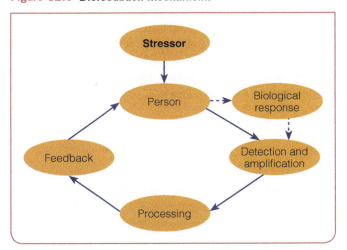

GLOSSARY

Biofeedback A stress management technique in which a person learns to influence physiological responses that are not typically under voluntary control or responses that typically are regulated but for which regulation has broken down as a result of injury, trauma, or illness.

Progressive muscle relaxation A stress management technique that involves sequential contraction and relaxation of muscle groups throughout the body.

Steps to Progressive Muscle Relaxation

Follow these steps to practice a complete sequence of progressive muscle relaxation:

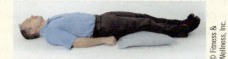

© Fitness & Wellness, Inc.

1. Point your feet, curling the toes downward. Study the tension in the arches and the top of the feet. Hold, continue to note the tension, and then relax. Repeat once.

2. Flex the feet upward toward the face and note the tension in your feet and calves. Hold and relax. Repeat once.

3. Push your heels down against the floor as if burying them in the sand. Hold and note the tension at the back of the thigh. Relax. Repeat once.

4. Contract the right thigh by straightening the leg, gently raising the leg off the floor. Hold and study the tension. Relax. Repeat with the left leg. Hold and relax. Repeat each leg.

5. Tense the buttocks by raising your hips ever so slightly off the floor. Hold and note the tension. Relax. Repeat once.

6. Contract the abdominal muscles. Hold them tight and note the tension. Relax. Repeat once.

7. Suck in your stomach. Try to make it reach your spine. Flatten your lower back to the floor. Hold and feel the tension in the stomach and lower back. Relax. Repeat once.

8. Take a deep breath, hold it, and then exhale. Repeat. Note your breathing becoming slower and more relaxed.

9. Place your arms at the sides of your body and clench both fists. Hold, study the tension, and relax. Repeat.

10. Flex the elbows by bringing both hands to the shoulders. Hold tight and study the tension in the biceps. Relax. Repeat.

11. Place your arms flat on the floor, palms up, and push the forearms hard against the floor. Note the tension on the triceps. Hold and relax. Repeat.

12. Shrug your shoulders, raising them as high as possible. Hold and note the tension. Relax. Repeat.

13. Gently push your head backward. Note the tension in the back of the neck. Hold and relax. Repeat.

14. Gently bring the head against the chest, push forward, hold, and note the tension in the neck. Relax. Repeat.

15. Press your tongue toward the roof of your mouth. Hold, study the tension, and relax. Repeat.

16. Press your teeth together. Hold, and study the tension. Relax. Repeat.

17. Close your eyes tightly. Hold them closed and note the tension. Relax, leaving your eyes closed. Do this one more time.

18. Wrinkle your forehead and note the tension. Hold and relax. Repeat.

Though completing the entire sequence will yield the best results, if you run out of time, do only the exercises specific to the areas that feel most tense to help relax those areas.

Breathing Techniques for Relaxation

How often do you pay attention to your breathing? Breathing is among the many physiological functions affected by stress, but even when minimal stress is present, few people maintain a habit of breathing fully and properly. On average, only one-third of an adult's lung capacity is required in normal breathing. Proper breathing is vital to optimal health because the process of inhaling air feeds life-sustaining oxygen to the lungs, and in turn, the cardiovascular system feeds it to virtually every part of the body, revitalizing organs, cells, and tissues. A pattern of shallow, quick breathing in reaction to stress restricts the body and brain from receiving the amount of oxygen required for healthy function.

Breathing fully and deeply has been shown to ease anxiety and pain, improve asthma symptoms, burn calories more efficiently, lower blood pressure, strengthen the immune system, and help people with diabetes control blood sugar. Students who practice deep breathing meditation significantly increase academic learning and achievement. One study in particular found that college students who practiced deep-breathing exercises before an exam reported decreased levels of anxiety, nervousness, and loss of concentration.[13] This improvement occurs as deep breathing raises oxygen saturation in cells, increasing energy, cognitive function, and heart-rate variability.

Breathing exercises engage one of your body's most powerful mechanisms for naturally reducing stress. These exercises have been used for centuries in the Orient and India to improve mental, physical, and emotional stamina. In breathing exercises, the person concentrates on "breathing away" the tension and inhaling a large amount of air with each breath. Breathing exercises can be learned in only a few minutes and require considerably less time than the progressive muscle relaxation exercises.

As with any other relaxation technique, these exercises should be done in a quiet, pleasant, well-ventilated room.

> **!**
> ### Critical Thinking
> List the three most common stressors that you face as a college student. What techniques have you used to manage these situations, and in what way have they helped you cope?

Three Breathing Exercises to Try

Try any of the three examples of breathing exercises presented here to help relieve tension induced by stress.

1. **Deep breathing.** Lie with your back flat against the floor and place a pillow under your knees. Feet are slightly separated, with toes pointing outward. (The exercise also may be done while sitting in a chair or standing straight.) Place one hand on your abdomen and the other hand on your chest.

   Slowly breathe in and out so that the hand on your abdomen rises when you inhale and falls as you exhale. The hand on the chest should not move much. Repeat the exercise about 10 times. Next, scan your body for tension and compare your present tension with the tension you felt at the beginning of the exercise. Repeat the entire process once or twice.

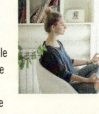

2. **Sighing.** Using the abdominal breathing technique, breathe in through your nose to a specific count (e.g., 4, 5, or 6). Now exhale through pursed lips to double the intake count (e.g., 8, 10, or 12, respectively). Repeat the exercise 8 to 10 times whenever you feel tense.

3. **Complete natural breathing.** Sit in an upright position or stand straight. Breathing through your nose, gradually fill your lungs from the bottom up. Hold your breath for several seconds. Now exhale slowly by allowing your chest and abdomen to relax, and try to empty your lungs completely. Repeat the exercise 8 to 10 times.

HOEGER KEY TO WELLNESS

Breathing exercises engage one of your body's most powerful mechanisms for naturally reducing stress. Before an exam, practice breathing fully and deeply to decrease levels of anxiety and nervousness and increase concentration and academic performance.

Visual Imagery

Visual or mental **imagery** has been used as a healing technique for centuries in various cultures around the world. In Western medicine, the practice of imagery is relatively new and not widely accepted among health care professionals.

Research is now being done to study the effects of imagery on the treatment of conditions such as cancer, hypertension, asthma, chronic pain, and obesity. Imagery induces a state of relaxation that rids the body of the stress that leads to illness. It improves circulation and increases the delivery of healing antibodies and white blood cells to the site of illness.[14] Imagery also helps a person increase self-confidence; regain control and power over the body; and lessen feelings of hopelessness, fear, and depression.

Visual imagery involves the creation of relaxing visual images and scenes in times of stress to elicit body and mind relaxation. Imagery works by offsetting the stressor with the visualization of relaxing scenes: a sunny beach, a beautiful meadow, a quiet mountaintop, lying in a hammock in a quiet backyard, soaking in a hot tub, or some other peaceful setting. If you are ill, you can also visualize your white blood cells attacking an infection or a tumor. Imagery is also used in conjunction with breathing exercises, meditation, and yoga.

As with other stress management techniques, imagery should be performed in a quiet and comfortable environment. You can either sit or lie down for the exercise. If you lie down, use a soft surface and place a pillow under your knees. Be sure that your clothes are loose and that you are as comfortable as you can be.

Steps to Visual Imagery

1. To start the exercise, close your eyes and take a few breaths using one of the breathing techniques previously described.

2. You then can proceed to visualize one of your favorite scenes in nature. Place yourself into the scene, and visualize yourself moving about and experiencing nature to its fullest. Enjoy the people, the animals, the colors, the sounds, the smells, and even the temperature in your scene.

3. After 10 to 20 minutes of visualization, open your eyes and compare the tension in your body and mind at this point with how you felt prior to the exercise. You can repeat this exercise as often as you deem necessary when you are feeling tension or stress.

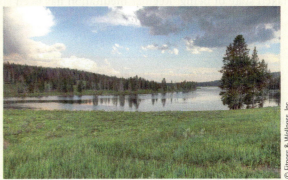

GLOSSARY

Breathing exercises A stress management technique wherein the individual concentrates on "breathing away" the tension and inhaling fresh air to the entire body.

Imagery Mental visualization of relaxing images and scenes to induce body relaxation in times of stress or as an aid in the treatment of certain medical conditions, such as cancer, hypertension, asthma, chronic pain, and obesity.

You may not always be able to find a quiet and comfortable setting in which to sit or lie down for 10 to 20 minutes. If you think imagery works for you, however, you can perform this technique while standing or sitting in an active setting. If you are able, close your eyes, disregard your surroundings for a short moment, and visualize one of your favorite scenes. Once you feel that you have regained some control over the stressor, open your eyes and continue with your assigned tasks.

Autogenic Training

Autogenic training is a form of self-suggestion in which people place themselves in an autohypnotic state by repeating and concentrating on feelings of heaviness and warmth in the extremities. This technique was developed by Johannes Schultz, a German psychiatrist, who noted that hypnotized individuals developed sensations of warmth and heaviness in the limbs and torso. The sensation of warmth is caused by dilation of blood vessels, which increases blood flow to the limbs. Muscular relaxation produces the feeling of heaviness.

The autogenic training technique is more difficult to master than any of those mentioned previously. The person should not move too fast through the entire exercise because this may interfere with learning and relaxation. Each stage must be mastered before proceeding to the next.

Meditation

Meditation helps people draw attention inward and calm the mind. It is a mental exercise that brings about mental, spiritual, and physical benefits, including stress reduction and a feeling of well-being. It encompasses a combination of techniques such as thoughts, breathing, sounds, postures, visualization, and/or movement that help achieve a relaxed state of being. Regular meditation has been shown to decrease blood pressure, stress, anger, anxiety, fear, negative feelings, and chronic pain as well as increase activity in the brain's left frontal region—an area associated with positive emotions.[15] The objective of meditation is to gain control over one's attention by clearing the mind and blocking out the stressor(s) responsible for the higher tension.

Basic meditation techniques can be learned rather quickly, but first-time users often drop out before reaping benefits because they feel intimidated, confused, bored, or frustrated. In such cases, a group setting is best to get started. Many colleges, community programs, health clubs, and hospitals offer classes.

Initially, the person who is learning to meditate should choose a room that is comfortable, quiet, and free of all disturbances (including telephones). After learning the technique, the person will be able to meditate just about anywhere. A time block of approximately 10 to 15 minutes is adequate to start, but as you become more comfortable with meditation, you can lengthen the time to 30 minutes or longer. To use meditation effectively, meditate daily—just once or twice per week may not provide noticeable benefits.

Mindfulness Meditation

Mindfulness can be defined as a mental state of heightened awareness of the present moment. In mindfulness meditation, you focus on becoming fully aware and accepting living in the present, paying particular attention to your feelings, thoughts, sensations, and emotions without passing judgment, dwelling in the past, or projecting yourself into the future. Mindfulness meditation adheres to three basic tenets: observe, accept, and let go. Important during mindfulness meditation is not to worry about things that you have no control over. To live in the present, you must understand

---

Steps to Autogenic Training

In this technique, the person lies down or sits in a comfortable position, eyes closed; concentrates progressively on six fundamental stages; and says (or thinks) the following:

1. **Heaviness**

   My right (left) arm is heavy.
   Both arms are heavy.
   My right (left) leg is heavy.
   Both legs are heavy.
   My arms and legs are heavy.

2. **Warmth**

   My right (left) arm is warm.
   Both arms are warm.

My right (left) leg is warm.
Both legs are warm.
My arms and legs are warm.

3. **Heart**

   My heartbeat is calm and regular. (Repeat four or five times.)

4. **Respiration**

   My body breathes itself. (Repeat four or five times.)

5. **Abdomen**

   My abdomen is warm. (Repeat four or five times.)

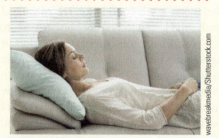

wavebreakmedia/Shutterstock.com

6. **Forehead**

   My forehead is cool. (Repeat four or five times.)

Steps to Meditation

Of the several forms of meditation, the following routine is recommended to get started:

1. Sit in a chair in an upright position with the hands resting either in your lap or on the arms of the chair. Close your eyes and focus on your breathing. Allow your body to relax as much as possible. Do not try to consciously relax because trying means work. Rather, assume a passive attitude and concentrate on your breathing.

2. Allow the body to breathe regularly, at its own rhythm, and repeat in your mind the word "one" every time you inhale, and the word "two" every time you exhale. Paying attention to these two words keeps distressing thoughts from entering your mind.

3. Continue to breathe in this way for about 15 minutes. Because the objective of meditation is to bring about a hypometabolic state leading to body relaxation, do not use an alarm clock to remind you that the 15 minutes have expired. The alarm will only trigger your stress response again, defeating the purpose of the exercise. Opening your eyes once in a while to

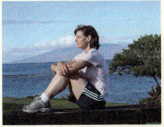

© Fitness & Wellness, Inc.

keep track of the time is fine, but do not rush or anticipate the end of the session. This time has been set aside for meditation, and you need to relax, take your time, and enjoy the exercise.

---

that the most significant event that you have control over is *your attitude*. While your confidence may be shaken because of life's challenges and stressors, you can control your attitude. Having a clear understanding that the "storm will pass" and that "there is light at the end of every tunnel" will allow you to navigate through life's stressors and ultimately overcome challenges and enjoy happiness while living in the present.

Example of Mindfulness in Life Let's look at an example. Your roommate agreed to clean up his 3-day mess in the kitchen that evening. When you get home from the library that night, the kitchen looks worse and your roommate is sound asleep in the bedroom. You are extremely disappointed and upset. Your thoughts turn to the past and how much worse it may get in the future. The fight-or-flight mechanism kicks in, and you are ready to wake your roommate up and let him have it. Your stress level rises with every thought of the past, present, and potential future. If you act on your impulses, the situation and your relationship with your roommate may only get worse.

Now put yourself in the same situation, but stay in the present moment. Don't dwell in the past or worry about the future. Instead of allowing greater anger to build up, choose to stay with the uncomfortable feeling of disappointment for a moment. Recognize it, feel it, and acknowledge the disappointment. Maybe your roommate has a valid reason for not getting it done. Perhaps tomorrow you could tell your roommate about your disappointment, but after a night's rest you may choose not to do so. Now turn your attention to another task in the present moment. Eat a healthy meal and savor every bite, listen to your favorite music and enjoy the melody, go for a walk and appreciate the surroundings and beauty of the night, or take a moment to relish your good health. You can now pay attention to your breathing and notice the fresh air and your breathing pattern for a few minutes. Before retiring to bed, conduct your nightly audit

and plan the next day's activities. At this point, notice that stress and the fight-or-flight mechanism have dissipated, and the disappointment of the unclean kitchen, over which you had no control, would not have been worth the frustration and anger that you could have experienced. A few years from now, you can have a healthy laugh over the incident.

Instead of Reacting, Respond Intentionally Rather than simply reacting, mindfulness helps people better recognize their thoughts and emotions so they can choose to respond intentionally. Mental training to work mindfully, eat mindfully, and enjoy daily life mindfully aims to prevent vulnerability to stress and illness through conscious living. Mindfulness has been successfully used in helping people adhere to medical treatment, improve hypertension and insomnia, more effectively handle pain, and manage anxiety and depression associated with illness. Athletes who practice mindfulness have shown increased adaptability in stressful situations, potentially enhancing performance and improving the ability to cope with the challenges of daily living.[16] In college students, mindfulness helps to improve intellectual and academic performance, including better knowledge retention during lectures.[17]

GLOSSARY

Autogenic training A stress management technique using a form of self-suggestion, wherein an individual is able to place himself or herself in an autohypnotic state by repeating and concentrating on feelings of heaviness and warmth in the extremities.

Meditation A stress management technique used to gain control over attention by clearing the mind and blocking out the stressor(s) responsible for the increased tension.

Mindfulness A mental state of heightened awareness of the present moment.

How these health benefits were attained on a molecular level through mindfulness and relaxation therapy was just discovered in recent years. Researchers have now determined that the relaxation response that counteracts the negative effects of stress can directly affect genes linked to mitochondrial function, energy metabolism, the immune system, and the secretion of insulin.[18] Gene expression is what governs health or illness and is highly susceptible to influences from our environment, diet, and thoughts. Relaxation techniques enhance the expression of those genes, improving the mitochondria and their supporting cell pathways while simultaneously suppressing pathways that channel chronic inflammation, trauma, stress, and cancer. These new findings suggest that in addition to the outward physiological and psychological benefits you enjoy when you practice mindfulness, you can effectively change yourself on the cellular level by means of healthy gene expression.

HOEGER KEY TO WELLNESS

To live in the present, understand that the most significant event that you have control over is your attitude. It is not life's stressors that cause distress, but the way you react to them which leads to illness and disease. A positive attitude is key for maintaining a healthy stress (eustress) level.

12.12 *Which Technique Is Best?*

Because each person reacts to stress differently, the best coping strategy depends mostly on what works for each individual. You may want to experiment with several or all of the techniques presented here to find out which works best for you. Many choose a combination of two or more.

All of the coping strategies discussed here help to block out stressors and promote mental and physical relaxation by diverting the attention to a different, nonthreatening action. Some of the techniques are easier to learn and may take less time per session. As a part of your class experience, you may participate in a stress management session (see Activity 12.8). Regardless of which technique you select, the time spent doing stress management exercises (several times a day, as needed) is well worth the effort when stress becomes a significant problem in life. After completing your stress management experience, use Activity 12.9 to conduct a self-assessment of the impact of stress in your life and ways that you can personally counteract or avoid stress-inducing events.

Keep in mind that most individuals need to learn to relax and take time for themselves. Stress is not what makes people ill; it's the way they react to the stress-causing agent. Individuals who learn to be diligent and take control of themselves find they enjoy a better, happier, and healthier life.

Assess Your Behavior

1. Are you able to channel your emotions and feelings to exert a positive effect on your mind, health, and wellness?

2. Do you use time management strategies on a regular basis?

3. Do you use stress management techniques, and do they allow you to be in control over the daily stresses of life?

Assess Your Knowledge

1. Positive stress is also referred to as
   a. eustress.
   b. posstress.
   c. functional stress.
   d. distress.
   e. physiostress.

2. Which of the following is *not* a stage of the GAS?
   a. alarm reaction
   b. resistance
   c. compliance
   d. exhaustion and recovery
   e. All are stages of the GAS.

3. The behavior pattern of highly stressed individuals who do not seem to be at higher risk for disease is known as type
   a. A.
   b. B.
   c. C.
   d. E.
   e. X.

4. Effective time managers
   a. delegate.
   b. learn to say "no."
   c. avoid boredom.
   d. set aside overtimes.
   e. All of the choices are correct.

5. Hormonal changes that occur during a stress response
   a. decrease heart rate.
   b. sap the body's strength.
   c. diminish blood flow to the muscles.
   d. induce relaxation.
   e. increase blood pressure.

6. Physical activity decreases stress levels by
   a. deliberately diverting stress to various body systems.
   b. metabolizing excess catecholamines.
   c. diminishing muscular tension.
   d. stimulating alpha-wave activity in the brain.
   e. All of the choices are correct.

7. Biofeedback is
   a. the interaction with the interior self.
   b. the biological response to stress.
   c. the nonspecific response to a stress-causing agent.
   d. used to identify biological factors that cause stress.
   e. most readily achieved while in a state of self-hypnosis.

8. The technique in which a person breathes in through the nose to a specific count and then exhales through pursed lips to double the intake count is known as
   a. sighing.
   b. deep breathing.
   c. meditation.
   d. autonomic ventilation.
   e. release management.

9. During autogenic training, a person
   a. contracts each muscle to about 70 percent of capacity.
   b. concentrates on feelings of warmth and heaviness.
   c. visualizes relaxing scenes to induce body relaxation.
   d. learns to reliably influence physiological responses.
   e. notes the positive and negative impacts of frequent stressors on various body systems.

10. Yoga exercises have been successfully used to
    a. stimulate ventilation.
    b. increase metabolism during stress.
    c. aid rehabilitation after stroke.
    d. decrease body awareness.
    e. All of the choices are correct.

Correct answers can be found at the back of the book.

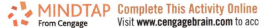

MINDTAP **Complete This Activity Online**
From Cengage   Visit **www.cengagebrain.com** to access MindTap, a complete digital course that includes interactive quizzes, videos, and more.

Activity 12.8   Stress Management Experience

Name _____ Date _____

Course _____ Section _____ Gender _____ Age _____

I. Stage of Change for Stress Management

Using Figure 2.7 and Table 2.3 (page 73), identify your current stage of change for a stress management program:

[   ]

II. Stress Management

Instructions: The class should be divided into groups of about five students per group. Each group should select and go through a minimum of two of the following stress management techniques outlined in this chapter:

1. Progressive Muscle Relaxation   3. Visual Imagery   5. Meditation
2. Breathing Techniques for Relaxation   4. Autogenic Training

Choose a group leader who will lead the chosen stress management techniques. Gather everyone into a comfortable room that is as free of noise as possible, and conduct the exercises according to the instructions provided for each relaxation technique in this chapter. If trained personnel or a recording for progressive muscle relaxation exercises is available, the entire class may participate in this experience at once. Institutions that have biofeedback equipment may use it in this activity as well.

After completing this activity, answer the following four questions:

1. Indicate the two relaxation techniques used in your class:

A. [   ]   B. [   ]

2. In your own words, relate your feelings as you were going through exercises A and B above:

Exercise A: _____

_____

Exercise B: _____

_____

3. Indicate how you felt mentally, emotionally, and physically after participating in this experience:

_____

_____

4. Are there situations in your daily life in which you think you would benefit from practicing the selected stress management exercises?

_____

_____

5. Number of daily steps: [   ]   Activity category (see Table 1.2, page 13): [   ]

© Fitness & Wellness, Inc.

Activity 12.9   Self-Assessment Stress Evaluation

Name _____ Date _____

Course _____ Section _____ Gender _____ Age _____

1. Do you currently perceive stress to be a problem in your life? ☐ Yes   ☐ No

2. Do you experience any of the typical stress symptoms listed in the box on page 470? If so, which ones?

3. Indicate any specific events in your life that trigger a stress response.

   _____

   _____

   _____

   _____

4. Write specific objectives to either avoid or help you manage the various stress-inducing events listed above, including one or more stress management techniques.

   _____

   _____

   _____

   _____

5. Do you have any behavior patterns you would like to modify? List those you would like to change.

   _____

   _____

   _____

   _____

6. List specific techniques of change you will use to change undesirable behaviors (see Table 2.2, page 72).

   _____

   _____

   _____

   _____

© Fitness & Wellness, Inc.

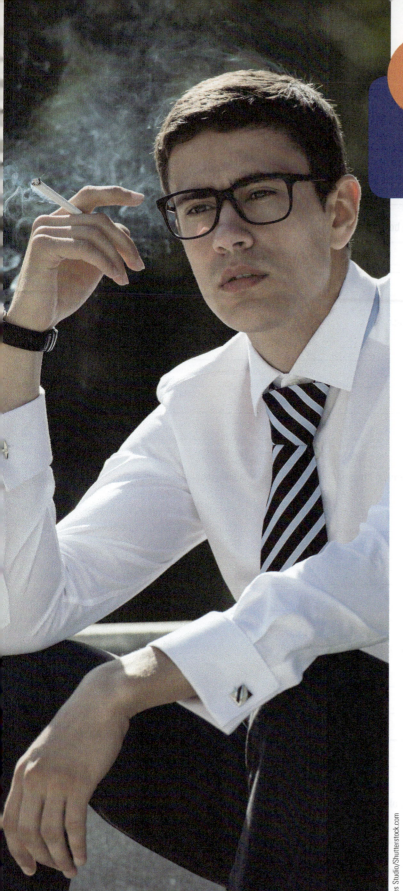

Milles Studio/Shutterstock.com

13

Addictive Behavior

Addictive behaviors are lifetime nightmares that focus on immediate self-gratification without thought or concern for one's wellbeing or that of others—ultimately taking away the control the person has over life itself.

Objectives

13.1 **Address** the detrimental effects of addictive substances, including caffeine, prescription drugs, inhalants, marijuana, cocaine, methamphetamine, MDMA (Ecstasy), heroin, new psychoactive substances (NPS), and alcohol.

13.2 **List** the detrimental health effects of tobacco use.

13.3 **Recognize** cigarette smoking as the largest preventable cause of premature illness and death in the United States.

13.4 **Enumerate** the reasons people smoke.

13.5 **Explain** the benefits and the significance of a smoking-cessation program.

13.6 **Learn** how to implement a smoking-cessation program to help yourself (if you smoke) or someone else go through the quitting process.

13.7 **Plan** for a drug-free future (including freedom from tobacco use).

FAQ

What is drug addiction, and how quickly can someone become addicted to drugs?

Drug addiction (addictive behavior, substance abuse, or chemical dependency) is a complex brain disease that, over time, can alter brain structure and function. It is characterized by compulsive and uncontrollable drug cravings with serious negative consequences. Because there are vast individual differences in sensitivity to different drugs, how quickly addictive behavior develops cannot be predicted.

Psychological and physiological factors, as well as the type of drug used, influence a person's response to the drug and subsequent addiction to it. Whereas one individual may use a certain drug several times without harmful effects, someone else may seriously overdose the first time the same drug is used. All drugs have potentially damaging effects, and some have life-threatening consequences. One moment of weakness, or caving in to peer pressure, can easily result in a lifetime nightmare, not just for users but for everyone around them as well.

How can I tell if someone is addicted to drugs?

People with addictive behavior compulsively seek and use drugs despite potential serious repercussions, such as physical and family problems, loss of a job, or problems with the law. Some individuals realize that they need to cut down on their drinking or drug use, or they are told to do so by others. At times, they crave alcohol or drugs when they first get up in the morning, and they feel bad or guilty about their addictive behavior. If you see any of these signs in someone you know, that person most likely has an addiction.

How is drug addiction treated?

In the early stages of substance abuse, most people believe that they can stop using the drug(s) on their own. Most of these attempts, however, fail to achieve long-term abstinence. Long-term drug use results in altered brain functions that linger long after the person stops using drugs. Effective treatment of drug addiction is rarely accomplished without professional help. Treatment modalities are behavioral-based therapies, oftentimes combined with medication to help the body detoxify and effectively manage symptoms of withdrawal. Responses to these therapies vary among individuals, and several courses of rehab may be necessary to overcome the problem. For some individuals, it becomes a lifetime battle, and relapses are possible even after prolonged periods of abstinence.

REAL LIFE STORY | Steve's Experience

In high school, I used to get teased and bullied a lot. It was so bad that I hated being the person I was, and I wanted to become somebody else. The way I tried to do that was through drugs. I started out drinking and doing marijuana. When I was drunk or high, I felt calm, confident, and popular. My self-doubts and self-hatred would go away for a while. The problem was, the bad feelings always came back. Eventually, some friends offered me meth, so I tried it. For me, the effects of meth were very intense. When I was using it, I felt like the king of the world. As soon as it wore off, I felt so horrible; I would do pretty much anything just to feel better again. That began a period of a couple years where meth crowded out everything else in my life. I stopped caring about school and about any goals I had for the future. I didn't care if I disappointed my parents or my friends. I didn't even care anymore about my younger brother, and he has always been my best friend and one of the people I love most in the world. Meth just completely took over my life. I dropped out of school and left home for several months. I camped out with several other addicts where we set up our own meth lab. We lived in really filthy conditions. Eventually I got disgusted with the way I was living, and I became terrified by the fact that I needed bigger and bigger doses of meth for a high that lasted only a fraction of the amount of time it used to. No matter how much I used, I was miserable much more often than I felt good. I finally moved back home and reached out for help to overcome my addiction. At first, I attended 12-step meetings almost constantly, and I finally managed to get clean. Now, the fact that I was able to go back and get my high school diploma, and now am in college, is a miracle to me. I have a second chance to make something of my life. That chance could easily have been lost forever due to drugs.

Renars Jurkovskis/Shutterstock.com

PERSONAL PROFILE: Addictive Behavior Survey

I. Have you ever suffered from addiction to any legal or illicit drug? What helped you overcome the addictive behavior? If you have not yet overcome it, are you ready to do so? Do you know where to turn for assistance?

II. Do you regularly—weekly or nearly weekly—exceed the recommended one to two alcoholic beverages per day? Do you understand potential health, personal, and family implications associated with alcohol abuse?

III. Have you decided to forgo instant gratification and peer pressure by saying "no" to substance abuse (legal or

illicit) that may or will harm your health and long-term life satisfaction? What led to this decision, and how long ago did you make this choice?

IV. What are your feelings about tobacco use in general and exposure to secondhand smoke?

V. If you smoked cigarettes, have you quit? If you never smoked, have you helped someone else successfully quit smoking? If so, what approach did you use and why were you successful in accomplishing this goal?

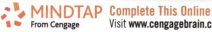 **MINDTAP** From Cengage **Complete This Online** Visit **www.cengagebrain.com** to access MindTap, a complete digital course that includes interactive quizzes, videos, and more.

Substance abuse remains one of the most serious health problems afflicting society. Chemical dependency is extremely destructive, damaging and ending millions of lives. When addictive behaviors are an issue, education is vital—more, perhaps, than with any other unhealthy behavior. Becoming educated about addiction and the risks of substance abuse will help you make more informed decisions when offered harmful substances. The time to make healthy choices is *now*.

13.1 *Addiction*

Psychotherapists have described **addiction** as a problem of imbalance or unease within the body and mind. Addictions are marked by incessant dependence on a particular behavior or substance despite continual negative physical and emotional consequences. Addictions bring about compulsive and uncontrollable behavior(s) or use of substance(s).

Although most people tend to associate addiction with drug and alcohol abuse, addiction can extend to many areas. Almost anything can be addicting. Of the many types of addiction, some addictive behaviors are more detrimental than others. The most serious form is chemical dependency on illicit and prescription drugs, tobacco, and alcohol. Less serious are addictions to work, coffee, shopping, and even exercise.

People who are addicted to food eat to release stress or boredom or to reward themselves for every small personal achievement. Technological innovation has also brought on addictions to television, digital devices, online gaming, and social networks. When career pursuits consume a person's life, even work can become an unhealthy behavior.

Even though exercise enhances health and quality of life, a relatively small number become obsessed with exercise, which has the potential for overuse and addiction. Compulsive exercisers feel guilty and uncomfortable when they miss a day's workout. Often, they continue to exercise even when they have injuries and sicknesses that require proper rest for adequate recovery. People who exceed the recommended guidelines to develop and maintain fitness (see Chapters 6–9) are exercising for reasons other than health—including addictive behavior.

13.2 *How Addiction Develops*

Although addictive behaviors cover a wide spectrum, they have factors in common that predispose people to addiction. Among these factors are the following[1]:

- The behavior is reinforced.
- The addiction is an attempt to meet basic human needs, such as physical needs, the need to feel safe, the need to belong, the need to feel important, or the need to reach one's potential.
- The addiction seems to relieve stress temporarily.
- The addiction results from peer pressure.
- The addiction can be present within the person's value system (e.g., a person whose values wouldn't let him or her shoot heroin may be able to rationalize compulsive eating or obsessive playing of computer games).
- A serious physical illness is present, and the addiction may provide escape from pain or fear of disfigurement.
- The addict feels pressured to perform or succeed.
- The addict has self-hate.
- A genetic link is present. Heredity might dictate susceptibility to some addictions.
- Society allows addiction. Advertising even encourages it (you can sleep better with a pill, snacking helps you enjoy life more fully, parties and sports are more fun with alcohol, shop 'til you drop, and so on).

The same general traits and behaviors are involved in all kinds of addictions, whether they involve food, sex, gambling, shopping, or drugs.

Even when an addiction is clear to people around them, most addicts deny that they are addicted, and often react with anger, excuses, and blame on others. In some cases, addicts admit their problem but fail to take any steps to change.

If you are uncertain about addictive behavior(s) in your life, the Addictive Behavior Questionnaire in Activity 13.1 can help you identify a potential problem.

GLOSSARY

Addiction Compulsive and uncontrollable behavior(s) or use of substance(s).

Activity 13.1   Addictive Behavior Questionnaire

Name _____ Date _____

Course _____ Section _____ Gender _____ Age _____

Could you be an addict?

I. Recognizing Addictive Behavior

The following questionnaire has been designed to identify possible addictive behavior (chemical dependency). This test is not designed to determine if you have an addictive disease, but rather to help recognize potential addictive behavior in yourself or the people around you. The term "drug" may imply illicit substances or drugs (such as marijuana, cocaine, heroin, Ecstasy, or methamphetamine), misuse of prescription drugs (painkillers, sleeping pills), or alcohol abuse.

		Yes	No
1.	Are you a compulsive person?	☐	☐
2.	Are you a person of excesses?	☐	☐
3.	Do you depend heavily on others?	☐	☐
4.	Do you spend a lot of time thinking about a drug(s)?	☐	☐
5.	Do you use drugs other than for medical reasons?	☐	☐
6.	Do you misuse prescription drugs?	☐	☐
7.	Are you unable to stop using drugs or limit their use to required situations only?	☐	☐
8.	Can you get through a week without misusing drugs?	☐	☐
9.	Do friends or relatives sense or mention that you have a drug problem?	☐	☐
10.	Has drug misuse ever created a problem between you and friends or relatives?	☐	☐
11.	Have family members or friends ever sought help for problems associated with your misuse of drugs?	☐	☐
12.	Have you ever sought help for drug misuse?	☐	☐
13.	Do you deny or lie about the misuse of drugs?	☐	☐
14.	Do you tend to associate with people who exhibit the same behaviors or take the same drugs you do?	☐	☐
15.	Do you get angry at people who try to keep you from getting the drugs you desire?	☐	☐
16.	Do you have a difficult time stopping the use of a drug when you start misusing it?	☐	☐
17.	Do you experience withdrawal symptoms if you do not take the drugs you wish to have?	☐	☐
18.	Has the misuse of drugs affected the way you function in life (school, work, recreation, etc.)?	☐	☐
19.	Have you put yourself or others at risk by your actions while misusing drugs?	☐	☐
20.	Have you unsuccessfully tried to cut back or stop the misuse of drugs?	☐	☐

Interpretation

If you answered "yes" to five or more of these questions, you may have an addictive behavior and should seek further evaluation by a physician, your institution's counseling center, or contact a local mental health clinic for a referral. You may also contact the National Center for Substance Abuse Treatment at 1-800-662-4357 for 24-hour substance abuse treatment centers in your area. Depending on the question (e.g., 7, 8, 12, 15, 16, 17, 18, 20), note that even fewer than five "yes" answers may already be indicative of chemical dependency.

II. Stage of Change for Addictive Behavior

If chemical dependency is a problem in your life, use Figure 2.7 and Table 2.3 (page 73) to identify your current stage of change for participation in a treatment program for addictive behavior.

III. Changing Addictive Behavior

On a separate sheet of paper indicate the steps that you are going to take to correct addictive behavior(s) and identify people or organizations that you will contact to help you get started.

© Fitness & Wellness, Inc.

13.3 *Drug Misuse and Abuse*

A drug is any substance that alters the user's ability to function. Drugs encompass over-the-counter drugs, prescription medications, and illegal substances. Many drugs lead to physical and psychological dependence.

Any drug can be misused and abused. "Drug misuse" implies the intentional and inappropriate use of over-the-counter or prescribed medications.[2] Examples include taking more medication than prescribed, mixing drugs, not following prescription instructions, or discontinuing a drug prior to a physician's approval. "Drug abuse" is the intentional and inappropriate use of a drug, resulting in physical, emotional, financial, intellectual, social, spiritual, or occupational consequences of the abuse.[3] Many substances, if used in the wrong manner, can be abused.

When drugs are used regularly, they integrate into the body's chemistry, increasing the user's tolerance to the drug and forcing the user to increase the dosage constantly to obtain similar results. Drug abuse leads to serious health problems, and more than half of all adolescent suicides are drug related. Often, drug abuse opens the gate to other illegal activities. According to the National Center on Addiction and Substance Abuse, the majority of convicted criminals—about 85 percent of federal and state inmates—have abused drugs.

The U.S. Department of Education warns that today's drugs are stronger and more addictive, and they pose a greater risk than ever before. Alcohol, tobacco, and illegal drug use lead to many negative health-related consequences—including cancers, cardiovascular diseases, stroke, bacterial endocarditis, fatal and nonfatal overdose, and susceptibility to sexually transmitted infections. Substance abuse is also linked to increased risk of intentional and unintentional injuries, complications in pregnancy and delivery, and psychiatric disturbances, ranging from acute panic attacks to chronic mood disturbances. Furthermore, illegal drug use is associated with negative effects on employment, school achievement, socioeconomic status, and family stability—primarily because illegal drug use, once detected, can lead to school suspension or expulsion and to arrest, conviction, and incarceration for drug-related crimes.[4]

According to the 2015 National Survey on Drug Use and Health (NSDUH) by the U.S. Department of Health and Human Services, more than 27 million Americans use illicit drugs, including marijuana, prescription-type psychotherapeutics used non-medically, cocaine, hallucinogens, inhalants, and heroin[5] (Figure 13.1). North America has the world's largest illicit drug market and, for most drugs, has use rates much higher than the global average.

Recognizing that all forms of addiction are unhealthy, this chapter focuses on some of today's most self-destructive addictive substances: caffeine, prescription drugs, inhalants, marijuana, cocaine, methamphetamine, MDMA (Ecstasy), heroin, new psychoactive substances (NPS), alcohol, and tobacco.

Caffeine

Caffeine is the most widely consumed psychoactive drug, and according to the Food and Drug Administration (FDA),

Figure 13.1 Numbers of past month illicit drug users among people aged 12 or older: 2015.

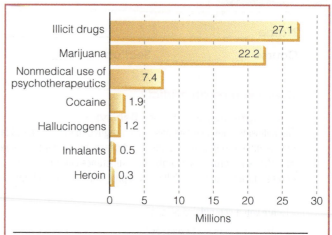

	Millions
Illicit drugs	27.1
Marijuana	22.2
Nonmedical use of psychotherapeutics	7.4
Cocaine	1.9
Hallucinogens	1.2
Inhalants	0.5
Heroin	0.3

SOURCE: Center for Behavioral Health Statistics and Quality, "Behavioral health trends in the United States: Results from the 2015 National Survey on Drug Use and Health," 2015, retrieved from http://www.samhsa.gov/, January 2017.

80 percent of adults in the United States consume caffeine daily. Caffeine is now advertised as an energy booster and is added to a variety of other food items such as energy bars, candy, gum, waffles, syrup, and even oatmeal. Pure caffeine powder—which is sold online virtually unregulated—contains as much caffeine in one teaspoon as the amount in about 28 cups of coffee! The accessibility of this product has been quite alarming to the FDA, which has recently taken measures to warn consumers and distributors about the dangers of the powerful powder. Individuals who are caffeine sensitive should read all food labels for potential caffeine in everyday food items and understand the risks of consuming high-caffeine products.

The caffeine content of drinks varies according to the product. In 8 ounces of coffee, for example, the content varies from 93 mg in instant coffee to as high as 133 mg in brewed coffee. Soft drinks, mainly colas, range in caffeine content from about 58 to 90 mg per 20-ounce bottle. The FDA states that 400 mg of caffeine per day—the amount in about four to five cups of coffee—is safe as a stimulant for most healthy adults.

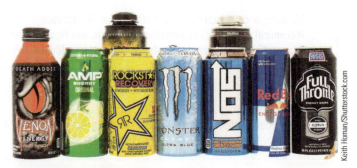

Young adults who consume energy drinks report higher rates of illicit drug, alcohol, and cigarette use.

Keith Homan/Shutterstock.com

For energy drinks, the FDA requires caffeine to be listed on the label, but it does not mandate that the amount of caffeine be specified. Energy drink manufacturers state that the products are safe when used as directed; however, the potential for excessive use is real because these products are not regulated by the FDA. Many popular energy drinks (Red Bull, Sobe Adrenaline Rush, Full Throttle, Rip It Energy Fuel, Monster) contain about 80 mg or more of caffeine per 8-ounce cup. Larger 16-ounce cans contain two servings and twice the amount of caffeine. If you drink two 16-ounce cans, you'll end up with upward of 300 mg of caffeine through these drinks alone. Popular 2- to 2.5-ounce 5-Hour Energy shots range from 78 to 242 mg per serving,[6] which, on the high end, is about the amount of caffeine in two cups of coffee. You may also have to consider additional caffeine intake from other beverages that you routinely consume during the day (coffee, tea, sodas). As with most addictive substances, invariably a sugar and caffeine rush is likely to end up in a physiological crash, requiring a subsequent larger intake to obtain a similar "physical high," thus augmenting the risk for adverse and life-threatening effects.

Teens who consume energy drinks—about one-third of adolescents in the United States—report higher rates of drug, alcohol, and cigarette use.[7] Among college students, research indicates that consumption of energy drinks is linked to precarious behaviors such as illicit drug use, violence, smoking, prescription drug use, and sexual risk taking.

Mixing energy drinks with alcohol is also a concerning college trend. A common misconception among young people is that energy drinks allow them to consume more alcohol because the energy drinks keep them awake longer. High consumption of caffeine can conceal the sedative effects of intoxication, making people who mix energy drinks with alcohol more likely to drive while drunk. Some erroneously believe that caffeine can help counteract the effects of drinking, making it safe to drive. Data also indicate that men are more likely to mix energy drinks with alcohol and illicit drugs, whereas women mix alcohol with pharmaceuticals.

Effects on the Body

Addiction to caffeine can have undesirable side effects. Too much caffeine can cause jitteriness and insomnia and induce symptoms of anxiety, depression, nervousness, and dizziness. In some individuals, caffeine doses in excess of 200 to 500 mg can also cause rapid heart rate (palpitations and tachycardia), ischemia (lack of blood flow to the heart muscle), chest pain, abnormal heart rhythms, higher blood pressure, paraesthesia (tingling or numbing of the skin), and increased secretion of gastric acids, leading to stomach problems and possible birth defects in offspring.

Most seriously, high caffeine intake has been linked to heart attacks and sudden cardiac deaths. In the past decade, deaths linked to the accidental overdose of highly caffeinated products—including 5-Hour Energy drinks and pure caffeine powder—has prompted the FDA to warn consumers and take action against several product distributors.

Nonmedical Use of Prescription Drugs

America's drug problem has been expanding to not only include illicit drug use, but also abuse of prescription drugs. As a result, the Centers for Disease Control and Prevention (CDC) has classified prescription drug abuse in the United States as an epidemic. Nearly 70 percent of Americans are on one or more prescription drugs, and 20 percent take five or more pills per day. Americans consume 80 percent of the world's prescription painkillers, though the United States makes up less than 5 percent of the global population. Psychotherapeutic drugs include any prescription pain reliever, tranquilizer, stimulant, or sedative (but not over-the-counter drugs). Currently, 6.4 million Americans abuse prescription drugs, with thousands dying of drug overdose each year. Drug poisoning is now the second-leading cause of unintentional injury deaths in the United States, killing more Americans than car accidents. In 2015, overdose deaths from opioids (pain relievers and heroin) reached an all-time high of 47,000 deaths, an increase of 14 percent over the previous year. This figure represents a 200 percent increase in opioid deaths since the year 2000.

The most commonly abused prescription medications are:

- *Opioids*, commonly prescribed to treat pain. These include codeine, morphine, oxycodone (OxyContin), and hydrocodone (Vicodin).
- *Central nervous system depressants*, used to treat anxiety and sleep disorders. Examples include Mebaral, Nembutal, Valium, Xanax®, Ambien, and Lunesta.
- *Stimulants*, prescribed to treat the sleep disorder narcolepsy, attention-deficit hyperactivity disorder (ADHD), and obesity. Examples include Dexedrine, Adderall, Ritalin, and Concerta®.

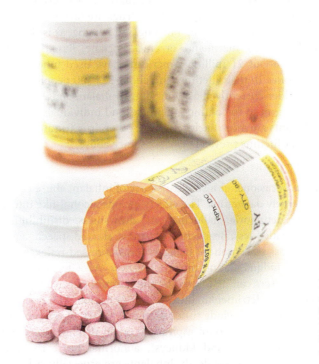

Accidental overdose deaths from prescription pain relievers have quadrupled over the past decade.

Ken Weinrich/Shutterstock.com

Most individuals, particularly young people, obtain these drugs with or without consent from friends and family members. A major concern is that many abusers believe these substances are safer than illicit drugs because they are prescribed by a health care professional and dispensed by a pharmacist and cause no serious or life-threatening consequences.

Effects on the Body

The risks associated with psychotherapy drug misuse or abuse vary depending on the drug. Some of the risks include respiratory depression or cessation, decreased or irregular heart rate, high body temperature, seizures, and cardiovascular failure. Abuse of prescription drugs, or using them in a manner other than exactly as prescribed, can lead to addiction.

HOEGER KEY TO WELLNESS

The United States makes up less than 5 percent of the global population, yet Americans consume 80 percent of the world's prescription painkillers. Nearly 70 percent of Americans are on one or more prescription drugs, and 20 percent take five or more pills per day.

Inhalant Abuse

Inhalant abuse involves common household products—including whipped cream canisters, cooking sprays, deodorant and hair sprays, glues, nail polish remover, spray paints, gasoline, and lighter and cleaning fluids—whose vapors or aerosol gases are inhaled to get high. Also referred to as "huffing" or "sniffing glue," these drugs are taken by volatilization and not following burning and heating, as is the case with tobacco, marijuana, or crack cocaine. Based on estimates, about 21 million Americans have used inhalants at least once in their lifetime, and about 527,000 people age 12 and older currently abuse inhalants.[8] Inhalant abuse leads to a strong need to continue their use, and individuals abusing inhalants are more likely to initiate other drug use and have a higher lifetime prevalence of substance abuse.

Effects on the Body

Even occasional or a single instance of inhalant abuse can be extremely dangerous. The effects include alcohol-like intoxication, euphoria, hallucinations, drowsiness, disinhibition, lightheadedness, headaches, dizziness, slurred speech, agitation, loss of sensation, belligerence, depressed reflexes, impaired judgment, and unconsciousness. As with other drug abuse, users can be injured by the harmful effects of the vapors and detrimental intoxication behavior. More serious consequences include suffocation due to lack of oxygen supply, pneumonia, vomit aspiration, organ damage (including the brain, liver, and kidneys), abnormal heart rhythms, and sudden cardiac death. Inhalants are especially risky because they can be deadly at any time, *even the very first time they are used.*

Marijuana

Marijuana (pot, grass, or weed as it is commonly called) is the most widely used illegal drug in the United States, and the number of people using marijuana has increased in recent years. There are now more college students who smoke marijuana daily than drink alcohol daily (see Figure 13.2). An estimated 22.2 million Americans aged 12 and older currently use marijuana.[9] Most users smoke loose marijuana that has been rolled into a joint or packed into a pipe. Other users bake it into foods such as brownies or use it to brew a tea. Marijuana cigarettes are often laced with other drugs, such as crack cocaine.

In small doses, marijuana has a sedative effect. Larger doses produce physical and psychological changes. Studies in the 1960s indicated that the potential effects of marijuana were exaggerated and that the drug was relatively harmless. The drug as it is used today, however, is much stronger than when the initial studies were conducted.

The main and most active psychoactive constituent in marijuana is delta-9-tetrahydrocannabinol (THC), a naturally

Figure 13.2 Marijuana use among full-time college students is on the rise.

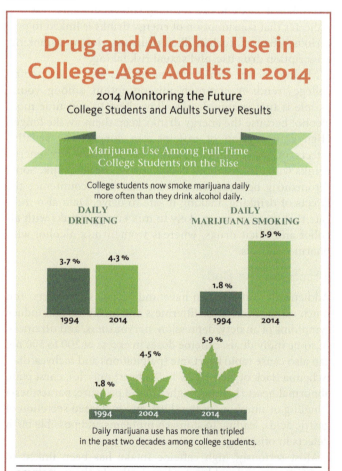

SOURCE: L. D. Johnson, P. M. O'Malley, J. G. Bachman, J. E. Schulenberg, and R. A. Miech, *Monitoring the Future National Survey Results on Drug Use, 1975–2014: Volume 2, College students and adults ages 19–55* (Ann Arbor, MI: Institute for Social Research, The University of Michigan, 2015), available at http://www.drugabuse.gov/related-topics/trends-statistics/infographics /drug-alcohol-use-in-college-age-adults-in-2014, downloaded January 2017

occurring compound in the *Cannabis sativa* plant from which marijuana is derived. In the 1960s, THC content in marijuana ranged from 0.02 to 2 percent. Users called the latter "real good grass." Today's THC content averages 11 percent, although it has been reported as high as 27 percent. The average potency has tripled over the past three decades.

THC reaches the brain within a few seconds after marijuana smoke is inhaled, and the psychic and physical changes reach their peak in about 2 or 3 minutes. THC then is metabolized in the liver to waste metabolites, but 30 percent of it remains in the body a week after the marijuana was smoked. THC is not completely eliminated until 30 days or more after an initial dose of the drug. The drug always remains in the system of regular users.

One of the most common myths about marijuana use is that it is not addictive; however, scientific evidence shows that regular users of marijuana do develop physical and psychological dependence. As with cigarette smokers, when regular users go without the drug, they crave the substance, go through mood changes, are irritable and nervous, and develop an obsession to get more. More than half of illicit drug users begin experimenting with marijuana.

Effects on the Body

Some short-term effects of marijuana are **tachycardia**, dryness of the mouth, reddened eyes, stronger appetite, decrease in coordination and tracking (the eyes' ability to follow a moving stimulus), difficulty in concentration, intermittent confusion, impairment of short-term memory and continuity of speech, interference with the physical and mental learning process during periods of intoxication, and increased risk for heart attack for a full day after smoking the drug. Another common effect is the **amotivational syndrome**. This syndrome persists after periods of intoxication but usually disappears a few weeks after the individual stops using the drug.

Long-term harmful effects include atrophy of the brain (leading to irreversible brain damage), less resistance to infectious diseases, chronic bronchitis, lung cancer (marijuana smoke may contain as much as 50 to 70 percent more cancer-producing hydrocarbons than cigarette smoke), and possible sterility and impotence. Recent research has also linked regular and heavy use of marijuana, particularly when the brain matures in adolescent years, to a lowered IQ and changes that can cause deterioration in the orbitofrontal cortex—the area of the brain involved in decision making and motivation.

The use of marijuana for medical purposes appears to be beneficial in selected conditions such as neuralgia, convulsive disorders, emaciation, and post-traumatic stress disorder (PTSD). Additional research is necessary, however, before we can fully understand its medicinal use.

Legalization of Marijuana

Though the sale and possession of marijuana continues to be illegal under federal law, the government has allowed states to amend possession offenses and decriminalize or legalize marijuana under individual state laws. As of 2017, marijuana has been legalized in some form in 26 states—with seven states making it legal for both medical and recreational use.

The legalization of marijuana for recreational use in these states has fueled a rapidly expanding market for marijuana-infused foods and edibles. "Cannabis cuisine"—from baked treats, ice cream, and sodas, to hot dogs and frozen burritos—has become a popular commodity among licensed marijuana dispensaries and food vendors. Relaxed regulatory laws combined with the vast variety and availability of marijuana-laced edibles has led to a decreased perceived risk of marijuana use, particularly among kids and teens. When marijuana can be legally sold in lollipops, sodas, and cookies, it's not surprising that more than 68 percent of high school seniors don't believe the use of natural marijuana is harmful.[10]

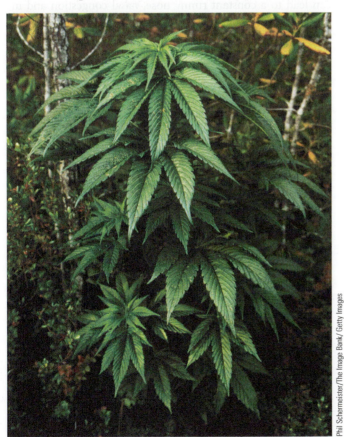

Cannabis sativa.

Phil Schermeister/The Image Bank/Getty Images

> **! Critical Thinking**
>
> The legalization of marijuana is being heatedly debated across the United States. Do you think this decision should rest with the government, medical personnel, or the individuals themselves?

GLOSSARY

Marijuana A psychoactive drug prepared from a mixture of crushed leaves, flowers, small branches, stems, and seeds from the hemp plant *Cannabis sativa*; also called pot, grass, or weed.

Tachycardia Faster-than-normal heart rate.

Amotivational syndrome A condition characterized by loss of motivation, dullness, apathy, and no interest in the future.

Because potency amounts vary greatly in marijuana-infused foods, it's far easier to overconsume high amounts of the drug through edibles than it is through smoking. The potential risk of marijuana-infused edibles among youth has received greater attention as accidental consumption of candy and baked goods containing marijuana has led to a higher incidence of emergency room visits, hospitalization, and deaths in young students, children, and even toddlers who consumed edibles purchased by their parents. As a result, some states have enacted laws to prohibit the sale of marijuana-infused treats that appeal strongly to children and require that edibles clearly indicate serving sizes and potency on product packaging.

Cocaine

Similar to marijuana, **cocaine** was thought for many years to be relatively harmless. This misconception came to an abrupt halt when, in 1986, two well-known athletes in their 20s—Len Bias (basketball) and Don Rogers (football)—died suddenly following cocaine overdoses. Over the years, cocaine has been given several different names, including, among others, coke, C, snow, blow, nose candy, toot, flake, Peruvian lady, white dragon, and happy dust. This drug can be sniffed or snorted, smoked, or injected.

When cocaine is snorted, it is absorbed quickly through the mucous membranes of the nose into the bloodstream. The drug is usually arranged in fine powder lines 1 to 2 inches long. Each line stimulates the autonomic nervous system for about 30 minutes. When cocaine is injected intravenously, larger amounts of cocaine can enter the body in a shorter time. The popularity of cocaine is based on the almost universal guarantee that users find themselves in an immediate state of euphoria and well-being. The addiction begins with a desire to get high, often at social gatherings and usually with the assurance that "occasional use is harmless." Many of these first-time users will become addicted, and for most, it is the beginning of a lifetime nightmare.

Animal research with cocaine has shown that all laboratory animals can become compulsive cocaine users. Animals work more persistently at pressing a bar for cocaine than bars for other drugs, including opiates. In one instance, an addicted monkey pressed the bar almost 13,000 times until it finally got a dose of cocaine. People respond in a similar way. Cocaine addicts prefer drug usage to any other activity and use the drug until the supply or the user is exhausted. Chronic users who constantly crave the drug often turn to crime, including murder, to sustain their habit. Some users view suicide as the only solution to this sad syndrome.

Cocaine users also exhibit unusual behaviors compared with their previous conduct, even to the point at which a user has been known to sell a child to obtain more cocaine. It is an expensive drug—$1,000 to $2,600 per ounce for powdered cocaine. Cocaine use is common in upper-middle-class communities and professions—daily habits can cost addicts hundreds to thousands of dollars, with binges in the $20,000 to $50,000 range. Cocaine addiction can lead to loss of a job and career, loss of family, bankruptcy, and death. Though intervention in the chain

of supply of cocaine by law enforcement has helped to considerably decrease cocaine use in the past decade, the United States remains the world's largest cocaine market.

Crack Cocaine

Crack cocaine is a smokable form of cocaine that is processed with baking soda or ammonia to make it into a more concentrated and solid "rock" form. The name comes from the cracking sound it makes when heated and smoked. Crack cocaine is many times more potent than powdered or injected cocaine and is highly addictive. Two-thirds of users in the United States who are addicted to cocaine use crack. Because it is so potent, crack doses are smaller and, therefore, less expensive ($8 to $40 each), although users still spend hundreds of dollars a day to support their addiction. The crack high lasts about 12 minutes, which is shorter than the high from snorted or injected cocaine. Choosing to use cocaine in this form heightens the risk for emphysema and heart attack.

Effects on the Body

Cocaine seems to alleviate fatigue and raise energy levels, as well as lessen the need for food and sleep. Following the high comes a "crash," a state of physiological and psychological depression, often leaving the user with the desire to get more. This can produce a constant craving for the drug. Similar to alcoholics, cocaine users recover only by abstaining completely from the drug. A single backslide can result in renewed addiction.

Light to moderate cocaine use is typically associated with feelings of pleasure and well-being. Sustained cocaine snorting can lead to a constant runny nose, nasal congestion and inflammation, and perforation of the nasal septum. Long-term consequences of cocaine use include loss of appetite, digestive disorders, weight loss, malnutrition, insomnia, confusion, anxiety, and cocaine psychosis, characterized by paranoia and hallucinations. In one type of hallucination, referred to as formication, or "coke bugs," the chronic user perceives imaginary insects or snakes crawling on or underneath the skin.

High doses of cocaine can cause nervousness, dizziness, blurred vision, vomiting, tremors, seizures, strokes, angina, cardiac arrhythmias, and high blood pressure. As with smoking marijuana, there is an increased risk for heart attack following

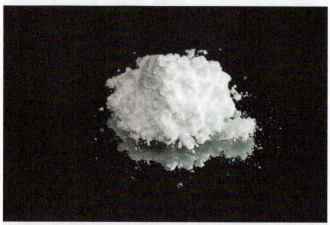

Powdered cocaine.

HamsterMan/Shutterstock.com

cocaine use. The user's risk may be 24 times higher than normal for up to 3 hours following cocaine use. Almost one-third of cocaine users who incurred a heart attack had no symptoms of heart disease prior to taking cocaine. In addition, users are at risk for hepatitis, HIV, and other infectious diseases because of the risky behaviors they engage in to obtain the drug.

Large overdoses of cocaine can precipitate sudden death from respiratory paralysis, cardiac arrhythmias, and severe convulsions. If individuals lack an enzyme used in metabolizing cocaine, as few as two to three lines of cocaine may be fatal.

Methamphetamine

Methamphetamine, or meth, is a more potent form of amphetamine. **Amphetamines** in general are part of a large group of synthetic agents used to stimulate the central nervous system. A powerfully addictive drug, methamphetamine falls under the same category of psychostimulant drugs as amphetamines and cocaine. It is also known as a "club drug," a group of illegal substances used at dance clubs, rock concerts, and raves (all-night dance parties). Other club drugs include MDMA, LSD, GHB, Rohypnol, and ketamine.

Methamphetamine is typically a white, odorless, and bitter-tasting powder that dissolves readily in water or alcohol. The drug is a potent central nervous system stimulant that produces a general feeling of well-being, decreases appetite, increases motor activity, and decreases fatigue and the need for sleep.

Unlike most other drugs, methamphetamine reaches rural and urban populations alike. Young people especially prefer methamphetamine because of its low cost and long-lasting effects—up to 12 hours following use.

In the past, methamphetamine was easily manufactured in clandestine meth "labs" using over-the-counter pseudo-ephedrine, typically found in cold medications. To reduce the accessibility of methamphetamine ingredients, in March 2006 the federal Combat Methamphetamine Epidemic Act of 2005 was signed into law. This law requires retailers to keep cold medications behind the counter, and consumers are limited as to the amount they can purchase.

Despite legislative efforts, reports of methamphetamine labs within the United States remain common as faster ways to produce the drug in smaller batches allow for increased proliferation. Methamphetamine labs are set up almost anywhere, including garages, basements, or hotel rooms. The abundance of potential meth lab sites makes it difficult for drug enforcement agencies to locate many of these facilities. The risk of injury in a meth lab, however, is high because potentially explosive environmental contaminants are discarded during production of the drug.

In recent years, cheaper and purer meth distributed through Mexican cartels has supplanted meth made in home labs. Mexico is the primary foreign source of methamphetamine for the United States.

Effects on the Body

Methamphetamine can be snorted, swallowed, smoked, or injected. It is commonly referred to as "speed" or "crystal" when

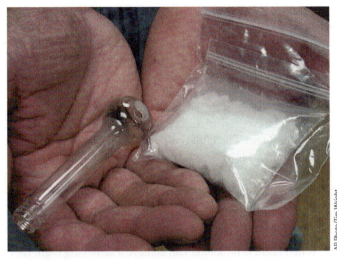

"Ice," so named for its appearance, is a smokable form of methamphetamine.

snorted or taken orally, as "ice" or "glass" when smoked, and as "crank" when injected. Depending on how it is taken, methamphetamine affects the body differently. Smoked or injected methamphetamine provides an immediate intense, pleasurable rush that lasts only a few minutes. Nonetheless, negative effects can continue for several hours. When the drug is snorted or taken orally, the user does not experience a rush but develops a feeling of euphoria that lasts up to 16 hours.

Users of methamphetamine experience increases in body temperature, blood pressure, heart rate, and breathing rate; a decrease in appetite; hyperactivity; tremors; and violent behavior. High doses produce irritability, paranoia, irreversible damage to blood vessels in the brain (causing strokes), and risk for sudden death from hypothermia and convulsions if not treated at once.

Chronic abusers experience insomnia, confusion, hallucinations, inflammation of the heart lining, schizophrenia-like mental disorder, and brain cell damage similar to that caused by a stroke. Physical changes to the brain may last months or perhaps become permanent. Over time, methamphetamine use may reduce brain levels of **dopamine**, which can lead to symptoms similar to those of Parkinson's disease. In addition, users frequently are involved in violent crime, homicide, and suicide. Using methamphetamine during pregnancy may cause prenatal complications, premature delivery, and abnormal physical and emotional development of the child.

GLOSSARY

Cocaine 2-beta-carbomethoxy-3-betabenozoxytropane, the primary psychoactive ingredient derived from coca plant leaves.

Methamphetamine A potent form of amphetamine; also called meth.

Amphetamines A class of powerful central nervous system stimulants.

Dopamine A neurotransmitter that affects emotional, mental, and motor functions.

Similar to other stimulants, methamphetamine is often used in a binge cycle. Addiction takes hold quickly because the person develops tolerance to methamphetamine within minutes of using it. The high disappears long before blood levels of the drug drop significantly. The user then attempts to maintain the pleasurable feelings by taking in more of the drug, and a binge cycle ensues.

The binge cycle, which can last for a couple of weeks, consists of several stages. The initial rush lasts 5 to 30 minutes. During this stage, heart rate, blood pressure, and metabolism increase, and the user receives a great sense of pleasure. The high follows, lasting up to 16 hours. During this stage, users become arrogant and more argumentative. The binge stage sets in next and lasts between 2 and 14 days. Addicts continue to use the drug in an attempt to maintain the high as long as possible.

When addicts no longer can achieve a satisfying high, they enter the tweaking stage, the most dangerous stage in the cycle. At this point, users may have gone without food for several days and without sleep anywhere from 3 to 15 days. They become paranoid, irritable, and violent. Tweakers crave more of the drug, but no amount of amphetamines restores the pleasurable, euphoric feelings they achieved during the high. Thus, the addicts become increasingly frustrated, unpredictable, and dangerous to those around them (including police officers and medical personnel) and to themselves. Once they finally crash, they are no longer dangerous. The users now become lethargic and sleep for 1 to 3 days.

Following the crash, addicts fall into a 1- to 3-month period of withdrawal. During this stage, they can be paranoid, aggressive, fatigued, depressed, suicidal, and filled with an intense craving for another high. Reuse of the drug relieves these feelings. Therefore, the incidence of relapse in users who seek treatment is high.

MDMA (Ecstasy)

MDMA, also known as Ecstasy, became popular among teenagers and young adults in the United States in the mid-1980s, when it evolved into the most common club drug. Although its use already constituted a serious drug problem in Europe, MDMA was not illegal in the United States until 1985. Prior to 1985, few Americans abused this drug. In the 1970s, some therapists used MDMA as a tool to help patients open up and feel at ease. MDMA is named for its chemical structure: 3,4-methylenedioxymethamphetamine. Street names for the drug are X-TC, E, Adam, and love drug. Typically, dealers push the drug as a way to increase energy, pleasure, and self-confidence.

In recent years, MDMA use has increased dramatically in a powder or capsule form known as Molly, marketed as a pure crystalline MDMA that is purportedly safer and purer than Ecstasy, which is routinely mixed with other drugs and contaminants. Molly has been glamorized in current music and pop culture, making it a popular drug with teens and college students at raves, dance clubs, and music festivals. Its claim to be a "pure" or "organic" MDMA has bolstered the drug into reaching a broader demographic of users—the U.S. Drug Enforcement Administration (DEA) has reported that Molly's newest users are middle-aged professionals. Law enforcement officials warn users to beware of claims that Molly offered to them is pure MDMA. Molly most often contains a toxic mixture of other drugs and lab-created chemicals that users ingest unknowingly when they take the drug. The DEA has found that only a small percentage of Molly seized in recent years actually contained any MDMA.

Although MDMA usually is swallowed in the form of one or two pills in doses of up to 120 mg per pill, it can also be smoked, snorted, or, occasionally, injected. Because the drug often is prepared with other substances, users have no way of knowing the exact potency of the drug or additional substances found in each pill. Furthermore, many users combine MDMA with alcohol, marijuana, or other drugs, which makes it even more dangerous.

MDMA shares characteristics with stimulants and hallucinogens. Its chemical structure closely parallels the hallucinogen **methylenedioxyamphetamine (MDA)** and methamphetamine, both manmade stimulants that damage the brain. The addictive properties of MDMA and stimulation of hyperactivity have been compared to stimulants such as amphetamines and cocaine. The chemical structure of MDMA and its appeal, however, are similar to those of hallucinogens, but with milder psychedelic effects.

Effects on the Body

Among young people, MDMA has a reputation for being fun and harmless as long as it is used sensibly, but it is not a harmless drug. Research is uncovering many negative side effects. The pleasurable effects peak about an hour after a pill is swallowed and last for 2 to 6 hours. Users claim to feel enlightened and introspective, accepting of themselves, and trustful of others. Because they tend to act and feel closer to, or more intimate with, the people around them, some believe this drug to be an aphrodisiac, even though MDMA actually hampers sexual ability. MDMA also acts as a stimulant by increasing brain activity and making users feel more energetic.

Like most addictive drugs, the effects of MDMA are said to diminish with each use. MDMA users may experience rapid eye movement, faintness, blurred vision, chills, sweating, nausea, muscle tension, and teeth grinding. Users often bring infant pacifiers to raves to combat the latter side effect. Individuals with heart, liver, or kidney disease or high blood pressure are especially at risk because MDMA increases blood pressure, heart rate, and body temperature. Thus, its use may lead to seizures, kidney failure, a heart attack, or a stroke. The hot, crowded atmosphere at raves and dance clubs also heightens the risk to the user. Deaths are more likely when water is unavailable because the crowded atmosphere, combined with the stimulant effects of MDMA, causes dehydration (bottled water is often sold at inflated prices at raves). Other evidence suggests that a pregnant woman using MDMA may find long-term learning and memory difficulties in her child.

The damaging effects of the drug can be long lasting and are possible after only a few uses. Long-term side effects, lasting for weeks after use, include confusion, depression, sleep disorders,

Figure 13.3 Heroin use is part of a larger substance abuse problem.

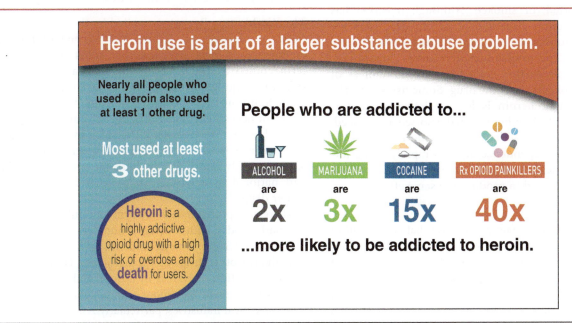

Heroin use is part of a larger substance abuse problem.

Nearly all people who used heroin also used at least 1 other drug.

Most used at least **3** other drugs.

Heroin is a highly addictive opioid drug with a high risk of overdose and **death** for users.

People who are addicted to...

ALCOHOL	MARIJUANA	COCAINE	Rx OPIOID PAINKILLERS
are	are	are	are
2x	**3x**	**15x**	**40x**

...more likely to be addicted to heroin.

SOURCE: National Survey on Drug Use and Health (NSDUH), 2011-2013, available at http://www.cdc.gov/vitalsigns/heroin/infographic.html, downloaded January 2017

anxiety, aggression, paranoia, and impulsive behavior. Questions still remain about other potential long-term effects. Verbal and visual memory may be significantly impaired for years after prolonged use. Researchers are focusing on these lasting side effects, which may be the result of depleted serotonin, a neurotransmitter that is released with each dose of MDMA. The short-term effect of serotonin release is increased brain activity. Serotonin helps regulate sleep cycles, pain, emotion, and appetite. Because MDMA may damage the neurons that release serotonin, long-term effects could be dangerous.

Heroin

Heroin use has increased in recent years. Although the most common users are those in suburban, middle-class neighborhoods and lower-income populations, its use is starting to appear in more affluent communities as well. Common nicknames for heroin include diesel, dope, dynamite, white death, nasty boy, china white, H. Harry, gumball, junk, brown sugar, smack, tootsie roll, and chasing the dragon.

In 2005, a heroin-based recreational drug referred to as cheese became popular among middle and high school students and has since attracted a wider base of older users. Cheese is a combination of heroin with crushed tablets of over-the-counter medications that contain acetaminophen and the antihistamine diphenhydramine. Law enforcement has dubbed the drug "starter" or "gateway" heroin.

Most recently, Mexican drug dealers have found a way to produce a purer (and therefore more potent) form of heroin known as Mexican tar heroin or black tar. Named after its black, gooey consistency, this ultrapotent form of heroin (reported as high as 60 to 80 percent potency) is known to kill unsuspecting users before they even have a chance to remove

the syringe or are done snorting the substance. The potency and cheap price of the drug have broadened its appeal, resulting in an increase in both use and reports of overdose among a wide range of users.

Heroin is classified as a narcotic drug. It is synthesized from morphine, a natural substance found in the seedpod of several types of poppy plants. In its purest form, heroin is a white powder, but on the streets, it is typically available in yellow or brown powders. The latter colors are attained when pure heroin is combined with other drugs or substances, such as sugar, cornstarch, chalk, brick dust, or laundry soap. Heroin also is sold in a hardened or solid form (black tar), which usually is dissolved with other liquids for use in injectable form. Many users combine heroin with cocaine, a risky process commonly called "speedballing."

Today's heroin is more pure, powerful, and affordable than ever before. Highly dangerous, heroin is a significant health threat to users in that they have no way of determining the strength of the drug purchased on the street, which places them at a constant risk for overdose and death. Heroin is highly addictive and classified as a "hard" drug that users often evolve to after first abusing one or more other drugs (see Figure 13.3).

GLOSSARY

MDMA 3,4-methylenedioxy-methamphetamine, a synthetic hallucinogenic drug with a chemical structure that closely resembles MDA and methamphetamine; also known as Ecstasy.

Methylenedioxy-amphetamine (MDA) A hallucinogenic drug that is structurally similar to amphetamines.

Heroin A potent drug that is a derivative of opium.

Heroin can be injected intravenously or intramuscularly, sniffed or snorted, or smoked. Although injection has been the predominant method of heroin use, users are turning from intravenous injections because of the risk for HIV infection. The availability of relatively low-priced, high-purity heroin further contributes to the number of people who smoke or snort the drug. Some users have the misconception that heroin is less addictive when it is snorted or smoked. Whether injected, snorted, or smoked, heroin is an extremely addictive drug, and both physical and psychological dependence develop rapidly. Drug tolerance sets in quickly, and each time the drug is used, a higher dose is required to produce the same effects.

Effects on the Body

Use of heroin induces a state of euphoria that comes within seconds of intravenous injection or within 5 to 15 minutes with other methods of administration. Because the drug is a sedative, during the initial rush people have a sense of relaxation and do not feel any pain. In users who inhale the drug, however, the rush may be accompanied by nausea, vomiting, intense itching, and, at times, severe asthma attacks. As the rush wears off, users experience drowsiness, confusion, slowed cardiac function, and decreased breathing rate.

A heroin overdose can cause convulsions, coma, and death. During an overdose, heart rate, breathing, blood pressure, and body temperature drop dramatically. These physiological responses can induce vomiting and tight muscles and cause breathing to stop. Death is often the result of lack of oxygen or choking to death on vomit.

About 4 to 5 hours after taking the drug, withdrawal sets in. Heroin withdrawal is painful and usually lasts up to 2 weeks—but it could go on for several months. Symptoms of short-term use include red or raw nostrils, bone and muscle pains, muscle spasms and cramps, sweating, hot and cold flashes, runny nose and eyes, drowsiness, sluggishness, slurred speech, loss of appetite, nausea, diarrhea, restlessness, and violent yawning. Heroin use can also kill a developing fetus or cause a spontaneous abortion.

Symptoms of long-term use of heroin include hallucinations, nightmares, constipation, sexual difficulties, impaired vision, reduced fertility, boils, collapsed veins, and a significantly elevated risk for lung, liver, and cardiovascular diseases, including bacterial infections in blood vessels and heart valves. The additives used in street heroin can clog vital blood vessels because these additives do not dissolve in the body, leading to infections and death of cells in vital organs. Sudden infant death syndrome (SIDS) also is seen more frequently in children born to heroin-addicted mothers.

Heroin addiction is treated with behavioral therapies and pharmaceutical agents. Medication suppresses withdrawal symptoms, which makes it easier for patients to stop using heroin. The combination of these two treatment modalities helps people learn to lead a more stable, productive, and drug-free lifestyle.

New Psychoactive Substances

The World Drug Report, compiled by the United Nations Office on Drugs and Crime, has warned of the rapid emergence of **new psychoactive substances (NPS)**, a term coined by the Commission on Narcotic Drugs to refer to unregulated substances of abuse whose effects are made to mimic that of controlled drugs.[11] The term "new" does not necessarily mean that the substance itself is new, but rather that the misuse of the substance or mixture of substances is newly introduced to a specific market. NPS are commonly referred to by both the general population and national associations as "synthetic drugs" or "designer drugs."

There are approximately 500 synthetic substances sold on the market today, with the largest numbers of NPS identified in the United States. Among students, NPS use is more common than all other drugs except marijuana. Though the highest concentration of NPS is in Europe and North America, most NPS originate in regions with advanced chemical and pharmaceutical industries, particularly Asia.

Widespread access to drug formulas via the Internet has allowed increased creativity in the preparation of synthetic substances or spinoffs by dealers in order to escape legislation. In July 2012, the U.S. Congress signed into law the Synthetic Drug Abuse Prevention Act (SDAPA), which identified 26 substances as Schedule I controlled substances, establishing drug codes for enforcement. Despite legislative efforts, however, small alterations in formulas by drug designers consistently outpace efforts to control or ban NPS.

Until they are placed under regulatory control, these substances are often marketed as legal alternatives to controlled drugs, said to be "legal highs" or "herbal highs," to emphasize a seemingly safe and natural origin. They are often labeled by dealers as "research chemicals" that are not for human consumption to avoid prosecution. Substances are also masked under the name of ordinary household products to imply that they are both harmless and legal, such as bath salts, plant food, herbal incense, potpourri, or jewelry cleaner. In truth, some of these substances are so potent that an amount as small as a grain of salt can produce adverse effects.

Because of the vast quantity of NPS that can each contain a mixture of many substances, it's difficult to determine or speculate on the long-term health implications of NPS use. NPS include a broad range of synthetic and plant-based psychoactive substances, including synthetic cannabinoids (synthetic marijuana and Spice), synthetic cathinones (mephedrone sold as bath salts, plant food, or meow meow), piperazines ("Ecstasy substitutes"), phenethylamines (4-MMA and methyl-MA), ketamine (Special K, vitamin K, and jet), and other plant-derived substances such as kratom, khat, and *Salvia divinorum*. The most prevalent forms of NPS in the United States are synthetic cannabinoids.

Synthetic Cannabinoids (Fake Pot or Spice)

Synthetic cannabinoids are currently the most widely used NPS in the United States and worldwide.[12] More commonly known as "fake pot," synthetic cannabinoids are manmade chemicals that contain compounds similar to the chemical THC found in the natural *Cannabis sativa* plant used for marijuana, though synthetic versions are generally more potent. Users claim that the substances provide a marijuana-like high and are popular among teenagers and young adults. The 2016 Monitoring the Future survey of youth drug-use trends found that 3.5 percent of high school seniors used synthetic cannabinoids in the past year, placing it as the second most common illicit drug used by seniors after marijuana.[13]

Synthetic cannabinoids are often sprayed onto a mixture of herbs and are sold as Spice, K2, Moon Rocks, Skunk, Kind, Genie, Summit, potpourri, herbal incense, Yucatan Gold, Purple Passion, Train Wreck, or Ultra (among other names).

Effects on the Body

According to the federal DEA, the adverse effects of synthetic cannabinoids are far more dangerous than the side effects of marijuana, and include seizures, high blood pressure, anxiety attacks, hallucinations, nausea, loss of consciousness, and chemical dependency. Some samples tested have been shown to be 100 times more potent than marijuana.

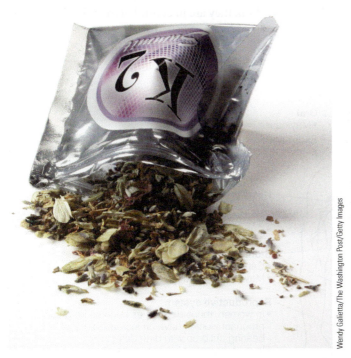

Synthetic cannabinoids, known as "fake pot," are often sprayed onto a mixture of herbs and sold as Spice, K2, potpourri, or other names.

13.4 *Alcohol*

Drinking **alcohol** has been a socially acceptable behavior for centuries—as an accompaniment at parties, ceremonies, dinners, sport contests, the establishment of kingdoms or governments, and the signing of treaties between nations. Alcohol has also been used for medical reasons as a mild sedative or as a painkiller for surgery.

For a short period of 14 years, from 1920 to 1933, by constitutional amendment, the sale and use of alcohol were declared illegal in the United States. This amendment was repealed because drinkers and nondrinkers alike questioned the right of government to pass judgment on individual moral standards. In addition, organized crime activities to smuggle and sell alcohol illegally expanded enormously during this period.

Alcohol is the most abused substance in the United States and the cause of one of the most significant health-related drug problems in the country today. Nearly 88,000

What Constitutes a Standard Drink?

In the United States, a drink is considered to be 0.6 fluid ounces (14 grams or 1.2 tablespoons) of pure alcohol, or the equivalent of:

- 5 ounces of wine (12 percent alcohol)
- 12 ounces of beer (5 percent alcohol)
- 8 ounces of malt liquor (7 percent alcohol)
- 1.5 ounces of 80-proof liquor or distilled spirits (40 percent alcohol)

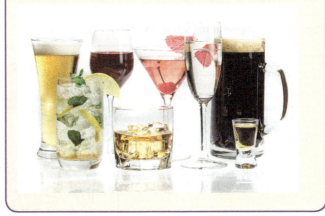

GLOSSARY

New psychoactive substances (NPS) Unregulated substances of abuse whose effects are made to mimic that of controlled drugs, often called "designer" or "synthetic" drugs.

Alcohol Ethyl alcohol, a depressant drug that affects the brain, slows central nervous system activity, and has strong addictive properties.

yearly deaths in the United States are due to excessive drinking.[14]

The 2015 *National Survey on Drug Use and Health* (NSDUH) reports that more than 138.3 million people 12 years and older (51.7 percent) used alcohol within a month of the survey, and 66.7 million (48 percent of current drinkers) participated in binge drinking at least once in the 30 days prior to the survey. About 39 percent of young adults age 18 to 25 were binge drinkers, or about 2 out of 5. Alcohol drinkers are also more likely to misuse other drugs. More than half of lifetime drinkers have used one or more illicit drugs at some time in their lives, compared with less than 10 percent of lifetime nondrinkers.

HOEGER KEY TO WELLNESS

Although alcohol is often touted in the press as "a vice that's good for you," the modest benefits of alcohol can be equated to those obtained by taking a small daily dose of aspirin (about 81 mg per day, or the equivalent of a baby aspirin) or eating a few nuts each day. Aspirin or a few nuts do not lead to impaired judgment or actions that you may later regret or have to live with for the rest of your life.

Effects on the Body

The effects of alcohol intake include impaired peripheral vision, decreased visual and hearing acuity, slower reaction time, reduced concentration and motor performance (including increased swaying), and impaired judgment of distance and speed of moving objects. Furthermore, alcohol alleviates fear, increases risk taking, stimulates urination, and

induces sleep. A single large dose of alcohol also may decrease sexual function. More serious consequences of alcohol abuse are increased risks of accidents and violent behavior. Excessive drinking has been linked to more than half of all deaths from car accidents. The risk for rape, domestic violence, child abuse, suicide, and murder also increases with alcohol abuse.

One of the most unpleasant, dangerous, and life-threatening effects of drinking is the **synergistic action** of alcohol when combined with other drugs, particularly central nervous system depressants. Each person reacts to a combination of alcohol and other drugs in a different way. The effects range from loss of consciousness to death.

Long-term effects of alcohol abuse are serious and often life threatening (Figure 13.4). Some of these detrimental effects are lower resistance to disease; **cirrhosis** of the liver; higher risk for breast, oral, esophageal, larynx, stomach, colon, and liver cancer; **cardiomyopathy**; irregular heartbeat; elevated blood pressure; greater risk for stroke; osteoporosis; inflammation of the esophagus, stomach, small intestine, and pancreas; stomach ulcers; sexual impotence; birth defects; malnutrition; brain cell damage leading to loss of memory; depression; psychosis; and hallucinations.

Addictive and Social Consequences of Alcohol Abuse

Alcohol is not for everyone. **Alcoholism** seems to have both a genetic and an environmental component. The reasons some people can drink for years without becoming addicted, whereas others follow the downward spiral of alcoholism, are not understood. The addiction to alcohol develops slowly. Most people think they are in control of their drinking habits

Figure 13.4 Long-term risks associated with alcohol abuse.

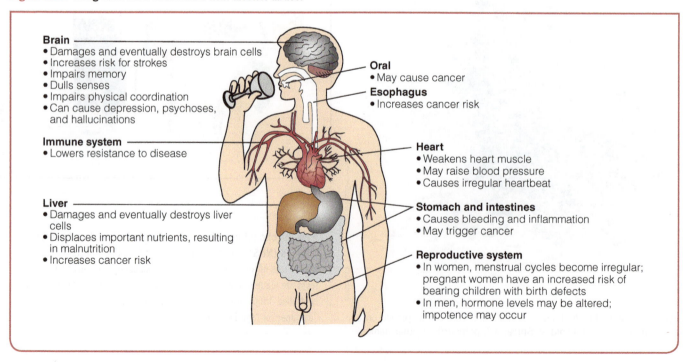

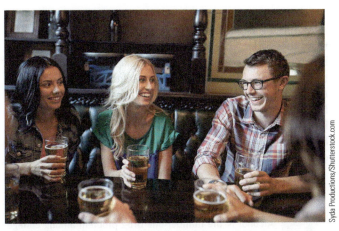

Approximately 14 million Americans will develop a drinking problem during their lifetime.

and do not realize they have a problem until they become alcoholics, when they find themselves physically and emotionally dependent on the drug. This addiction is characterized by excessive use of, and constant preoccupation with, drinking. Alcohol abuse, in turn, leads to mental, emotional, physical, and social problems.

The Risks of College Drinking

The statistics are sobering. Each year, for college students between the ages of 18 and 24,

- 1,825 die from alcohol-related unintentional injuries.
- Almost 700,000 are assaulted by another student who had been drinking.
- 599,000 are unintentionally injured under the influence of alcohol.
- More than 150,000 develop alcohol-related health problems.
- About 97,000 are victims of alcohol-related sexual assault or date rape.
- 400,000 have unprotected sex.
- More than 100,000 were too intoxicated to know whether they'd consented to having sex.
- Almost 3.4 million drive under the influence of alcohol.

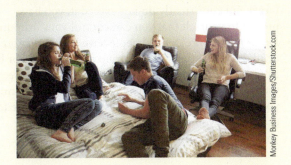

SOURCE: "A Snapshot of Annual High-risk College Drinking Consequences," available at http://www.collegedrinkingprevention.gov/statssummaries/snapshot.aspx, downloaded January 2017.

Heavy drinking contributes to decreased performance at work and school because drinkers are more likely to arrive late, make more mistakes, leave assignments incomplete, encounter problems with fellow workers or students, get lower grades and job evaluations, and flunk out of school or lose jobs. Alcohol abuse also leads to social problems that include loss of friends and jobs, separation of family members, child abuse, domestic violence, divorce, and problems with the law. Finally, alcohol abuse worsens financial concerns because drinkers have less money for needed items such as food and clothing; they often fail to pay bills; and they tend to incur additional medical expenses, insurance premiums, and fines.

Alcohol on Campus

Alcohol is the number-one drug problem among college students. According to national surveys, about 60 percent of full-time college students report using alcohol within the past month, and 39 percent have engaged in binge drinking (consumed five or more drinks in a row). Alcohol is a factor in about 25 percent of all college dropouts, and of the more than 18 million college students in the United States, between 2 and 3 percent eventually will die from alcohol-related causes.

In terms of academic work, a national survey involving about 94,000 college students from 197 colleges and universities conducted over 3 years showed that grade point average (GPA) was related to average number of drinks per week (Figure 13.5).[15] Students with a D- or F-level GPA reported a

Figure 13.5 **Average number of drinks by college students per week by GPA.**

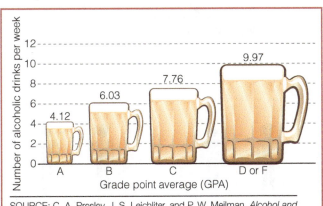

SOURCE: C. A. Presley, J. S. Leichliter, and P. W. Meilman, *Alcohol and Drugs on American College Campuses: Findings from 1995, 1996, and 1997 (A Report to College Presidents)* (Carbondale, IL: Southern Illinois University, 1999).

GLOSSARY

Synergistic action The effect of mixing two or more drugs, which can be much greater than the sum of two or more drugs acting by themselves.

Cirrhosis A disease characterized by scarring of the liver.

Cardiomyopathy A disease affecting the heart muscle.

Alcoholism A disease in which an individual loses control over drinking alcoholic beverages.

weekly consumption of almost 10 drinks. Students with A-level GPAs consumed about four drinks per week.

The National Institute on Alcohol Abuse and Alcoholism states that about one-quarter of college students report having academic problems due to alcohol abuse, including missing classes, falling behind, and receiving lower grades on exams and papers. Students tend to be most susceptible to drinking during the first 6 weeks of their freshman year when they encounter new social and academic pressures. In fact, college students enrolled full-time have higher rates of alcohol use, binge and heavy drinking, and driving under the influence than their peers ages 18 to 22 who are part-time students or who don't attend college (see Figure 13.6). College students who develop habits of heavy and binge drinking in their first year put their health and academic potential at risk during their college years and into early adulthood.

Another major concern is that more than half of college students participate in games that involve heavy drinking (consuming five or more drinks in one sitting). Often, students take part because of peer pressure and fear of rejection. Some students even binge drink three days in a row on weekends.

Excessive drinking can also precipitate unplanned and unprotected sex (risking HIV infection), date rape, and alcohol poisoning. When some young people turn 21, they "celebrate"

by having 21 drinks. Unaware of the risks of excessive alcohol intake in a relatively short period, drinking friends then try to let them "sleep it off," only to find that they never wake up but rather suffer death from alcohol poisoning. Each year, thousands of college students are taken to the emergency room for alcohol poisoning, which can result in permanent brain damage or death. Signs of alcohol poisoning include inability to wake or rouse a person, vomiting, slow or irregular breathing, low body temperature or hypothermia, bluish or pale skin, or mental confusion.

HOEGER KEY TO WELLNESS

Alcohol is the number-one drug problem among college students. Of the more than 18 million college students in the United States, 2 to 3 percent eventually will die from alcohol-related causes.

How to Cut Down on Drinking

To find out whether drinking is a problem in your life, refer to the questionnaire in Activity 13.2. A "yes" answer to any of these questions can be regarded as a warning sign to potential future problems. If you have answered three or more of them with a "yes," your drinking habits can be harmful to your well-being and may indicate that you are alcohol dependent or an alcoholic. An evaluation by a health care professional is highly recommended.

If a person is determined to control the problem, it is not that difficult. The first and most important step is to want to cut down. If you want to do this but cannot seem to do so, you need to accept the probability that alcohol is becoming a serious problem for you, and you should seek guidance from your physician or from an organization such as Alcoholics Anonymous. The next few suggestions also may help you cut down your alcohol intake:

- *Set reasonable limits for yourself.* Decide not to exceed a certain number of drinks on a given occasion, and stick to your decision. No more than two beers or two cocktails a day is a reasonable limit. If you set a target and consistently do not exceed it, you have proven to yourself that you can control your drinking.
- *Learn to say "no."* Many people have "just one more" drink because others in the group are doing this or because someone puts pressure on them, not because they want a drink. When you reach the sensible limit you have set for yourself, politely but firmly refuse to exceed it. If you are being the generous host, pour yourself a glass of water or juice "on the rocks." Nobody will notice the difference.
- *Drink slowly.* Don't gulp a drink. Choose your drinks for their flavor, not their "kick," and savor the taste of each sip.

Figure 13.6 Heavy alcohol use is higher in college students than in non-college peers.

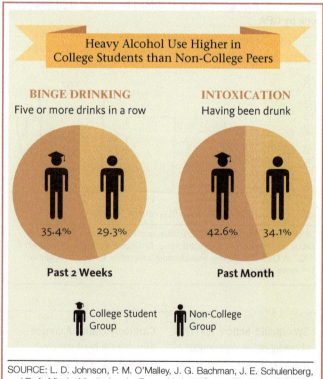

Heavy Alcohol Use Higher in College Students than Non-College Peers

BINGE DRINKING
Five or more drinks in a row

INTOXICATION
Having been drunk

35.4%   29.3%   42.6%   34.1%

Past 2 Weeks   **Past Month**

College Student Group   Non-College Group

SOURCE: L. D. Johnson, P. M. O'Malley, J. G. Bachman, J. E. Schulenberg, and R. A. Miech, *Monitoring the Future National Survey Results on Drug Use, 1975–2014: Volume 2, College students and adults ages 19–55* (Ann Arbor, MI: Institute for Social Research, The University of Michigan, 2015), available at http://www.drugabuse.gov/related-topics/trends-statistics/infographics/drug-alcohol-use-in-college-age-adults-in-2014, downloaded January 2017.

Behavior Modification Planning

When Your Date Drinks

- Don't make excuses for his/her behavior, no matter how embarrassing.
- Don't allow embarrassment to put you in a situation with which you are uncomfortable.
- Do be sure that body language and tone of voice match verbal messages you send.
- Do leave as quickly as you can, without your date. Don't stop to argue. Intoxicated people can't listen to reason.

- Do call a cab, a friend, or your parents. Don't ride home with your date.
- Do make your position clear. "No!" is much more effective than "Please stop!" or "Don't!"
- Do make it clear that you will call the police if rape is attempted.

Try It

In your online journal or class notebook, write down strategies you can incorporate today to ensure your health and wellness.

- *Dilute your drinks.* If you prefer cocktails to beer, try tall drinks: Instead of downing gin or whiskey straight or nearly so, drink it diluted with a mixer such as tonic water or soda water in a tall glass. That way, you can enjoy both the flavor and the act of drinking but take longer to finish each drink. Also, you can make your two-drink limit last all evening or switch to the mixer by itself.
- *Do not drink on your own.* Confine your drinking to social gatherings. You may have a hard time resisting the urge to pour yourself a relaxing drink at the end of a hard day, but many formerly heavy drinkers have found that a soft drink satisfies the need as well as alcohol did. What may help you really unwind, even with no drink, is a comfortable chair, loosened clothing, and perhaps soothing music, a television program, a good book to read, or even some low- to moderate-intensity physical activity.
- *Try a smartphone app to help control your drinking.* More and more smartphone applications are being developed that offer great tools to help you monitor and control drinking habits. Some features include tracking tools to help calculate blood alcohol levels as you drink, the ability to set up messaging from your personal support team to check your progress, profiles from a network of peers also trying to cut down to provide motivation, and links to helpful resources about addiction and recovery. One recent study found that recovery patients who used a smartphone app after treatment for alcohol abuse were 12 percent more likely to abstain from alcohol and also have fewer relapses.[16]

13.5 *Treatment of Addictions*

Recovery from any addiction is more likely to be successful with professional guidance and support. The first step is to recognize the reality of the problem. The Addictive Behavior Questionnaire in Activity 13.1 will help you recognize

possible addictive behavior in yourself (or someone you know). If the answers to five or more of these questions are positive, you may have a problem, in which case you should contact a physician, your institution's counseling center, or the local mental health clinic for a referral.

You also may contact the Substance Abuse and Mental Health Services Administration at 1-800-662-HELP (1-800-662-4357) for referral to 24-hour substance abuse treatment centers in your local area. All information discussed during a phone call to this center is kept strictly confidential. Information is also available online at http://www.samhsa.gov. The national center provides printed information on drug abuse and addictive behavior.

Among intervention and treatment programs for addiction are psychotherapy, medical care, and behavior modification. If addiction is a problem in your life, you need to act upon it without delay. Addicts do not have to resign themselves to a lifetime of addiction. The sooner you start, and the longer you stay in treatment, the better your chances of recovering and leading a healthier and more productive life.

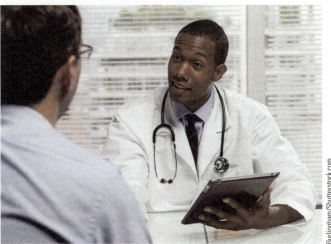

The sooner treatment for addiction is started, and the longer the user stays in treatment, the better the chances for recovery and a more productive life.

Activity 13.2   Alcohol Use Questionnaire

Name _____ **Date** _____

Course _____ **Section** _____ **Gender** _____ **Age** _____

I. Alcohol Abuse

This questionnaire can help you determine if your drinking (alcohol) patterns are a problem for you. If you do not consume alcohol, skip this questionnaire, as drinking does not interfere with your health and well-being.

	Yes	No
1. Do you consume more than one (women) or two (men) drinks per day?	☐	☐
2. Does drinking interfere with your short- or long-term goals?	☐	☐
3. Does drinking interfere with your school or work productivity?	☐	☐
4. Have you missed school or work because of drinking?	☐	☐
5. Do you skip workouts because of drinking?	☐	☐
6. Do you drink to increase self-confidence?	☐	☐
7. Do you drink to feel more at ease with others?	☐	☐
8. Do you drink to be socially accepted by others?	☐	☐
9. Are you annoyed by other people's comments about your drinking habits?	☐	☐
10. Are you untruthful about the number of drinks you have had when questioned by others?	☐	☐
11. Do you associate with people that negatively influence you, or that you don't normally relate to, only because they drink?	☐	☐
12. Do you drink alone?	☐	☐
13. At social gatherings, do you actively look for a refill before being offered one?	☐	☐
14. Do you frequently serve yourself a more generous drink than the "going" amount for others?	☐	☐
15. Do you drink to relieve stress, forget worries, or life's problems?	☐	☐
16. Has drinking affected your reputation?	☐	☐
17. Have you missed appointments due to drinking?	☐	☐
18. Do you participate in binge drinking episodes?	☐	☐
19. Do you have difficulty remembering what you have done because of drinking?	☐	☐
20. Does drinking affect your family life or relationships?	☐	☐
21. Are you ever abusive to others when drinking?	☐	☐
22. Have you experienced financial difficulties as a result of drinking?	☐	☐
23. Do you feel physically deprived if you cannot drink daily?	☐	☐
24. Do you need a drink early in the day to get going?	☐	☐
25. Do you need a drink at certain times of the day?	☐	☐
26. Has drinking disrupted your sleeping pattern?	☐	☐
27. Do you ever feel that you need to cut down on drinking?	☐	☐
28. Do you ever feel bad or guilty about your drinking pattern?	☐	☐
29. Have you been treated by a physician or health professional for drinking?	☐	☐
30. Have you ever been treated in a hospital or other institution for drinking?	☐	☐

A "yes" answer to any of these questions can be regarded as a warning sign to potential future problems. If you have answered three or more of them with a "yes", your drinking habit can be harmful to your well-being and may indicate that you are alcohol dependent or an alcoholic. An evaluation by a healthcare professional is highly recommended.

© Fitness & Wellness, Inc.

13.6 *Tobacco*

People throughout the world have used tobacco for hundreds of years. Before the 18th century, they smoked tobacco primarily in the form of pipes or cigars. Cigarette smoking per se did not become popular until the mid-1800s, and its use started to increase dramatically in the 20th century.

When tobacco leaves are burned, hot air and gases containing **tar** (chemical compounds) and **nicotine** are released in the smoke. More than 7,000 chemicals, hundreds of them toxic, have been found in tobacco smoke. About 70 are proven carcinogens. The harmful effects of cigarette smoking and tobacco use in general were not exactly known until the early 1960s, when research began to show a link between tobacco use and disease.

In 1964, the U.S. Surgeon General issued the first major report presenting scientific evidence that cigarettes were a major health hazard in American society. More than 40 percent of the U.S. adult population smoked cigarettes at the time. Since the report in 1964, more than 15 million premature deaths in the United States alone are attributed to smoking.

Every day more than 3,200 Americans under age 18 smoke their first cigarette, and 2,100 will become daily smokers. Young people who smoke are also more likely to abuse other illicit drugs. Smokers between the ages of 12 and 17 are nine times more likely to use drugs than nonsmokers in this same age group.

Types of Tobacco Products

Many tobacco users are aware of the health consequences of cigarette smoking but may fail to realize the risks of pipe smoking, cigar smoking, and tobacco chewing. As depicted in Figure 13.7, tobacco use in general declines with education. Today, an estimated 64 million Americans age 12 and older use tobacco products, including 52 million cigarette smokers, 12.5 million cigar smokers, 9 million using smokeless tobacco, and 2.3 million pipe smokers.[17]

Pipes and Cigars

As a group, pipe and cigar smokers have lower risks for heart disease and lung cancer than cigarette smokers. Nevertheless, blood nicotine levels in pipe and cigar smokers have been shown to approach those of cigarette smokers because nicotine is still absorbed through the membranes of the mouth. Therefore, these tobacco users still have a higher risk for heart disease than nonsmokers do.

Cigarette smokers who substitute pipe or cigar smoking for cigarettes usually continue to inhale the smoke, which results in more nicotine and tar being brought into their lungs than they inhale through cigarette smoke. Consequently, the risk for disease is even higher if pipe or cigar smoke is inhaled. The risk and mortality rates for lip, mouth, and larynx cancer for pipe smoking, cigar smoking, and tobacco chewing are higher than those for cigarette smoking.

Figure 13.7 Tobacco use among adults age 18 or older, 2015.

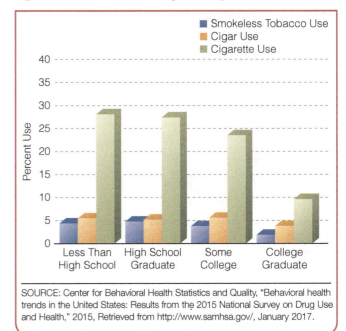

SOURCE: Center for Behavioral Health Statistics and Quality, "Behavioral health trends in the United States: Results from the 2015 National Survey on Drug Use and Health," 2015, Retrieved from http://www.samhsa.gov/, January 2017.

Smokeless Tobacco

Smokeless tobacco has been promoted in the past as a safe alternative to cigarette smoking. However, the Advisory Committee to the U.S. Surgeon General has stated that smokeless tobacco represents a significant health risk and is just as addictive as cigarette smoking.

Close to 9 million Americans use smokeless tobacco. The greatest concern is the increase in use of smokeless tobacco among young people. The average starting age for smokeless tobacco use is 10 years old.

Using smokeless tobacco can lead to gingivitis and periodontitis. It carries a fourfold increase in oral cancer and, in some cases, even premature death. People who chew or dip also have a higher rate of cavities, sore gums, bad breath, and stained teeth. Their senses of smell and taste diminish; consequently, they tend to add more sugar and salt to food. These practices alone increase the risk for being overweight and having high blood pressure. Nicotine addiction and its related health risks also hold true for smokeless tobacco users. Nicotine blood levels approach those of cigarette smokers, increasing the risk for diseases of the cardiovascular system. Furthermore, research has revealed changes in heart rate and blood pressure similar to those of cigarette smokers.

Using tobacco in any form can be addictive and poses a serious threat to health and well-being. Eliminating its use is the most important lifestyle change a tobacco user can make to improve health, quality of life, and longevity.

GLOSSARY

Tar A chemical compound that forms during the burning of tobacco leaves.

Nicotine An addictive compound found in tobacco leaves.

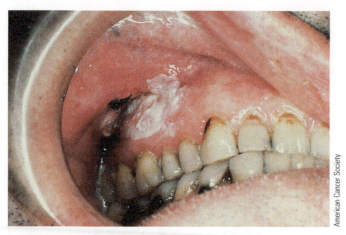

Smokeless tobacco can lead to gum and tooth damage as well as oral cancer (pictured).

Critical Thinking

Do you think the government should outlaw the use of tobacco in all forms, or does the individual have the right to engage in self-destructive behavior?

Cigarettes

Cigarette smoking is the largest preventable cause of illness and premature death in the United States. Death rates from heart disease, cancer, stroke, aortic aneurysm, chronic bronchitis, emphysema, and peptic ulcers all increase with cigarette smoking.

In pregnant women, cigarette smoking has been linked to retarded fetal growth, higher risk for spontaneous abortion (miscarriage), and prenatal death. Smoking is also the most prevalent cause of injury and death from fire. The average life expectancy for chronic smokers is 10 years shorter than that for nonsmokers, and the death rates among chronic smokers during their most productive years of life, between ages 25 and 65, is twice the national average. If we consider all related deaths, smoking is responsible for more than 480,000 U.S. deaths each year—enough deaths to wipe out the entire population of Miami in a single year. For every tobacco-related death, there are 30 others, or 16 million people in the United States, who suffer from at least one serious illness associated with cigarette smoking. More deaths are caused each year by tobacco use than by all deaths from HIV, illegal drug use, car accidents, alcohol use, suicides, and murders combined.

Based on a report by U.S. government physicians, each cigarette shortens life by 7 to 11 minutes. This figure represents 5.5 million years of potential life that Americans lose to smoking each year.

Effects on the Cardiovascular System

Each year, approximately one-third of coronary heart disease deaths are attributed to cigarette smoking. The CDC states that smoking increases the risk of coronary heart disease two- to fourfold. The mortality rate following heart attacks is higher for smokers because their attacks usually are more severe and their risk for deadly arrhythmias is much greater.

Cigarette smoking affects the cardiovascular system by increasing heart rate, blood pressure, and susceptibility to atherosclerosis, blood clots, coronary artery spasm, cardiac arrhythmia, and arteriosclerotic peripheral vascular disease. Evidence also indicates that smoking decreases high-density lipoprotein (HDL) cholesterol, the "good" cholesterol that lowers the risk for heart disease. Smoking further increases the amount of fatty acids, glucose, and various hormones in the blood. The carbon monoxide in smoke hinders the capacity of the blood to carry oxygen to body tissues. Both carbon monoxide and nicotine can damage the inner walls of the arteries and thereby encourage the buildup of fat on them. Smoking also causes increased adhesiveness and clustering of platelets in the blood, decreases platelet survival and clotting time, and increases blood thickness. Any of these effects can precipitate a heart attack.

HOEGER KEY TO WELLNESS

More than 7,000 chemicals, hundreds of them toxic, have been found in tobacco smoke. About 70 are proven carcinogens.

Smoking and Cancer

The American Cancer Society reports that 80 percent of lung cancer is attributable to smoking. Lung cancer is the leading cancer killer, accounting for approximately 155,870 deaths in the United States, or about one in four of all deaths from cancer.[18] In addition to lung cancer, cigarette smoking increases the risk for oral cavity, lip, nasopharynx, nasal cavity and paranasal sinus, pharynx, larynx, esophagus, stomach, colorectum, pancreas, uterine cervix, ovary, kidney, bladder, liver, and acute myeloid leukemia cancers. Cigarette smoking also leads to chronic lower respiratory disease, the third-leading cause of death in the United States (see also Chapter 1). Figure 13.8 illustrates normal and diseased **alveoli** and Figure 13.9 details the risks to health from smoking.

Figure 13.8 Normal and diseased alveoli in lungs.

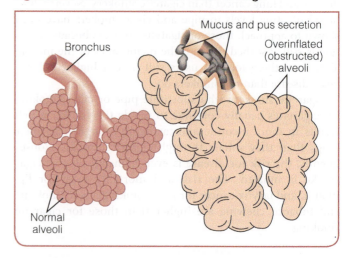

Figure 13.9 The health effects of smoking.

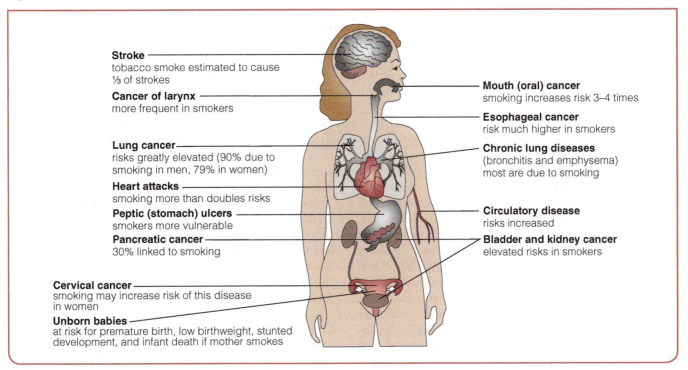

Stroke
tobacco smoke estimated to cause
⅓ of strokes

Cancer of larynx
more frequent in smokers

Lung cancer
risks greatly elevated (90% due to
smoking in men, 79% in women)

Heart attacks
smoking more than doubles risks

Peptic (stomach) ulcers
smokers more vulnerable

Pancreatic cancer
30% linked to smoking

Cervical cancer
smoking may increase risk of this disease
in women

Unborn babies
at risk for premature birth, low birthweight, stunted
development, and infant death if mother smokes

Mouth (oral) cancer
smoking increases risk 3–4 times

Esophageal cancer
risk much higher in smokers

Chronic lung diseases
(bronchitis and emphysema)
most are due to smoking

Circulatory disease
risks increased

Bladder and kidney cancer
elevated risks in smokers

Effects of Secondhand Smoke

The most common carcinogenic exposure in the workplace is cigarette smoke. Both fatal and nonfatal cardiac events are increased greatly in people who are exposed to passive smoke. About 42,000 additional deaths result each year in the United States from secondhand smoke (also known as environmental tobacco smoke, or ETS), which include deaths from cardiovascular diseases, lung cancer, and SIDS.[19] Furthermore, almost 22 million children between the ages of 3 and 11 are exposed to secondhand smoke, and approximately 30 percent of the indoor workforce is not protected by smoke-free workplace policies. According to the U.S. Surgeon General, the evidence clearly shows that there is no risk-free level of exposure to secondhand smoke, prompting Dr. Richard Carmona, former U.S. Surgeon General, to state: *"Based on the science, I wouldn't allow anyone in my family to stand in a room with someone smoking."*[20]

—GLOSSARY—

Alveoli Air sacs in the lungs where gas exchange (oxygen and carbon dioxide) takes place.

Adverse Effects of Secondhand Smoke

- Increases coronary heart disease risk by 30 percent (some adverse effects begin within minutes to hours of exposure).
- Increases blood clotting, enhancing the risk of heart attacks and strokes.
- Lowers HDL (good) cholesterol.
- Increases oxidation of LDL cholesterol, enhancing atherosclerosis.
- Increases oxygen-free radicals.
- Decreases levels of antioxidants.
- Increases chronic inflammation.
- Increases insulin resistance, leading to higher blood sugar levels and risk for diabetes.
- Increases lung and overall cancer risk.

- Increases risk for pulmonary diseases.
- Increases risk for adverse effects during pregnancy.
- Increases sudden infant death syndrome (SIDS) risk.

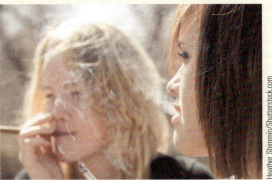

Heather Shimmin/Shutterstock.com

Two large-scale reviews of research studies on American, Canadian, and European communities that have passed laws to curb secondhand smoke by banning it in public places, including bars and restaurants, have shown an average drop of 17 percent in heart attacks in the first year compared to levels in communities without such a ban. There is a further 26 percent decline in heart attacks for at least 3 years each year thereafter.

Within 20 minutes of secondhand smoke inhalation, chemical changes can be detected in the body's blood clotting mechanism, increasing the risk for heart attack or stroke. Research also indicates that lifetime exposure to secondhand smoke (which, in adults, is defined as 20 years or more for home exposure or 10 years or more of work exposure) increases the risk of stillbirth, miscarriage, or tubal ectopic pregnancy in women regardless of whether they ever smoked personally. Nonsmokers exposed to secondhand smoke at home or at the office have up to a 30 percent greater risk of suffering a heart attack. Furthermore, exposure to thirdhand smoke—tobacco smoke contamination that saturates carpets, wallpaper, paint, fabrics, and furniture upholstery—also increases the risk of cancer and is particularly damaging for infants and young children who have the most contact with floors, surfaces, furniture, toys, and other objects in the home.

Critical Thinking

You are in a designated nonsmoking area and the person next to you lights up a cigarette. What can you say to this person to protect your right to clean air?

Health Care Costs of Smoking

Heavy smokers use the health care system, especially hospitals, twice as much as nonsmokers do. The American Cancer Society reports that for every time smokers purchase a pack of cigarettes in the United States at an average price of $6.36, they create $35 of future health-related costs for themselves. The yearly cost to a given company has been estimated to be up to $6,000 per smoking employee. This cost includes employee health care, absenteeism, additional health insurance, morbidity or disability and early mortality, on-the-job time lost, property damage or maintenance and depreciation, workers' compensation, and the impact of secondhand smoke.

If every U.S. smoker were to give up cigarettes, in one year alone, sick time would drop by approximately 90 million days; heart conditions would decrease by 280,000; chronic bronchitis and emphysema would number 1 million fewer cases; and total death rates from cardiovascular disease, cancer, and peptic ulcers would fall off drastically.

Morbidity and Mortality

Tobacco use in all its forms is considered a significant threat to life. Up to half of tobacco users will die from its use. World Health Organization estimates indicate that 10 percent of the 7 billion people presently living will die as a result of smoking-related illnesses, which kill more than 6 million people each year. A total of 100 million tobacco-related deaths occurred in the 20th century, and based on estimates, there will be 1 billion deaths in the 21st century. To gain some perspective on the seriousness of the tobacco problem, CDC statistics indicate that drug overdoses kill more than 50,000 people per year in the United States. By comparison, tobacco, a legal drug, kills almost ten times as many people as all illegal drugs combined.

Smoking kills more Americans in a single year than died in battle during World War II and the Vietnam War combined. Think of the public outrage if 480,000 Americans were to die annually in a meaningless war. What if a single nonprescription drug were to cause more than 160,000 deaths from cancer and 180,000 deaths from heart disease? The U.S. public would not tolerate these situations. We would mount an intense fight to prevent the deaths. If cigarettes were invented today, the tobacco industry would be put on trial for mass murder.

HOEGER KEY TO WELLNESS

Cigarette smoking is the largest preventable cause of illness and premature death in the United States. More deaths are caused each year by tobacco use than by all deaths from HIV, illegal drugs, car accidents, alcohol, suicides, and murders combined.

Trends Against Tobacco

Though the fight against all forms of tobacco use is stronger than ever, this was not always the case. It has been difficult to fight an industry that wields such enormous financial and political influence as does the tobacco industry in the United States. Almost $25 million is spent every day in cigarette advertising and promotions, and tobacco is one of the top ten cash crops in the United States.

The FDA Drug Abuse Advisory Committee has taken a strong stance against the use of all forms of tobacco products. Although the American Heart Association (AHA) commends the work initiated by the FDA, the AHA has further stated that the FDA and the federal government have an obligation to take regulatory action against the national problem of nicotine addiction and abuse of cigarettes and tobacco products in general. The U.S. Surgeon General has stated that health education combined with social, economic, and regulatory approaches is imperative to offset the tobacco industry's marketing and to promote nonsmoking environments.

Fortunately, the federal Clean Air Act and state regulatory laws have come a long way in providing more nonsmoking environments. Smoking is prohibited in most public places as a result of nonsmokers and ex-smokers alike fighting for their rights to clean air and health. Cigarette smoking is no longer acceptable in most social circles.

13.7 *Why Smoking Is Addicting*

The American Psychiatric Association and the National Institute on Drug Abuse have indicated that nicotine is perhaps the most addictive drug known to humans. The U.S. Surgeon General has concluded that[21]

- Cigarettes and other forms of tobacco are addicting.
- Nicotine is the drug responsible for the addictive behavior.
- Pharmacological and behavioral traits that determine addiction to tobacco are similar to those that determine addiction to drugs such as heroin and cocaine.

Smoking only three packs of cigarettes can lead to physiological addiction and a tolerance to nicotine and tobacco smoke. Within seconds of inhalation, nicotine affects the central nervous system and can act simultaneously as a tranquilizer and a stimulant. The stimulating effect produces strong physiological and psychological dependency. The physical addiction to nicotine is six to eight times more powerful than the addiction to alcohol and greater than that of some illegal drugs.

Psychological dependency develops over a longer time. People smoke to aid relaxation, and they gain a certain amount of pleasure from the ritual of smoking. Smokers automatically associate many activities of daily life with cigarettes—coffee drinking, alcohol drinking, being part of a social gathering, relaxing after a meal, talking on the phone, driving, reading, and watching television. In many cases, the social rituals of smoking are the most difficult to eliminate. The dependency is so strong that years after people have stopped smoking, they may still crave cigarettes when they engage in certain social activities.

Why Do You Smoke? Test

Although the remaining information in this chapter is written directly to smokers, nonsmokers will gain a better understanding of smoking addiction and how to help others stop smoking by reading it.

Most people smoke for a variety of reasons. To find out why people smoke, the National Clearinghouse for Smoking and Health developed the simple Why Do You Smoke? Test. This test, contained in Activity 13.3, lists some statements by smokers describing what they get out of smoking cigarettes. Smokers are asked to indicate how often they have the feelings described in each statement when they are smoking.

The scores obtained on this test assess smokers for each of six factors that describe individuals' feelings when they smoke. The first three highlight the positive feelings that people derive from smoking. The fourth factor relates to reducing tension and relaxing. The fifth reveals the extent of dependence on cigarettes. The sixth factor differentiates habit smoking and purely automatic smoking. Each of the remaining factors fits one of the six reasons for smoking discussed next. A score of 11 or above on any factor indicates that smoking is an important source of satisfaction for you. The higher you score (15 is the highest), the more important a given factor is in your smoking, and the more useful a discussion of that factor can be in your attempt to quit.

If you do not score high on any of the six factors, chances are that you do not smoke much or have not been smoking for long. If so, giving up smoking, and staying off, should be easier.

1. *Stimulation.* If you score high or fairly high on the stimulation factor, you are among those smokers stimulated by the cigarette. You think it helps wake you up, organize your energies, and keep you going. If you try to give up smoking, you may want a safe substitute—a brisk walk or moderate exercise, for example—whenever you feel the urge to smoke.
2. *Handling.* Handling things can be satisfying, but you can keep your hands busy in many ways without lighting up or playing with a cigarette. Why not toy with a pen or pencil? Try doodling. Play with a coin, a piece of jewelry, or some other harmless object.
3. *Pleasure.* Finding out whether you use the cigarette to feel good—you get real, honest pleasure from smoking—or to keep from feeling bad (factor 4) is not always easy. About two-thirds of smokers score high or fairly high on accentuation of pleasure, and about half of those also score as high or higher on reduction of negative feelings. Those who get real pleasure from smoking often find that honest consideration of the harmful effects of their habit is enough to help them quit. They substitute social and physical activities and find that they do not seriously miss cigarettes.
4. *Crutch: Tension Reduction.* Many smokers use cigarettes as a crutch during moments of stress or discomfort. Ironically, the heavy smoker—the person who tries to handle severe personal problems by smoking many times a day—is apt to discover that cigarettes do not help deal with problems effectively. This kind of smoker may stop smoking readily when everything is going well but may be tempted to start again in a time of crisis. Again, physical exertion or social activity may be a useful substitute for cigarettes, especially in times of tension.
5. *Craving: Psychological Addiction.* Quitting smoking is difficult for people who score high on this factor. The craving for a cigarette begins to build the moment the previous cigarette is put out, so tapering off is not likely to work. Such smokers must go **cold turkey**. If you are dependent on cigarettes, you might try smoking more than usual for a day or two to spoil your taste for cigarettes and then isolating yourself from cigarettes until the craving is gone.

---GLOSSARY---

Cold turkey Eliminating a negative behavior all at once.

6. *Habit.* If you are smoking from habit, you no longer get much satisfaction from cigarettes. You light them frequently without even realizing you are doing it. You may have an easy time quitting and staying off if you can break the habitual patterns you have built up. Cutting down gradually may be effective if you change the way you smoke cigarettes and the conditions under which you smoke them. The key to success is to become aware of each cigarette you smoke. You can do this by asking yourself, "Do I really want this cigarette?" You might be surprised at how many you do not want.

13.8　*How to Quit*

Even though giving up smoking is not easy, it is by no means impossible, as attested by the many people who have quit. During the past four decades, cigarette smoking in the United States has declined gradually among smokers of all ages.

In 1964 (when the U.S. Surgeon General first reported the link between smoking and increased risk for disease and mortality), 40 percent of the adult population—53 percent of men and 32 percent of women—smoked. Today, only 25.6 percent of adult men and 20.4 percent of adult women smoke. Almost 50 million Americans have given up cigarettes, and more than 91 percent have been able to do it on their own, either by quitting cold turkey or by using self-help kits from organizations such as the American Cancer Society, the AHA, and the American Lung Association. Smokers' information and treatment centers can be readily found online.

Do You Want to Quit? Test

A person's sincere desire to quit is the most important factor in quitting successfully. Surveys have shown that approximately 70 percent of all smokers would like to quit. Although a few light or casual smokers can quit easily, for heavy smokers, quitting is typically a difficult battle that will take several attempts. Annually, only about 20 percent of smokers who try to quit the first time succeed. Even though many do not succeed the first time, the odds of quitting are better for those who repeatedly try to stop.

If you are a smoker and want to find how ready you are to quit, the Do You Want to Quit? Test, developed by the National Clearinghouse for Smoking and Health and contained in Activity 13.4, will measure your attitude toward the four primary reasons you want to quit smoking. The results indicate whether you are ready to start the program. On this test, the higher you score in any category, say, the Health category, the more important that reason is to you. A score of 9 or above in one of these categories indicates that this is one of the most important reasons you may want to quit.

1. *Health.* Many people have successfully stopped smoking after learning about the harmful consequences of cigarettes. If your score on the Health factor is 9 or above, the health hazards of smoking may be enough to make you want to quit now. If your score on this factor is low (6 or below), consider learning more about the added risk of disease and premature death that come from smoking.

2. *Example.* Some people stop smoking because they want to set a good example for others. Parents quit to make it easier for their children to resist starting to smoke. Doctors quit so that they can be role models for their patients. Teachers quit to discourage their students from smoking. Sports stars want to set an example for their young fans. Husbands quit to influence their wives to quit, and vice versa. Examples have a significant influence on behavior. Surveys show that almost twice as many high school students smoke if both parents are smokers compared with those whose parents are nonsmokers or former smokers. If your score is low (6 or lower), consider how important your example could be to others.

3. *Aesthetics.* People who score high (9 or above) in this category recognize and are disturbed by some of the unpleasant aspects of smoking. The smell of stale smoke on your clothing, bad breath, and stains on your fingers and teeth might be reason enough to consider quitting.

4. *Mastery.* If you score 9 or above on this factor, you are bothered by knowing that you cannot control your desire to smoke. You are not your own master. Awareness of this challenge to your self-control may make you want to quit.

Seven Steps to Break the Habit

Use the following seven-step plan as a guide to help you quit smoking. You should complete the total program in four weeks or less. Steps 1 through 4 combined should take no longer than two weeks. A maximum of 2 additional weeks is allowed for the rest of the program.

Step 1

Decide positively that you want to quit. Avoid negative thoughts of how difficult this can be. Think positive. You can do it.

Now prepare a list of the reasons you smoke and the reasons you want to quit (see Activity 13.5). Make several copies of the list, and keep them in places where you commonly smoke. Frequently review the reasons for quitting, because this will motivate and prepare you psychologically to quit.

When the reasons for quitting outweigh the reasons for smoking, you will have an easier time quitting. Read as much information as possible on the detrimental effects of tobacco and the benefits of quitting.

Step 2

Initiate a personal diet and exercise program. About one-third of the people who quit smoking gain weight. This could be caused by one or a combination of the following reasons:

1. Food becomes a substitute for cigarettes.
2. Appetite increases.
3. Basal metabolism may slow.

If you start an exercise and weight-control program prior to quitting smoking, weight gain should not be a problem. If anything, exercise and lower body weight create more awareness of healthy living and strengthen the motivation for giving up cigarettes.

Even if you gain some weight, the harmful effects of cigarette smoking are much more detrimental to human health than a few extra pounds of body weight. Experts have indicated that as far as the extra load on the heart is concerned, giving up one pack of cigarettes a day is the equivalent of losing between 50 and 75 pounds of excess body fat.

Step 3

Decide on the approach you will use to stop smoking. You may quit cold turkey or gradually cut down the number of cigarettes you smoke daily. Base your decision on your scores obtained on the Why Do You Smoke? Test. If you score 11 points or higher in either the Crutch: Tension Reduction or the Craving: Psychological Addiction category, your best chance for success is quitting cold turkey. If your highest scores occur in any of the other four categories, you may choose either approach.

People still argue about which approach is more effective. Quitting cold turkey may cause fewer withdrawal symptoms than tapering off gradually. When you are cutting down slowly, the fewer cigarettes you smoke, the more important each one becomes. Therefore, you have a greater chance for relapse and returning to the original number of cigarettes you smoked. But when the cutting-down approach is accompanied by a definite target date for quitting, the technique has been shown to be quite effective. Smokers who taper off without a target date for quitting are the most likely to relapse.

Step 4

Keep a daily log of your smoking habit for a few days. This will help you understand the situations that trigger your desire to smoke. Make copies of Activity 13.6 or develop your own form to keep with you, and every time you smoke, record the required information. Keep track of the number of cigarettes you smoke, times of day you smoke them, events associated with smoking, amount of each cigarette smoked, and a rating of how badly you needed that cigarette. Rate each cigarette from 1 to 3:

1 = desperately needed
2 = moderately needed
3 = no real need

This daily log will assist you in three ways:

1. You will get to know your habit.
2. It will help you eliminate cigarettes you do not crave.
3. It will help you find positive substitutes for situations that trigger your desire to smoke.

Step 5

Set the target date for quitting. If you are going to taper off gradually, read the instructions in the "Cutting Down Gradually" section before you proceed to step 6. When you set the target date, choose a special date to add extra incentive. An upcoming birthday, anniversary, vacation, graduation, family reunion—all are examples of good dates to free yourself from smoking. Dates when you are going to be away from events and environments that trigger your desire to smoke may be especially helpful. Once you have set the date, don't allow anyone or anything to interfere with this date.

Let your friends and relatives know of your intentions and ask for their support. Consider asking someone else to quit with you. That way, you can support each other in your efforts to stop. Avoid anyone who will not support you in your effort to quit. When you are attempting to quit, other people can be a prime obstacle. Many smokers are intolerable when they first stop smoking, so some friends and relatives prefer that they continue to smoke.

Step 6

Stock up on low-calorie foods—carrots, broccoli, cauliflower, celery, popcorn (butter and salt free), fruits, sunflower seeds (in the shell), sugarless gum, and so on—and drink plenty of water. Keep the food handy on the day you stop and the first few days following cessation. Substitute this food for a cigarette when you want one.

Step 7

Do not keep cigarettes handy. Stay away from friends and events that trigger your desire to smoke, and drink a lot of water and fruit juices. To replace the old behavior with new behavior, replace smoking time with new, positive substitutes that make smoking difficult or impossible.

When you want a cigarette, take a few deep breaths and then occupy yourself by doing any of a number of things, such as talking to someone else, washing your hands, brushing your teeth, eating a healthy snack, chewing on a straw, doing dishes, playing sports, going for a walk or a bike ride, or going swimming. Engage in activities that require the use of your hands. Try gardening, sewing, writing letters, drawing, doing household chores, or washing the car. Visit nonsmoking places such as libraries, museums, stores, and theaters. Plan an outing or a trip away from home. Any of these activities can keep your mind off cigarettes. Record your choice of activity or substitute under the Remarks/Substitutes column in Activity 13.6.

Activity 13.3   "Why Do You Smoke?" Test

Name _____ Date _____

Course _____ Section _____ Gender _____ Age _____

	Always	Fre-quently	Occa-sionally	Seldom	Never
A. I smoke cigarettes to keep myself from slowing down.	5	4	3	2	1
B. Handling a cigarette is part of the enjoyment of smoking it.	5	4	3	2	1
C. Smoking cigarettes is pleasant and relaxing.	5	4	3	2	1
D. I light up a cigarette when I feel angry about something.	5	4	3	2	1
E. When I have run out of cigarettes, I find it almost unbearable until I can get them.	5	4	3	2	1
F. I smoke cigarettes automatically without even being aware of it.	5	4	3	2	1
G. I smoke cigarettes for stimulation, to perk myself up.	5	4	3	2	1
H. Part of the enjoyment of smoking a cigarette comes from the steps I take to light up.	5	4	3	2	1
I. I find cigarettes pleasurable.	5	4	3	2	1
J. When I feel uncomfortable or upset about something, I light up a cigarette.	5	4	3	2	1
K. I am very much aware of the fact when I am not smoking a cigarette.	5	4	3	2	1
L. I light up a cigarette without realizing I still have one burning in the ashtray.	5	4	3	2	1
M. I smoke cigarettes to give me a "lift."	5	4	3	2	1
N. When I smoke a cigarette, part of the enjoyment is watching the smoke as I exhale it.	5	4	3	2	1
O. I want a cigarette most when I am comfortable and relaxed.	5	4	3	2	1
P. When I feel "blue" or want to take my mind off cares and worries, I smoke cigarettes.	5	4	3	2	1
Q. I get a real gnawing hunger for a cigarette when I haven't smoked for a while.	5	4	3	2	1
R. I've found a cigarette in my mouth and didn't remember putting it there.	5	4	3	2	1

Scoring Your Test:

Enter the numbers you have checked on the test questions in the spaces provided below, putting the number you have circled to question A on line A, to question B on line B, and so on. Add the three scores on each line to get a total for each factor. For example, the sum of your scores over lines A, G, and M gives you your score on "Stimulation"; lines B, H, and N give the score on "Handling." Scores can vary from 3 to 15. Any score 11 and above is high; any score 7 and below is low.

A [_____] + G [_____] + M [_____] = [_____] Stimulation
B [_____] + H [_____] + N [_____] = [_____] Handling
C [_____] + I [_____] + O [_____] = [_____] Pleasure/Relaxation
D [_____] + J [_____] + P [_____] = [_____] Crutch: Tension Reduction
E [_____] + K [_____] + Q [_____] = [_____] Craving: Psychological Addiction
F [_____] + L [_____] + R [_____] = [_____] Habit

From *A Self-Test for Smokers*, U.S. Department of Health and Human Services, 1983.

© Fitness & Wellness, Inc.

MINDTAP From Cengage   **Complete This Online**
Visit **www.cengagebrain.com** to access MindTap, a complete digital course that includes interactive quizzes, videos, and more.

Activity 13.4	"Do You Want to Quit?" Test

Name _____ Date _____

Course _____ Section _____ Gender _____ Age _____

	Strongly Agree	Mildly Agree	Mildly Disagree	Strongly Disagree
A. Cigarette smoking might give me a serious illness.	4	3	2	1
B. My cigarette smoking sets a bad example for others.	4	3	2	1
C. I find cigarette smoking to be a messy kind of habit.	4	3	2	1
D. Controlling my cigarette smoking is a challenge to me.	4	3	2	1
E. Smoking causes shortness of breath.	4	3	2	1
F. If I quit smoking cigarettes, it might influence others to stop.	4	3	2	1
G. Cigarettes cause damage to clothing and other personal property.	4	3	2	1
H. Quitting smoking would show that I have willpower.	4	3	2	1
I. My cigarette smoking will have a harmful effect on my health.	4	3	2	1
J. My cigarette smoking influences others close to me to take up or continue smoking.	4	3	2	1
K. If I quit smoking, my sense of taste or smell will improve.	4	3	2	1
L. I do not like the idea of feeling dependent on smoking.	4	3	2	1

How to Score: (See page 508, "Do You Want to Quit?" Test, to interpret your results.)

Write the number you have checked after each statement on the test in the corresponding space to the right. Add the scores on each line to get your totals. For example, the sum of your scores A, E, and I gives you your score for the Health factor. Scores can vary from 3 to 12. Any score of 9 or over is high; any score 6 or under is low.

A [_____] + E [_____] + I [_____] = [_____] Health

B [_____] + F [_____] + J [_____] = [_____] Example

C [_____] + G [_____] + K [_____] = [_____] Aesthetics

D [_____] + H [_____] + L [_____] = [_____] Mastery

From *A Self-Test for Smokers,* U.S. Department of Health and Human Services, 1983.

© Fitness & Wellness, Inc.

MINDTAP From Cengage **Complete This Online**
Visit **www.cengagebrain.com** to access MindTap, a complete digital course that includes interactive quizzes, videos, and more.

Activity 13.5 Reasons for Smoking Versus Quitting

Name _____ Date _____

Course _____ Section _____ Gender _____ Age _____

Make several copies of this list and keep them in places where you commonly smoke. Frequently review the reasons for quitting to help motivate and prepare you psychologically to quit.

Reasons for Smoking Cigarettes

1. _____
2. _____
3. _____
4. _____
5. _____
6. _____
7. _____
8. _____
9. _____
10. _____

Reasons for Quitting Cigarette Smoking

1. _____
2. _____
3. _____
4. _____
5. _____
6. _____
7. _____
8. _____
9. _____
10. _____

© Fitness & Wellness, Inc.

Activity 13.6　Daily Cigarette Smoking Log

Name _____ **Date** _____

Course _____ **Section** _____ **Gender** _____ **Age** _____

> Make copies of this form. Keep one copy with you every day and, every time you smoke, record the required information. This log will help you get to know your habit, eliminate cigarettes you really do not crave, and find positive substitutes for situations that trigger your desire to smoke.

Today's Date: _____ **Quit Date:** _____ **Decision Date:** _____

Cigarettes to be smoked today: _____ **Brand:** _____

No.	Time	Activity	Amount Smoked[a]	Rating[b]	Remarks/Substitutes
1.					
2.					
3.					
4.					
5.					
6.					
7.					
8.					
9.					
10.					
11.					
12.					
13.					
14.					
15.					
16.					
17.					
18.					
19.					
20.					

[a]Amount smoked: entire cigarette, two thirds, half, etc.
[b]Rating:　1 = desperately needed, 2 = moderately needed, 3 = no real need

Additional comments, list of friends and/or activities to avoid. Continue on a separate sheet of paper as needed.

_____
_____
_____
_____
_____

© Fitness & Wellness, Inc.

MINDTAP From Cengage　**Complete This Online**
Visit **www.cengagebrain.com** to access MindTap, a complete digital course that includes interactive quizzes, videos, and more.

HOEGER KEY TO WELLNESS

The U.S. Surgeon General has identified that the nation's current top health goals are exercise, increased consumption of fruits and vegetables, *smoking cessation*, and the practice of safe sex.

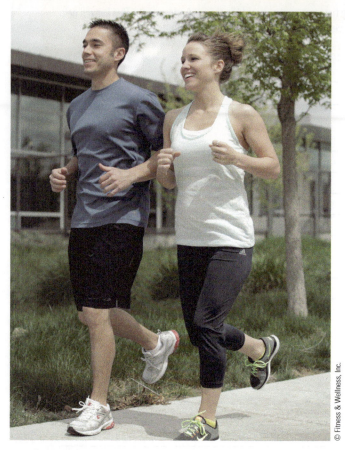

© Fitness & Wellness, Inc.

Starting an exercise program prior to giving up cigarettes encourages cessation and helps with weight control during the process.

Quitting Cold Turkey

Many people have found that quitting all at once is the easiest way to stop smoking. Most smokers have tried this approach at least once. Even though it might not work the first time, they don't allow themselves to get discouraged, and they eventually succeed. Many times, after several attempts, all of a sudden they are able to overcome smoking without too much difficulty.

On average, as few as three smokeless days are sufficient to break the physiological addiction to nicotine. The psychological addiction may linger for years but will get weaker as time goes by.

Cutting Down Gradually

Tapering off cigarettes can be done in several ways:

1. Eliminate cigarettes you do not strongly crave (those ranked 3 and 2 on your daily log).

2. Switch to a brand lower in nicotine, tar, or both every few days.
3. Smoke less of each cigarette.
4. Smoke fewer cigarettes each day.

Most people prefer a combination of these four suggestions.

Before you start cutting down, set a target date for quitting. Once the date is set, don't change it. The total time until your quit date should be no longer than 2 weeks. Reduce the total number of cigarettes you smoke each day by 10 to 25 percent. As you smoke less, be careful not to take more puffs or inhale more deeply as you smoke, because this offsets the principle of cutting down.

As an aid in tapering off, make several copies of Activity 13.6. By now, you should have completed the first daily log of your smoking habit—see step 4 under "Seven Steps to Break the Habit" on pages 508–509. Start a new daily log, and every night review your data and set goals for the following day.

Decide and record which cigarettes will be easiest to give up, what brand you will smoke, the total number of cigarettes to be smoked, and how much of each you will smoke. Log any comments or situations you want to avoid, as well as any substitutes you could use to help you in the program. For example, if you always smoke while drinking coffee, substitute juice for coffee. If you smoke while driving, arrange for a ride or take a bus to work. If you smoke with a certain friend at lunch, avoid having lunch with that friend for a week or so. Continue using this log until you have stopped smoking completely.

Nicotine-Substitution Products

Nicotine-substitution drug products such as nicotine transdermal patches and nicotine gum were developed to help people kick the tobacco habit. These products are thought to be most effective when used in a physician-supervised cessation program. As with tapering off, these products gradually decrease the amount of nicotine used until their users no longer crave the drug.

Nicotine Patches

Nicotine patches supply a steady dose of nicotine through the skin. According to a nicotine-replacement patch website, the program consists of a 10-week plan with three levels of nicotine patches. The person is asked to stop smoking before beginning the program; otherwise, the individual ends up with a very high blood nicotine level. A 21-mg patch is used during the first 6 weeks of the program, followed by a 14-mg patch for 2 weeks, and a final 7-mg patch for the last 2 weeks. The intent is to simulate a gradual weaning from the nicotine with fewer side effects. The instructions are specific, and the individual must carefully follow the instructions for the program to be effective. The site is clear that the program only works if the person is committed to quit the habit because the patch does not override the mind.

At present, evidence shows that patches are not more effective for quitting smoking than doing so without patches. However, one study showed that patches are more effective when used in conjunction with exercise.[22] About eight out of ten smokers who exercised along with the use of nicotine-replacement therapy successfully quit smoking.

Nicotine-replacement patches are available in various dosages, delivering anywhere from about 5 to 21 mg of nicotine in a 24-hour period. The retail cost for a 10-week program ranges from $100 to $200, significantly cheaper than smoking a pack a day for 10 weeks. Public safety concerns regarding the use of nicotine patches, including indications, precautions, warnings, contraindications, potential abuse, and marketing and labeling issues, are monitored and regulated by the FDA. People contemplating their use should pay careful attention to contraindications and potential side effects. Pregnant and lactating women and people with heart disease or high blood pressure or who have had a recent heart attack should check with their physician prior to using nicotine-substitution products. Skin redness, swelling, or rashes are sometimes associated with the use of nicotine patches. Other undesirable side effects are listed on the label and should be monitored closely.

Electronic Cigarettes

Electronic cigarettes, more commonly known as e-cigarettes, personal vaporizers, or simply VP, were introduced to the U.S. market nearly a decade ago as alternative devices to simulate the act of tobacco smoking. The electronic inhaler heats up a liquid nicotine solution into an aerosol mist that smokers inhale. Although e-cigarettes don't produce secondhand smoke, they do produce secondhand vapor. Because the vapor can contain many of the same toxic chemicals found in cigarette smoke, there is a growing national trend to regulate the devices. E-cigarettes have been banned on aircrafts and in many cities and restaurants where traditional smoking is not allowed. E-cigarettes are marketed as safer alternatives because they have far fewer of the toxic chemical compounds found in cigarette smoke. The amount of nicotine an e-cigarette delivers depends on the strength of the liquid nicotine cartridge a smoker installs, which can contain nicotine comparable to light or ultra light cigarettes, or as much nicotine as regular cigarettes or more. Some cartridges also contain liquid without nicotine to help users continue to experience the sensation of smoking without the detrimental effects.

Though distributors are not allowed to market e-cigarettes as aids to smoking cessation, e-cigarettes are commonly being used as an alternative to nicotine patches and as aids to help reduce the frequency of smoking or replace traditional cigarettes. Some recent studies have found that e-cigarette use is actually linked to significantly *lower* rates of smoking cessation. The CDC reports that one-fifth of traditional-cigarette adult smokers had tried e-cigarettes. The real concern is that if smokers use both traditional and

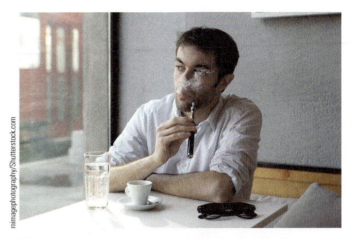

Electronic cigarettes, more commonly known as e-cigarettes, personal vaporizers, or simply VP, were introduced to the U.S. market in 2007 as alternative devices to simulate the act of tobacco smoking.

e-cigarettes, rather than using e-cigarettes to quit cigarettes completely, the health consequences could be exponentially greater.

The FDA warns of potential addiction and abuse of e-cigarettes, and in August 2016, officially restricted sales of e-cigarettes to minors under age 18. Nicotine can damage the developing brain of teens while also leading to addiction. Authorities also fear candy-flavored e-cigarettes may cause young people to use the devices as a "gateway" to conventional cigarettes. Federal surveys show that 17 percent of high school seniors currently use e-cigarettes, and teens are more likely to use e-cigarettes than traditional cigarettes.[23] In fact, the Surgeon General reported in 2016 that e-cigarette use among high school students had increased 900 percent from 2011 to 2016 to become the most commonly used form of tobacco among American youth, surpassing cigarettes, cigars, chewing tobacco, and hookahs.[24]

> **!**
> ### Critical Thinking
>
> If you ever smoked or now smoke cigarettes, discuss your perceptions of how others accepted your behavior. If you smoked and have quit, how did you accomplish the task, and has it changed the way others view you? If you never smoked, how do you perceive smokers?

13.9 *Life after Cigarettes*

When you first quit smoking, you can expect a series of withdrawal symptoms for a few days; among them are lower heart rate and blood pressure, headaches, gastrointestinal discomfort, mood changes, irritability, aggressiveness, and difficulty sleeping.

Figure 13.10 Benefits of quitting smoking.

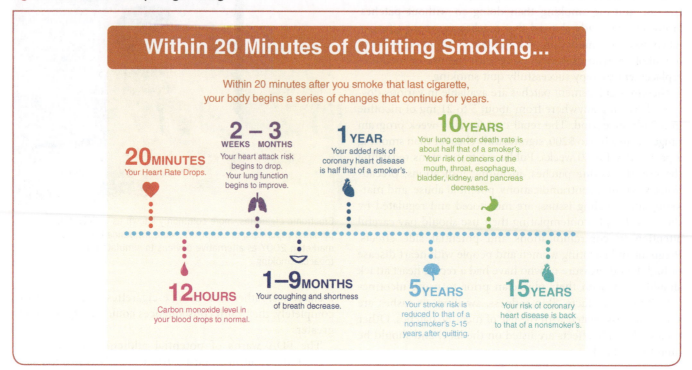

Within 20 Minutes of Quitting Smoking...

Within 20 minutes after you smoke that last cigarette, your body begins a series of changes that continue for years.

20 MINUTES
Your Heart Rate Drops.

2–3 WEEKS MONTHS
Your heart attack risk begins to drop. Your lung function begins to improve.

1 YEAR
Your added risk of coronary heart disease is half that of a smoker's.

10 YEARS
Your lung cancer death rate is about half that of a smoker's. Your risk of cancers of the mouth, throat, esophagus, bladder, kidney, and pancreas decreases.

12 HOURS
Carbon monoxide level in your blood drops to normal.

1–9 MONTHS
Your coughing and shortness of breath decrease.

5 YEARS
Your stroke risk is reduced to that of a nonsmoker's 5-15 years after quitting.

15 YEARS
Your risk of coronary heart disease is back to that of a nonsmoker's.

Don't let this discourage you! Know that the physiological addiction to nicotine is broken only 3 days following your last cigarette and the physical cravings will subside as time goes on.

For the habitual smoker, the psychological dependency could be the most difficult to break. The first few days probably will not be as difficult as the first few months. Any of the activities of daily life that you have associated with smoking—either stress or relaxation, joy or unhappiness—may trigger a relapse even months, or at times years, after quitting. To help break the psychological dependency, instead of thinking about how miserable you may feel without a cigarette, try the opposite: Think of the immediate health benefits you are experiencing from having quit the habit.

Enjoy Immediate Health Benefits

It is never too late to enjoy the improved health that comes with quitting cigarettes. The risk for premature death and illness starts to decrease the moment you stop smoking. You will have fewer sore throats and sores in the mouth, less hoarseness, no more cigarette cough, and a lower risk for peptic ulcers. Circulation to the hands and feet will improve, as will gastrointestinal and kidney and bladder functions.

The ex-smoker's risk for stroke approaches that of a lifetime nonsmoker 5 years following cessation (see Figure 13.10). Everything will taste and smell better. You will have more energy, and you will gain a sense of freedom, pride, and well-being. You no longer will have to worry whether you have enough cigarettes to last through a day, a party, a meeting, a weekend, or a trip.

Think of Yourself as a Non-Smoker

If you have been successful and stopped smoking, a lot of events can still trigger your urge to smoke. When confronted with these events, some people rationalize and think, "One cigarette won't hurt. I've been off for months (years in some cases)" or "I can handle it. I'll smoke just today." It won't work. Before you know it, you will be back to the habit. Be prepared to take action in those situations by finding substitutes, such as those provided in the "Tips to Help Stop Smoking" box that begins on page 517.

Start thinking of yourself as a nonsmoker—no "butts" about it. Remind yourself how difficult it has been and how long it has taken you to get to this point. If you have come this far, you certainly can resist brief moments of temptation. It will get easier as time goes on.

Behavior Modification Planning

Tips to Help Stop Smoking

Check the suggestions that may work for you and incorporate them into your own retraining program.

I PLAN TO

I DID IT

Preparing to Quit

❑ ❑ Create a personal list of reasons to quit. Keep the list handy, review it frequently, and add to it as needed.

❑ ❑ Know what to expect. Information is available from government sources, health organizations, doctors, hospitals, or on the web. Talk with people who have quit or contact a local group or a hotline.

❑ ❑ Review any past attempts to quit. Determine what worked and what didn't work for you.

❑ ❑ Get a physical examination and discuss your desire to quit smoking with your doctor. Ask whether medication may help you quit.

❑ ❑ Create a stop-smoking plan customized to your personality, preferences, and schedule. If you are tapering off, set intermediate goals. Make sure to plan for times of intense desire for a cigarette. Be prepared and determine what you can use as a substitute for that cigarette. Is there anyone you can call for assistance or to help you distract your mind? Do not forget to include rewards for your success. Sign a contract and ask a friend to sign it as a witness.

❑ ❑ Determine your quit day. Choose a special day, such as a birthday, an anniversary, or a holiday. Select a day on which you will not feel a strong temptation to smoke—for instance, a stressful work day. Once you pick a date, do not alter this date.

❑ ❑ Enlist the support of friends, loved ones, team members, coworkers—as many people as you can. Ask others not to smoke around you or leave cigarettes in view. If you can, find someone else who wants to quit with you.

❑ ❑ Inquire about counseling. Individual, group, and telephone counseling can improve your chances of success.

❑ ❑ Consider starting a weight loss and exercise program before you quit. Such positive action will increase your confidence in your ability to quit and can keep you from gaining weight when you stop smoking.

❑ ❑ Stage a farewell activity to cigarettes and smoking; perhaps by overindulging so that the idea of smoking is no longer appealing, or with a ceremony to destroy all cigarettes, lighters, and ashtrays.

❑ ❑ Change your environment. Clean your room or house, clothes, and car to remove the scent of tobacco smoke. Rearrange the furniture, paint the walls a different color, open windows to freshen the air, and buy plants or flowers.

❑ ❑ Plan changes in your routine. Reschedule regular activities, use different routes to get to places you normally go, go to bed earlier and get up earlier, avoid being rushed.

❑ ❑ Start a new hobby or other activity; for example, dancing, making videos, painting, acting, or learning to cook ethnic foods—something enjoyable that you've wanted to do for a long time.

❑ ❑ Stock up on healthy, low-calorie snacks.

While Tapering Off

❑ ❑ Make cigarettes as hard to get as possible. Leave them with someone else, lock them up, or wrap them up like gifts with lots of tape or ribbon.

❑ ❑ Don't store cigarettes—wait until one pack is finished before buying another.

❑ ❑ Never carry matches or a lighter.

❑ ❑ Each time you want to smoke, write down what you are doing and feeling and how important the cigarette is to you—before you light up.

❑ ❑ Smoke only in uninteresting or uncomfortable places.

❑ ❑ Put off the first cigarette of the day for as long as possible.

❑ ❑ Smoke just half a cigarette.

After Quitting

❑ ❑ To help prevent relapse, rather than saying "I quit smoking," say "I don't want to smoke."

❑ ❑ Get plenty of sleep.

❑ ❑ Eat regular, healthy, appetizing meals; pay attention to the flavors and textures of the foods.

❑ ❑ Be mindful of negative thoughts and replace them with positive actions—from "I can't stand this" to "What else can I do right now to keep my mind off cigarettes?" for example.

❑ ❑ Spend time in places where smoking is not allowed—libraries, museums, churches, malls, and movie theaters.

❑ ❑ Tune in to the sights and scents around you.

❑ ❑ Drink plenty of water and other low-calorie drinks (but avoid caffeine).

❑ ❑ Deal with 1 minute, 1 hour, and 1 day at a time.

❑ ❑ Plan something that will bring you pleasure every day.

❑ ❑ Be aware of life stressors and plan a variety of ways to relax without cigarettes.

(continued)

Behavior Modification Planning (continued)

- ❑ ❑ Avoid situations in which you used to smoke, including being with people who smoke.
- ❑ ❑ Be wary of alcohol: Drinking lowers your chances of success.
- ❑ ❑ Use your lungs more by increasing daily physical activity and sports participation. Try to notice how clean the air feels flowing in and out of your lungs.
- ❑ ❑ Celebrate and reward yourself for each success.
- ❑ ❑ Visit your dentist and have your teeth cleaned and whitened.
- ❑ ❑ Calculate how much money you are saving and use this money to reward yourself or someone else with a small luxury.
- ❑ ❑ Consult your doctor if you are concerned about your physical or emotional feelings.
- ❑ ❑ If you gain weight, don't attempt to lose the weight until after you get over the craving for cigarettes.

Instead of Smoking a Cigarette

- ❑ ❑ Take several deep breaths, focusing on your breathing and the fresh air that you are inhaling.
- ❑ ❑ Tell yourself to wait three minutes; redirect your thoughts by visualizing a serene landscape or planning a dream vacation or weekend away from home.
- ❑ ❑ Go for a walk. If you have a dog, take the dog for a walk.
- ❑ ❑ Chew gum or suck on hard, sugarless candy—always carry some with you.

- ❑ ❑ Talk to someone you can easily reach for support.
- ❑ ❑ Munch on carrots, celery sticks, or other healthy snacks.
- ❑ ❑ Use your hands: wash dishes, sweep the floor, brush your teeth, write in a journal, sketch a cartoon, play a musical instrument.
- ❑ ❑ Go swimming or take a shower.

If You Relapse

- ❑ ❑ Don't be discouraged—most people try several times before they are finally able to kick the habit.
- ❑ ❑ Instead of berating yourself, remember your successes and recommit to quitting.
- ❑ ❑ Re-evaluate your smoking-cessation plan and modify it as necessary.
- ❑ ❑ Remember that relapse doesn't mean failure. Failure comes to those who give up. Instead, learn from your mistake and reach once more for your goal.

Try It

Nicotine is believed to be the most addictive drug we know. Smokers who are trying to kick the habit need behavioral change strategies to enhance their rate of success. From the above strategies, prepare a list of those that may work for you. Conduct nightly audits on how well you have done that day. Every third day, review all of the above strategies and make changes to your list as necessary.

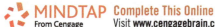 **Complete This Online**
Visit **www.cengagebrain.com** to access MindTap, a complete digital course that includes interactive quizzes, videos, and more.

Assess Your Behavior

1. Is your life free of addictive behavior? If not, will you commit right now to seek professional help at your institution's counseling center? Addictive behavior destroys health and lives— don't let it waste yours.

2. Are you prepared to walk away, even at the peril of losing close friendships and relationships, if you are put in a situation in which you are pressured to drink, smoke, or engage in any other form of drug (legal or illegal) abuse?

Assess Your Knowledge

1. Which of the following substances is not an object of chemical dependency?
   a. Ecstasy
   b. Alcohol
   c. Cocaine
   d. Heroin
   e. All choices are objects of chemical dependency.

2. The most widely used illegal drug in the United States is
   a. marijuana.
   b. alcohol.
   c. cocaine.
   d. heroin.
   e. Ecstasy.

3. Cocaine use
   a. causes lung cancer.
   b. leads to atrophy of the brain.
   c. can lead to sudden death.
   d. causes amotivational syndrome.
   e. All of the choices are correct.

4. Methamphetamine
   a. is less potent than amphetamine.
   b. increases fatigue.
   c. helps a person relax.
   d. is a central nervous system stimulant.
   e. increases the need for sleep.

5. Ecstasy
   a. is currently only popular among teenagers.
   b. is a relatively harmless drug.
   c. is used primarily by African American males.
   d. increases heart rate and blood pressure.
   e. All of the choices are correct.

6. Treatment of chemical dependency is
   a. accomplished primarily by the individual alone.
   b. most successful when there is peer pressure to stop.
   c. best achieved with the help of family members.
   d. seldom accomplished without professional guidance.
   e. usually done with the help of friends.

7. Cigarette smoking is responsible for about ___ deaths in the United States each year.
   a. 12,000
   b. 87,000
   c. 255,000
   d. 480,000
   e. 850,000

8. Cigarette smoking increases death rates from
   a. heart disease.
   b. cancer.
   c. stroke.
   d. aortic aneurysm.
   e. All of the choices are correct.

9. The percentage of lung cancer attributed to cigarette smoking is
   a. 25 percent.
   b. 43 percent.
   c. 58 percent.
   d. 64 percent.
   e. 80 percent.

10. Smoking cessation results in
    a. a decrease in sore throats.
    b. improved gastrointestinal function.
    c. a decrease in risk for sudden death.
    d. a heightened sense of taste.
    e. All of the choices are correct.

Correct answers can be found at the back of the book.

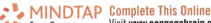 **Complete This Online**
Visit **www.cengagebrain.com** to access MindTap, a complete digital course that includes interactive quizzes, videos, and more.

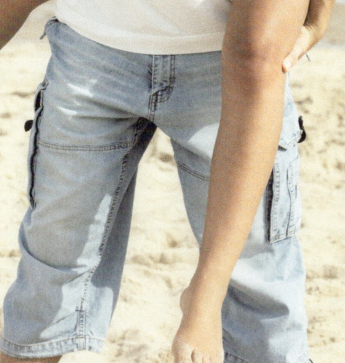

14

Preventing Sexually Transmitted Infections

Anyone who has unprotected sexual contact can acquire a sexually transmitted infection (STI). More than half of all Americans will be infected during their lifetime. Infections are most common among teens and young adults, with about half of all infections occurring in people younger than 25. One in four college students has had or has an STI. Multiple sex partners and unsafe sexual practices greatly increase the risk of acquiring an STI.

Objectives

14.1 **Name** and describe the most common sexually transmitted infections (STIs).

14.2 **Outline** the health consequences of STIs.

14.3 **Define** the difference between human immunodeficiency virus (HIV) and acquired immune deficiency syndrome (AIDS).

14.4 **Explain** the seriousness of the AIDS epidemic in the United States and worldwide.

14.5 **Describe** ways to prevent acquiring STIs.

14.6 **Evaluate** your risk of HIV/AIDS.

oliverong/Shutterstock.com

FAQ

What is the difference between a sexually transmitted infection (STI) and a sexually transmitted disease (STD)?

Health experts are beginning to replace the acronym STD with STI. The concept of disease implies a clear medical condition that manifests itself through signs or symptoms that define a specific disease. In terms of STIs, once infected, a person may or may not develop signs or symptoms indicative of disease. The unfortunate reality is that in the early stages of infection, many individuals with STIs exhibit no signs or symptoms or ones that are so mild that they are often ignored.

What is "safe" sex?

Safe sex means taking precautions during sexual intercourse or other forms of sexual contact that are designed to prevent the exchange of blood, semen, vaginal fluids, or breast milk and that can keep you or your partner from getting an STI. These infections include chlamydia, gonorrhea, syphilis, trichomoniasis, human papillomavirus (HPV)/genital warts, genital herpes, hepatitis, and human immunodeficiency virus (HIV). When unsure about your partner, use a lubricated latex condom from start to finish for each sexual act. If you think you should use a condom but your partner refuses to do so, say "no" to sex with that person. While a condom definitely reduces the risk for infection, you need to realize that, even with condom use, you may acquire an STI. Condoms may not totally cover surrounding infected areas, and sometimes they rupture.

How does HIV damage the immune system?

Upon HIV infection, the virus attacks and starts killing CD4 cells in the immune system. CD4 cells are a special type of white blood cell that fights off infections (viral, fungal, and parasitic). Initially, the body can make more CD4 cells to replace the cells damaged by HIV. Eventually, however, the body is unable to replace all damaged cells. As the number of CD4 cells decreases, the immune system weakens and the person is more susceptible to illness and infections, including the development of acquired immune deficiency syndrome (AIDS).

Am I at risk for contracting HIV in a medical or dental office?

Though there have been a few documented cases of patients becoming infected with HIV in a health care setting, these occurrences are extremely rare. All health care providers are required by law to implement strict anti-infection procedures to protect both patients and health professionals from any blood-borne illnesses like HIV. These universal precautions for infection control include disposing of all used needles, thorough hand washing, proper sterilization and disinfection of equipment before use with other patients, adequate facial protection through surgical masks and eyewear, and routine environmental cleaning of frequently touched surfaces. The implementation of highly sensitive HIV screenings by the U.S. Public Health Service has also dramatically reduced HIV transmission through blood transfusions since the 1980s, lowering the risk to about one in 1.5 million today. The CDC has also mandated that all organ donors be screened for HIV within a week of the donor operation.

REAL LIFE STORY | Annalisa's Experience

I started dating Seth my freshman year of college. He had sex before; I was a virgin. When we started sleeping together, he didn't really want to wear a condom, and I decided it wasn't necessary. After all, I was in love with him. Seth had never been tested for STIs, but I remember thinking, "He's on the cross-country team. Nobody who manages to run that many miles a week could possibly be sick or have a disease." However, it turned out that I was wrong—he was actually infected with chlamydia, and he passed it on to me. I was infected for several years before I found out. It wasn't until my senior year, when I took a health class and we were advised to get tested for STIs, that I learned I had chlamydia. During the time it had gone untreated, the disease did permanent damage to my reproductive system. I'll probably never be able to have kids now, and that was something I really wanted to do someday. Seth and I broke up not long after the diagnosis. Part of me was very angry and wanted to blame him for the whole thing, but the fact is, I had heard my whole life that you have to have "safe sex" and use a condom. Yet I made justifications for why that didn't apply to me. I made the wrong choice, and now I have to live with the results. As traumatic as it was for me to have chlamydia, the truth is that I was lucky. Because 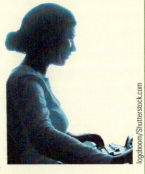 I engaged in unprotected sex, I could have contracted HIV. Then while everyone else was planning for graduation and their new lives, I would be worrying about dying of AIDS.

logoboom/Shutterstock.com

PERSONAL PROFILE: STIs Survey

I. Have you ever been screened for, diagnosed with, or treated for a sexually transmitted infection?

II. Are you aware of the primary ways STIs are transmitted, and which of more than 30 STIs are curable and incurable?

III. Can you explain the difference between HIV infection and AIDS?

IV. Do you understand the concept of "safe sex" and guidelines to follow to prevent STIs?

V. If you choose not to have sex, have you thought out an appropriate response in the event that you are asked or are pressured to have sex?

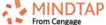

MINDTAP From Cengage **Complete This Online**
Visit **www.cengagebrain.com** to access MindTap, a complete digital course that includes interactive quizzes, videos, and more.

Based on estimates by the World Health Organization, more than 1 million people worldwide are infected daily with **sexually transmitted infections (STIs)**.[1] STIs have also reached epidemic proportions in the United States. According to the American Sexual Health Association, more than half of all Americans will acquire at least one STI in their lifetime.

Each year, about 20 million Americans are newly infected with STIs, half of which affect young people between the ages of 15 and 24 (see Figure 14.1).[2] Young people are most at risk because they are more likely to have multiple sex partners. According to estimates, one in four college students has had or has an STI. To avoid embarrassment, stigma, or concerns about confidentiality, young people are often reluctant to discuss their risky sexual behavior with a physician. Though the private nature of STIs makes people less willing to talk about them openly, early education about STI prevention and honest communication between sexual partners is crucial for both individual health and the health of the nation.

Though the infection rate is about the same among young men and young women, the health consequences of untreated STIs for women are more serious, including infertility. More than 20,000 women in the United States become infertile each year because of an STI they may not have even known they had.[3] Because the majority of STIs do not cause obvious symptoms, a person can have an STI that goes unnoticed for years. Most STIs do not cause significant harm, but if not diagnosed or treated early, some STIs can lead to

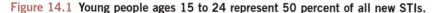

Figure 14.1 Young people ages 15 to 24 represent 50 percent of all new STIs.

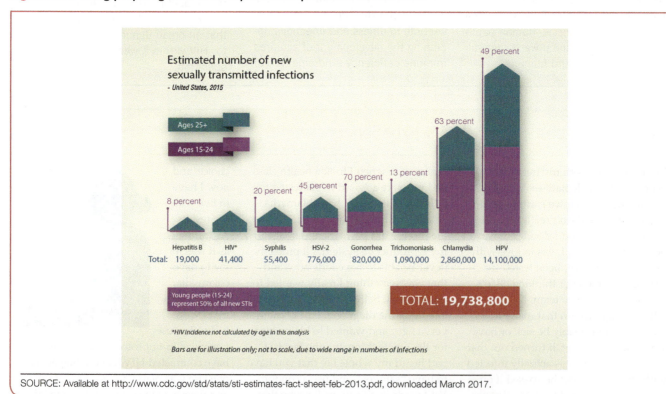

SOURCE: Available at http://www.cdc.gov/std/stats/sti-estimates-fact-sheet-feb-2013.pdf, downloaded March 2017.

Centers for Disease Control and Prevention's (CDC) STI Screening Recommendations

If you are sexually active, getting tested for STIs is one of the most important things you can do to protect your health. Make sure you have an open and honest conversation about your sexual history and STI testing with your doctor and ask whether you should be tested for STIs. If you are not comfortable talking with your regular health care provider about STIs, there are many clinics that provide confidential and free or low-cost testing. Here is a brief overview of STI testing recommendations.

- All adults and adolescents from ages 13 to 64 should be tested at least once for HIV.

- Annual chlamydia screening of all sexually active women younger than 25 years, as well as older women with risk factors such as new or multiple sex partners, or a sex partner who has a sexually transmitted infection.

- *Annual gonorrhea screening for all sexually active women younger than 25 years,* as well as older women with risk factors such as new or multiple sex partners, or a sex partner who has a sexually transmitted infection.

- *Syphilis, HIV, chlamydia, and hepatitis B screening for all pregnant women,* and gonorrhea screening for at-risk pregnant women starting early in pregnancy, with repeat testing as needed, to protect the health of mothers and their infants.

- *Screening at least once a year for syphilis, chlamydia, and gonorrhea for all sexually active gay, bisexual, and other men who have sex with men (MSM).* MSM who have multiple or anonymous partners should be screened more frequently for STIs (i.e., at 3- to 6-month intervals).

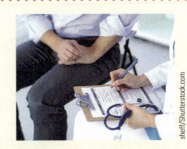

sheff/Shutterstock.com

- *Anyone who has unsafe sex or shares injection drug equipment should get tested for HIV at least once a year.* Sexually active gay and bisexual men may benefit from more frequent testing (e.g., every 3 to 6 months).

SOURCE: Available at https://www.cdc.gov/std/prevention /screeningreccs.htm, downloaded March 2017.

---

serious health problems, including cervical cancer, pelvic inflammatory disease, ectopic pregnancy, and an increased risk of HIV. As early detection is critical, the Centers for Disease Control and Prevention (CDC) has released general screening recommendations for all sexually active people.

14.1 *Types and Causes of Sexually Transmitted Infections*

Of the more than 30 known pathogens that are transmitted through sexual contact—including bacteria, parasitical organisms, fungi, protozoa, and viruses—eight are responsible for most STIs. Four of those eight infections are caused by bacteria and other parasitical organisms and can be readily treated and cured if diagnosed early: chlamydia, gonorrhea, syphilis, and trichomoniasis. The other four infections are caused by viruses and currently have no cure: human papillomavirus (HPV)/genital warts, genital herpes (HSV), hepatitis B (HBV), and human immunodeficiency virus (HIV). These viral infections are often referred to as the four "H"s.

14.2 *Four Most Common Bacterial STIs*

Currently, the United States has the highest rate of STIs of any country in the industrialized world. A press release from the CDC reported an unprecedented rise in all new cases of chlamydia, gonorrhea, and syphilis in 2015—the total number of cases representing the highest ever reported in the United States[4] The majority of new cases continue to disproportionately affect young people, women, and gay and bisexual men. Because STIs are preventable, early screening, education, and prevention methods are critical to reduce the number of new infections. Bacterial STIs can be readily treated and cured if diagnosed early and are often treated with antibiotics. The next section focuses on the symptoms, diagnosis, and treatments of the four most common bacterial STIs reported in the United States: chlamydia, gonorrhea, syphilis, and trichomoniasis.

Chlamydia

Chlamydia is a bacterial infection that spreads during vaginal, anal, or oral sex or from the vagina to a newborn baby during childbirth. It is the most commonly reported bacterial STI. In any given year, there may be as many as 2.86 million cases of chlamydia in the United States; however, a large number of cases go unreported because most people are unaware of their infection.[5] Sexually active young people are especially at risk. Among sexually active females aged 14 to 24, estimates show 1 in 20 has chlamydia.

GLOSSARY

Sexually transmitted infections (STIs) Communicable diseases spread through sexual contact.

Chlamydia An STI, caused by a bacterial infection, that can significantly damage the reproductive system. The most common bacterial STI in the United States.

Eight Most Common STIs

Bacterial/parasitical (can be cured)

- Chlamydia
- Gonorrhea
- Syphilis
- Trichomoniasis

Viral (known as the four "H"s—no current cure)

- HPV—human papillomavirus/genital warts
- HSV—genital herpes
- HBV—hepatitis B
- HIV—human immunodeficiency virus

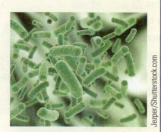

Jezper/Shutterstock.com

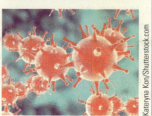

Kateryna Kon/Shutterstock.com

Symptoms

Chlamydia can seriously damage the reproductive system. This infection is considered a major factor in male and female infertility. Because symptoms are usually mild or absent, three out of four people with the infection don't know they're ill until the infection has become quite serious. Testing is frequently skipped because patients are mistreated for symptoms that mimic other STIs. Infertility often occurs "silently" because the individual is unaware of the infection until it is too late to prevent the irreversible damage. Symptoms of serious infection include abdominal pain, fever, nausea, vaginal bleeding, and arthritis.

Diagnosis and Treatment

The CDC recommends that sexually active women age 25 or younger be tested every year for chlamydia and that all women who are pregnant be tested at their first prenatal visit. Untreated chlamydia in pregnant women can lead to pre-term delivery, conjunctivitis, and pneumonia in the newborn baby. Chlamydia that goes untreated may also increase the chance of transmitting or acquiring HIV. Although chlamydia can be treated successfully with oral antibiotics, damage that may have occurred to the reproductive system is irreversible. Those treated for chlamydia should be tested again after 3 months, even if their sex partner was also treated, because it is common to be reinfected with chlamydia.

Gonorrhea

One of the oldest STIs, **gonorrhea** is the second most reported bacterial STI in the United States. Gonorrhea is transmitted through contact with the vagina, penis, anus, or mouth of an infected person. Mothers can also pass the infection to their babies during childbirth. According to the CDC, approximately 820,000 individuals get new gonorrheal infections each year in the United States, less than half of the cases are reported, and about 570,000 are in the 15 to 24 age group.[6]

Symptoms

Typical symptoms in men include a pus-like secretion from the penis and painful urination. In women, gonorrhea can be hard to detect and is often mistaken for bladder or vaginal infections. Infected women may have vaginal discharge, bleeding, and painful urination as well; however, most women with gonorrhea don't experience any symptoms until the infection has become fairly serious. At this stage, women can develop a fever, severe abdominal pain, and pelvic inflammatory disease (discussed next).

Diagnosis and Treatment

If untreated, gonorrhea can produce widespread bacterial infection, infertility, heart damage, and arthritis in men and women, as well as blindness in children born to infected women. Anyone experiencing genital discharge, sores, rash, or burning during urination should abstain from sex and be examined by a health care provider. If a person is diagnosed with gonorrhea, he or she should inform all recent sex partners (within the past 60 days) so they can be tested and treated.

At present, gonorrhea is treated with antibiotics, but these will not repair any damage already done. People treated for gonorrhea should return to be reevaluated if symptoms persist more than a few days because the infection is becoming more difficult to treat successfully. Gonorrhea has progressively developed antimicrobial resistance over the years and has now grown resistant to every drug used in treatment, including penicillin and several other antibiotics that had been successful previously. The CDC now recommends dual therapy medication (using two drugs) to treat gonorrhea and continues to combatively revise its treatment guidelines in response to widespread drug resistance in recent years. However, the latest CDC surveillance data report that it is "only a matter of time" before strains grow resistant to the few remaining antibiotic treatment options.[7]

Pelvic Inflammatory Disease

In the United States about 2.5 million women live with a condition known by the umbrella term **pelvic inflammatory disease (PID)**.[8] PID is not an STI but, rather, refers to complications resulting from STIs, especially chlamydia and gonorrhea. PID often develops when the STI spreads to the fallopian tubes, uterus, and ovaries. Sexually active women are at higher risk for developing PID—especially those younger than age 25, because the cervix is not yet fully matured, increasing the risk for STIs that lead to PID. The more sex partners a woman has, the greater the risk for PID.

Complications associated with PID typically include scarring and obstruction of the fallopian tubes (which may lead to infertility), ectopic pregnancies, and chronic pelvic pain. If a woman with PID becomes pregnant, she could have an ectopic (tubal) pregnancy, which destroys the embryo and can be fatal to the mother. Thousands of women in the United States become infertile each year as a result of PID.

Typical symptoms of PID are fever, nausea, vomiting, chills, spotting between menstrual periods, heavy bleeding during periods, and pain in the lower abdomen during sexual intercourse, between menstrual periods, or during urination. Many times, however, women do not know they have PID because these symptoms are not always present. PID is treated with antibiotics, bed rest, and sexual abstinence. Furthermore, surgery may be required to remove infected or scarred tissue or to repair or remove the fallopian tubes or uterus.

HOEGER KEY TO WELLNESS

 Many STIs have no symptoms and are often mistaken for other conditions. If you have been sexually active, consider being tested even if you or your partner don't appear infected. Certain STIs can be treated and cured before they do irreversible damage.

Syphilis

Syphilis is another common type of STI caused by bacterial infection. It is referred to as "the great imitator" because its signs and symptoms are often indistinguishable from those of other diseases.

Once on the verge of elimination, syphilis began reappearing as a public health threat in the last fifteen years. More than 74,000 new cases are reported each year.[9] The incidence is highest in men between 20 and 29 years of age, with over 80 percent of primary and secondary stage syphilis (see following discussion) cases occurring among men who have sex with men.

Symptoms

Syphilis is transmitted through direct contact with a syphilis sore during vaginal, anal, or oral sex. In the primary stage, between 10 and 90 days following infection (average of 21 days), a painless sore appears where the bacteria entered the body (sometimes multiple sores appear). A sore also can appear on the lips or in the mouth and can infect another person through kissing. This sore disappears on its own in 3 to 6 weeks. If untreated, the infection progresses to the secondary stage.

During the secondary stage, as the initial sore is healing or for several weeks thereafter, skin rashes and mucous membrane lesions appear. A rough, reddish-brown rash can be seen on the palms of the hands and the bottoms of the feet, although types of rashes can appear on other parts of the body. Additional sores may also appear within 6 months of the initial outbreak. Signs and symptoms of the secondary stage disappear with or without treatment. Untreated, the infection progresses into the latent stage.

A latent stage, during which the victim is not contagious, may last up to 30 years, lulling victims into thinking they are healed. During the last stage of the infection, some people develop paralysis, crippling, gradual blindness, heart disease, brain and organ damage, or dementia; others die as a direct result of the infection. Syphilis can also spread from an infected mother to her unborn baby in pregnancy and cause serious health issues in a developing fetus, including premature birth and stillbirth.

Diagnosis and Treatment

Syphilis is diagnosed by microscopic examination of material from a sore or through a simple blood test. One of the oldest known STIs, syphilis once killed its victims, but now penicillin and other antibiotics are used to treat it. A single injection of penicillin cures individuals who have been infected for less than a year. Additional treatments are necessary for people infected longer than a year. Antibiotics are also available for individuals allergic to penicillin. People infected with syphilis must abstain from sexual activity until all syphilis sores have disappeared. Sexual partners must be informed of potential infection so that they can seek treatment if necessary.

Trichomoniasis

Although not as well known as other STIs, **trichomoniasis** or "trich" is a very common STI caused by infection with a protozoan parasite called *Trichomonas vaginalis*. Although symptoms of the disease vary, most women and men who have the parasite cannot tell they are infected. It is considered the most common curable STI. About 3.7 million people in the United States are infected, about 70 percent do not have any signs or symptoms of infection, and the incidence is greater in women than men.

Symptoms

Presently, it is unknown why some people with the infection get symptoms while others don't. Most likely it is related to the person's age and overall health. Asymptomatic infected individuals can still pass the infection on to others.

Men with trichomoniasis can experience itching or irritation inside the penis, a burning sensation after urination or ejaculation, or discharge from the penis. Women may also feel itching or burning, redness or soreness of the genitals,

---

GLOSSARY

Gonorrhea An STI caused by a bacterial infection.

Pelvic inflammatory disease (PID) An infection of the female reproductive system caused primarily by chlamydia and gonorrhea.

Syphilis An STI caused by a bacterial infection.

Trichomoniasis An STI caused by a parasitical infection.

uncomfortable urination, or an unusual discharge that can be clear, white, yellowish, or greenish. Having trichomoniasis can make sex quite uncomfortable. Without treatment, the infection can last for months or even years. Trichomoniasis also increases the risk of getting or spreading other STIs. For example, trichomoniasis can cause genital inflammation that makes it easier to become HIV-infected or to pass the virus on to others.

Diagnosis and Treatment

Trichomoniasis can be cured with a single dose of prescription antibiotics, either metronidazole or tinidazole. Pregnant women can also be treated with these medications. Drinking alcohol within 24 hours of taking the medication can lead to uncomfortable side effects.

People who have been treated for trichomoniasis can get reinfected. About 20 percent of people get infected again within 3 months of antibiotic treatment. To avoid reinfection, be sure that all sex partners get treated as well, and do not engage in sexual activity until all of your symptoms have disappeared (about a week). See your physician if the symptoms return.

HOEGER KEY TO WELLNESS

Successful treatment of an STI does not guarantee immunity. After you have been treated and cured of an STI, be vigilant and always practice safe sex. It is common to be reinfected if your partner has not been treated.

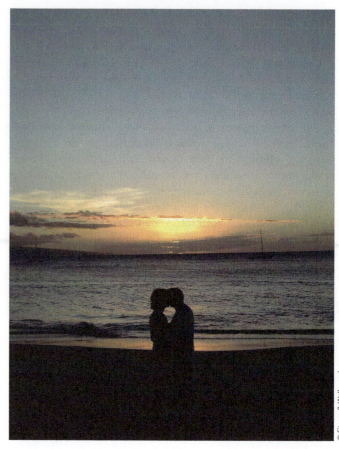

More than 30 infections are spread through sexual contact, and more than half of all Americans will have an STI at some point in their lifetime.

© Fitness & Wellness, Inc.

14.3 *Four Most Common Viral STIs*

This section focuses on the symptoms, diagnosis, and treatments of the four most common viral STIs reported in the United States: human papillomavirus (HPV)/genital warts, genital herpes (HSV), hepatitis B (HBV), and human immunodeficiency virus (HIV). These viral infections are often referred to as the four "H"s, and currently have no cure. HBV and HPV are the only two STIs that can be prevented if a person is vaccinated before being exposed to the virus, though for HIV, some evidence has shown that early antiretroviral drug therapy may help reduce the chance of infection even after exposure (see HIV treatment). Symptoms from all viral STIs can be alleviated with corresponding forms of treatment.

Human Papillomavirus (HPV) and Genital Warts

Human papillomavirus is the most common STI in the United States. There are more than 100 strains of HPV, and about 40 are sexually transmitted. "Low-risk" strains are wart causing, whereas "high-risk" are cancer causing. Some strains of HPV infect the genital area, including the skin of the penis, vulva, anus, lining of the vagina, cervix, and rectum, but they can also infect the mouth and throat as well. Others are known as "high-risk" types and can lead to cancers of the cervix, vulva, vagina, anus, or penis.

Approximately 14 million new cases of HPV are reported each year, and at least 79 million Americans are currently infected.[10] Most sexually active people acquire HPV infection during their lifetime. Infection is spread through genital or oral contact. Because most people have no signs or symptoms, they are unaware of the infection and can transmit the virus to a sex partner.

Symptoms

Most HPVs have no signs or symptoms, and the body's immune system clears them up within 2 years of infection without any form of treatment, while some forms persist. Presently, experts do not know why that is the case. When the body's immune system can't clear up a high-risk HPV infection, over time it turns normal cells into abnormal cells and subsequently cancer. Thirteen HPV types can cause cancer of the cervix; one of these types can cause cancers of the vulva, vagina, penis, and anus and certain head and neck cancers (specifically, the oropharynx, which includes the back of the throat, base of the tongue, and tonsils).

HPV is estimated to be responsible for more than 90 percent of cervical and anal cancers, 70 percent of oropharyngeal cancers, 70 percent of vaginal and vulvar cancers, and 60 percent of penile cancers.

One of the potential health problems associated with HPV is **genital warts**, which show up between weeks and months after exposure. These warts may be flat or raised and usually are found on the penis or around the vulva and the vagina. They also can appear in the mouth, throat, or rectum; on the cervix; or around the anus. Based on data from the CDC, about one in 100 sexually active adults have genital warts at any given time in the United States.

Health problems associated with genital warts include increased risk for cancers of the cervix, vulva, vagina, anus, and penis, and enlargement and spread of the warts, leading to obstruction of the urethra, vagina, and anus. Because babies born to infected mothers commonly develop warts over their bodies, cesarean section is recommended for childbirth.

Diagnosis and Treatment

Genital warts are usually diagnosed by an examination from a health care provider. Most women are diagnosed with HPV through an abnormal Pap test. Treatment requires completely removing all warts. This can be done by freezing them with liquid nitrogen, dissolving them with chemicals, or removing them through electrosurgery or laser surgery. Infected patients may have to be treated more than once because genital warts can recur.

Prevention of HPV infection is best accomplished through a mutually monogamous sexual relationship with an uninfected partner. It is difficult to know, however, if a person who has been sexually active in the past is currently infected.

HPV Vaccines Can Help Prevent Cervical Cancer

Two HPV vaccines, Gardasil and Cervarix, are available to prevent cervical cancer and other diseases caused by HPV. Both vaccines protect against HPV types 16 and 18, which cause most cervical cancers. Additionally, Gardasil protects against HPV types 6 and 11 and most genital warts. Gardasil 9 has been approved by the FDA to protect against an additional five strains of HPV (for a total of nine). Studies have shown Gardasil 9 to be up to 97 percent effective against those added HPV strains, which are associated with 20 percent of cervical cancers.[11]

The HPV vaccines have surpassed all expectations in terms of disease prevention and are considered "anti-cancer" vaccines. Since the introduction of the vaccines in 2006, vaccine-type HPV prevalence decreased 56 percent among female teenagers 14 to 19 years of age. According to CDC Director Tom Frieden, "This report shows that HPV vaccine works well, and the report should be a wake-up call to our nation to protect the next generation by increasing HPV vaccination rates. Unfortunately only one-third of girls aged 13 to 17 have been fully vaccinated with HPV vaccine. Countries such as Rwanda have vaccinated more than 80 percent of their teen girls. Our low vaccination rates represent 50,000 preventable

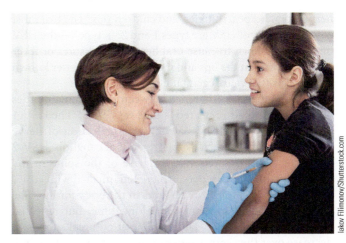

Over the past decade, vaccine-type HPV prevalence has decreased 56 percent among females aged 14 to 19 years.

Iakov Filimonov/Shutterstock.com

tragedies—50,000 girls alive today will develop cervical cancer over their lifetime that would have been prevented if we reach 80 percent vaccination rates. For every year we delay in doing so, another 4,400 girls will develop cervical cancer in their lifetimes."[12]

The CDC recommends that all boys and girls ages 11 or 12 years get vaccinated. To derive the benefits provided, a two-dose series of HPV vaccinations given at least six months apart is routinely recommended for 11- and 12-year-old girls and boys, and is highly recommended in a three-dose series for all teens and young adults between ages 15 and 26 if they did not receive all doses when they were younger.

To get the full benefits of the vaccine, people should get vaccinated before they become sexually active. The vaccines are most effective in women who have not been infected with any of the HPV types covered. Few women, however, are infected with all HPV types; thus, vaccination still offers protection against those viruses that have not been acquired. The vaccine has not been widely tested in people older than 26. Licensing for this group may become available if the vaccine proves to be safe and effective for the older age group as well.

Genital Herpes

One of the most common STIs, **genital herpes** is caused by the herpes simplex virus (HSV). There are several types of HSV that produce different ailments, including genital

---

GLOSSARY

Human papillomavirus (HPV) A group of viruses with strains that spread through sexual contact and can cause genital warts and several cancers; HPV can be prevented through vaccination.

Genital warts An STI caused by a viral infection of HPV.

Genital herpes An STI caused by a viral infection of HSV-1 or HSV-2. The virus can attack different areas of the body but typically causes blisters on the genitals.

herpes, oral herpes, shingles, and chicken pox. The two most common forms of HSV are types 1 and 2. In type 1—the HSV most often known to cause oral herpes—cold sores or fever blisters appear on the lips and mouth. HSV-2 is better known as the virus that causes genital herpes.

The fundamental difference between the two main types of HSV lies in their preferred "site of residence." The HSV-1 virus typically establishes latency in a collection of nerve cells near the ear known as the trigeminal ganglion. HSV-2 usually establishes latency at the base of the spine in the sacral ganglion. Once a person has been infected with either HSV-1 or HSV-2, the virus remains in the body for life. The virus can remain dormant for a long time, but repeated outbreaks are common. The number of outbreaks tends to decrease over the years. Excessive fatigue, stress, cold, wind, wetness, heat, sun, sweating, rubbing, chafing, and friction—as well as lack of sleep, illness, restrictive clothing, and diet—can precipitate new outbreaks. Some foods such as popcorn, coffee, peanuts, chocolate, and alcohol may trigger outbreaks.

Unknown to most people, HSV-1 also causes genital herpes, and an increasing number of cases of genital herpes caused by HSV-1 have been found worldwide. Approximately 100 million Americans older than the age of 12 are infected with HSV-1. Most of these individuals acquired the virus as children. By age 50, more than 80 percent of the population has been exposed to HSV-1. One out of six people 14 to 49 years old is infected with the type 2 virus.[13]

Symptoms

HSV is a highly contagious virus. Victims are most contagious during an outbreak, but the virus can also spread through virus-containing secretions. A few days following infection, a tingling sensation and lesions appear on the infected areas—most notably the mouth, genitals, and rectum—but can also surface on other parts of the body. Lesions can be somewhat painful.

Individuals infected with oral HSV-1 may shed the virus about 5 percent of the time, when they have no other symptoms of infection or visible lesions. Persons with asymptomatic HSV-2 infections can shed the virus up to 10 percent of days when they show no symptoms. At present, HSV-2 transmission most often occurs from an infected person who does not have a visible sore and may not even be aware of such an infection.

In conjunction with the lesions, victims usually have mild fever, swollen glands, and headaches. The symptoms disappear within a few weeks, causing some people to believe they are cured. Presently, though, herpes is incurable, and its victims remain infected for life.

Cold Sores/Fever Blisters Can Cause Genital Herpes

Society has typically labeled HSV-1 infection (cold sores) an "acceptable" viral infection, whereas infection with HSV-2 is viewed as a "bad" infection. The social stigma and emotional perspective of genital herpes make it difficult to objectively compare it with an oral infection, labeled as "just a cold sore" and acceptable to most people. HSV types 1 and 2, nonetheless, both cause oral and genital herpes. People who have an outbreak of oral herpes should not touch their own or someone else's genitals after touching the oral cold sores. Doing so can lead to a herpes infection of the genitals (genital HSV-1 infection). Oral sex can also result in transmission of HSV from the lips to the genitals. Thirty percent of *all new cases* of genital herpes result from HSV-1 infection.

This startling finding is a result of changing beliefs in what constitutes "safe" sex. The primary mode of HSV-1 transmission is by direct contact. College students assume that oral sex is safer and thus have vaginal intercourse and oral sex at about the same rate, giving HSV-1 a greater opportunity to spread.

> **!** **Critical Thinking**
>
> A "cold sore" or "fever blister" caused by an HSV-1 infection is highly contagious and can lead to the development of genital herpes either by direct contact through oral sex or if the person with the outbreak touches the sore and then his or her own or his or her partner's genitals. Thirty percent of genital herpes cases result from HSV-1 infection, and once infected, the virus remains in the body for life. What can you do to protect yourself, loved ones, and others from a wider spread of the virus?

The opposite is true as well: Oral sex with a genital HSV-2-infected person can cause oral HSV-2 infection (although there seems to be some degree of immunity against oral HSV-2 in people already infected with oral HSV-1). People with oral or genital sores should take care not to touch these sores. Following hand contact with cold or herpes sores, individuals should carefully wash themselves with soap. Avoid touching the eyes as such can cause vision damage as well.

During an outbreak, genital lesions may appear in areas that can be covered by a latex condom, but they can also appear in areas that cannot be covered. Use of a latex condom may protect against genital herpes only when the infected area is completely covered. Condoms, however, may not cover all infected areas. Thus, genital herpes infections still occur.

Diagnosis and Treatment

Blood tests are available to determine HSV infection. Individuals with HSV infection should abstain from sexual activity when lesions or other herpes symptoms are present. Sex partners of infected individuals should always be informed that they may become infected even if no lesions or symptoms are present. Though there is no cure for herpes, it is not life-threatening, and medications are available to help prevent outbreaks and relieve symptoms. The best preventive approach is a mutually monogamous sexual relationship with an uninfected partner.

Hepatitis

Hepatitis is a general term that means inflammation of the liver, but it also refers to a group of viruses (A, B, C, D, and E) that cause liver inflammation through infection. Viral hepatitis is the leading cause of liver cancer and the need for liver transplants. About 4.4 million Americans live with chronic hepatitis and don't know they are infected.

Hepatitis viruses spread through physical contact with the blood or bodily fluid of an infected person. Of the five viruses, B and C are the two most frequently transmitted through sexual activity, with hepatitis B being the most prevalent. Most people don't think of hepatitis as an STI; however, it is estimated that as much as 30 percent of infections result from sexual transmission.

Hepatitis B (HBV) is the world's most common liver infection, affecting 240 million people chronically worldwide. HBV is reported to be 50 to 100 times more infectious than HIV. Hepatitis B is transmitted when blood, semen, or other bodily fluid enters the body through kissing and vaginal, anal, or oral sex. HBV can also be passed from an infected mother to her baby during pregnancy or through blood contact via intravenous drug use, body piercings, and tattoos.

Symptoms

Hepatitis viruses travel through infected tissue into the blood and then to the liver, where they cause inflammation and cell damage. Hepatitis B can cause both acute and chronic liver inflammation. Only 50 percent of newly acquired infections produce symptoms, which include yellow coloration of the skin or eyes (jaundice), fever, abdominal pain, loss of appetite, tiredness, and nausea. The initial (acute) phase of infection lasts only a few weeks and then clears for the majority of people. Those who recover from the initial infection develop immunity to HBV, protecting them from future infection. Only a small number of people who do not recover from the infection develop chronic inflammation that can lead to disease, including cancer, in the liver.

Diagnosis and Treatment

Infection from HBV can be diagnosed by laboratory tests detecting the virus or antibodies against the virus in the blood. Hepatitis B is one of only two STIs that can be successfully prevented through vaccination. Since 1990, implementation of routine vaccination at birth has resulted in a drastic 82 percent decline in rates of acute hepatitis B, especially among children. The vaccine is administered in a three-dose series of injections to the muscle tissue of the shoulder over a period of months. It is recommended that all babies be vaccinated at birth, as well as at-risk groups, including sexually active men and women, illicit drug

users, health care workers, adoptees from countries where hepatitis B is common, international travelers, and welfare volunteers.

Critical Thinking

Many individuals who have STIs withhold this information from potential sexual partners. Do you think it should be considered a criminal action if an individual knowingly transmits an STI to someone else?

HIV and AIDS

Of all STIs, **human immunodeficiency virus (HIV)** infection is the most frightening because in most cases it is fatal and it has no known cure. **AIDS**—which stands for **acquired immune deficiency syndrome**—is the end stage of infection by HIV. In Activity 14.1, you have the opportunity to evaluate your basic understanding of HIV and AIDS.

HIV is a chronic infectious disease that is passed from one person to another through blood-to-blood and sexual contact. The virus spreads most commonly among individuals who engage in risky behavior, such as having unprotected sex or sharing hypodermic needles. When a person becomes infected with HIV, the virus multiplies, then attacks and destroys white blood cells. These cells are part of the immune system, and their function is to fight off infections and diseases in the body.

As the number of white blood cells that are killed increases, the body's immune system gradually breaks down or may be destroyed. Without an immune system, a person becomes susceptible to various **opportunistic infections** and to cancers.

Transmission of HIV

HIV is transmitted by the exchange of four body fluids, listed in order of highest concentration of the virus: blood, semen, vaginal secretions, and maternal milk. The concentration of HIV found in other body fluids including tears,

---

GLOSSARY

Hepatitis B (HBV) An STI caused by a viral infection that damages the liver and can be prevented through vaccination.

Human immunodeficiency virus (HIV) A virus that leads to acquired immune deficiency syndrome (AIDS).

Acquired immune deficiency syndrome (AIDS) Any of a number of diseases that arise when the body's immune system is compromised by HIV; the final stage of HIV infection.

Opportunistic infections Infections that arise in the absence of a healthy immune system, which would fight them off in healthy people.

Activity 14.1   Self-Quiz on HIV and AIDS

Name _____   Date _____

Course _____   Section _____   Gender _____   Age _____

> Indicate whether the following statements are true or false, then turn the page to see how well you understand HIV and AIDS.

	True	False
1. AIDS—acquired immune deficiency syndrome—is the end stage of infection caused by the human immuno-deficiency virus, HIV.	☐	☐
2. HIV is a chronic infectious disease that spreads among individuals who choose to engage in risky behavior such as unprotected sex or the sharing of hypodermic needles.	☐	☐
3. AIDS is completely curable.	☐	☐
4. Abstaining from sex is the only 100 percent sure way to protect yourself from HIV infection through sexual activity.	☐	☐
5. A person infected with HIV can look and feel healthy.	☐	☐
6. Condoms are 100 percent effective in protecting you against HIV infection.	☐	☐
7. Using drugs and alcohol makes a person less likely to use a condom and use it correctly.	☐	☐
8. If you're sexually active, latex condoms provide the best protection against HIV infection.	☐	☐
9. Using drugs and alcohol can make you more likely to have unplanned and unprotected sex.	☐	☐
10. A pregnant woman who has HIV can transmit the virus to her baby during childbirth.	☐	☐
11. You can become HIV-infected by donating blood.	☐	☐
12. HIV can be transmitted by spending time with or through casual contact (shaking hands, hugging) with an infected person.	☐	☐
13. The only means to determine whether someone has HIV is through an HIV antibody test.	☐	☐
14. HIV can completely destroy the immune system.	☐	☐
15. The HIV virus may live in the body 10 years or longer before AIDS symptoms develop.	☐	☐
16. People infected with HIV have AIDS.	☐	☐
17. HIV infection is preventable.	☐	☐
18. Early treatment can reduce the symptoms of HIV-infected people.	☐	☐
19. Drugs are now available that can lengthen the life of an HIV-infected person.	☐	☐
20. Antiretroviral drugs delay the progress of HIV infection and can keep many people from developing AIDS.	☐	☐

(continued)

Selected items on this questionnaire are adapted from *Test Your Survival Smarts: Self-Quiz on Drugs and AIDS*, National Institute on Drug Abuse, U. S. Department of Health & Human Services.

Activity 14.1 **Self-Quiz on HIV and AIDS** *(continued)*

Answers:

1. True. AIDS is the term used to define the manifestation of opportunistic diseases and cancers that occur as a result of HIV infection (also referred to as "HIV disease").

2. True. People do not get HIV because of who they are, but because of what they do. Almost all of the people who get HIV do so because they choose to engage in risky behaviors.

3. False. There is no cure for AIDS, although some medications are now available that delay the progress of HIV and keep some people from developing AIDS.

4. True. Abstinence will protect you from HIV infection. But you may still get the virus by sharing hypodermic needles.

5. True. The symptoms of HIV are often not noticeable until several years after a person has been infected. That's why—no matter who your partner is—it is important to always protect yourself against HIV and the risk of developing AIDS, either by abstaining from sex or by *always* practicing safe sex.

6. False. Only abstaining from sex gives you 100 percent protection, but condoms, if used correctly, are effective in protecting against HIV infection.

7. True. People who are drunk or high are less likely to use condoms because, under the influence, they forget or believe that nothing "bad" can happen.

8. True. Proper use is necessary to minimize the risk of infection, but condoms are not 100 percent foolproof as sometimes they break.

9. True. Otherwise-prudent people often act irrationally and engage in risky behaviors when they are under the influence of drugs and alcohol.

10. True. HIV transmission can occur between a pregnant woman and her baby during childbirth. A baby can also be infected through breastfeeding, although this occurs less frequently.

11. False. A myth regarding HIV is that it can be transmitted by donating blood. People cannot get HIV from giving blood. A brand-new needle is used by health professionals every time they draw blood. These needles are used only once and are destroyed and thrown away immediately after each individual has donated blood.

12. False. HIV is transmitted by the exchange of cellular body fluids, including blood and other body fluids containing blood, semen, vaginal secretions, and maternal milk. These fluids are most often exchanged during sexual intercourse, by using hypodermic needles previously used by infected individuals, or by contact with open wounds, cuts, or sores.

13. True. Not you, not a nurse, not even a doctor, can tell without an HIV antibody test. On HIV infection, the immune system's line of defense against the virus is the formation of antibodies that bind to the virus. On average it takes three months for the body to manufacture enough antibodies to show positive in an HIV antibody test. Sometimes it takes 6 months or longer.

14. True. The virus multiplies, then attacks and destroys white blood cells. These cells are part of the immune system, and their function is to fight off infections and diseases in the body. As the number of white blood cells killed increases, the body's immune system gradually breaks down or may be completely destroyed.

15. True. Ten years or longer may go by before the person develops AIDS.

16. False. Being HIV-positive does not necessarily mean that the person has AIDS. It may be 10 years or longer following infection before the individual develops the symptoms that fit the case definition of AIDS. From that point on, the person may live another two to three years. In essence, from the point of infection, the individual may endure a chronic disease for about 12 or more years.

17. True. The best prevention technique is abstaining from sex until the time comes for a mutually monogamous sexual relationship (two people having a sexual relationship only with each other). That one behavior will almost completely remove you from any risk of HIV infection or developing any other sexually transmitted disease.

18. True. The sooner treatment is initiated, the better the prognosis is for a longer life.

19. True. Available antiretroviral drugs can delay the progress of infection.

20. True. Antiretroviral drugs allow HIV infected individuals to live healthier and longer lives and even keep some people from developing AIDS. However, these drugs do not cure HIV or AIDS.

© Fitness & Wellness, Inc.

MINDTAP From Cengage **Complete This Online**
Visit **www.cengagebrain.com** to access MindTap, a complete digital course that includes interactive quizzes, videos, and more.

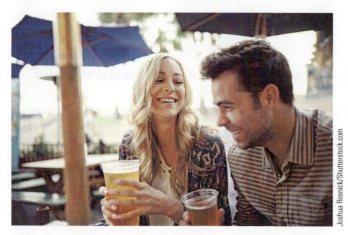

Stay sober in dating situations. Drug and alcohol use can impair your ability to make responsible choices regarding potential sexual activity.

sweat, feces, or urine is too minimal to be infectious. This means that it is virtually impossible to become infected with the virus through casual contact with a person infected with HIV. HIV cannot be transmitted by spending time with, shaking hands with, or hugging an infected person; from a toilet seat, dishes, or silverware used by an HIV patient; or by sharing a drink, food, a towel, or clothes with a person who has HIV. Because the virus can only live within body cells and fluids, once exposed to air, HIV cannot survive outside the body longer than a few minutes. The only way for HIV to be transmitted through skin-to-skin contact with a surface contaminated with infected bodily fluid is if it comes in direct contact with an access point into the bloodstream through an open cut or wound or through vaginal, anal, or oral sex.

Three Primary Routes of HIV Transmission

There are three primary routes that allow HIV transmission:

1. **Having unprotected vaginal, anal, or oral sex with an HIV-infected person.** Unprotected sex means having sex without using a condom properly. A person should select only latex (rubber or prophylactic) condoms that state "disease prevention" on the package. Although you might have unprotected sex with an infected person and not get the virus, you can get it by having unprotected sex only once with an infected individual.

   Rubbing during sexual intercourse often damages mucous membranes and causes unseen bleeding (even in the mouth). During vaginal, anal, or oral sexual contact, infected blood, semen, or vaginal fluids can penetrate the mucous membranes that line the vagina, the penis, the rectum, the mouth, or the throat. From the membrane, HIV then travels into the previously uninfected person's blood.

   Health experts believe that unprotected anal sex is the riskiest type of sex. Even though bleeding is not visible in most cases, anal sex almost always causes tiny tears and bleeding in the rectum. This happens because the rectum does not stretch easily, the mucous membrane is quite thin, and small blood vessels lie directly beneath the membrane. Condoms also are more likely to break during anal intercourse because more friction is produced in a smaller cavity. All of these factors greatly enhance the risk of transmitting HIV.

   Although latex condoms, if used correctly, provide for "safer" sex, they are not foolproof. Abstaining from sex is the only 100 percent assurance that you are protecting yourself from HIV infection and other STIs.

2. **Direct contact with infected blood through sharing hypodermic needles or other drug paraphernalia.** Following an injection, a small amount of blood remains in the needle and sometimes in the syringe. If the person who used the syringe is infected with HIV and you use that same syringe to shoot up, regardless of the drug used (legal or illegal), that small amount of blood is sufficient to spread the virus. All used syringes should be destroyed and disposed of immediately.

   In addition, you must be cautious when getting acupuncture, getting a tattoo, or having the ears or other body parts pierced. If the needle was used previously on an HIV-infected person and was not disinfected properly, you risk getting HIV.

   Though it is possible for HIV to be transmitted through accidents in health care settings, today, the risk of being infected with HIV from a blood transfusion or other blood products is slight. Prior to 1985, several cases of HIV infection came from blood transfusions because the blood had been donated by HIV-infected individuals. Now, all individuals who donate blood are first tested for HIV. To be absolutely safe, people who are planning to have surgery might consider storing their own blood in advance, so safe blood will be available if a transfusion becomes necessary.

3. **Contact from mother to baby before or during childbirth or through breastfeeding.** HIV can be passed from mother to child right before or during childbirth (though cesarean delivery can sometimes reduce the risk of transmission) and also through breast milk. Though breast milk has a lower concentration of HIV as compared to blood, semen, and vaginal fluid, and therefore doesn't pose as large of a threat to adults, it is still a primary mode of transmission to infants.

Myths about HIV Transmission

Education on how HIV transmission occurs and how it does not occur is important to reduce both the spread of the virus and misinformation about its transmittal.

Kissing Because the concentration of HIV in saliva is too minimal to transmit the virus, you cannot get HIV by engaging in dry kissing with an individual who is infected with HIV. However, if two people have open cuts on the lips or in the mouth or gums, HIV could potentially be transmitted through open-mouth kissing. Prolonged open-mouth kissing can damage the mouth or lips and allow HIV to be transmitted from an infected person to a partner through cuts or sores in the mouth. These cases, however, are rare.

Exercise and Perspiration HIV cannot be transmitted through perspiration. Using the same exercise equipment as an infected individual or participating in sporting activities with no physical contact pose no risk to uninfected individuals unless they both have open wounds through which blood from an infected person can come in direct contact with the open wound of the uninfected person. The skin is an excellent line of defense against HIV. Blood from an infected person cannot penetrate the skin except through an opening in the skin. As an extra precaution, a person should use vinyl or latex gloves when performing work that requires direct contact with someone else's blood or open wound.

Health Care and Donating Blood Infection during medical check-ups and procedures is extremely rare. Health care workers are mandated by law to protect themselves and their patients from HIV transmission through universal precautions for infection control. Because health professionals must use a brand-new needle every time they withdraw blood from a person, the risk of HIV transmission from donating blood is virtually nonexistent.

Insects and Animals Another myth regarding HIV transmission is that you can get it from insects or animals. The H in HIV stands for "human." Though there are some types of immunodeficiency viruses that specifically affect animals, these viruses are not generally considered a risk to humans, and studies have shown that contracting HIV through insect bites is virtually impossible.

Symptoms

HIV is a progressive infection. At first, people who become infected with HIV might not know they are infected. An incubation period of weeks, months, or years may pass during which no symptoms appear. The virus may live in the body 10 years or longer before disease symptoms emerge. HIV infection can produce neurological abnormalities, leading to depression, memory loss, slower mental and physical response time, and sluggishness in limb movements that may progress to a severe disorder known as HIV dementia. The earliest symptoms of AIDS include unexplained weight loss, constant fatigue, mild fever, swollen lymph glands, diarrhea, and sore throat. Advanced symptoms include loss of appetite, skin diseases, night sweats, and deterioration of mucous membranes.

HIV Testing

The only means to determine whether someone has HIV is through an HIV antibody test. A person can be tested for HIV in several ways. You may look up your local Public Health Department or AIDS Information Service (or related names) on the Internet or visit the student health clinic at your local educational institution. Testing results are kept confidential. Many states also conduct anonymous testing. Your name is never recorded.

You can call several toll-free hotlines or access the CDC website (www.cdc.gov/hiv) for more information on anonymous testing, treatment programs, support services, and information about HIV, AIDS, and STIs in general. All information discussed during a phone call to these hotlines is kept confidential. The numbers to call are:

- National AIDS Hotline: 1-800-CDC-INFO (1-800-232-4636) in English and Spanish
- National AIDS Hotline for the hearing impaired (TTY): 1-888-232-6348
- STI Hotline: 1-800-227-8922

Information on local testing facilities is also available online at http://www.hivtest.org.

The CDC recommends HIV testing for all patients in health care settings ages 15 to 64, including pregnant women during the routine panel of prenatal screening tests. The recommendations further include annual screening for people at high risk for infection. Consent for HIV

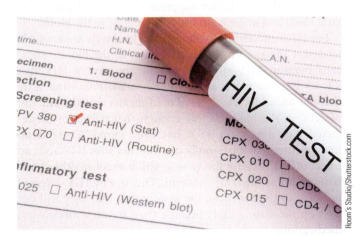

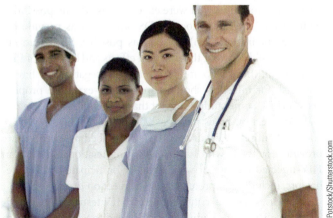

If HIV infection is suspected, seek medical attention immediately. Early detection is critical to improve long-term prognosis.

testing is now included in the general consent form for medical care. Patients, however, can decline testing if they choose to do so.

Diagnosis

Being HIV-positive does not mean that the person has AIDS. When the infection progresses to a point at which certain diseases develop, the person is said to have AIDS. HIV itself doesn't kill. Nor do people die from AIDS. "AIDS" is the term designating the final stage of HIV infection, and death is the result of a weakened immune system that is unable to fight off opportunistic infections.

Most of the illnesses that AIDS patients develop are harmless and rare in the general population but are fatal to AIDS victims. Two of the fatal conditions in AIDS patients, for example, are *Pneumocystis jiroveci* pneumonia (a parasitic infection of the lungs) and Kaposi's sarcoma (a type of skin cancer). HIV also attacks the nervous system, causing damage to the brain and spinal cord. An unsettling finding is that brain damage is seen even in patients who are on drug therapy. The brain appears to provide a haven for HIV where drugs cannot follow, leading to a selective destruction pattern of brain regions that control motor, language, and sensory functions. This finding may explain why individuals often display slower reflexes and disruption of balance and gait in the early stages of AIDS. Patients also frequently exhibit mild vocabulary loss, judgment problems, and difficulty planning.

On becoming infected, the immune system forms antibodies that bind to the virus. Most infected individuals will show these antibodies within 3 months of infection, the average being 25 days. In rare cases, they are not detectable until after 6 months or longer.

PEP and PrEP

If HIV infection is suspected, seek medical attention *immediately*. Some evidence indicates that an immediate course of antiretroviral drugs reduces the chances that a person will be infected. This is referred to as post-exposure prophylaxis (PEP) and is frequently used to prevent transmission in health care workers injured by needles. Less information is available about the effectiveness of PEP for people exposed to HIV through sexual activity or drug-use injections, but it also appears to be effective. If you think you were exposed, discuss the possibility with an HIV specialist (local AIDS organizations provide the most recent information) as soon as possible. Sexual assault victims should consider the potential effects and benefits of PEP. In addition, those who are currently HIV-negative but have a high risk for infection should consider pre-exposure prophylaxis (PrEP). Some studies suggest that PrEP can reduce the risk of HIV infection by as much as 90 percent.[14] This preventive course of antiretroviral drugs can be prescribed by a health care provider for those who have an ongoing relationship with an HIV-infected partner or who regularly participate in risky behaviors, including unprotected sex or injection drug use.

Following an initial consultation for HIV testing with a medical specialist, an individual may still need to wait 3 months to be tested. If the test is negative and the person still suspects infection, the test should be repeated 3 months later. During this time, and from then on, individuals should refrain from further endangering themselves and others through risky behaviors. Some people are tested to reassure themselves that their behaviors are acceptable. Even if the test turns up negative for HIV, this does not represent a "license" to continue risky behaviors.

No one has to become infected with HIV. At present, once infected, with the exception of a handful of rare cases, a person cannot become uninfected. There is no second chance. Everyone must protect himself or herself against this chronic infection. If people do not—and harbor the belief that it cannot happen to them—they are putting themselves and their partners at risk.

New therapies are preventing AIDS from developing in a growing number of HIV-infected individuals. Professionals, however, disagree as to how many HIV carriers actually will develop AIDS. Even if individuals have not developed AIDS, they can pass on the virus to others, who then could easily develop AIDS.

Treatment

Although AIDS still has no known cure, antiretroviral drugs are available that delay the progress of HIV infection and even keep many people from developing AIDS. Antiretroviral drugs have turned HIV infection from an almost imminent predecessor of death to a lifelong chronic disease. Thanks to advances in the development of these drugs, many HIV-infected people can now look forward to decades of life. In fact, people who are diagnosed early and begin receiving therapy immediately and consistently can now enjoy a life expectancy close to that of the uninfected population. The sooner the treatment is initiated, the better the prognosis for a longer life. This success in long-term suppression of the virus to extremely low levels in adults who have been treated immediately after diagnosis gives researchers hope that a "functional cure" for HIV may be possible in the future. HIV-infected individuals, however, must take the drugs every day for the rest of their lives. In most cases, failure to do so results in the virus coming back with full strength. The drugs don't eradicate HIV but rather suppress the virus (decrease the viral load) and make it almost undetectable in the blood.

For HIV-infected individuals, viral load tests are available to detect the amount of virus present in the blood. These tests measure HIV ribonucleic acid, the part of HIV that knows how to make more of the virus. Following drug therapy, an undetectable viral load means that the amount of HIV in the blood is low enough that it cannot be detected, but doesn't mean it has been cured. There is no known cure, so the person is still infected with HIV and can infect others because the virus is still present in other body tissues and in the lymph system. This is why HIV-infected individuals cannot make the assumption that they will not pass on the virus simply because they are on antiretroviral medications.

The Success of Early Antiretroviral Drug Therapy: A Look at the Data

Studies have proven that early treatment with antiretroviral drugs is critical to decrease the transmission risk of HIV. A breakthrough study sponsored by the National Institutes of Health that was set to conclude in 2015 was stalled early in May 2011 when a data review by a federal monitoring agency called for immediate release of its findings because of its significance in the prevention of HIV transmission. The study found that early treatment with antiretroviral drugs, at the time of HIV diagnosis, greatly decreased the risk of transmitting the virus to an uninfected partner. The research was conducted on 1,763 couples in nine countries throughout the world. Only one of the partners in each couple was infected with HIV. The results showed a 96 percent reduction in HIV infection risk only among patients who received the early drug treatment. (All couples in the study were urged to use condoms, which are still critical for protection.)

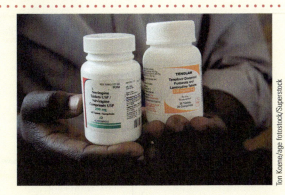

The value of early treatment has been further substantiated with two cases of newborn babies whose infections were effectively suppressed for several years by early and aggressive drug therapy that began just hours after birth. Though both children eventually suffered relapses after living years without medication, the stunning success of the two cases nonetheless fueled international measures to revise recommended treatment methods for infected newborns. The World Health Organization (WHO) currently recommends all infants born to HIV-positive mothers be treated as soon as possible after birth.

SOURCE: M.S. Cohen et al., "Prevention of HIV-1 Infection with Early Antiretroviral Therapy," *New England Journal of Medicine,* 2011. doi:10.1056 /NEJMoa1105243.

Medications that suppress HIV are usually used in combinations, commonly referred to as highly active antiretroviral therapy or "AIDS cocktails." Because the virus mutates rapidly and because some individuals don't tolerate some of the drugs, physicians often switch drug combinations to keep HIV under control.

Though many approaches to an AIDS vaccine continue to be explored, the development of a vaccine to prevent HIV infection or AIDS seems highly unlikely in the near future. People should not expect a medical breakthrough, although researchers are cautiously optimistic about finding a cure. The best advice at this point is to take a preventive approach. Treatment modalities, however, continue to improve and allow HIV-infected individuals and AIDS patients to live longer and more productive lives.

How Common Are HIV Infection and AIDS?

People do not get HIV because of who they are but, rather, because of the choices they make. The majority of new cases of HIV infection occur because of the choice to engage in risky behaviors. Nobody is immune to HIV. HIV and AIDS can threaten anyone of any age or race.

- Globally, close to 37 million people are currently living with HIV, and more than 2.1 million are infected each year.
- 1.8 million children are living with HIV worldwide; most were infected by their HIV-positive mothers during pregnancy, childbirth, or breastfeeding.

- In the United States, about 1.2 million people are infected with HIV, and almost 13 percent are unaware of the infection.
- One in every four newly reported cases are in youth ages 13 to 24, and because most don't know they are infected, they are not receiving treatment and have a high risk of passing the virus to others unknowingly.
- The average cost in the United States to treat one infected individual over his or her lifetime is $379,668.
- Blacks/African Americans, Hispanics, and gay and bisexual men of all races remain the most disproportionately affected by HIV.
- Although men who have sex with men (MSM) represent only 4 percent of American males, the rate of new HIV diagnoses among them is more than 44 times that of other men.
- The first five cases of HIV were reported in 1981. Now, an estimated 35 million people worldwide have died from AIDS since the 1981 epidemic began.

The most recent data available on HIV infection diagnoses among young adults and adolescents in the United States by race/ethnicity are given in Figure 14.2.

The percentage of adults and adolescents currently living with a diagnosis of HIV infection, by gender and transmission category, are provided in Figure 14.3.

Figure 14.2 **Diagnoses of HIV infection among adolescents and young adults ages 13 to 24, by race or ethnicity, 2009–2014, United States and six U.S.-dependent areas.**

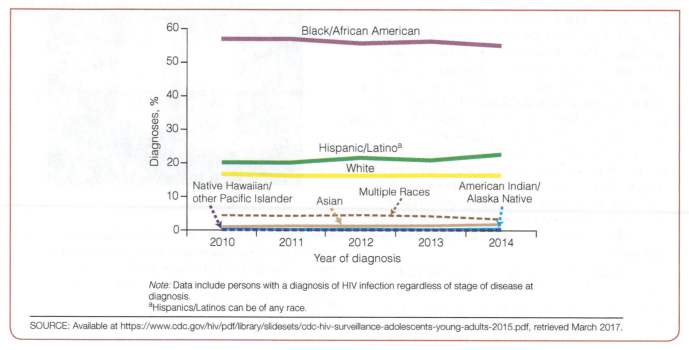

Note: Data include persons with a diagnosis of HIV infection regardless of stage of disease at diagnosis.
[a]Hispanics/Latinos can be of any race.

SOURCE: Available at https://www.cdc.gov/hiv/pdf/library/slidesets/cdc-hiv-surveillance-adolescents-young-adults-2015.pdf, retrieved March 2017.

Figure 14.3 **Adolescents and young adults ages 13 to 24 living with diagnosed HIV infection, by sex and transmission category, year-end 2014, United States and six dependent areas.**

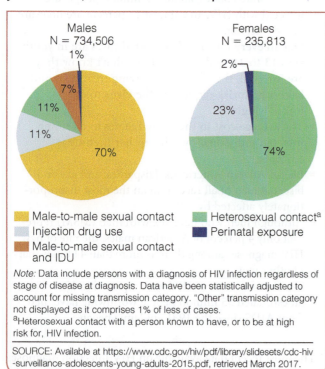

Note: Data include persons with a diagnosis of HIV infection regardless of stage of disease at diagnosis. Data have been statistically adjusted to account for missing transmission category. "Other" transmission category not displayed as it comprises 1% of less of cases.
[a]Heterosexual contact with a person known to have, or to be at high risk for, HIV infection.

SOURCE: Available at https://www.cdc.gov/hiv/pdf/library/slidesets/cdc-hiv-surveillance-adolescents-young-adults-2015.pdf, retrieved March 2017.

Though annual AIDS diagnoses and deaths within the United States and dependent areas have subsided since their peak in the early 1990s (Figure 14.4), the number of people living with AIDS in the United States continues to increase over time, escalating the need for better treatment methods and assistance for those that are victimized by the disease.

14.4 Preventing Sexually Transmitted Infections

The good news is that you can do things to prevent the spread of STIs and take precautions to keep yourself from becoming a victim. The CDC recommends sexual abstinence in dating followed by a long-term mutually monogamous relationship with an uninfected partner as the most reliable way to avoid STI infection.[15]

Wise Dating

With the advent of the Internet, it has become common to search for sex partners online. Surveys have shown that people who seek sex partners over the Internet are at greater risk of contracting an STI. These people also are more likely to have characteristics that increase their chances of transmitting STIs.

Dating and getting to know other people are normal aspects of life. Dating, however, does not mean the same thing as having sex. Sexual intercourse as a part of dating can be risky, and one of the risks is infection. You can't tell whether someone you are dating or would like to date has been exposed to HIV or other STIs. Avoiding sexual activity in dating keeps you virtually risk free from STI infection.

Figure 14.4 **Stage 3 (AIDS) classifications, deaths, and persons living with HIV infection ever classified as stage 3 (AIDS) 1985–2013—United States and six U.S.-dependent areas.**

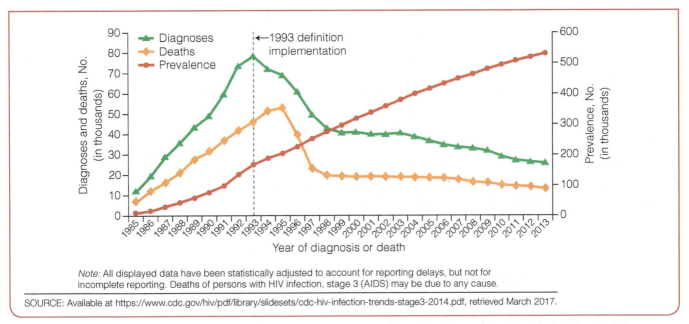

Note: All displayed data have been statistically adjusted to account for reporting delays, but not for incomplete reporting. Deaths of persons with HIV infection, stage 3 (AIDS) may be due to any cause.

SOURCE: Available at https://www.cdc.gov/hiv/pdf/library/slidesets/cdc-hiv-infection-trends-stage3-2014.pdf, retrieved March 2017.

HOEGER KEY TO WELLNESS

A mutually monogamous sexual relationship with an uninfected partner will prevent nearly 100 percent of STIs. If you choose to have multiple partners, although not 100 percent foolproof, commit to "safe sex" by using latex condoms during all types of intercourse, mutually discussing your sexual past, and avoiding drinking and drugs in sexual situations.

Monogamous Sexual Relationship

The facts are in: The best long-term prevention technique is a mutually monogamous sexual relationship. Mutual **monogamy** means both you and your partner agree to only have sex with each other. Committing to this one behavior removes you almost completely from any risk for developing an STI in your lifetime.

Unfortunately, in today's society, trust is elusive. You may be led to believe you are in a safe, monogamous relationship when your partner actually (1) may cheat on you and get infected, (2) has a one-night stand with someone who is infected, (3) got infected several years ago before the current relationship and still doesn't know about the infection, (4) may choose not to tell you about the infection, or (5) shoots up drugs and becomes infected. In any of these cases, an STI, including HIV, can be passed on to you.

Because your future and your life are at stake, and because you may never know if your partner is infected, you should give serious and careful consideration to postponing sex until you believe you have found an uninfected person with whom you can have a lifetime monogamous relationship. In doing so, you do not have to live with the fear of catching HIV or other STIs or deal with an unplanned pregnancy.

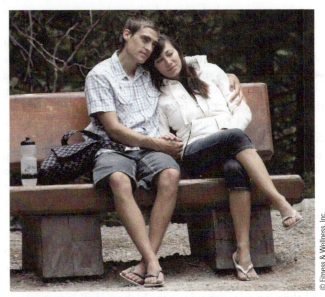

A monogamous sexual relationship almost completely removes people from risking HIV infection and the danger of developing other STIs.

Many people postpone sexual activity until they are married. This is the best guarantee against HIV. Young people should understand that married life provides plenty of time for fulfilling and rewarding sex.

If you choose to delay sex, don't let peers pressure you into changing your mind. Some people would have you believe that you aren't a "real" man or woman if you don't

GLOSSARY

Monogamy A sexual relationship in which two people have sexual relations only with each other.

Behavior Modification Planning

Protecting Yourself and Others from STIs

Are you sexually active? If you are not, read the following items to better educate yourself regarding intimacy. If you are sexually active, continue through all the following questions.

- Do you plan ahead before you get into a sexual situation?

- Do you know whether your partner now has or has ever had an STI? Are you comfortable asking your partner this question?

- Are you in a mutually monogamous sexual relationship, and do you know that your partner does not have an STI?

- Do you have multiple sexual partners? If so, do you *always* practice safe sex?

- Do you avoid alcohol and drugs in situations where you may end up having planned or unplanned sex?

- Do you abstain from sexual activity if you know or suspect that you have an STI? Do you seek medical care and advice as to when you can safely resume sexual activity?

Try It

Taking chances during sexual contact is not worth the risk of an STI. Sex lasts a few minutes; the STI can last a lifetime, with potentially fatal consequences. Think ahead, know the facts, and don't place yourself in a situation where you may no longer be able to or have the desire to say "no." Keep in mind that more than half of all Americans will acquire at least one STI in their lifetime. A few minutes of sexual pleasure can have consequences you may regret for the rest of your life.

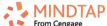 **MINDTAP** **Complete This Online**
From Cengage   Visit **www.cengagebrain.com** to access MindTap, a complete digital course that includes interactive quizzes, videos, and more.

have sex. Manhood and womanhood are proven not during sexual intercourse but, instead, through mature, responsible, and healthy choices.

Other people may lead you to believe that love doesn't exist without sex. Sex in the early stages of a relationship is not the product of love. It is simply the fulfillment of a physical, and often selfish, drive. A loving relationship develops over a long time with mutual respect for each other.

Having sexual encounters with multiple partners may be considered commonplace by peers or even encouraged to gain popularity. The reality is that nearly 50 percent of young women and more than 40 percent of young men ages 15 to 19 years old have not had any sexual partners, with about 20 percent reporting only one sexual partner between the ages of 20 and 24.[16]

Teenagers are especially susceptible to peer pressure leading to premature sexual intercourse. The result? More than 249,000 girls under age 20 get pregnant each year in the United States. Presently, the U.S. teen pregnancy, teen birth, and abortion rates are among the highest of all industrialized nations. Too many young people wish they had postponed sex and silently admire those who do. Sex lasts only a few minutes. The consequences of irresponsible sex may last a lifetime, and in some cases, they are fatal!

Sexual promiscuity never leads to a trusting, loving, and lasting relationship. Mature people respect others' choices. If someone doesn't respect your choice to wait, he or she certainly doesn't deserve your friendship—or anything else.

There is no greater sex than that between two loving and responsible individuals who mutually trust, admire, and love each other. Contrary to many beliefs, these relationships are possible when built on unselfish attitudes and behaviors.

As you look around, you will find that many people hold these values. Seek them out, and build your friendships and

future around people who respect you for who you are and what you believe. You don't have to compromise your choices or values. In the end, you will reap the greater rewards of a lasting relationship free of HIV and other STIs.

Also, be prepared so that you know your course of action before you get into an intimate situation. Look for common interests, and work together toward them. Express your feelings openly: "I'm not ready for sex; I just want to have fun, and kissing is fine with me." If your friend doesn't accept your answer and isn't willing to stop the advances, be prepared with a strong response. Statements like, "Please stop" or "Don't!" are mostly ineffective. Use a firm statement such as, "No, I'm not willing to have sex" or "I've already thought about this and I'm not going to have sex." If this still doesn't work, inform them that their forceful behavior is considered rape and say, "This is rape, and I'm going to call the police."

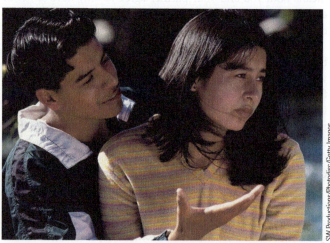

If someone does not respect your choice to wait, he or she does not deserve your friendship—or anything else.

! **Critical Thinking**

Discuss how the information presented in this chapter has affected your feelings and perceptions about sex. What impact will this information have on your wellness lifestyle?

Avoiding risky behaviors that destroy quality of life and life itself is crucial to a healthy lifestyle. Learning the facts and acting upon your personal values so that you can make responsible choices can protect you and those around you from painful, embarrassing, startling, unexpected, or fatal conditions.

20 Ways to Reduce Your Risk

Taking the following precautions can reduce your risk for STIs and HIV infection:

1. *Postpone sex* until you and your uninfected partner are prepared to enter into a lifetime monogamous relationship.

2. *Practice safer sex every time* you have sex, and don't have sexual contact with anyone who doesn't practice safe sex. Unless you are in a monogamous relationship and you know your partner isn't infected (which you may never know for sure), this means you should use a latex condom from start to finish for each sexual act. Take a few minutes and list at least three ways you might bring up the subject of condoms with your partner. If your partner refuses to use a condom, your answer should be quite simple: "No condom, no sex."

3. *Use a dental dam or condom during oral sex* to prevent the spread of STIs through semen, blood, saliva, or other bodily fluids.

4. *Wash immediately and thoroughly after sexual activity.* Although washing your hands with hot, soapy water does not guarantee safety against STIs, it can prevent you from spreading certain germs on your fingers and might wash away bacteria and viruses that have not entered the body yet. Also consider washing your genitals.

5. *Avoid casual sexual encounters and limit your number of sexual partners.* The days are gone when sex was thought to be safe with anonymous encounters at a party or a singles bar. Having only one partner lowers your chances of becoming infected. Although you can still become infected by having unprotected sex with one person only, the more partners you have, the greater your chances for infection.

6. *Determine the conditions under which you will allow sex.* Know your partner well and be sure the relationship has met your standards of trust and respect before agreeing to sex. Ask yourself: "Am I willing to have sex with this person?" If you decide to have sex, practice safer sex. There is no reason to accept anything else.

7. *Plan before you get into a sexual situation.* Discuss STIs with the person you are contemplating having sex with before you do so. Even though talking about STIs might be awkward, the short-lived embarrassment of addressing intimate questions can keep you from contracting or spreading infection.

8. *Negotiate safer sex.* Focus on the problem, not the person. Describe your feelings about the problem, using "I" or "we" instead of "you." For example, you might say, "I'm feeling awkward and uncomfortable. The only way I can feel comfortable is by using a condom." You also can offer options and provide alternative solutions. You might indicate to your partner, "We can work this out together. Let's go for a drive and get a condom. We'll feel better about what we're doing."

9. *Stay sober in dating situations* and avoid risky behavior that puts you at high risk for infection. Drug and alcohol use can impair your ability to make responsible choices regarding potential sexual activity. Otherwise prudent people often act irrationally and engage in risky behaviors when they are under the influence of drugs. Getting high can make you willing to have sex when you didn't plan to—thereby running the risk of contracting HIV.

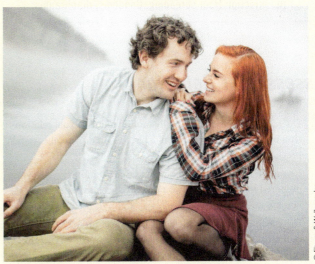

© Fitness & Wellness, Inc.

(continued)

20 Ways to Reduce Your Risk *(continued)*

10. *Schedule regular physical checkups if you are sexually promiscuous.* You can easily get exposed to an STI from a person who does not have any symptoms and who is unaware of the infection. Sexually promiscuous men and women between ages 15 and 35 are a particularly high-risk group for developing STIs.

11. *Avoid sexual contact with anyone who has had sex with one or more individuals at risk for getting HIV,* even if they are now practicing safer sex.

12. *Avoid exchanging body fluids* if you have sex with someone whose history is unknown to you or who might be infected with HIV.

13. *Don't share toothbrushes, razors, or other implements* that could become contaminated with blood with anyone who is, or who might be, infected with HIV.

14. *If you suspect that your partner is infected with an STI, ask.* He or she may not be aware of the infection, so look for signs, such as sores, redness, inflammation, a rash, growths, warts, or a discharge. If you are unsure, abstain.

15. *Be responsible enough to abstain from sexual activity if you know you have an infection.* Go to a physician or a clinic for treatment, and ask your doctor when you can safely resume sexual activity. Abstain until it is safe. Just as you want to be protected in a sexual relationship, you should want to protect your partner. If you are diagnosed with an STI and you believe you know the person who gave it to you, think of ways you might bring up the subject of STIs with this person. You need to take responsibility and discuss this matter with your partner. As a result of your conversation, medical treatment can be initiated and other people can be protected from infection. You can also use other "barrier" methods of contraception to help prevent the infection from spreading. Condoms, diaphragms,

spermicidal suppositories, foams, and jellies can all deter the spread of certain STIs.

16. *Wear loose-fitting clothes made from natural fibers.* Tight-fitting clothing made from synthetic fibers (especially underwear and nylon pantyhose) can create conditions that encourage the growth of bacteria and can actually aggravate STIs.

17. *Consider abstaining from sexual relations if you have any kind of illness or disease, even a common cold.* Any kind of illness makes you more susceptible to other illnesses, and lower immunity can make you more vulnerable to STIs. The same holds true for times when you are under extreme stress, fatigued, or overworked. Drugs and alcohol also can lower your resistance to infection.

18. *Be cautious regarding procedures in which needles or other nonsterile instruments may be used repeatedly to pierce the skin or mucous membranes* (e.g., acupuncture, tattooing, and ear piercing). These procedures are safe if proper sterilization methods are followed or disposable needles are used. Before undergoing the procedure, ask what precautions are being taken.

19. *Insist that frozen sperm be obtained from a laboratory that tests all donors for infection with HIV if you plan to undergo artificial insemination.* Donors should be tested twice before the lab accepts the sperm—once at the time of donation and again a few months later.

20. *Consider donating blood for your own use if you know you will be having surgery soon, and if you are able.* This eliminates the already small risk of contracting HIV through a blood transfusion. It also eliminates the more substantial risk for contracting other blood-borne diseases, such as hepatitis, from a transfusion.

Assess Your Behavior

1. Do you believe that a mutually monogamous sexual relationship is the best way to prevent STIs? If not, do you always take precautions to practice safer sex?

2. If you are not prepared to have a sexual relationship, are you prepared to say so? Have you prepared exactly what to say if you are asked to have sex?

3. Have you carefully considered the consequences of engaging in a sexual relationship, including the risk for STIs, HIV infection, your partner being untruthful about his or her

sexual history and STIs, and the potential of an unplanned pregnancy?

4. Are you capable of discussing your and your partner's sexual history prior to engaging in a sexual relationship that could bring about detrimental consequences for the rest of your life?

5. If you have an STI or a history of STIs, are you sufficiently responsible to have an open and honest discussion with a potential partner about the risk for infection and consequences thereof?

Assess Your Knowledge

1. What percentage of Americans will develop at least one STI in their lifetime?
   a. 30 to 40 percent
   b. 20 to 30 percent
   c. More than 50 percent
   d. 15 to 20 percent
   e. 40 to 50 percent

2. Which of the following STIs is not caused by a bacterial infection?
   a. Chlamydia
   b. Genital warts
   c. Syphilis
   d. Gonorrhea
   e. All of the choices are caused by bacterial infections.

3. Chlamydia
   a. can cause damage to the reproductive system that cannot be reversed by treatment.
   b. is the most common bacterial STI in the United States.
   c. may occur without symptoms.
   d. may cause arthritis.
   e. All of the choices are correct.

4. Gonorrhea can cause
   a. widespread bacterial infection.
   b. infertility.
   c. heart damage.
   d. arthritis.
   e. All of the choices are correct.

5. Genital warts are treated
   a. by dissolving the warts with chemicals.
   b. with electrosurgery.
   c. by freezing the warts with liquid nitrogen.
   d. All of the choices are correct.
   e. None of the choices are correct.

6. Herpes
   a. is incurable.
   b. causes sores that are treated with electrosurgery.
   c. requires antibiotics for successful treatment and cure.
   d. is caused by a bacterial infection.
   e. is not a serious STI because the person becomes uninfected once the sores heal.

7. Cold sores or fever blisters
   a. can cause genital herpes.
   b. are not highly contagious.
   c. are treatable if caused by a bacterial infection.
   d. All of the choices are correct.
   e. None of the choices are correct.

8. The only way to determine whether someone is infected with HIV is through
   a. an AIDS outbreak.
   b. a physical exam by a physician.
   c. a bacterial culture test.
   d. an HIV antibody test.
   e. All of the choices are correct.

9. HIV
   a. attacks and destroys white blood cells.
   b. readily multiplies in the human body.
   c. breaks down the immune system.
   d. increases the likelihood of developing opportunistic infections and cancers.
   e. All of the choices are correct.

10. The best way to protect yourself against STIs is
    a. through the use of condoms for all sexual acts.
    b. by knowing about the people who have previously had sex with your partner.
    c. through a mutually monogamous sexual relationship.
    d. by having sex only with an individual who has no symptoms of STIs.
    e. All of the choices provide equal protection against STIs.

Correct answers can be found at the back of the book.

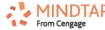 **Complete This Online**
Visit **www.cengagebrain.com** to access MindTap, a complete digital course that includes interactive quizzes, videos, and more.

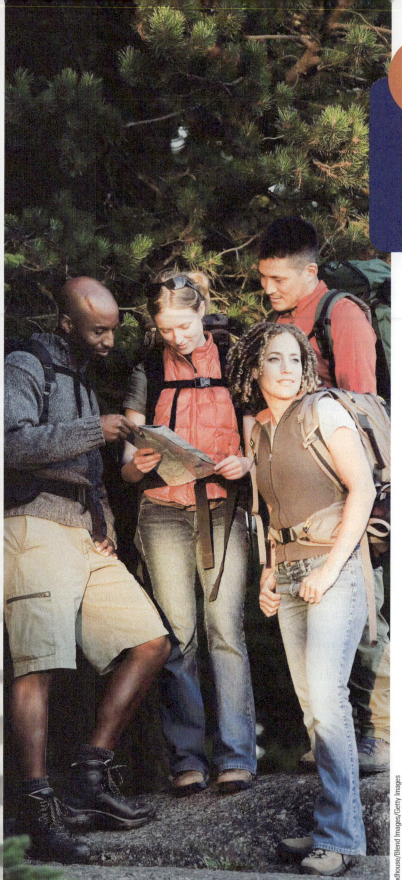

Jeremy Woodhouse/Blend Images/Getty Images

15

Lifetime Fitness and Wellness

The human body is extremely resilient during youth—not so during middle and older age. Thus, lifestyle choices you make today will affect your health, well-being, and quality of life tomorrow.

Objectives

15.1 Understand the effects of a healthy lifestyle on longevity.

15.2 Learn to differentiate between physiological and chronological age.

15.3 Estimate your life expectancy and determine your real physiological age.

15.4 Learn about complementary and alternative medicine practices.

15.5 Understand factors to consider when selecting a health or fitness club.

15.6 Know how to select appropriate exercise equipment.

15.7 Review health and fitness accomplishments and chart a wellness program for the future.

15.8 Evaluate how you have changed and plan for a healthy future.

FAQ

How does regular physical activity affect chronological age versus physiological age?

Chronological age is your actual age—that is, how old you are. Physiological age is used in reference to your functional capacity to perform physical work at any stage of your life. Data on individuals who have taken part in systematic physical activity throughout life indicate that these people maintain a higher level of functional capacity and do not experience the declines typical in later years. From a functional point of view, typical sedentary people in the United States are about 25 years older than their chronological age indicates. Thus, an active 60-year-old person can have a physical capacity similar to that of an inactive 35-year-old person. Similarly, a sedentary 20-year-old college student most likely has the physical capacity of a 45-year-old active individual.

What are the differences among conventional medicine, complementary and alternative medicine (CAM), and integrative medicine?

Conventional medicine implies the practice of traditional medicine by medical doctors, osteopaths, and allied health professionals, such as registered nurses, physical therapists, and psychologists. CAM comprises a group of diverse medical and health care systems, practices, and products that are not presently considered part of conventional medicine. The safety and effectiveness of many of these practices have not been rigorously tested through well-designed scientific studies. Integrative medicine is a growing trend among health care providers that uses a combination of conventional medicine and CAM treatments for which there is some scientific evidence of safety and effectiveness.

What is the greatest benefit of a lifetime wellness lifestyle?

There are many benefits derived from an active wellness lifestyle, including greater functional capacity, good health, less sickness, lower health care expenses and time under medical supervision, and a longer and more productive life. Without question, these benefits together translate into one great benefit: an optimum quality of life; that is, the combined benefit is the freedom to live life to its fullest without functional and health limitations. Most people go through life merely wishing that they could live without such limitations. But the power to do so is within each of us. It is accomplished only by taking action today and living a wellness way of life for the rest of our lives.

REAL LIFE STORY | Ken's Experience

Over the course of the fitness and wellness class I took last year, I made changes to my habits for the better. I started exercising regularly and eating better, and I even tried meditation. I can honestly say that by the end of the class, I was feeling as good and healthy as I ever have before. However, I have a history of going back and forth between being fit and being out of shape. When I was younger, I ran track, and when I was training and racing during the school year, I would be in excellent shape. Then when summer came, I would mostly stop running, eat whatever junk food I wanted, gain weight, and be a couch potato. When the new school year started, I would have to start from the very beginning to try to get back in shape. When I started college, I was no longer involved in track, so I followed the earlier pattern of letting myself go. It wasn't until my junior year, when I took the fitness class, that I started exercising again. So as the class was ending, I was concerned that I would no longer have the motivation to work out and be healthy, once I didn't have my teacher and classmates there to reinforce the healthy habits. But I thought about it, and I realized that my reasons for being healthy shouldn't just be because of external factors, like doing well at track or getting a good grade in class and keeping up with my classmates. I wanted to be healthy for myself, so I can live a long, high-quality life where I look and feel great. So when my class ended, rather than forgetting about fitness, I set new SMART goals for myself, and made a commitment to stick with it. Now, almost 6 months later, rather than turning back into a couch potato, I have become even more fit than I was when class ended. I intend to continue my healthy diet and exercise habits for a lifetime.

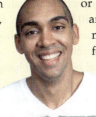
© Fitness & Wellness, Inc.

PERSONAL PROFILE: My Lifetime Fitness and Wellness

I. Have you considered how long you would like to live and what type of health and well-being you desire to enjoy throughout life? Explain lifestyle habits you have implemented to help meet your goals.

II. Do you understand the difference between chronological and physiological age? What is your current physiological age? ____ years   Consider changes that you can still work on to add years to your life and life to your years.

III. Have you ever sought complementary or alternative medical treatment? If so, were you happy with your results?

IV. Have you ever been the victim of quackery and fraud? If so, how were you entrapped? Can you discuss precautions that a person can take to prevent such occurrences?

V. Have you planned and written out short-term and long-range SMART goals to work on now that you are about to finish this course? What arrangements have you made to maintain your exercise program and healthy lifestyle habits? What can you do to stay up-to-date on fitness and wellness concepts and future developments in the field?

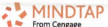 **MINDTAP** **Complete This Online**
From Cengage   Visit **www.cengagebrain.com** to access MindTap, a complete digital course that includes interactive quizzes, videos, and more.

Better health, higher quality of life, and longevity are the three most important benefits derived from a lifetime fitness and wellness program. You have learned that physical fitness in itself does not always lower the risk for chronic diseases and ensure better health. Implementation of healthy behaviors is the only way to attain your highest potential for well-being. The real challenge comes now that you are about to finish this course: maintaining your lifetime commitment to fitness and wellness. Adhering to a program in a structured setting is a lot easier, but from now on, you will be on your own.

15.1 *Chronological versus Physiological Age*

Aging is a natural process, but some people seem to age better than others. Most likely, you know someone who looks younger than his or her **chronological age** indicates, and vice versa—that is, someone who appears older than his or her chronological age indicates. For example, you may have an instructor who you would have guessed was about 40 but in reality is 52 years old. On the other hand, you may have a relative who looks 60 but is actually 50 years old. Why the differences?

During the aging process, natural biological changes occur within the body. Although no single measurement can predict how long you will live, the rate at which aging changes take place depends on a combination of genetic and lifestyle factors. Your lifestyle habits determine to a great extent how your genes affect your aging process. Hundreds of research studies point to critical lifestyle behaviors that determine your statistical chances of dying at a younger age or living a longer life. Research also shows that lifestyle behaviors have a far greater impact on health and longevity than genes alone.

In this chapter, you have an opportunity to evaluate how well you are adhering to health-promoting behaviors and how these behaviors affect your **physiological age** and length of life. You will also learn how to chart a personal wellness program for the future.

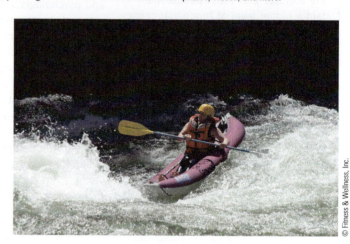

Good physical fitness provides freedom to enjoy many of life's recreational and leisure activities without limitations.

Research data indicate that healthy (and unhealthy) lifestyle actions you take today have an impact on health and quality of life in middle and advanced age. Whereas most young people don't seem to worry much about health and longevity, you may want to take a closer look at the quality of life of your parents or other middle-aged and older friends and relatives that you know. Though you may have a difficult time envisioning yourself at that age, their health status and **functional capacity** may help you determine how you would like to live when you reach your fourth, fifth, and subsequent decades of life.

Critical Thinking

Have you examined the quality of life that older people around you have, and have you considered what life will be like for you at that age?

Although previous research has documented declines in physiological function and motor capacity as a result of aging, no hard evidence at present proves that large declines in

Figure 15.1 Relationships among physical work capacity, aging, and lifestyle habits.

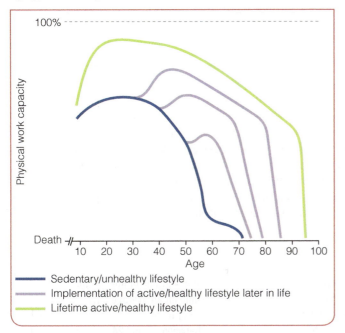

- ⸺⸺ Sedentary/unhealthy lifestyle
- ⸺⸺ Implementation of active/healthy lifestyle later in life
- ⸺⸺ Lifetime active/healthy lifestyle

physical work capacity are related primarily to aging alone. Lack of physical activity—a common phenomenon in today's society as people age—is accompanied by decreases in physical work capacity that are far greater than the effects of aging.

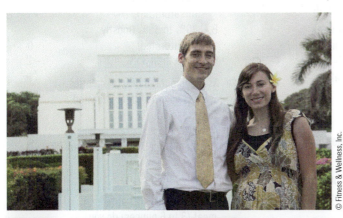

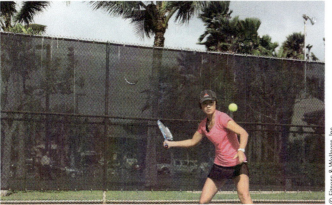

A healthy lifestyle enhances functional capability, quality of life, and longevity.

Unhealthy behaviors precipitate premature aging. For sedentary people, any type of physical activity is seriously impaired by age 40 and productive life ends before age 60. Most of these people hope to live to be age 65 or 70 and often must cope with serious physical ailments. These people "stop living at age 60 but are buried at age 70" (see the theoretical model in Figure 15.1).

Scientists believe that a healthy lifestyle allows people to live a vibrant life—a physically, intellectually, emotionally, socially active, and functionally independent existence—to age 95. Such are the rewards of a wellness way of life. When death comes to active people, it usually is rather quick and not a result of prolonged illness. In Figure 15.1, note the low, longer slope of the "sedentary/unhealthy lifestyle" before death.

HOEGER KEY TO WELLNESS

 Unhealthy behaviors precipitate premature aging and impair physical function before age 60. Many people "stop living at age 60 but are buried at age 70." A healthy lifestyle, nonetheless, can allow you to live a vibrant life to age 95.

15.2 Life Expectancy

Are your lifestyle habits accelerating or decelerating the rate at which your body is aging? The **life expectancy** and physiological age prediction questionnaire provided in Activity 15.1 can help answer this question. By looking at 48 critical genetic and lifestyle factors, you will be able to estimate your life expectancy and your real physiological age to determine how long and how well you may live the rest of your life. Most of these factors are under your control, and you can do something to make them work for you instead of against you.

Be honest with yourself as you fill out the questionnaire. Your life expectancy and physiological age prediction are based on your present lifestyle habits, should you continue those habits for life. Using the questionnaire, you will review factors you can modify or implement in daily living that may add years and health to your life. The questionnaire is not a precise scientific instrument, but rather an estimated life

GLOSSARY

Chronological age Calendar age.

Physiological age The biological and functional capacity of the body as it should be in relation to the person's maximal potential at any given age in the lifespan.

Functional capacity The ability to perform ordinary and unusual demands of daily living without limitations and excessive fatigue or injury.

Life expectancy How many years a person is expected to live.

Activity 15.1   Life Expectancy and Physiological Age Prediction Questionnaire

Name _____   Date _____

Course _____   Section _____   Gender _____   Age _____

INSTRUCTIONS

Circle the points to the correct answer to each question. At the end of each page, obtain a net score for that page. Be completely honest with yourself. Your age prediction is based on your lifestyle habits, should you continue those habits for life. Using this questionnaire, you will learn about factors that you can modify or implement that can add years and health to your life. The scoring system is provided at the end of the questionnaire. Please note that the questionnaire is not a precise scientific instrument, but rather an estimated life expectancy analysis according to the impact of lifestyle factors on health and longevity. This questionnaire is not intended to substitute for advice and tests conducted by medical and healthcare practitioners.

Questionnaire

1. What is your current health status?
   A. Excellent   +2
   B. Good   +1
   C. Average   0
   D. Fair   −1
   E. Poor   −2
   F. Bad   −3

2. How many days per week do you accumulate 30 minutes of moderate-intensity physical activity (at least 40 percent of heart rate reserve—see Chapter 6)?
   A. 6 or 7   +3
   B. 3 to 5   +1
   C. 1 or 2   0
   D. Less than once per week   −3

3. How often do you participate in a vigorous-intensity cardio-respiratory exercise (more than 60 percent of heart rate reserve – see Chapter 6) for at least 20 minutes?
   A. 3 or more times per week   +2
   B. 2 times per week   +1
   C. Once per week   −1
   D. Less than once per week   −2

4. How often do you perform strength-training exercises per week (a minimum of 8 exercises using 8 to 12 repetitions to near-fatigue on each exercise)?
   A. 1–2 times   +2
   B. Less than once or less than 8 exercises with 8 to 12 reps per session   0
   C. Do not strength train   −1

5. How many times per week do you perform flexibility exercises (at least 2–3 days, with daily being ideal)?
   A. 3 or more   +1
   B. 1 to 3 times   +.5
   C. 1 time   0
   D. Do not perform flexibility exercises   −.5

6. How many servings of fruits and vegetables do you eat on a daily basis?
   A. 9 or more   +3
   B. 6 to 8   +2
   C. 5   +1
   D. 3 or 4   0
   E. 2 or less   −2

7. How many grams of fiber do you consume on an average day?
   A. 25 or more   +1
   B. Between 13 and 24   0
   C. 10 to 12 or don't know   −1
   D. Less than 10   −2

8. As a percentage of total calories, what is your average fat intake daily?
   A. 30% or less (mostly unsaturated)   +1
   B. 30% to 35% (mostly unsaturated)   0
   C. More than 35%   −2

9. As a percentage of total calories, what is your average saturated fat intake daily?
   A. 5% or less   +1
   B. More than 5% but less than 7%   0
   C. Don't know   −1
   D. More than 7%   −2

10. How many servings of red meat (3 to 6 ounces) do you consume weekly?
    A. 1 or none   +1
    B. 2 or 3   0
    C. 4 to 7   −2
    D. More than 7   −3

Page score: [   ]

SOURCE: Fitness & Wellness, Inc., Boise, Idaho, ©2017. Reprinted with permission.

Activity 15.1 Life Expectancy and Physiological Age Prediction Questionnaire (continued)

11. How many servings of omega-3-rich fish (3 to 6 ounces) do you consume weekly?
    A. 2 or more — +2
    B. 1 — 0
    C. None — −1

12. As a percentage of total calories, what is your average daily trans fatty acid intake?
    A. No trans fat intake — +1
    B. Less than 1% — 0
    C. 1% to 2% — −1
    D. More than 2% — −2

13. How many alcoholic drinks (a 5-ounce glass of wine, 12-ounce can of beer, 8-ounce bottle of malt liquor, or 1.5-ounce shot of 80-proof liquor/spirits) do you consume per day?
    A. Men 2 or less, women 1 or none — +1
    B. None — 0
    C. Men 3–4, women 2–4 — −1
    D. 5 or more — −3

14. How many milligrams of vitamin C do you get from food daily?
    A. Between 250 and 500 — +1
    B. More than 90 but less than 250 — +.5
    C. Less than 90 — −1

15. How many micrograms of selenium do you get daily (preferably from food)?
    A. Between 100 and 200 — +1
    B. Between 50 and 99 — +.5
    C. Less than 50 — −1

16. How many milligrams of calcium and how many international units of vitamin D do you get from food and supplements on an average day?
    A. Calcium = 1,200, vitamin D = 1,000 or more — +1
    B. Calcium = 1,200, vitamin D = less than 1,000 — +.5
    C. Calcium = 800 to 1,200, vitamin D = less than 1,000 — 0
    D. Calcium = less than 800, vitamin D = less than 1,000 — −1

17. How many times per week do you eat breakfast?
    A. 7 — +1
    B. 5 or 6 — +.5
    C. 3 or 4 — 0
    D. Less than 3 — −.5

18. How many cigarettes do you smoke each day?
    A. Never smoked cigarettes or more than 15 years since giving up cigarettes — +2
    B. None for 5 to 14 years — +1
    C. None for 1 to 4 years — 0
    D. None for 0 to 1 year — −1
    E. Smoker, less than 1 pack per day — −3
    F. Smoker, 1 pack per day — −5
    G. Smoker, up to 2 packs per day — −7
    H. Smoker, more than 2 packs per day — −10

19. Do you use tobacco products other than cigarettes?
    A. Never have — 0
    B. Less than once per week — −1
    C. Once per week — −2
    D. 2 to 6 times per week — −3
    E. More than 6 times per week — −5

20. How often are you exposed to secondhand smoke or other environmental pollutants?
    A. Less than 1 hour per month — 0
    B. Between 1 and 5 hours per month — −1
    C. Between 5 and 29 hours per month — −2
    D. Daily — −3

21. Do you use addictive drugs, other than tobacco or alcohol?
    A. None — 0
    B. 1 — −3
    C. 2 or more — −5

22. What is the age of your parents (or how long did they live)?
    A. Both older than 76 — +3
    B. Only one older than 76 — +1
    C. Both are still alive and younger than 76 — 0
    D. Only one younger than 76 — −1
    E. Neither one lived past 76 — −3

23. What is your body composition classification (see Table 4.11 on page 156)?
    A. Excellent — +2
    B. Good — +1
    C. Average — 0
    D. Overweight — −1
    E. Obese — −2

24. What is your blood pressure?
    A. 120/80 or less (both numbers) — +2
    B. 120–140 or 80–90 (either number) — −1
    C. Greater than 140/90 (either number) — −3

25. What is your HDL cholesterol?
    A. Men greater than 45, women greater than 55 — +2
    B. Men 35 to 44, women 45 to 54 — 0
    C. Don't know — −1
    D. Men less than 35, women less than 45 — −2

26. What is your LDL cholesterol?
    A. Less than 100 — +2
    B. 100 to 130 — 0
    C. 130 to 159 — −1
    D. 160 or higher — +2
    E. Don't know — −2

27. Do you floss and brush your teeth regularly?
    A. Every day — +.5
    B. 3 to 6 days per week — 0
    C. Less than 3 days per week — −.5

28. Are you a diabetic?
    A. No — 0
    B. Yes, well-controlled — −1
    C. Yes, poorly or not controlled — −3

Page score: ☐

Activity 15.1 Life Expectancy and Physiological Age Prediction Questionnaire *(continued)*

29. How often do you get 10 to 20 minutes of unprotected ("safe") sun exposure between 10:00 a.m. and 4:00 p.m.?
    A. Almost daily — +3
    B. 4 to 5 times per week — +1
    C. 3 times per week — 0
    D. 1 to 2 times per week — −1
    E. Less than once per week — −3

30. How often do you tan (sun and/or tanning bed)?
    A. Not at all — +1
    B. Less than 3 times per year — −1
    C. More than 3 times per year — −2

31. How often do you wear a seat belt?
    A. All the time — +1
    B. Most of the time — −.5
    C. Less than half the time — −1

32. How fast do you drive?
    A. Always at or less than the speed limit — 0
    B. Up to 5 mph above the speed limit — −.5
    C. Between 5 and 10 mph above the speed limit — −1
    D. More than 10 mph above the speed limit — −2

33. Do you drink and drive?
    A. Never — 0
    B. Yes (even if only once) — −5

34. Do you suffer from addictive behavior (misuse or abuse of alcohol, prescription and/or hard drugs)?
    A. No — 0
    B. Yes — −10

35. In terms of your sexual activity:
    A. I am not sexually active or I am in a monogamous sexual relationship — +1
    B. I have more than one sexual partner but I always practice safe sex — −1
    C. I have multiple sexual partners and I do not practice safe sex techniques — −3

36. What is your marital status?
    A. Happily married — +1
    B. Single and happy — 0
    C. Single and unhappy — −.5
    D. Divorced — −1
    E. Widowed with a belief in life hereafter — −1
    F. Widowed — −2
    G. Married and unhappy — −2

37. On the average, how many hours of sleep do you get each night?
    A. 8 — +2
    B. 7 to 8 — 0
    C. 6 to 7 — −1
    D. Less than 6 — −2

38. Your stress rating according to the Stress Events Scale (see Activity 12.1, page 454) is:
    A. Excellent — +1
    B. Good — 0
    C. Average — −.5
    D. Fair — −1
    E. Poor — −2

39. Your Type A behavior rating (see Chapter 12) is:
    A. Low — 0
    B. Medium — −1
    C. High — −2

40. When under stress (distress), how often do you practice stress management techniques?
    A. Always — +1
    B. Most of the time — +.5
    C. Not applicable (don't suffer from stress) — 0
    D. Sometimes — −1
    E. Never — −2

41. Do you suffer from depression?
    A. Not at all — 0
    B. Mild depression — −1
    C. Severe depression — −2

42. How often do you associate with people who have a positive attitude about life?
    A. Always — +.5
    B. Most of the time — 0
    C. About half of the time — −.5
    D. Less than half the time — −1

43. Do you have close family or personal relationships whom you can trust and rely on for help in times of need?
    A. Yes — +1
    B. No — −1

44. Do you feel loved and can you routinely give affection and love?
    A. Yes — +1
    B. No — −1

45. Do you have a good sense of humor?
    A. Yes — +1
    B. No — −1

46. How satisfied are you with your schoolwork?
    A. Satisfied — +.5
    B. It's okay — 0
    C. Not satisfied — −.5

47. How do you rate your present job satisfaction?
    A. Love it — +1
    B. Like it — 0
    C. It's okay — −.5
    D. Don't like it — −1
    E. Hate it — −2
    F. Not applicable — 0

48. How do you rate yourself spiritually?
    A. Very spiritual — +1
    B. Spiritual — 0
    C. Somewhat spiritual — −.5
    D. Not spiritual at all — −1

Page score: [   ]

Net score for all questions: [   ]

Activity 15.1 Life Expectancy and Physiological Age Prediction Questionnaire *(continued)*

How to Score

To estimate the total number of years that you will live, (a) determine a net score by totaling the results from all 48 questions, (b) obtain an age change score by multiplying the net score by the age correction factor given next, and (c) add or subtract this number from your base life expectancy age (77 for men and 81 for women—the current life expectancies in the United States). For example, if you are a 20-year-old male and the net score from the answers to all questions is −16, your estimated life expectancy would be 71.2 years (age change score = −16 × .3 = −4.8, life expectancy = 77 − 4.8 = 72.2).

You also can determine your real physiological age by subtracting a positive age-change score or adding a negative age-change score to your current chronological (calendar) age. For instance, in the previous example, the real physiological age would be 24.8 years (20 + 4.8). If the age change score had been +4.8, the real physiological age would have been 15.2 years (20 − 4.8). Thus, a healthy lifestyle will always make your physiological age younger than your chronological age. Your real physiological age will have much greater significance in middle and older age, when real-age reductions of 10 to 25 years occur in people who lead healthy lifestyles. Thus a 50-year-old person could easily have a real physiological age of 30.

Age Correction Factor (ACF)*

Age	ACF
≤30	.3
31–40	.4
41–50	.5
51–60	.6
61–70	.6
71–80	.5
81–90	.4
≥9	.3

*Adapted from M. F. Roizen, *RealAge*
(New York: Cliff Street Books, 1999).

Age Change Score (ACS) = [_____] (net score) × [_____] (ACF) = [_____]

Life Expectancy

Men = 77 ± [_____] (ACS) = [_____] years

Women = 81 ± [_____] (ACS) = [_____] years

Real Physiological Age**

Men = [_____] (your age) ± [_____] (ACS) = [_____] years

Women = [_____] (your age) ± [_____] (ACS) = [_____] years

**Subtract a positive ACS from, or add a negative ACS to, your current age.

Behavior Modification

State your feelings about the experience of taking this questionnaire, analyze your results, and list lifestyle factors that you can work on that will positively affect your health and longevity.

_____

_____

_____

_____

_____

_____

_____

_____

_____

_____

© Fitness & Wellness, Inc.

expectancy analysis according to the impact of lifestyle factors on health and longevity. Also, the questionnaire is not intended as a substitute for advice and tests conducted by medical and health care practitioners.

HOEGER KEY TO WELLNESS

 From a functional point of view, typical sedentary people in the United States are about 25 years older than their chronological age. A sedentary 20-year-old college student can have the physical capacity of a 45-year-old active individual, and an active 60-year-old can have the physical capacity of an inactive 35-year-old.

15.3 *Conventional Western Medicine*

Conventional Western medicine, also known as allopathic medicine, has seen major advances in care and treatment modalities during the past few decades. Conventional medicine is based on scientifically proven methods, wherein medical treatments are tested through rigorous scientific trials. In addition to a **primary care physician** (medical doctor), people seek advice from other practitioners of conventional medicine, including **osteopaths**, **dentists**, **oral surgeons**, **orthodontists**, **ophthalmologists**, **optometrists**, **physician assistants**, and **nurses**.

Finding a Physician

Invariably there are times when you will need medical attention. Finding the right physician can be a challenging task because there are few resources available to assist you to do so. Preventive health care professionals caution that you should shop for a doctor the same way you do research to shop for other items and get the best quality care for your investment. It is important to establish a relationship with your doctor while you are in good health to get the best possible care when needed. Attempting to get an appointment on short notice is often difficult for new patients, and the choices can be limited.

Most people select a physician by a referral from family and friends, but your search requires more than that. You ought to be comfortable with your doctor, and a few questions and skepticism on your part may help. If you trust your doctor, you can be completely open about your health care concerns. If a follow-up consultation is needed, your physician can help direct you to the appropriate specialist to coordinate your care.

First, determine your medical needs, and then start your search by taking a look at the list of doctors in your health care plan and cross-checking the list with the top doctors in the area where you live. Location and hospital affiliations are important to consider as well. Having to travel a long distance discourages patients from seeking medical care when recommended or needed. Next, inquire about education, qualifications, skills,

residency, and experience so that they meet your expectations. Because your association with your physician may become a lifetime relationship, you also want to make sure that your personalities agree.

Other considerations include gender and age. Many women prefer female physicians for certain conditions, whereas men are generally more open to either gender. Older physicians are typically more experienced, while younger ones may be more in tune with recent advances and new medical procedures and technologies. You need to decide for yourself about your comfort zone and potential treatment options for your condition.

Finally, researching online can provide valuable information about the physician's practice, friendliness, and availability to patients. Some sites provide information regarding board certification and possible disciplinary actions. Once you have narrowed your search, an introductory phone conversation is fully within your right. Most physicians are open to such a conversation. A physician's choice not to do so gives you information about the doctor's personality, time constraints, or openness with patients.

HOEGER KEY TO WELLNESS

 Only about 20 percent of conventional treatments have been proven to be clinically effective in scientific trials. Preventive health care professionals caution that it is best to shop for a doctor the way you shop for other items; do your research to get the best quality care for your investment.

Searching for a Hospital

Another point to consider is the choice of hospital if a medical procedure is needed. An alarming statistic in the United States is that medical errors are the third leading cause of death after heart disease and cancer, causing 250,000 deaths per year.[1] Selecting the appropriate facility is just as important as finding a good physician. Research has shown that in some hospitals patients get better medical care, experience fewer medical complications, and receive better attention for their needs. To decide on a hospital, follow these simple steps:

1. ***Does the hospital routinely handle your medical procedure?*** Check the hospital's record of treating patients with your condition in a safe and effective way. As with the physician of your choice, the more experienced the staff is with your procedure, the better the outcome for you.
2. ***Is the hospital accredited by The Joint Commission?*** The Joint Commission is an independent foundation that administers accreditation programs for hospitals and other health care organizations.
3. ***Does your doctor have privileges at the hospital (is he/she permitted to admit patients)?***

4. *Is the hospital covered by your health care plan?*

5. *What is the hospital readmission or bounce back rate?* The "bounce back rate" is a medical term used to look at how many patients require rehospitalization within 30 days of the procedure. The higher the rate, the higher the risk for post-medical care complications. At present, one in five admissions results in readmission within 30 days. You can find out about the hospital bounce back rating at http://www.medicare.gov/hospitalcompare.

6. *How well does the hospital check and improve its own safety record?* Hospitals with effective staff communication, good team work, and regular patient care discussions have lower rates of infection than hospitals with a poor culture of safety. Although such data aren't readily available to the consumer, you can ask the hospital staff if they would trust their health care to their place of employment. Don't just accept a "yes" response, but evaluate the behavior, character, and choice of words in their response.

7. *Have you discussed with former patients, family members, and friends their experience at the hospital?* They can provide information on the treatment, response, friendliness, care, and helpfulness of the personnel, as well as the privacy, comfort, and condition of the hospital.

8. *Do you have a choice of procedures?* If you do, always select a minimally invasive procedure. Discuss with your doctor all available options. If needed, opt for a second opinion. About one-third of second opinions differ from the initial diagnosis. Minimally invasive procedures have a lower risk of infection and involve shorter hospital stays and less pain.

9. *What is the surgeon's experience?* Consider asking how *many* times the surgeon has performed the procedure in the past year. Death rates for any given surgical procedure are greatly reduced by the surgeon's experience with the procedure.

10. *Is the facility a teaching hospital with medical interns and residents?* If so, inquire as to who will provide and oversee your care. If possible, avoid teaching hospitals during the month of July, when new interns and residents arrive and your medical care may not be as safe and efficient as the rest of the year.

11. *Is the hospital a for-profit or not-for-profit hospital?* For-profit hospitals may discharge you early or skip out on proper treatment because you are either uninsured or your health care plan only allows a certain amount of time in the hospital. If such is an issue, some consumer groups feel that you should think twice before going to a for-profit hospital.

12. *Have you obtained a copy of your medical records?* Request a copy of the physician's notes taken during your visit or procedure. Reviewing the notes can help clarify a diagnosis and the prescribed follow-up treatment. It will also allow you to correct any errors in information you provided your doctor. Under federal law, you have the right to obtain your records.

15.4 Complementary and Alternative Medicine

Despite modern technological and scientific advancements, many medical treatments either do not improve a patient's condition or cause other ailments. Only about 20 percent of conventional treatments have proved to be clinically effective in scientific trials.[2] More than 30 percent of adults (Figure 15.2) and 12 percent of children in the United States are turning to **complementary and alternative medicine**, or **CAM** (also called "unconventional," "nonallopathic," or "integrative" medicine) in search of answers to their health problems.[3] Unconventional medicine is referred to as "complementary" if it is used in conjunction with their conventional medical care, or "alternative" if it is used as a replacement for conventional practices.

The reasons for seeking complementary and alternative treatments are diverse. Among the reasons commonly given by patients who seek unconventional treatments are lack of progress in curing illnesses and disease, frustration and dissatisfaction with physicians, lack of personal attention, testimonials about the effectiveness of alternative treatments, and

GLOSSARY

Conventional Western medicine A traditional medical practice based on methods that are tested through rigorous scientific trials; also called allopathic medicine.

Primary care physician A medical practitioner who provides routine treatment of ailments; typically, the patient's first contact for health care.

Osteopath A medical practitioner with specialized training in musculoskeletal problems who uses diagnostic and therapeutic methods of conventional medicine in addition to manipulative measures.

Dentists Practitioners who specialize in diseases of the teeth, gums, and oral cavity.

Oral surgeons Dentists who specialize in surgical procedures of the oral-facial complex.

Orthodontists Dentists who specialize in the correction and prevention of tooth irregularities.

Ophthalmologists Medical specialists concerned with diseases of the eye and prescription of corrective lenses.

Optometrists Health care practitioners who specialize in the prescription and adaptation of lenses.

Physician assistants Health care practitioners trained to treat most standard cases of care.

Nurses Health care practitioners who assist in the diagnosis and treatment of health problems and provide many services to patients in a variety of settings.

Complementary and alternative medicine (CAM) A group of diverse medical and health care systems, practices, and products that are not presently considered part of conventional medicine; also called unconventional, nonallopathic, or integrative medicine.

Figure 15.2 Complementary and alternative medicine use by age, United States.

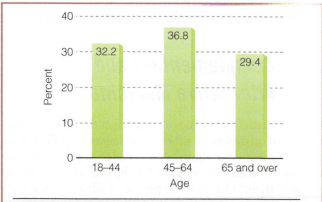

SOURCE: T. C. Clarke, L. I. Black, B. J. Stussman, et al., "Trends in the Use of Complementary Health Approaches Among Adults: United States, 2002–2012," *National Health Statistics Reports*, no. 79. Hyattsville, MD: National Center for Health Statistics, 2017.

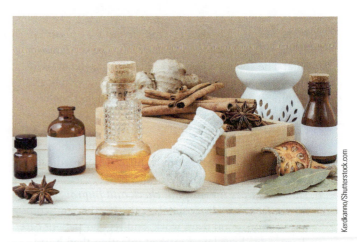

Interest in natural products and remedies has grown considerably in recent decades.

rising health care costs. People who use CAM are shown to have higher income and education levels, and believe that body, mind, and spirit all contribute to good health.

The National Center for Complementary and Integrative Health (NCCIH) was established under the National Institutes of Health (NIH) to examine methods of healing previously unexplored by science. CAM includes treatments and health care practices not widely taught in medical schools, not generally used in hospitals, and not usually reimbursed by medical insurance companies. Many physicians now endorse complementary and alternative treatments, and an ever-increasing number of medical schools are offering courses in this area.

The NCCIH classifies CAM therapies into two broad categories:[4]

1. *Natural products.* This includes the use of a variety of herbal medicines (also known as botanicals), vitamins, and minerals. Many are sold over-the-counter as dietary supplements. (Some uses of dietary supplements—for example, taking a multivitamin to meet minimum daily nutritional requirements or taking calcium to promote bone health—are not considered CAM.) CAM natural products include probiotics—live microorganisms (usually bacteria) that are similar to microorganisms normally found in the human digestive tract.

   Interest in and use of CAM natural products have grown considerably in recent decades. Approximately 17.7 percent of American adults use a nonvitamin or nonmineral natural product. The most commonly used product was fish oil or omega-3 fatty acids, as reported among all adults who said they use natural products.

2. *Mind and body practices.* This category encompasses a broad and diverse group of techniques, healing philosophies, and procedures that are taught by trained practitioners. Meditation, yoga, and hypnotherapy are practices that focus on the interactions among the brain, mind, body, and behavior, with the intent to use the mind to affect physical functioning and promote health.

Spinal manipulation and massage therapy focus on the structures and systems of the body, including the bones and joints, soft tissues, and circulatory and lymphatic systems. Spinal manipulation is performed by chiropractors and by other health care professionals such as physical therapists, osteopaths, and some conventional medical doctors. Practitioners use their hands or a device to apply a controlled force to a joint of the spine, moving it beyond its passive range of motion: The amount of force applied depends on the form of manipulation used. Spinal manipulation is among the treatment options used by people with low-back pain—a very common condition that can be difficult to treat.

Massage therapists manipulate the muscles and other soft tissues of the body. People use massage for a variety of health-related purposes, including to relieve pain, rehabilitate sports injuries, reduce stress, increase relaxation, address anxiety and depression, and aid general well-being.

Types of CAM Practices

Of the many CAM practices, those most often associated with nonallopathic medicine are **acupuncture, chiropractics, herbal medicine, homeopathy, naturopathic medicine, Ayurveda, magnetic therapy,** and **massage therapy**. The most popular among adults in the United States are deep breathing exercises, yoga/tai chi/qi gong, chiropractics, meditation, and massage therapy (see Figure 15.3).[5] Other practices include healing touch, progressive muscle relaxation, guided imagery, and various types of movement therapies. Each of these practices offers a different approach to treatments based on its beliefs about the body, some of which are hundreds or thousands of years old.

Many CAM practitioners believe that their modality aids the body as it performs its natural healing process. Because of their approach, alternative treatments usually take longer than conventional allopathic medical care. Nonallopathic treatments are usually less harsh on the patient, and practitioners tend to avoid surgery and extensive use of medications.

Figure 15.3 10 most common complementary health approaches among adults—2012.

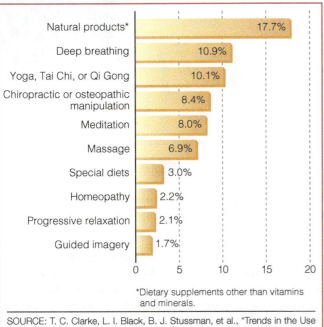

Approach	Percentage
Natural products*	17.7%
Deep breathing	10.9%
Yoga, Tai Chi, or Qi Gong	10.1%
Chiropractic or osteopathic manipulation	8.4%
Meditation	8.0%
Massage	6.9%
Special diets	3.0%
Homeopathy	2.2%
Progressive relaxation	2.1%
Guided imagery	1.7%

*Dietary supplements other than vitamins and minerals.

SOURCE: T. C. Clarke, L. I. Black, B. J. Stussman, et al., "Trends in the Use of Complementary Health Approaches Among Adults: United States, 2002–2012," *National Health Statistics Reports*, no. 79. Hyattsville, MD: National Center for Health Statistics, 2017.

Unconventional therapies are frequently viewed as "holistic," implying that the practitioner looks at all dimensions of wellness when evaluating a person's condition. Practitioners often persuade patients to adopt healthier lifestyle habits that not only help improve current conditions, but also prevent other ailments. CAM also allows patients to better understand treatments, and patients are often allowed to administer self-treatment.

Costs for CAM

Costs for CAM practices are typically lower than conventional medicine costs. With the exception of acupuncture and chiropractic care, most nonallopathic treatments are not covered by health insurance. Typically, patients pay directly for these services. Estimates indicate that $30.2 billion is spent out-of-pocket a year on complementary and alternative medical treatments. These costs account for about 9.2 percent of total out-of-pocket health care expenses in the United States.[6] If you are considering alternative medical therapies, consult with your health care insurance provider to determine which therapies are reimbursable.

CAM Shortcomings

Alternative medicine practices have not gone through the same standard scrutiny as conventional medicine. Nonallopathic treatments are often based on theories that have not been scientifically proven. This does not imply that unconventional medicine practices do not help people. Many people have found relief from ailments or been cured through

unconventional treatments. In due time, however, these theories will need to be investigated using scientific trials similar to those in conventional medicine.

Because CAM does have shortcomings, anyone researching alternative forms of treatment should consider the following:

1. Many practitioners do not have the years of education given to conventional medical personnel and often know less about physiological responses that occur in the body.
2. Some practices are devoid of science; hence, the practitioner can rarely explain the specific physiological benefits of the treatment used. Much of the knowledge is based on experiences with previous patients.
3. The practice of CAM is not regulated like that of conventional medicine. The training and certification of practitioners, malpractice liability, and evaluation of tests and methods used in treatments are not routinely standardized. Many states, however, license practitioners in the areas of chiropractic services, acupuncture, naturopathy, homeopathy, herbal therapy, and massage therapy. Other therapies are usually unmonitored.
4. Unconventional medicine lacks regulation of natural and herbal products. The word "natural" does not imply that the product is safe. Many products, including some herbs, can be toxic in large doses.
5. About one-third of all adults in the United States combine multivitamins, antacids, and other herbal and dietary supplements with their prescriptions.[7] Combinations such as these can yield undesirable side effects. Therefore, individuals should always let their health care practitioners know which medications and alternative (including vitamin and mineral) supplements are being taken in combination.

GLOSSARY

Acupuncture A Chinese medical system that requires body piercing with fine needles during therapy to relieve pain and treat ailments and diseases.

Chiropractics A health care system that proposes many diseases and ailments are related to misalignments of the vertebrae and emphasizes manipulation of the spinal column.

Herbal medicine An unconventional system that uses herbs to treat ailments and disease.

Homeopathy A system of treatment based on the use of minute quantities of remedies that in large amounts produce effects similar to the disease being treated.

Naturopathic medicine An unconventional system of medicine that relies exclusively on natural remedies to treat disease and ailments.

Ayurveda A Hindu system of medicine based on herbs, diet, massage, meditation, and yoga to help the body boost its natural healing process.

Magnetic therapy Unconventional treatment that relies on magnetic energy to promote healing.

Massage therapy The rubbing or kneading of body parts to treat ailments.

Herbal medicine has been around for centuries. Through trial and error, by design, or by accident, people have found that certain plant substances have medicinal properties. Today, products that are safer and more effective and have fewer negative side effects have replaced many of these plant products. Although science has found the mechanisms whereby some herbs work, much research remains to be done.

Many herbs or herbal remedies are not safe for human use and continue to meet resistance from the scientific community. One of the main concerns is that active ingredients in drug therapy must be administered in accurate dosages. With herbal medicine, the potency cannot always be adequately controlled.

Also, some herbs produce undesirable side effects. For example, ephedra (ma huang), a popular weight loss and energy supplement, can cause high blood pressure, rapid heart rate, tremor, seizures, headaches, insomnia, stroke, and even death. About 1,400 reports of adverse effects linked to herbal products containing ephedra, including 81 ephedra-related deaths, prompted its removal from the marketplace. Saint-John's-wort, commonly taken as an antidepressant, can produce serious interactions with drugs used to treat heart disease. Ginkgo biloba impairs blood clotting; thus, it can cause bleeding in people already on regular blood-thinning medication or aspirin therapy. Other herbs, like yohimbe, kava, chaparral, comfrey, and jin bu huan, have been linked to adverse events.

Finding a CAM Practitioner

Conventional health care providers are becoming more willing to refer patients to someone who is familiar with alternative treatments, but you need to be an informed consumer. Ask your primary care physician to obtain valid information regarding the safety and effectiveness of a particular treatment.

Nonetheless, the medical community at times resists and rejects unconventional therapies. If your physician is unable or unwilling to provide you with valid information about a treatment, medical, college, or public libraries and popular bookstores are good places to search for this information. You need to educate yourself about the advantages and disadvantages of alternative treatments, risks, side effects, expected results, and length of therapy.

Information on a range of medical conditions or specific diseases can also be obtained by calling the NIH at 1-301-496-4000. Ask the operator to direct you to the appropriate NIH office. The NCCIH office also provides a website (https://nccih.nih.gov/) with access to federal databases hosting hundreds of thousands of bibliographic records of research published on CAM during the past four decades.

When you select a primary care physician or a nonallopathic practitioner, consult local and state medical boards, other health regulatory boards and agencies, and consumer affairs departments for information about a given practitioner's education, accreditation, and license and about complaints that

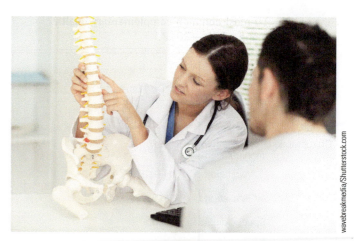

Chiropractics and osteopathic manipulation are among the most common CAM practices in the United States.

may have been filed against this health care provider. Many unconventional medical fields also have a national organization that provides guidelines for practitioners and health consumers. These organizations can guide you to the appropriate regulatory agencies within your state where you can obtain information regarding a specific practitioner.

You may also talk to individuals who have undergone similar therapies and learn about the competence of the practitioner in question. Keep in mind, however, that patient testimonials do not adequately assess the safety and effectiveness of alternative treatments. Whenever possible, search for results of controlled scientific trials of the therapy in question and use this information in your decision process.

When undergoing any type of treatment or therapy, always disclose this information with all of your health care providers, whether conventional or unconventional. Adequate health care management requires that health care providers be informed of all concurrent therapies so that they have a complete picture of the treatment plan. Lack of knowledge by one health care provider regarding treatments by another provider can interfere with the healing process or even worsen a given condition.

Millions of Americans have benefited from CAM practices. You may also benefit from such services, but you need to make careful and educated decisions about the available options. By finding well-trained (and preferably licensed) practitioners, you increase your chances for recovery from ailments and disease.

> **! Critical Thinking**
>
> Have you or someone you know ever used complementary or alternative medicine treatments? What experiences did you have with these treatment modalities, and would you use them in the future?

15.5 *Integrative Medicine*

Integrative medicine involves a combination of the practices and methods of conventional Western medicine and of CAM. Physicians and other health care professionals may use an integrative approach to help patients manage symptoms or improve the effectiveness of a conventional treatment. For example, many cancer treatment centers have instituted integrative programs that offer acupuncture, massage, meditation, and other forms of counseling or therapies to ease pain and side effects from conventional treatments like chemotherapy.

Integrative medicine is a preventative and proactive approach to health and wellness that encompasses all aspects of the individual's lifestyle, taking into account the whole person, not just the disease or illness. It is based on a partnership between the patient and the doctor, where the ultimate goal is to treat the body, mind, and spirit. It can further involve principles of preventive medicine and therapies not accepted as typical medical practice, including prayer, meditation, social support, and recreation.

Many patients are turning to integrative medicine because of dissatisfaction with their health care providers, reporting scheduling frustrations, unclear communication, lack of involvement in treatment decisions, or limited time with physicians to adequately discuss health concerns. As a result, integrative medicine has become a growing trend among physicians and health care systems within the United States, with integrative medicine departments being instituted at several universities, hospitals, and various treatment centers. The concept is not without its critics as the practice is driven by market forces that tout benefits that may or may not be backed by reliable scientific data, making it hard for patients to make informed decisions about using integrative care options.

15.6 *Quackery and Fraud*

The growth of the fitness and wellness industry during the past few decades has spurred the promotion of fraudulent products that deceive consumers into supposedly miraculous, quick, and easy ways to achieve total well-being. **Quackery and fraud** have been defined as the conscious promotion of unproven claims for profit.

Today's market is saturated with "special" foods, diets, supplements, pills, cures, equipment, books, and videos that promise quick, dramatic results. Advertisements for these products often are based on testimonials, unproven claims, secret research, half-truths, and quick-fix statements that the uneducated consumer wants to hear. In the meantime, the organization or enterprise making the claims stands to reap a large profit from consumers' willingness to pay for astonishing and spectacular solutions to problems related to their unhealthy lifestyles.

Deception in Advertising

Television, social media, magazine, online, and newspaper advertisements are not necessarily reliable. For instance, one piece of equipment sold through television and newspaper advertisements promised to "bust the gut" through 5 minutes of daily exercise that appeared to target the abdominal muscle group. This piece of equipment consisted of a metal spring attached to the feet on one end and held in the hands on the other end. According to handling and shipping distributors, the equipment was "selling like hotcakes," and companies could barely keep up with consumer demands.

Three problems became apparent to the educated consumer: First, there is no such thing as spot reducing; therefore, the claims could not be true. Second, 5 minutes of daily exercise burn hardly any calories and therefore have no effect on weight loss. Third, the intended abdominal (gut) muscles were not really involved during the exercise. The exercise engaged mostly the gluteal and lower back muscles. This piece of equipment could then be found at garage sales for about a tenth of its original cost.

Although people in the United States tend to be firm believers in the benefits of physical activity and positive lifestyle habits as a means to promote better health, most do not reap these benefits because they simply do not know how to put into practice a sound fitness and wellness program that gives them the results they want. Unfortunately, many uneducated wellness consumers are targets of deception by organizations making fraudulent claims for their products.

Deception in the Media

Deception is not limited to advertisements. Deceit is all around us: in newspaper and magazine articles, the Internet, trade books, radio, and television shows. To make a profit, popular magazines occasionally exaggerate health claims or leave out pertinent information to avoid offending advertisers. Some publishers print books on diets or self-treatment approaches that have no scientific foundation. Consumers should even be cautious about news reports of the latest medical breakthroughs. Reporters have been known to overlook important information or give certain findings greater credence than they deserve. To research the credibility of a claim or study that has been featured in the news, you can search the U.S. National Library of Medicine's web page "Behind the Headlines," which publishes impartial reviews of health-related stories (see http://www.ncbi.nlm.nih.gov/pubmedhealth/behindtheheadlines).

GLOSSARY

Integrative medicine The combination of the practices and methods of alternative medicine with conventional Western medicine.

Quackery and fraud The conscious promotion of unproven claims for profit.

Tips to Avoid Unreliable Information Online

Precautions must also be taken when seeking health advice online. The Internet is full of both credible and dubious information. The following tips can help as you conduct an online search:

- *Look for government, university, non-profit, or well-known medical school websites.* Sites ending in ".gov" are produced and maintained by federal agencies and typically publish information based on the most reliable and up-to-date research. University and non-profit websites typically end in ".edu" or ".org," respectively. Be aware, however, that sites containing these endings in their web addresses may not always be reputable as scammers often set up deceptive sites with addresses that look credible to target consumers.

- *Look for credentials of the person or organization sponsoring the site.* Ensure those authoring the site's content are listed clearly, and research their names to be certain they are recognized authorities in the field.

- *Check when the site was last updated.* Look for signs that the information might be out-of-date, including broken links or old dates on pages and documents. Credible sites are updated often.

- *Check the appearance of the information on the site.* It should be presented in a professional manner. If every sentence ends with an exclamation point, you have a good cause for suspicion.

- *Exercise caution if the site's sponsor is trying to sell a product.* If so, be leery of opinions posted on the site. They could be biased, given that the company's main objective is to sell a product. Credible companies trying to sell a product online usually reference their sources of health information and provide additional links that support their product.

- *On informational sites that don't sell a product but contain advertisements, check the source of supporting funds, whether they are donated, public, or provided by commercial ventures.* Sponsorships should be disclosed, and advertisements should be labeled clearly.

- *Compare a site's content to other credible sources.* The content should be similar to that of other reputable sites or publications.

- *Note the address and contact information for the company.* A reliable company lists more than a P.O. box, an 800 number, and the company's e-mail address. When only the latter information is provided, consumers may never be able to locate the company for questions, concerns, or refunds.

- *Be on the alert for companies that claim to be innovators while criticizing competitors or the government for being closed minded or trying to keep them from doing business.*

- *Watch for advertisers that use valid medical terminology in un irrelevant context or use vague pseudomedical jargon to sell their product.*

- *Look for medical research presented in the information.* Give more credence to reliable scientific evidence than opinions and testimonials.

How to Research and Report Consumer Fraud

Not all people who promote fraudulent products, however, know they are doing so. Some may be convinced that the product is effective. If you have questions or concerns about a health product, you can search the Federal Trade Commission's website at www.consumer.ftc.gov under the topic "Health & Fitness" to get credible information on the latest market claims concerning healthy living, treatment and

---

Reliable Health Websites

- American Cancer Society:
  http://www.cancer.org
- American College of Sports Medicine:
  http://www.acsm.org
- American Heart Association:
  http://www.heart.org
- Centers for Disease Control and Prevention:
  http://www.cdc.gov
- Clinical Trials Listing Service:
  http://www.centerwatch.com
- Food and Drug Administration:
  http://www.fda.gov
- Healthfinder—Your Guide to Reliable Health Information:
  http://www.healthfinder.gov
- MedlinePlus—Trusted Health Information for You:
  http://www.medlineplus.gov
- National Cancer Institute:
  http://www.cancer.gov
- National Center for Complementary and Integrative Health:
  http://www.nccih.nih.gov
- National Institutes of Health:
  http://www.nih.gov
- National Library of Medicine:
  http://www.nlm.nih.gov
- National Women's Health Information Center:
  http://www.womenshealth.gov
- WebMD:
  http://www.webmd.com
- World Health Organization:
  http://www.who.int/en/

cures, weight loss, and fitness. As the FTC is the nation's consumer protection agency, you can also file a complaint about scams and/or dubious health claims at www.ftccomplaintassistant.gov, or by calling 1-877-382-4357.

Other consumer protection organizations also offer to follow up on complaints about quackery and fraud. The existence of these organizations, however, should not give the consumer a false sense of security. The overwhelming number of complaints made each year makes it impossible for these organizations to follow up on each case individually. The U.S. Food and Drug Administration's (FDA's) Center for Drug Evaluation Research, for example, has developed a priority system to determine which health fraud product it should regulate first. Products are rated on how great a risk they pose to the consumer. With this in mind, you can use the following list of organizations to make an educated decision before you spend your money. You can also report consumer fraud to these organizations:

- *Food and Drug Administration (FDA).* The FDA regulates safety and labeling of health products and cosmetics. You can search for the office closest to you in the federal government listings (blue pages) of the phone book or online at www.fda.gov.
- *Better Business Bureau (BBB).* The BBB can tell you whether other customers have lodged complaints about a product, a company, or a salesperson. You can find a listing for the local office in the business section of the phone book, or you can check the organization's website at www.bbb.com.
- *Consumer Product Safety Commission (CPSC).* This independent federal regulatory agency targets products that threaten the safety of American families. Unsafe products can be researched and reported on their website at http://www.cpsc.gov.
- *Your state Attorney General.* Attorneys General govern state consumer protection divisions to enforce local laws and investigate claims that protect consumers and businesses from deceptive acts and practices. Find a list of state Attorneys General at http://www.naag.org.
- *Your local Consumer Protection Office.* Find your local consumer protection office to report frauds and scams or get help with a consumer complaint at http://www.consumeraction.gov/state-consumer.

Another way to get informed before you make your purchase is to seek the advice of a reputable professional. Ask someone who understands the product but does not stand to profit from the transaction. As examples, a physical educator or an exercise physiologist can advise you regarding exercise equipment; a registered dietitian can provide information on nutrition and weight control programs; and a physician can offer advice on nutrition supplements. Also, be alert to those who bill themselves as "experts." Look for qualifications, degrees, professional experience, certifications, and reputation.

Keep in mind that if it sounds too good to be true, it probably is. Fraudulent promotions often rely on testimonials or

scare tactics and promise that their products will cure a long list of unrelated ailments; they use words like "quick fix," "time-tested," "newfound," "miraculous," "special," "secret," "all natural," "mail-order only," and "money-back guarantee." Deceptive companies move often so that customers have no way of contacting the company to ask for reimbursement.

When claims are made, ask where the claims are published. Refereed, or peer-reviewed, scientific journals are the most reliable sources of information. When a researcher submits information for publication in a refereed journal, at least two qualified and reputable professionals in the field conduct blind reviews of the manuscript. A blind review means the author does not know who reviewed the manuscript and the reviewers do not know who submitted the manuscript. Acceptance for publication is based on this input and relevant changes.

15.7 Looking at Your Fitness Future

Once you've decided to pursue a lifetime wellness program, you face several more decisions about exactly how to accomplish it. To stay up-to-date on fitness and wellness developments, you should buy a reputable and updated fitness and wellness book every 4 to 5 years. You may also subscribe to credible health, fitness, nutrition, or wellness newsletters to stay current.

Health and Fitness Club Memberships

You may want to consider joining a health or fitness facility. Or, if you have mastered the contents of this book and your choice of fitness activity is one you can pursue on your own (walking, jogging, cycling, etc.), you may not need to join a health club. Barring injuries, you may continue your exercise program outside the walls of a health club for the rest of your

---

Reliable Sources of Health, Fitness, Nutrition, and Wellness Information

Newsletter	Yearly Issues	Approx. Annual Cost
Consumer Reports on Health www.ConsumerReports.org/health 800-333-0663	12	$30
Environmental Nutrition www.environmentalnutrition.com 800-829-5384	12	$20
Tufts University Health & Nutrition Letter www.tuftshealthletter.com 800-274-7581	12	$24
University of California Berkeley Wellness Letter www.berkeleywellness.com 386-447-6328	12	$24

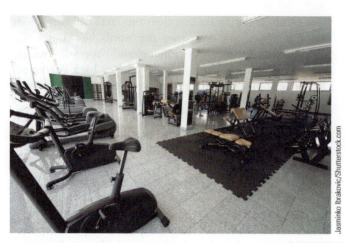

Jasminko Ibrakovic/Shutterstock.com

Exercising in a health or fitness center offers social support, professional guidance, and multiple exercise options.

life. You also can conduct strength-training and stretching programs in your home (see Chapters 7 and 8). Nonetheless, exercising in a health or fitness center provides not only social support but also professional guidance and multiple exercise choices—all three of which are strong motivators for exercise maintenance and adherence.

If you are contemplating membership in a fitness facility, do all of the following:

- *Make sure that the facility complies with the standards established by the American College of Sports Medicine (ACSM) for health and fitness facilities.* These standards are given in Figure 15.4.

- *Examine all exercise options in your community.* This includes health clubs and spas, YMCAs, gyms, colleges, schools, community centers, senior centers, and the like.

- *Check to see whether the facility's atmosphere is pleasant and nonthreatening to you.* Studies have found that the supportive environment offered by staff personnel can be a major factor in achieving your specific fitness goals and maintaining a healthy lifestyle. Will you feel comfortable with the instructors and other people who go there? Is it clean and well kept? If the answers are "no," this may not be the right place for you.

- *Analyze costs across facilities, equipment, and programs.* Take a look at your personal budget. Will you really use the facility? Will you exercise there regularly? Many people obtain memberships and permit dues to be withdrawn automatically from a credit card or local bank account, yet seldom attend the fitness center.

- *Find out what types of spaces and features are available.* Ask about the following: walking and running track; basketball, tennis, or racquetball courts; aerobic exercise room; strength-training room; pool, locker rooms; saunas; hot tubs; handicapped access; and so on.

- *Check the aerobic, strength-training, and stretching equipment available.* Does the facility have treadmills, bicycle ergometers, elliptical trainers, a swimming pool, free weights, and strength-training machines? Make sure that the features and equipment meet your activity interests.

- *Consider the location.* Is the facility close, or do you have to travel several miles to get there? Distance often discourages participation.

- *Check on times the facility is accessible.* Is it open during your preferred exercise time (e.g., early morning or late evening)?

- *Work out at the facility several times before becoming a member.* Does it have ample space amid all the equipment and people in the facility? Are people standing in line to use equipment, or is it readily available during your exercise time?

- *Evaluate the facility for cleanliness and hygiene.* Are the equipment and facility regularly cleaned and disinfected? Sweat and body fluids are great environments for bacterial growth. The facility should also provide hand sanitizers, paper towels, facial tissue, and clean towels for members.

- *Inquire about the instructors' knowledge and qualifications.* Do the fitness instructors have college degrees or professional training certifications from organizations such as the ACSM, the American Council on Exercise (ACE), the National Strength and Conditioning Association (NSCA), or the National Academy of Sports Medicine (NASM)? These organizations have rigorous standards to ensure professional preparation and quality of instruction.

- *Consider the approach to fitness (including all health-related components of fitness).* Is it well rounded? Do the instructors spend time with members, or do members have to seek them out constantly for help and instruction?

- *Ask about supplementary services.* Does the facility provide or contract out for regular health and fitness assessments (cardiovascular endurance, body composition, blood pressure, blood chemistry analysis, etc.)? Are wellness seminars (e.g., nutrition, weight control, and stress management) offered? Do these have hidden costs?

Figure 15.4 ACSM standards for health and fitness facilities.

1. A facility must have an appropriate emergency plan.
2. A facility must offer each adult member a preactivity screening that is relevant to the activities that will be performed by the member.
3. Each person who has supervisory responsibility must be professionally competent.
4. A facility must post appropriate signs in those areas of a facility that present potential increased risk.
5. A facility that offers services or programs to youth must provide appropriate supervision.
6. A facility must conform to all relevant laws, regulations, and published standards.

Adapted from ACSM's Health/Fitness Facility Standards and Guidelines (Champaign, IL: Human Kinetics, 2012).

Personal Trainers

The current way of life has opened an entire job market for personal trainers, who are presently in high demand by health and fitness participants. A **personal trainer** is a health or fitness professional who evaluates, motivates, educates, and trains clients to help them meet individualized healthy lifestyle goals. Rates typically range between $20 and $50 an hour, and trainers who are highly specialized or in high demand command even more. Some trainers offer reduced rates for extended packages or prepaid sessions. For most people, using the expertise of a personal trainer is an investment in fitness, health, and quality of life.

Exercise sessions are usually conducted at a health or fitness facility or at the client's home. Experience and the ability to design safe and effective programs based on the client's current fitness level, health status, and fitness goals are important. Personal trainers also recognize their limitations and refer clients to other health care professionals as necessary.

Popular reality shows featuring trainers using "tough love" and "no pain–no gain" approaches to exercise for weight loss have led to an increase in high-intensity programs such as CrossFit, boot camp, Insanity, and others. Though this type of training has its benefits, be aware that extreme, military-type conditioning programs can result in injury or adverse health problems for those unconditioned for high-intensity training. The ACSM recommends that personal trainers have prospective clients undergo pre-exercise screening to identify any cardiac or injury risk factors before enrolling in a new exercise program. When choosing a potential trainer who may use a challenging approach, be sure to discuss any health restrictions with your trainer to ensure you receive instruction that is both safe and well tailored to your personal fitness level.

Currently, anyone who prescribes exercise can make the claim to be a personal trainer without proof of education, experience, or certification. Although good trainers need to strive to maximize their health and fitness, a good physique and previous athletic experience do not certify a person as a personal trainer.

Because of the high demand for personal trainers, more than 200 organizations now certify fitness specialists. This has led to great confusion among clients on how to evaluate the credentials of personal trainers. Certification and a certificate are different. Certification implies that the individual has met educational and professional standards of performance and competence. A certificate typically is awarded to an individual who attended a conference or workshop but is not required to meet any professional standards.

Presently, no licensing body is in place to oversee personal trainers, making the process of becoming a personal trainer relatively easy. Some states have proposed bills that would require potential trainers to apply for a state-issued license before offering services to the public, though no legislation has yet been signed into law. At a minimum, personal trainers should have an undergraduate degree and certification from a reputable organization such as the ACSM, ACE, NSCA, or NASM. Undergraduate (and graduate) degrees should be conferred in

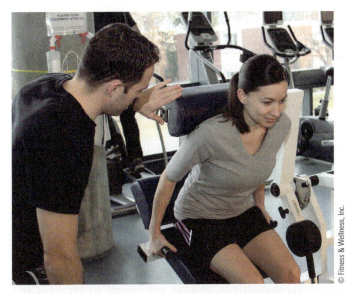

A personal trainer provides valuable guidance and helps motivate individuals to achieve fitness goals.

a fitness-related area such as exercise science, exercise physiology, kinesiology, sports medicine, or physical education. When looking for a personal trainer, always inquire about the trainer's education and certification credentials.

Before selecting a trainer, you must establish your program goals. Following are sample questions to ask yourself and consider when interviewing potential trainers prior to selecting one:

- *Can the potential personal trainer provide you with a résumé?*
- *What type of professional education and certification does the potential trainer possess?*
- *How long has the person been a personal trainer, and are references available upon request?*
- *Are you looking for a male or female trainer?*
- *What are the fees? Are multiple sessions cheaper than a single session? Can individuals be trained in groups? Are there cancellation fees if you are not able to attend a given session?*
- *How long will you need the services of the personal trainer: one session, multiple sessions, periodically, or indefinitely?*
- *What goals do you intend to achieve with the guidance of the personal trainer: weight loss, cardiorespiratory fitness, strength fitness, flexibility fitness, improved health, sport fitness conditioning, or a combination of these?*
- *What type of personality are you looking for in the trainer—a motivator, a hard-challenging trainer, a gentle trainer, or professional counsel only?*

When seeking fitness advice from a health or fitness trainer online, here's a final word of caution: Be aware that certain services cannot be provided over the Internet. An online

GLOSSARY

Personal trainer A health or fitness professional who evaluates, motivates, educates, and trains clients to help them meet individualized healthy lifestyle goals.

trainer is not able to directly administer fitness tests, motivate, observe exercise limitations, or respond effectively in an emergency situation (spotting or administering first aid or cardiopulmonary resuscitation [CPR]) and thus is not able to design the safest and most effective exercise program for you.

Purchasing Exercise Equipment

A final consideration is that of purchasing your own exercise equipment. First ask yourself: Do I really need this piece of equipment? Most people buy on impulse because of television advertisements or because a salesperson has convinced them it is a great piece of equipment that will do wonders for their health and fitness. Ignore claims that an exercise device or machine can provide "easy" or "no sweat" results in a few minutes only. Keep in mind that the benefits of exercise are obtained only if you do exercise. With some creativity, you can implement an excellent and comprehensive exercise program with little, if any, equipment (see Chapters 6–9).

Many people buy expensive equipment only to find they do not enjoy that mode of activity. They do not remain regular users. Stationary bicycles (lower body only) and rowing ergometers were among the most popular pieces of equipment a few years ago. Now, most of them are seldom used and have become "fitness furniture" somewhere in the garage or basement. Also be skeptical of testimonials and before-and-after pictures from "satisfied" customers. These results may not be typical, and it doesn't mean that you will like the equipment.

Exercise equipment has its value for people who prefer to exercise indoors, especially during winter months. It supports some people's motivation and adherence to exercise. The convenience of having equipment at home also allows for flexible scheduling. You can exercise before or after work or while you watch your favorite television show.

Behavior Modification Planning

24 Healthy Lifestyle Guidelines

1. Accumulate a minimum of 30 minutes of moderate-intensity physical activity at least 5 days per week.

2. Exercise aerobically in the proper cardiorespiratory training zone at least three times per week for a minimum of 20 minutes.

3. Accumulate at least 10,000 steps on a daily basis.

4. Strength-train at least once per week (preferably twice per week) using a minimum of eight exercises that involve all major muscle groups of the body.

5. Perform flexibility exercises that involve all major joints of the body at least two to three times per week.

6. Avoid excessive sitting throughout the day: Take intermittent 10-minute breaks for every hour that you are sitting (at the computer, studying, playing table games, or watching television).

7. Eat a healthy diet that is rich in 100 percent-whole-wheat grains, with ample amounts of fruits and vegetables; includes cold-water fish two to three times per week; and is low in saturated and trans fats.

8. Eat a healthy breakfast every day.

9. Minimize the consumption of refined foods, simple carbohydrates, sweets, and added sugars.

10. Include protein with each meal throughout the day.

11. Substitute unsaturated fats for saturated fat and trans fat in your daily diet.

12. Maintain healthy body weight (achieve a range between the high-physical fitness and health-fitness standards for percent body fat).

13. Do not use tobacco in any form and avoid secondhand smoke.

14. Avoid all forms of substance abuse.

15. Get 7 to 8 hours of sleep per night.

16. Practice safe sex every time you have sex and don't have sexual contact with anyone who doesn't practice safe sex.

17. Get 10 to 20 minutes of safe sun exposure on most days of the week.

18. Manage stress effectively.

19. Limit daily alcohol intake to two or less drinks per day if you are a man or one drink or less per day if you are a woman (or do not consume any alcohol at all).

20. Have at least one close friend or relative in whom you can confide and to whom you can express your feelings openly.

21. Be aware of your surroundings and take personal safety measures at all times.

22. Seek continued learning on a regular basis.

23. Subscribe to a reputable health/fitness/nutrition newsletter to stay up-to-date on healthy lifestyle guidelines.

24. Seek proper medical evaluations as necessary.

Try It

Now that you are about to complete this course, evaluate how many of the healthy lifestyle guidelines have become part of your personal wellness program. Prepare a list of those that you still need to work on, and use Activity 15.4 to write SMART goals and specific objectives that will help you achieve the desired behaviors. Remember that each one of the guidelines will lead to a longer, healthier, and happier life.

If you are going to purchase equipment, the best recommendation is to try it out several times before buying it. Ask yourself several questions: Did I enjoy the workout? Is the unit comfortable? Am I too short, tall, or heavy for it? Is it stable, sturdy, and strong? Do I have to assemble the machine? If so, how difficult is it to put together? How durable is it? Ask for references—people or clubs that have used the equipment extensively. Are they satisfied? Have they enjoyed using the equipment? Talk with professionals at colleges, sports medicine clinics, or health clubs.

Another consideration is to look at used units for signs of wear and tear. Quality is important. Cheaper brands may not be durable, so your investment would be wasted.

Finally, watch out for expensive gadgets. Monitors that provide exercise heart rate, work output, caloric expenditure, speed, grade, and distance may help motivate you, but they are expensive, need repairs, and do not enhance the actual fitness benefits of the workout. Look at maintenance costs and check for service personnel in your community.

15.8 Self-Evaluation and Behavioral Goals for the Future

The main objective of this book is to provide the information and experiences necessary to implement your personal fitness and wellness program. If you have implemented the programs in this book, including exercise, you should be convinced that a wellness lifestyle is the only way to attain a higher quality of life.

Most people who engage in a personal fitness and wellness program experience this new quality of life after only a few weeks of training and practicing healthy lifestyle patterns. In some instances, however—especially for individuals who have led a poor lifestyle for a long time—a few months may be required to establish positive habits and feelings of well-being. In the end, though, everyone who applies principles of fitness and wellness will reap the desired benefits.

Prior to the completion of this course, you need to identify community resources available to you that will support your path to lifetime fitness and wellness. Activity 15.2 provides a road map to initiate your search for this support.

Self-Evaluation

Throughout this course, you have had an opportunity to assess various fitness and wellness components and write goals to improve your quality of life. You should now take the time to evaluate how well you have achieved your goals. Ideally, if time allows and facilities and technicians are available, reassess the health-related components of physical fitness. If you are unable to reassess these components, determine subjectively how well you accomplished your goals. You will find a self-evaluation form in Activity 15.3.

Behavioral Goals for the Future

Realizing that you may not have achieved all of your goals during this course, or perhaps you need to reach beyond your current achievements, the Wellness Scale provided in Activity 15.3 will help you chart the future. This guide provides a list of various wellness components, each illustrating a scale from poor to excellent. Using the Wellness Scale, rate yourself for each component according to the following instructions:

1. Indicate with an "I" (I = Initial) the category from poor to excellent where you stood on each component at the beginning of the term. For example, if at the start of this course, you rated poor in cardiorespiratory endurance, place an "I" under the poor column for this component.
2. Mark with a "C" (C = Current) a second column (between poor and excellent) to indicate where you stand on each component at the current time. If your level of cardiorespiratory endurance improved to average by the end of the term, write a "C" under this column. If you were not able to work on a given component, simply make a "C" out of the "I."
3. Select one or two components you intend to work on in the next 2 months. Developing new behavioral patterns takes time, and trying to work on too many components at once most likely will lower your chances for success. Start with components in which you think you will have a high chance for success.

Next, place a "G" (G = Goal) under the intended goal column to accomplish by the end of this period. If your goal in the next 2 months is to achieve a "good" level of cardiorespiratory endurance, place a "G" under the good column for this component in the Wellness Scale.

Use Activity 15.4 to write the goals and actions for two components you intend to work on during the next two months. As you write and work on these goals and actions, review the goal-setting guidelines provided in Chapter 2, pages 73–74. Using these guidelines will help you design an effective plan of action to reach your goals. You are encouraged to keep this form (activity) in a place that you will remember so that you may review it in months and years to come.

At the end of your assignment, summarize your feelings about your past and present lifestyle, what you have learned in this course, and changes that you were able to successfully implement. Activity 15.5 can be used for this experience.

HOEGER KEY TO WELLNESS

People in the United States are firm believers in physical activity and positive lifestyle habits to improve and maintain good health. Most people, however, do not act on these beliefs. Fitness and wellness is a process and you will need to put forth a constant and deliberate effort to live in a manner that will enhance wellness and add quality years to your life.

Activity 15.2	Fitness and Wellness Community Resources

Name _____ Date _____

Course _____ Section _____ Gender _____ Age _____

NECESSARY LAB EQUIPMENT
None required.

OBJECTIVE
To identify community resources available for you to continue your path toward lifetime fitness and wellness.

INSTRUCTION
Using a community directory, identify a minimum of three fitness, recreational, or wellness facilities that will allow you to maintain and further develop your personal fitness and wellness program. Initially, contact all three facilities by phone to obtain the pertinent information (see Item I). On completion of this task, make an appointment to personally visit at least one of the facilities during a time when you would work out, and evaluate the equipment, equipment availability, personnel, and programs that would be available to you. Keep in mind that one of the options available to you may be your own campus health/fitness/recreation center. College alumni, for a fee, often have the option to continue to use such a facility.

I. Initial Contact

	Facility I	Facility II	Facility III
Facility Name:	_____	_____	_____
Address:	_____	_____	_____
Distance from home:	_____	_____	_____
Mode of transportation to the facility:	_____	_____	_____
Travel time to the facility:	_____	_____	_____
Monthly fee:	_____	_____	_____
Hours of operation:	_____	_____	_____
Cardio equipment:	_____	_____	_____
	_____	_____	_____
	_____	_____	_____
Strength training:	_____	_____	_____
	_____	_____	_____
	_____	_____	_____
Flexibility equipment:	_____	_____	_____
	_____	_____	_____
	_____	_____	_____
Personal trainers, availability and costs:	_____	_____	_____
Personal trainers' certifications:	_____	_____	_____
Fitness tests, availability and costs:	_____	_____	_____
Exercise classes:	_____	_____	_____
	_____	_____	_____
	_____	_____	_____
Other services (nutrition,	_____	_____	_____
stress management, smoking	_____	_____	_____
cessation, cardiac profiles, etc.):	_____	_____	_____
Free trial of facility available?	_____	_____	_____

Activity 15.2 **Fitness and Wellness Community Resources** (continued)

II. Facility Visit and Evaluation

1. Provide an overall impression of the facility:

_____

_____

2. Was the staff knowledgeable, accessible, and friendly? Why or why not?

_____

_____

3. Were you able to work out at the facility?   ____ Yes   ____ No
   If so, was the equipment available and suitable to your preferences?

_____

_____

   Did you feel comfortable with other individuals using the facility (please indicate why or why not)?

_____

_____

4. Provide an overall evaluation of the locker facilities and other amenities available to you.

_____

_____

5. Overall letter grade for the facility: A   B   C   D   F

III. Ongoing Educational Program

1. Are there any other community resources available to you that would benefit your personal health, fitness, and wellness lifestyle program? Please list:

_____

_____

2. Contact at least one reliable health, fitness, nutrition, or wellness newsletter that you may subscribe to (see page 557) for a free copy and list the newsletter in the space provided. Also indicate if there are any other fitness/wellness materials that have provided valuable information to you.

_____

_____

3. List at least three reliable and helpful websites that you accessed this term and indicate why these sites were useful to you.

_____

_____

© Fitness & Wellness, Inc.

Activity 15.3 — Self-Evaluation of Selected Wellness Components

Name _____ Date _____

Course _____ Section _____ Gender _____ Age _____

Enter I (for Initial) on the scale from poor to excellent to indicate where you rated in each Wellness Component category at the beginning of the term, C (for Current) to indicate where you rate yourself currently, and G (for Goal) in one or two components according to the rating you'd like to achieve within the next 2 months. See page 561 for full instructions.

Wellness Rating

Wellness Components	Poor	Fair	Average	Good	Excellent
Cardiorespiratory Endurance					
Muscular Fitness (Strength and Endurance)					
Muscular Flexibility					
Body Composition					
Nutrition					
Cardiovascular Disease Prevention					
Cancer Prevention					
Stress Control					
Tobacco Use					
Substance Abuse Control*					
Sexuality*					
Accident Prevention and Personal Safety					
Spirituality*					
Health Education					

Current Number of Daily Steps: _____   **Activity category** (see Table 1.2, page 13): _____

*These components are personal, and you are not required to reveal this information. If you think that counseling is necessary, you are encouraged to seek professional help.

© Fitness & Wellness, Inc.

MINDTAP From Cengage — **Complete This Online** Visit **www.cengagebrain.com** to access MindTap, a complete digital course that includes interactive quizzes, videos, and more.

Activity 15.4 — Goal Setting: Behavioral Goals for the Future

Name _____ Date _____

Course _____ Section _____ Gender _____ Age _____

Select two wellness components that you will work on during the next couple of months. Specify your SMART goals and write specific actions that will lead to your accomplishing these goals (you may not need six objectives; write only as many as you need).

Goal: _____

Actions:

1. _____
2. _____
3. _____
4. _____
5. _____
6. _____

Goal: _____

Actions:

1. _____
2. _____
3. _____
4. _____
5. _____
6. _____

Number of Daily Steps Goal: [_____]   Activity Category Goal: [_____]

© Fitness & Wellness, Inc.

MINDTAP From Cengage — **Complete This Online**
Visit **www.cengagebrain.com** to access MindTap, a complete digital course that includes interactive quizzes, videos, and more.

Activity 15.5   Wellness Lifestyle Self-Assessment

Name _____ Date _____

Course _____ Section _____ Gender _____ Age _____

On a separate sheet of paper, please answer all of the following questions.

I.   Explain the exercise program that you implemented in this course. Express your feelings about the outcomes of this program, and evaluate how well you accomplished your fitness goals.

_____

_____

_____

II.   List nutritional or dietary changes that you were able to implement this term and the effects of these changes on your body composition and personal wellness.

_____

_____

_____

III. What do you know about your family health history and, if applicable, do you know what may have led to any health issues encountered by members of your family?

_____

_____

_____

IV.   List other lifestyle changes that you were able to make this term that may decrease your risk for disease. In a few sentences, explain how you feel about these changes and their impact on your overall well-being.

_____

_____

_____

V.   Briefly evaluate this course and its impact on your quality of life. Indicate what you think you will need so that you are able to continue to adhere to an active and healthy lifestyle.

_____

_____

_____

© Fitness & Wellness, Inc.

!

Critical Thinking

Do you admire some people around you whom you would like to emulate in their wellness lifestyle? What behaviors do these people exhibit that would help you adopt a healthier lifestyle? What keeps you from emulating these behaviors, and how can you overcome these barriers?

15.9 *The Fitness and Wellness Experience: Patty's Success*

Patty Neavill is a typical example of someone who often tried to change her life but was unable to do so because she did not know how to implement a sound exercise and weight control program. At age 24 and at 240 pounds, she was discouraged with her weight, level of fitness, self-image, and quality of life in general. She had struggled with her weight most of her life. Like thousands of other people, she had made many unsuccessful attempts to lose weight.

Patty put her fears aside and decided to enroll in a fitness course. As part of the course requirement, a battery of fitness tests was administered at the beginning of the semester. Patty's cardiovascular endurance and muscular (strength) fitness ratings were poor, her flexibility classification was average, and her percent body fat was 41 percent.

Following the initial fitness assessment, Patty met with her course instructor, who prescribed an exercise and nutrition program like the one in this book. Patty fully committed to carry out the prescription. She walked or jogged five times a week. She enrolled in a weight-training course that met twice a week. Her daily caloric intake was set in the range of 1,500 to 1,700 calories.

Determined to increase her level of activity further, Patty signed up for recreational volleyball and basketball courses.

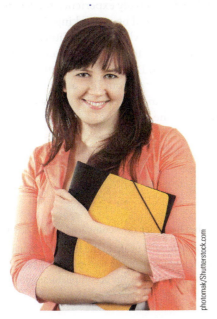

photomak/Shutterstock.com

Besides being fun, these classes provided 4 additional hours of activity per week.

She took care to meet the minimum required servings from the basic food groups each day, which contributed about 1,200 calories to her diet. The remainder of the calories came primarily from complex carbohydrates.

At the end of the 16-week semester, Patty's cardiovascular endurance, muscular fitness, and flexibility ratings had all improved to the good category, she had lost 50 pounds, and her percent body fat had decreased to 22.5 percent.

Patty was tall. At 190 pounds, most people would have thought she was too heavy. Her percent body fat, however, was lower than the average for college female physical education major students (about 23 percent body fat).

A thank-you note from Patty to the course instructor at the end of the semester read:

Thank you for making me a new person. I truly appreciate the time you spent with me. Without your kindness and motivation, I would have never made it. It is great to be fit and trim. I've never had this feeling before, and I wish everyone could feel like this once in their life.

Thank you,
Your trim Patty!

Patty had never been taught the principles governing a sound weight loss program. She not only needed this knowledge but, like most Americans who never have experienced the process of becoming physically fit, also needed to be in a structured exercise setting to truly feel the joy of fitness.

Even more significant was that Patty maintained her aerobic and strength-training programs. A year after ending her calorie-restricted diet, her weight increased by 10 pounds, but her body fat decreased from 22.5 to 21.2 percent. As you may recall from Chapter 5, this weight increase is related mostly to changes in lean tissue, which is lost during the weight-reduction phase.

In spite of only a slight drop in weight during the second year following the calorie-restricted diet, a 2-year follow-up revealed a further decrease in body fat, to 19.5 percent. Patty understood the new quality of life reaped through a sound fitness program, and at the same time, she finally learned how to apply the principles that regulate weight maintenance.

15.10 *A Lifetime Commitment to Fitness and Wellness*

If you have read and successfully completed all of the assignments set out in this book, including a regular exercise program, you should be convinced of the value of exercise and healthy lifestyle habits in achieving a new quality of life.

Perhaps this new quality of life was explained best by the late Dr. George Sheehan, when he wrote[8]:

For every runner who tours the world running marathons, there are thousands who run to hear the leaves and listen to

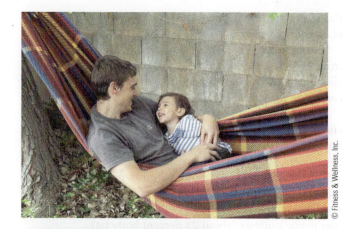

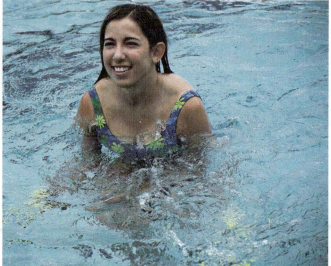

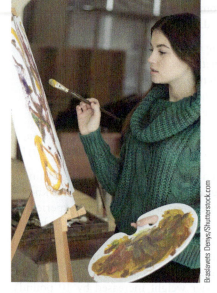

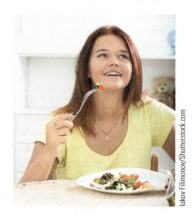

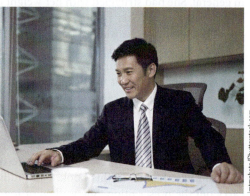

Fitness and healthy lifestyle habits lead to improved health, quality of life, and wellness.

the rain, and look to the day when it is all suddenly as easy as a bird in flight. For them, sport is not a test but a therapy, not a trial but a reward, not a question but an answer.

The real challenge comes now: a lifetime commitment to fitness and wellness. To make the commitment easier, enjoy yourself and have fun along the way. If you implement your program based on your interests and what you enjoy doing most, then adhering to your new lifestyle will not be difficult.

Your activities over the past few weeks or months may have helped you develop "positive addictions" that will carry on throughout life. If you truly experience the feelings Dr. Sheehan expressed, there will be no looking back. If you don't get there, you won't know what it's like. Fitness and wellness is a process, and you need to put forth a constant and deliberate effort to achieve and maintain a higher quality of life. Improving the quality of your life, and most likely your longevity, is in your hands. Only you can take control of your lifestyle and reap the benefits of wellness.

Assess Your Behavior

1. Has your level of physical activity increased compared with the beginning of the term?

2. Do you participate in a regular exercise program that includes cardiorespiratory endurance, muscular fitness, and muscular flexibility training?

3. Is your diet healthier now compared with a few weeks ago?

4. Are you able to take pride in the lifestyle changes that you have implemented over the past several weeks? Have you rewarded yourself for your accomplishments?

Assess Your Knowledge

1. From a functional point of view, typical sedentary people in the United States are about ___ years older than their chronological age indicates.
   a. 2
   b. 8
   c. 15
   d. 20
   e. 25

2. Which one of the following factors has the greatest impact on health and longevity?
   a. Genetics
   b. The environment
   c. Lifestyle behaviors
   d. Chronic diseases
   e. Gender

3. Your real physiological age is determined by
   a. your birthdate.
   b. lifestyle habits.
   c. amount of physical activity.
   d. your family's health history.
   e. your ability to obtain proper medical care.

4. Complementary and alternative medicine is
   a. also known as allopathic medicine.
   b. referred to as "Western" medicine.
   c. based on scientifically proven methods.
   d. a diverse group of unconventional health practices.
   e. All of the choices are correct.

5. Complementary and alternative medicine health care practices and treatments are
   a. not widely taught in medical schools.
   b. endorsed by many physicians.
   c. not generally used in hospitals.
   d. not usually reimbursed by medical insurance companies.
   e. All of the choices are correct.

6. In complementary and alternative medicine,
   a. practitioners believe that their treatment modality aids the body as it performs its natural healing process.
   b. treatments are usually shorter than with typical medical practices.
   c. practitioners rely extensively on the use of medications.
   d. patients are often discouraged from administering self-treatment.
   e. All of the choices are correct.

7. When the word "natural" is used with a product,
   a. it implies that the product is safe.
   b. the product cannot be toxic, even when taken in large doses.
   c. the product cannot yield undesirable side effects when combined with prescription drugs.
   d. there will be no negative side effects with the product's use.
   e. None of the choices are correct.

8. To protect yourself from consumer fraud when buying a new product,
   a. get as much information as you can from the salesperson.
   b. obtain details about the product from another salesperson.
   c. ask someone who understands the product but does not stand to profit from the transaction.
   d. obtain all research information from the manufacturer.
   e. All of the choices are correct.

9. Which of the following should you consider when looking to join a health or fitness center?
   a. Location
   b. Instructor's certifications
   c. Type and amount of equipment available
   d. Verification that the facility complies with ACSM standards
   e. All of the choices are correct.

10. When you purchase exercise equipment, the most important factor is
   a. to try it out several times before buying it.
   b. a recommendation from an exercise specialist.
   c. cost effectiveness.
   d. that it provides accurate exercise information.
   e. to find out how others like this piece of equipment.

Correct answers can be found at the back of the book.

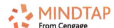 **Complete This Online**
From Cengage Visit **www.cengagebrain.com** to access MindTap, a complete digital course that includes interactive quizzes, videos, and more.

Appendix A: Physical Fitness and Wellness Profile

Fill out the following profile as you obtain the results for each fitness and wellness component. Attempt to determine the four fitness components (cardiorespiratory endurance, muscular fitness, muscular flexibility, and body composition) during the first 2 or 3 weeks of the term so that you may proceed with your exercise program. After determining each component, discuss with your instructor the goals to be accomplished and the date of completion.

Name: _____ Course: _____ Section: _____ Gender: _____ Age: _____

Item	Pre-Assessment			Goal[a]	Post-Assessment		
	Date	Test Results	Category		Date	Test Results	Category
Cardiorespiratory Endurance							
VO_{2max}							
Daily min. of phys. activity							
Total daily steps							
Muscular Fitness (Strength)							
Muscular Flexibility							
Body Composition							
Body Weight							
Percent body fat							
Lean Body Mass							
BMI							
Waist Circumference							
Waist-to-Height Ratio							
Cardiovascular Risk							
Cancer Risk							
Lung							
Colorectal							
Skin							
Breast[b]							
Cervical[b]							
Endometrial[b]							
Prostate							
Testicular							
Pancreatic							
Kidney and Bladder							
Oral							
Esophageal and Stomach							
Ovarian							
Thyroid							
Liver							
Leukemia							
Lymphomas							
Stress							
Stress Events Scale							
Vulnerability Questionnaire							
Tobacco Use[c]							

INSTRUCTOR'S SIGNATURE: _____ STUDENT'S SIGNATURE: _____

[a]Indicate goal to complete by end of the term.
[b]Women only.
[c]For test results, indicate type and amount smoked; for classification indicate smoker, ex-smoker, nonsmoker.

Answer Key

Chapter 1
1. c   2. e   3. d   4. a   5. e   6. d   7. c
8. b   9. a   10. b

Chapter 2
1. a   2. a   3. e   4. d   5. e   6. d   7. a
8. b   9. e   10. e

Chapter 3
1. b   2. e   3. c   4. d   5. d   6. e   7. a
8. c   9. a   10. e

Chapter 4
1. e   2. b   3. d   4. a   5. b   6. c   7. b
8. b   9. e   10. e

Chapter 5
1. b   2. c   3. e   4. a   5. b   6. e   7. a
8. c   9. d   10. e

Chapter 6
1. a   2. d   3. c   4. c   5. c   6. e   7. b
8. d   9. c   10. c

Chapter 7
1. c   2. d   3. a   4. b   5. d   6. a   7. c
8. c   9. e   10. e

Chapter 8
1. b   2. e   3. a   4. e   5. a   6. b   7. c
8. b   9. c   10. e

Chapter 9
1. a   2. e   3. d   4. c   5. d   6. e   7. b
8. a   9. e   10. e

Chapter 10
1. e   2. b   3. a   4. e   5. e   6. e   7. e
8. e   9. e   10. a

Chapter 11
1. b   2. a   3. a   4. e   5. e   6. e   7. b
8. e   9. b   10. e

Chapter 12
1. a   2. c   3. c   4. e   5. e   6. e   7. a
8. a   9. b   10. c

Chapter 13
1. e   2. a   3. c   4. d   5. d   6. d   7. d
8. e   9. e   10. e

Chapter 14
1. c   2. b   3. e   4. e   5. d   6. a   7. a
8. d   9. e   10. c

Chapter 15
1. e   2. c   3. b   4. d   5. e   6. a   7. e
8. c   9. e   10. a

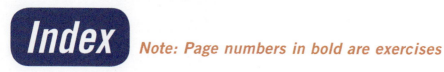

Index

Note: Page numbers in bold are exercises